Mechanisms of Injury, Protection and Repair of the Upper Gastrointestinal Tract

Mechanisms of Injury, Protection and Repair of the Upper Gastrointestinal Tract

Edited by

ANDREW GARNER

Department of Biochemistry, University College of Wales
Aberystwyth, UK

and

PAUL E. O'BRIEN

Monash University Department of Surgery, Alfred Hospital
Melbourne, Australia

JOHN WILEY & SONS

Chichester · New York · Brisbane · Toronto · Singapore

Other Wiley Editorial Offices

John Wiley & Sons, Inc., 605 Third Avenue,
New York, NY 10158-0012, USA

Jacaranda Wiley Ltd, G.P.O. Box 859, Brisbane,
Queensland 4001, Australia

John Wiley & Sons (Canada) Ltd, 22 Worcester Road,
Rexdale, Ontario M9W 1LI, Canada

John Wiley & Sons (SEA) Pte Ltd, 37 Jalan Pemimpin 05-04,
Block B, Union Industrial Building, Singapore 2057

*A catalogue record for this book is
available from the British Library*

ISBN 0 471 93078 4

Printed in Great Britain by Biddles Ltd, Guildford

CONTENTS

x   ACKNOWLEDGEMENTS

xi   CONTRIBUTORS

xxii   PREFACE

SECTION 1   -   LUMINAL FACTORS IN INJURY

1   Luminal acidity: role in ulceration and healing
        Richard H. Hunt

7   Pepsin induced mucosal damage compared to that with ethanol
        or hypertonic saline: the role of the adherent mucus barrier
        Adrian Allen, Andrea J. Leonard, J.P. Pearson,
        Lynda A. Sellers, Mark K. Bennett

19   Helicobacter pylori
        J.R. Lambert, S.K. Lin, M. Schembri

29   Inhibition of gastric bicarbonate secretion by NSAIDs:
        importance of luminal exposure
        John Crampton, Linda Gibbons, Wynne Rees

37   Acid secretory and mucosal ulcerogenic responses induced by
        lowering body temperature: a pathogenic importance of body
        temperature
        K. Takeuchi, H. Niida, K. Ueshima, S. Okabe

SECTION 2   -   EXPRESSION OF INJURY

47   Assessment of cell death in hypoxic cell injury
        Anna-Liisa Nieminen, Gregory J. Gores, Roberto Imberti,
        Brian Herman, John J. Lemasters

61   Role of 16,16 dmPGE$_2$ in gastric cell protection against bile salts
        Adam J. Dziki, John W. Harmon, Shmuel Batzri,
        Barbara L. Bass, Richard M. Ugarte

71   Role of gastric microvascular perfusion in mucosal protection
        against ethanol injury
        Gary M. Frydman, Angela G. Penney, Cathy Malcontenti,
        Paul E. O'Brien

81   Role of ambient Cl⁻ in the electrophysiologic response of
        amphibian gastric mucosa to injury
        J.B. Matthews, A. Garner

91   The relationship between alkaline secretion and mucosal
        permeability in duodenum
        Olof Nylander, Manaf Sababi

SECTION 3   -   ENDOGENOUS MEDIATORS OF INJURY

103   Role of sensory neuropeptides in gastric mucosal damage and
        protection
        **P. Holzer, H.E. Raybould, I.Th. Lippe, R. Amann, E.H. Livingston,
        B.M. Peskar, B.A. Peskar, Y. Tache, P.H. Guth**

115   Peripheral opioid-sensitive mechanisms of mucosal injury and
        protection
        J.V. Esplugues, B.J.R. Whittle

127   Role of the endogenous vasoactive mediators, nitric oxide,
        prostanoids and sensory neuropeptides in the regulation of gastric
        blood flow and mucosal integrity
        B.J.R. Whittle, B.L. Tepperman

139   Mediation of NSAID-induced gastropathy by leukocytes and
        leukocyte-derived mediators
        John Wallace, Catherine Keenan, Webb McKnight, Paula Vaananen

149   Ischemia-reperfusion induced changes in microvascular
        permeability
        M.A. Perry, D.N. Granger

159   Reactive oxygen metabolites: mediators of gastrointestinal injury
        Patrick M. Reilly, Gregory B. Bulkley

SECTION 4   -   SURFACE PROTECTION

175   Epithelial cell and membrane permeability to protons.
        Barry H. Hirst

187   Specialization of the apical surface of parietal cells: identification
        and characterization of a   -subunit of the gastric H,K-ATPase
        J.G. Forte, C.T. Okamoto, D.C. Chow, V.A. Canfield, R. Levenson

199   Is there a role for transcellular (apical membrane) diffusion of
        hydrogen ions in acute acid injury to rabbit esophageal
        epithelium?
        Roy C. Orlando, Edward J. Cragoe Jr., Nelia A. Tobey

207   Gastric mucosal hydrophobicity
        T.C. Northfield, P.M. Goggin

223   Neuroendocrine control of mucosa protective functions in the
        duodenum
        L. Fandriks, A. Hamlet, C. Jonson

237   Human duodenal mucosal bicarbonate secretion in health and
        disease
        Daniel L. Hogan, Jon I. Isenberg

SECTION 5 - INTRACELLULAR pH REGULATION

247 Regulation of intracellular pH (pHi) in oxynticopeptic cells: studies in intact amphibian gastric mucosa
A. Yanaka, K. Carter, P. Goddard, W. Silen

253 pHi-regulating ion transport systems in isolated rabbit parietal, chief and surface cells
U. Seidler, S. Roithmaier, V. Schusdziarra, M. Classen, W. Silen

271 Intracellular pH in acid-exposed gastric mucosa
E. Kivilaakso, T. Kiviluoto, H. Mustonen, H. Paimela

281 Intracellular pH regulation in the duodenal mucosa
M. Starlinger, M. Weinlich, R. Kinne

SECTION 6 - MICROVASCULATURE

291 Microvasculature of the gastric and duodenal mucosa
Bren Gannon

299 Physiological and pathological responses in the gastric mucosal blood flow
Nobuhiro Sato, Sunao Kawano, Shingo Tsuji, Tatsuo Ogihara, Hisato Kitagawa

309 Effects of aging on gastric secretion and blood flow in rats
Yutaka Masuda, Tomochika Ohno, Hiroshi Uramoto, Takafumi Ishihara

319 Role of increased blood flow after mucosal injury
K. Svanes, J.E. Gronbech

327 Quantitative histology in the assessment of gastric mucosal injury and protection.
Gary M. Frydman, Cathy Malcontenti, Angela G. Penney, P.E. O'Brien

SECTION 7 - MEDIATORS OF PROTECTION

343 Intercellular matrix in the gut: putative roles in gastric protection
O.W. Wiebkin, D. Hillen, S.C. Wiebkin, D.J.C. Shearman

357 Gastric adaptation to repeated administration of a necrotizing agent
A. Robert, C. Lancaster, A.S. Olafsson, W. Zhang

371   Local and referred protection in the gastric mucosa: prostaglandin-
       independent and prostaglandin-dependent mechanisms
       G.P. Morris, C.L. Donaldson, C.A. Holitzner,
       K.H. Tufts, T.E. Williamson

383   Intracisternal injection of calcitonin-gene related peptide
       inhibits experimental gastric ulcers
       Yvette Tache

SECTION 8   -   ACUTE RECOVERY

395   Chronic challenge with hyperosmolar salt protects the rat gastric
       mucosa against acute hemorrhagic lesions: response of antral
       mucous cells
       Eric R. Lacy, Kathryn S. Cowart, Jan S. King

403   Restitution in the intestine
       R. Schiessel, M. Riegler, W. Feil, E. Wenzl

413   Effects of nutrient HCO_3^- and luminal pH on restitution of
       colonic mucosa in vitro
       P.H. Rowe, Q. Zhang, D.C. Hanley, R.C. Mason

SECTION 9   -   GROWTH FACTORS

427   Chronic ulceration: role of gastrin
       F. Halter

435   Role of epidermal growth factor (EGF) and prostaglandins (PG) in
       the protection against stress-induced gastric ulceration
       S.J. Konturek, T. Brzozowski, P.K. Konturek, A. Dembinski

447   Vascular factors in mucosal injury, protection and ulcer healing
       S. Szabo, J. Folkman, R.E. Morales, P. Vattay, G. Pinkus, K. Kato

455   Effects of indomethacin and prednisolone on connective tissue
       at the base of acetic acid-induced gastric ulcers in rats
       Y. Ogihara, Y. Fuse, S. Okabe

SECTION 10   -   CLINICAL REALITIES

467   Gastric mucosal injury and haemostasis: effects of aspirin,
       smoking and prophylactic strategies
       C.J. Hawkey, A.T. Cole, A.B. Hawthorne, N. Hudson,
       Y.R. Mahida, S.G. Mann

479   Adaptation to nonsteroidal anti-inflammatory drug induced
gastroduodenal damage in man.   Studies of morphology,
histology and mucosal blood flow
C.J. Shorrock, W.D.W. Rees

491   Chronic duodenal ulcer: the abscopal model
R.H. Gompertz, A.S. Michalowski, J.H. Baron

503   The role of dietary prostaglandin precursors (essential fatty acids)
in the prevention of gastroduodenal mucosal injury
D. Hollander, A. Tarnawski

511   Utility of prostaglandins for prevention of nonsteroidal anti-
inflammatory drug-induced ulcers
David Y. Graham

521   Indomethacin impairs quality of experimental gastric ulcer
healing. A quantitative histological and ultrastructural analysis.
**A. Tarnawski, J. Stachura, T.G. Douglass, W.J. Krause,
H. Gergely, I.J. Sarfeh**

533   **Subject Index**

ACKNOWLEDGEMENTS

This book is based on the proceeding of an
international conference held in
Cairns, North Queensland in August 1990.

The Editors wish to gratefully acknowledge
the generous sponsorship of this conference
by the following Companies.

SANDOZ PHARMACEUTICALS LTD,
MINATO-KU, TOKYO, JAPAN

KANEBO LIMITED
OSAKA, JAPAN

NIPPON CHEMIPHAR CO. LTD.,
TOKYO, JAPAN

ZERIA PHARMACEUTICAL CO. LTD.
SAITAMA, JAPAN

MERCK SHARP & DOHME (AUSTRALIA) PTY. LTD.
AUSTRALIA

SEARLE LABORATORIES PTY. LTD.
AUSTRALIA

SMITH KLINE & FRENCH LABORATORIES (AUSTRALIA) PTY. LTD.
AUSTRALIA

THE BOOTS COMPANY
AUSTRALIA

CONTRIBUTORS

*Adrian Allen,
Department of Physiological Sciences,
Medical School,
Framlington Place,
Newcastle upon Tyne, UK

R. Amann,
Department of Experimental
& Clinical Pharmacology,
University of Graz,
Austria

J.H. Baron,
Royal Postgraduate Medical School,
University of London,
Hammersmith Hospital,
London W12 ONN, U.K.

Barbara L. Bass,
Department of Surgery,
V.A. Medical Center,
Washington D.C. 20422
U. S. A.

Shmuel Batzri,
Department of Surgery,
V.A. Medical Center,
Washington D.C. 20422
U. S. A.

Mark K. Bennett,
Department of Histopathology,
Freeman Hospital,
Newcastle upon Tyne, U.K.

T. Brzozowski,
Institute of Physiology,
Academy of Medicine,
Krakow,
Poland

*Gregory B. Bulkley,
The Department of Surgery,
The Johns Hopkins Medical
Institutions,
Baltimore,
Maryland, U.S.A.

V.A. Canfield,
Dept. of Cell Biology,
Yale Univ. School of Medicine,
New Haven,
Connecticut, U.S.A..

K. Carter,
Harvard Medical School,
Beth Israel Hospital,
Boston,
Massachusetts, U.S.A.

D.C. Chow,
Dept. of Cell & Molecular Biology,
University of California,
Berkeley,
California. U.S.A.

M. Classen,
II Med. Klinik der Techn.
Universitat,
Munich,
Germany

A.T. Cole,
Department of Therapeutics,
Queen's Medical Centre,
University Hospital,
Nottingham, U.K.

Kathryn S. Cowart,
Dept. of Anatomy & Cell Biology,
Medical University of
        South Carolina,
Charleston, SC. U.S.A.

Edward J. Cragoe,
2211 Oak Terrace Dr.
Lansdale,
Pennsylvania, U.S.A

John Crampton,
University of Cambridge,
School of Clinical Medicine,
Addenbrooke's Hospital,
Cambridge, CB2 2QQ, U.K.

* Conference Participant

A. Dembinski,
Institute of Physiology,
Academy of Medicine,
Krakow,
Poland

C.L. Donaldson,
Gastrointestinal Disease Research
Unit & Department of Biology,
Queen's University,
Kingston,
Ontario,
Canada

T.G. Douglass,
California State University,
Long Beach,
California. U.S.A.

Adam J. Dziki,
Department of Surgery,
V.A. Medical Center,
Washington D.C. 20422
U. S. A.

*J.V. Esplugues,
Department of Pharmacology,
University of Valencia,
Valencia,
Spain.

*L. Fändriks,
Department of Physiology,
University of Gothenburg,
P.O. Box 33031,
S-400 33 Gothenburg,
Sweden

W. Feil,
Clinic of Surgery 1,
University of Vienna,
Alserstrasse 4,
1090 Vienna,
Austria

J. Folkman,
Department of Surgery,
Children's Hospital Medical Center,
Harvard Medical School,
Boston,
Massachusetts 02115. U. S. A.

* J.G. Forte,
Department of Cell & Molecular
Biology,
University of California,
Berkeley,
California, U.S.A.

* Gary M. Frydman,
Monash University
Department of Surgery,
Alfred Hospital,
Melbourne. Australia

Y. Fuse,
Third Department of Internal
Medicine, Kyoto Prefectural
University of Medicine,
Kyoto, Japan

* Bren Gannon,
Department of Anatomy & Histology,
Flinders University of South Australia
Bedford Park,
South Australia

* A. Garner,
Department of Biochemistry,
University College of Wales,
Aberystwyth, U.K.

H. Gergely,
The University of California,
Irvine,
California. U.S.A.

Linda Gibbons,
Hope Hospital,
University of Manchester
School of Medicine,
Salford, U.K.

P. Goddard,
Harvard Medical School,
Beth Israel Hospital,
Boston,
Massachusetts, U.S.A.

P.M. Goggin,
Department of Medicine,
St. George's Hospital Medical School,
Cranmer Terrace,
Tooting,
London, U.K.

R.H. Gompertz,
Department of Surgery,
The Medical School,
Framlington Place,
Newcastle Upon Tyne, U.K.

Gregory J. Gores,
Dept. of Cell Biology & Anatomy,
School of Medicine,
University of North Carolina
    at Chapel Hill,
North Carolina, U.S.A.

*David Y. Graham,
Veterans Affairs Medical Center,
2002 Holcombe Blvd,
Houston,
Texas 77030, U.S.A.

D.N. Granger,
Department of Physiology and
Biophysics,
LSU Medical Centre,
Shreveport,
Louisiana, U.S.A

J.E. Grønbech,
Surgical Research Laboratory,
Department of Surgery,
University of Bergen,
Bergen, Norway

P.H. Guth,
Center for Ulcer
    Research & Education,
Wadsworth Veteran's
Administration Medical Centre,
Los Angeles,
California, 90073 U.S.A.

*F. Halter,
Gastrointestinal Unit,
University Hospital,
Inselspital,
Bern, Switzerland

A. Hamlet,
Department of Physiology,
University of Gothenburg,
S-400 33 Gothenburg,
Sweden

D.C. Hanley,
Department of Surgery,
Guy's Hospital,
London, U.K.

*John W. Harmon,
Department of Surgery,
V.A. Medical Center,
Washington D.C. 20422
U. S. A.

*C.J. Hawkey,
Department of Therapeutics,
Queen's Medical Centre,
University Hospital,
Nottingham, U.K.

A.B. Hawthorne,
Department of Therapeutics,
Queen's Medical Centre,
University Hospital,
Nottingham, U.K.

Brian Herman,
Dept. of Cell Biology & Anatomy,
School of Medicine,
University of North Carolina
    at Chapel Hill,
North Carolina, U.S.A.

D. Hillen,
Department of Medicine,
University of Adelaide,
Royal Adelaide Hospital,
Adelaide,
South Australia

*B.H. Hirst,
Department of Physiological Sciences,
University of Newcastle upon Tyne,
Newcastle upon Tyne, U.K.

*Daniel L. Hogan,
Division of Gastroenterology,
UCSD Medical Center,
University of California San Diego,
San Diego,
California. U.S.A.

C.A. Holitzner,
Gastrointestinal Disease Research
Unit & Department of Biology,
Queen's University,
Kingston,
Ontario, Canada

*D. Hollander,
Division of Gastroenterology,
College of Medicine,
University of California,
Irvine,
California, U.S.A.

*P. Holzer.
Dept. of Experimental & Clinical
Pharmacology,
University of Graz,
Austria

N. Hudson,
Department of Therapeutics,
Queen's Medical Centre,
University Hospital,
Nottingham, U.K.

*Richard H. Hunt,
Division of Gastroenterology,
McMaster University Medical Centre,
Hamilton,
Ontario, Canada

Roberto Imberti,
Dept. of Cell Biology & Anatomy,
School of Medicine,
University of North Carolina
    at Chapel Hill,
North Carolina, U.S.A.

Jon I. Isenberg,
Division of Gastroenterology,
UCSD Medical Center,
University of California San Diego,
San Diego,
California. U.S.A.

Takafumi Ishihara,
Laboratory of Experimental
Pharmacology,
Suntory Institute for Biomedical
Research,
Osaka, Japan

C. Jönson,
Department of Physiology,
University of Gothenburg,
P.O. Box 33031,
S-400 33 Gothenburg,
Sweden

K. Kato,
Takeda Chemical Industries Ltd.,
Osaka, Japan

Sunao Kawano,
The First Department of Medicine,
Osaka University Medical School,
Osaka, Japan

Catherine Keenan,
Gastrointestinal Research Group,
University of Calgary,
Calgary,
Alberta, Canada

Jan S. King,
Dept. of Anatomy & Cell Biology,
Medical University of South Carolina,
Charleston, SC. U.S.A.

R. Kinne,
Chirurgische Universitatsklinik
Tubingen and Max-Planck-Institut fur
Systemphysiologie,
Dortmund,
Germany.

Hisato Kitagawa,
The First Department of Medicine,
Osaka University Medical School,
Osaka, Japan

*Eero Kivilaakso,
II Department of Surgery,
Helsinki University Central Hospital,
SF-00290 Helsinki 29, Finland.

T. Kiviluoto,
II Department of Surgery,
Helsinki University Central Hospital,
SF-00290 Helsinki 29, Finland.

P.K. Konturek,
Institute of Physiology,
Academy of Medicine,
Krakow, Poland

*S.J. Konturek,
Institute of Physiology,
Academy of Medicine,
Krakow, Poland

W.J. Krause,
The University of Missouri,
Columbia,
Missouri, U.S.A.

*Eric R. Lacy,
Dept. of Anatomy & Cell Biology,
Medical University
of South Carolina,
Charleston, SC. U.S.A.

*John R. Lambert,
Monash University
Department of Medicine,
Prince Henry's Hospital,
Melbourne, Australia

C. Lancaster,
Safety Pharmacology,
The Upjohn Company,
Kalamazoo,
Missouri, U.S.A.

John J. Lemasters,
Dept. of Cell Biology & Anatomy,
School of Medicine,
University of North Carolina
at Chapel Hill,
North Carolina, U.S.A.

Andrea J. Leonard,
Department of Physiological Sciences,
Medical School,
Framlington Place,
Newcastle upon Tyne, U.K.

R. Levenson,
Department of Cell Biology,
Yale Univ. School of Medicine,
New Haven, CT. U.S.A.

S.K. Lin,
Monash University
Department of Medicine,
Prince Henry's Hospital,
Melbourne, Australia

I. Th. Lippe,
Department of Experimental &
Clinical Pharmacology,
University of Graz,
Austria

E.H. Livingston,
Center for Ulcer
Research & Education,
Wadsworth Veteran's Administration
Medical Centre,
Los Angeles,
California. 90073 U.S.A.

Y.R. Mahida,
Department of Therapeutics,
Queen's Medical Centre,
University Hospital,
Nottingham, U.K.

Cathy Malcontenti,
Monash University
Department of Surgery,
Alfred Hospital,
Melbourne. Australia

S.G. Mann,
Department of Therapeutics,
Queen's Medical Centre,
University Hospital,
Nottingham, U.K.

R.C. Mason,
Department of Surgery,
Guy's Hospital,
London, U.K.

Y. Masuda,
Laboratory of Experimental
Pharmacology,
Suntory Institute for
Biomedical Research,
Osaka, Japan

*J.B. Matthews,
Department of Surgery,
Beth Israel Hospital,
Boston,
Massachusetts, U.S.A.

Webb McKnight,
Gastrointestinal Research Group,
University of Calgary,
Calgary,
Alberta, Canada

A.S. Michalowski,
Royal Postgraduate Medical School,
University of London,
Hammersmith Hospital,
London W12 ONN, U.K.

R.E. Morales,
Department of Pathology,
Brigham & Women's Hospital,
75 Francis Street,
Boston,
Massachusetts 02115. U.S.A.

*G.P. Morris,
Gastrointestinal Disease Research
Unit & Department of Biology,
Queen's University,
Kingston,
Ontario, Canada

H. Mustonen,
II Department of Surgery,
Helsinki University Central Hospital,
SF-00290 Helsinki 29,
Finland.

*Anna-Liisa Nieminen,
Dept. of Cell Biology & Anatomy,
School of Medicine,
University of North Carolina
    at Chapel Hill,
North Carolina, U.S.A.

H. Niida,
Department of Applied Pharmacology,
Kyoto Pharmaceutical University,
Misasagi, Yamashina,
Kyoto, Japan

*T.C. Northfield,
Department of Medicine,
St. George's Hospital Medical School,
Cranmer Terrace,
Tooting,
London, U.K

*Olof Nylander,
Department of Physiology and
Medical Biophysics,
Biomedical Center,
Uppsala University,
Sweden

*Paul O'Brien,
Monash University
Department of Surgery,
Alfred Hospital,
Melbourne, Australia

Tatsuo Ogihara,
The First Department of Medicine,
Osaka University Medical School,
Osaka, Japan

Y. Ogihara,
Department of Applied Pharmacology,
Kyoto Pharmaceutical University,
Kyoto, Japan,

*Tomochika Ohno,
Laboratory of Experimental
Pharmacology, Suntory Institute for
Biomedical Research,
Osaka, Japan

*Susumu Okabe,
Department of Applied Pharmacology,
Kyoto Pharmaceutical University,
Misasagi, Yamashina,
Kyoto, Japan

C.T. Okamoto,
Dept. of Cell & Molecular Biology,
University of California,
Berkeley,
California. U.S.A.

A.S. Olafsson,
Safety Pharmacology,
The Upjohn Company,
Kalamazoo,
Missouri, U.S.A.

*Roy C. Orlando,
University of North Carolina
School of Medicine,
Department of Medicine,
Chapel Hill,
North Carolina, U.S.A.

CONTRIBUTORS

H. Paimela,
II Department of Surgery,
Helsinki University Central Hospital,
SF-00290 Helsinki 29,
Finland.

J.P. Pearson,
Department of Physiological Sciences,
Medical School,
Framlington Place,
Newcastle upon Tyne, UK

Angela Penny,
Monash University
Department of Surgery,
Alfred Hospital,
Melbourne. Australia

*****Michael A. Perry,**
School of Physiology and
Pharmacology,
University of New South Wales,
Sydney, Australia

B.A. Peskar,
Department of Pharmacology
    & Toxicology,
University of Bochum,
Germany.

B.M. Peskar,
Deptartment of Experimental
    Clinical Medicine,
University of Bochum,
Germany

G. Pinkus,
Department of Pathology,
Brigham & Women's Hospital,
75 Francis Street,
Boston
Massachusetts 02115, U.S.A.

H.E. Raybould,
Center for Ulcer
    Research & Education,
Wadsworth Veteran's Administration
Medical Centre,
Los Angeles,
California, U.S.A.

*****Wynne Rees,**
Hope Hospital,
University of Manchester
School of Medicine,
Salford, U.K.

Patrick M. Reilly,
The Department of Surgery,
The Johns Hopkins Medical
Institutions,
Baltimore,
Maryland, U.S.A.

M. Riegler,
Clinic of Surgery 1,
University of Vienna,
Alserstrasse 4,
1090 Vienna,
Austria

*****Andre Robert,**
Safety Pharmacology,
The Upjohn Company,
Kalamazoo,
Missouri, U.S.A.

S. Roithmaier,
II Med. Klinik der Techn.
Universitat,
Munich,
Germany

*****Paul H. Rowe,**
Eastbourne District General Hospital,
Kings Drive,
Eastbourne,
East Sussex, U.K.

Manaf Sababi,
Department of Physiology
    and Medical Biophysics,
Biomedical Center,
Uppsala University,
Sweden

I.J. Sarfeh,
DVA Medical Centre, Long Beach,
and The University of California,
Irvine,
California. U.S.A.

*Nobuhiro Sato,
The First Department of Medicine,
Osaka University Medical School,
Osaka, Japan

M. Schembri,
Monash University
Department of Medicine,
Prince Henry's Hospital,
Melbourne, Australia

*R. Schiessel,
Clinic of Surgery 1,
University of Vienna,
Alserstrasse 4,
1090 Vienna, Austria

V. Schusdziarra,
II Med. Klinik der Techn.
Universitat,
Munich,
Germany

*Ursula Seidler,
II Med. Klinik der Techn.
Universitat,
Munich,
Germany

Lynda A. Sellers,
Department of Physiological Sciences,
Medical School,
Framlington Place,
Newcastle upon Tyne, U.K.

*David J.C. Shearman,
Department of Medicine,
University of Adelaide,
Royal Adelaide Hospital,
Adelaide, South Australia

*C. J. Shorrock,
University Department of Medicine,
Queen Elizabeth Hospital,
Birmingham, U.K.

*W. Silen,
Harvard Medical School,
Beth Israel Hospital,
Boston,
Massachusetts, U.S.A.

J. Stachura,
The University of California,
Irvine,
California. U.S.A.

*Michael Starlinger,
Chirurgische Universitatsklinik
Tubingen and Max-Planck-Institut fur
Systemphysiologie,
Dortmund, Germany.

*Knut Svanes,
Surgical Research Laboratory,
Department of Surgery,
University of Bergen,
Bergen, Norway

*Sandor Szabo,
Department of Pathology,
Brigham & Women's Hospital,
75 Francis Street,
Boston,
Massachusetts 02115, U.S.A.

*Yvette Tache,
Center for Ulcer
   Research and Education,
VA Wadsworth Medical Center,
Department of Medicine & Brain
Research Institute, UCLA,
Los Angeles. U.S.A.

*K. Takeuchi,
Department of Applied Pharmacology,
Kyoto Pharmaceutical University,
Misasagi, Yamashina,
Kyoto, Japan

*A. Tarnawski
Division of Gastroenterology,
College of Medicine,
University of California,
Irvine,
California, U.S.A.

Barry L. Tepperman,
Department of Pharmacology,
Wellcome Research Laboratories,
Langley Court,
Beckenham,
Kent, U.K.

Neila A. Tobey,
University of North Carolina
School of Medicine,
Department of Medicine,
Chapel Hill,
North Carolina, U.S.A.

Shingo Tsuji,
The First Department of Medicine,
Osaka University Medical School,
Osaka, Japan

K.H. Tufts,
Gastrointestinal Disease Research
Unit & Department of Biology,
Queen's University,
Kingston,
Ontario, Canada

K. Ueshima,
Department of Applied Pharmacology,
Kyoto Pharmaceutical University,
Misasagi, Yamashina,
Kyoto, Japan

Richard M. Ugarte,
Department of Surgery,
V.A. Medical Center,
Washington D.C. 20422. U. S. A.

Hiroshi Uramoto,
Laboratory of Experimental
Pharmacology,
Suntory Institute for Biomedical
Research,
Osaka, Japan

Paula Vaananen,
Gastrointestinal Research Group,
University of Calgary,
Alberta, Canada

P. Vattay,
Department of Pathology,
Brigham & Women's Hospital,
75 Francis Street,
Boston
Massachusetts 02115, U.S.A.

*John Wallace,
Gastrointestinal Research Group,
University of Calgary,
Alberta, Canada

M. Weinlich,
Chirurgische Universitatsklinik
Tubingen and Max-Planck-Institut fur
Systemphysiologie,
Dortmund, Germany.

E. Wenzl,
Clinic of Surgery 1,
University of Vienna,
Alserstrasse 4,
1090 Vienna, Austria

*B.J.R. Whittle,
Department of Pharmacology,
Wellcome Research Laboratories,
Langley Court, Beckenham,
Kent, U.K.

O.W. Wiebkin.
Department of Medicine,
University of Adelaide,
Royal Adelaide Hospital,
Adelaide, South Australia

S.C. Wiebkin,
Department of Medicine,
University of Adelaide,
Royal Adelaide Hospital,
Adelaide, South Australia

T.E. Williamson,
Gastrointestinal Disease Research
Unit & Department of Biology,
Queen's University,
Kingston,
Ontario, Canada

A. Yanaka,
Harvard Medical School,
Beth Israel Hospital,
Boston,
Massachusetts, U.S.A.

Q. Zhang,
Department of Surgery,
Guy's Hospital,
London, U.K.

W. Zhang,
Safety Pharmacology,
The Upjohn Company,
Kalamazoo,
Missouri, U.S.A.

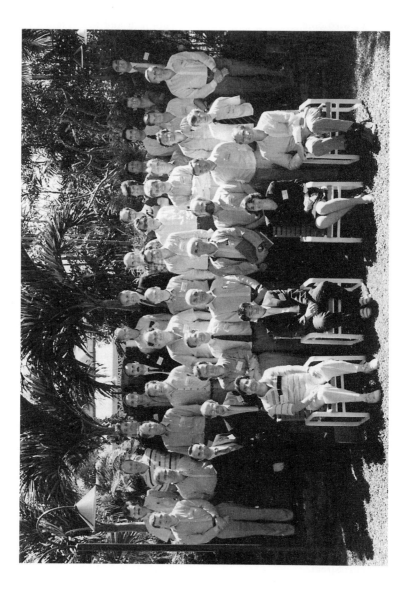

xxi

INVITED SPEAKERS

Back Row *(from left)*

Wynne Rees, Richard Hunt, Eric Lacy, John Wallace, Juan Esplugues,
Bill Silen, Gregory Bulkley, Sandor Szabo, Michael Starlinger, Andrew Garner,
Tomochika Ohno, Jeffrey Matthews, Christopher Shorrock, Koji Takeuchi.

Third Row *(from left)*

John Lambert, Eero Kivilaakso, Knut Svanes, Bren Gannon, Gary Frydman,
Timothy Northfield, Paul O'Brien, Fred Halter, Christopher Hawkey,
Olof Nylander, Barry Hirst, Lars Fandriks, Daniel Hogan.

Second Row *(from left)*

Roy Orlando, Andrew Robert, Adrian Allen, Peter Holzer,
Andrzej Tarnawski, Stanislaw Konturek, Gerald Morris, Rudi Schiessel, Michael Perry.

Front Row *(from left)*

Robert Breslier, Susumu Okabe, Yvette Tache, John Harmon

Speakers absent from photograph

John Forte, David Graham, Henry Gompertz, Daniel Hollander, Anna-Liisa Nieminen, Paul Rowe,
Nobuhiro Sato, Ursula Siedler, David Shearman, Brendan Whittle

PREFACE

Opportunity to organise this symposium was presented on the occasion of the 9th World Congress of Gastroenterology held in Sydney in August 1990. The symposium, entitled "Mechanisms of Injury, Protection and Repair of the Upper Gastrointestinal Tract", was an official satellite meeting of the World Congress. The meeting was addressed by over fifty leading research workers in the field, ranging from basic scientists to clinical gastroenterologists, and attended by a further seventy delegates. As befits a conference on mucosal barriers, the meeting was held in Cairns, North Queensland - the gateway to the Great Barrier Reef.

The topic of mucosal protection was the subject of innumerable symposia during the 1980s and has been reviewed at length in the scientific literature. Thus, in organising the present meeting, we saw little value in gathering together international experts simply to review their own and others' published data. Rather, the conference was based on short presentations of original data as reflected in the following contributions to this book. Such an approach provided an excellent stimulus for discussion at the meeting itself and should considerably enhance the value of the published proceedings to other workers in this field.

In planning the present symposium we wished to emphasise the changes which are occurring with respect to both laboratory and clinical research. It will be apparent to readers of this volume that progress has been made in identifying mediators of injury and protection, quantitative assessment of damage and repair, and understanding the basis of protection at the cellular and membrane levels. Changes have also occurred with the focus shifting to study of chronic processes rather than acute responses, the microvasculature and deeper mucosal elements rather than surface phenomena, and use of relevant pathophysiological means of inducing injury rather than nonspecific chemical necrotising agents.

Organising of scientific meetings is a complex and time-consuming task. Our special thanks go to Kathy Noble, Department of Surgery, Monash University School of Medicine, who handled the administrative responsibilities and local organisation of this symposium. Thanks are also due to Drs. Eric Lacy, Susumo Okabe, Wynne Rees, William Silen and Brendan Whittle who assisted in planning the scientific sessions and with raising financial support for the conference. Finally we acknowledge the co-operation of John Wiley & Sons for ensuring prompt publication of this volume which, we believe, represents the most comprehensive and up-to-date account of current work on the topic of gastrointestinal mucosal injury, protection and repair.

ANDREW GARNER   PAUL O'BRIEN

xxii

LUMINAL ACIDITY: ROLE IN ULCERATION AND HEALING

Richard H. Hunt

Division of Gastroenterology, McMaster University Medical Centre, Hamilton, Ontario, Canada

INTRODUCTION

The presence of acid is still considered a major factor in the causation of mucosal gastric injury in peptic ulcer disease. Peptic ulcer does not occur in patients who are achlorhydric and very rarely in those with a maximal acid output of <10 mmol per hour. Furthermore, suppression of gastric acid by surgical or a variety of pharmacological means provides the most effective and rapid ulcer healing. However, the exact relationship between gastric acid secretion and the occurrence of peptic ulceration or between acid suppression and ulcer healing has not been clearly established. This paper reviews the role of acid in experimental ulceration and new data indicating the appropriate level of acid suppression for ulcer healing.

ACUTE ULCERATION IN ANIMAL STUDIES

In experimental studies of acute ulceration, several authors have questioned the role of acid alone as a damaging agent. In classical studies conducted as far back as the 1940's Schiffrin and Warren demonstrated the importance of pepsin in addition to acid for ulceration to occur [1]. In studies in the cat, 12 hour perfusion of a loop of the jejunum with acid at pH 1.2-1.3 resulted in no bleeding, ulceration, or perforation. The mucosa presented a greyish necrotized appearance but histology revealed little damage to the villi. When a 3% solution of 1:3000 pepsin was added to the perfusate at the same pH bleeding and ulceration, and sometimes frank perforation occurred. Similarly, pepsin in an acid medium produced more damage in the duodenum and the stomach. However, the differences in the degree of damage between acid alone and acid with pepsin was less obvious in the stomach, but this was explained by the fact that acid perfusion alone of the stomach had acquired measurable peptic activity as it passed through the stomach. In the presence of pepsin, the optimum pH for ulceration in the jejunum was pH 1.1-1.5 and there was no digestion when the pH was 2.24.

Recent studies in the rat have questioned the functional importance of the mucus bicarbonate barrier in protecting the gastric mucosa against the injurious effects of acid and pepsin [2]. By minimizing the possible protective effects of a mucus stabilized pH gradient with continuous stirring, it was seen that acid at pH 1.3 or pH 0.8 rapidly dissipated this gradient. Exposure to acid alone or with the addition of the mucolytic agent N-acetylcysteine or pepsin did not damage the mucosa as assessed by

1

PD, macroscopically, histologically, or by measurement of the luminal protein concentration. However, disruption of the surface epithelium by 1M hypertonic saline rendered the mucosa significantly more susceptible to the damaging action of acid at pH 0.8. This capacity of damaging agents to initiate the damaging effects of concentrated acid is also seen with ethanol injury [3].

In this study, 40% ethanol alone resulted in focal hyperaemia of the mucosa with exfoliation of the surface epithelium and release of mucus. When 50 mM HCl (pH 1.3) was added, subsequent to the ethanol, black haemorrhagic areas were seen, platelet thrombi were destroyed, mucus dissipated, and the fibrin network broken down. This resulted in irreversible cell damage and exposure of the basal lamina. Furthermore, under normal circumstances with an intact gastric mucosal barrier some H+ back diffusion occurs during acid exposure in the lumen [4]. Disruption of the normal mucosal barrier leads to reflux of bicarbonate from the mucosa which neutralizes H+ locally, masking H+ back diffusion and protecting the mucosa. If the supply of HCO_3^- to the mucosa is blocked during exposure of the mucosa to acid at low pH together with a barrier breaking agent H+ back diffusion is unmasked and leads to extensive acidification and subsequent ulceration of the mucosa.

Studies such as these suggest that acid alone down to pH 0.8 is not in itself inherently damaging and that some additional injurious luminal factor or the failure of HCO_3^- release from the surface epithelium is responsible for irreversible damage to occur. However, these results come from a variety of animal studies of acute ulceration usually performed *in vitro*. It is difficult to extrapolate these findings to the clinical situation in patients with peptic ulcer disease where antisecretory agents are so effectively used to accelerate ulcer healing.

ROLE OF ACID SUPPRESSION IN ULCER HEALING

The relationship between intragastric acidity and peptic ulcer healing has aroused great interest since the early part of this century when Schwarz advocated "no acid - no ulcer" [5]. The development of potent and long acting antisecretory drugs such as the proton pump blockers and high affinity H2-receptor antagonists can almost totally abolish acid secretion depending on the dose prescribed. Furthermore, increased potency of acid suppression is associated with the highest observed healing rates, and a leftward shift of the healing, time curve [6]. However, such profound acid suppression has raised concerns about possible adverse effects [7].

Several attempts to define the degree of acid secretion to obtain ulcer healing have been described. A threshold secretion rate of 12 mmol/h for MAO to 15 mmol/h for PAO has been proposed by Baron from studies of stimulated acid secretion, and this is widely used as a target in surgical treatment and for the pharmacological control of patients with Zollinger Ellison syndrome [8]. More recently the relationship between acid suppression and duodenal ulcer healing has been extensively examined in two models using advanced meta-analysis techniques to correlate the suppression of 24 h intragastric acidity with weighted ulcer healing rates

[9,10]. Two similar meta-analyses have been undertaken to explore the relationship between acid suppression and gastric ulcer healing [11,12].

In the first duodenal ulcer analysis [9] it was shown for the first time that there is a clear and predictable linear relationship between acid suppression and the rate of duodenal ulcer healing. The results provided important information about the antisecretory drugs currently available for ulcer therapy. Analysis of the H2-receptor antagonists alone confirmed a highly significant relationship between four week healing rates and the suppression of night time acidity (r=0.926, p=0.0001). Furthermore, step-wise linear regression established that suppression of nocturnal acidity with this class of drugs was primarily responsible for the suppression of 24 h acidity and four week healing rates (r=0.681, p=0.0203). This phenomenon is due predominantly to the fact that the H2-receptor antagonists are very effective at inhibiting basal acid secretion and the night time is a prolonged period of basal acid secretion. During the day acid secretion is stimulated by the ingestion of food and drinks at meal times. The relationship of both nocturnal and 24h acid suppression to ulcer healing is linear in the range of suppression achieved by the H2-receptor antagonists between 60 and 95%, but the regression line does not predict 100% ulcer healing at four weeks even with complete suppression of intragastric acidity. When the data for an antacid, a prostaglandin, and four doses of omeprazole were included in the analysis with the H2-receptor antagonists, duodenal ulcer healing correlated better with the suppression of total 24h intragastric acidity (r=0.911,p<0.0001). This suggested that for some drugs suppression of daytime acidity might be an advantage or that the duration of time for which any given degree of acid suppression was achieved might be important. In this analysis the relative contribution of the suppression of daytime to night-time acidity with omeprazole was difficult to evaluate since this drug has a relatively prolonged duration of action over the 24h period [13].

This analysis emphasized the arbitrary nature of the time points chosen for the duration of treatment trials in duodenal ulcer. For example, omeprazole 60 mgm achieves 100% duodenal ulcer healing after four weeks treatment, an effect approached by single nocturnal doses of cimetidine 800 mgm hs or ranitidine 300 mgm hs after eight weeks treatment with healing rates of 96% and 95% respectively.

This analysis identified two important parameters of time: the duration for which acidity was suppressed during the 24h period and also the duration for which treatment was given.

A similar approach has been taken to examine the relationship between the suppression of intragastric acidity and gastric ulcer healing [11,12]. For a variety of antisecretory drug regimens there was a significant correlation between the suppression of 24 hour intragastric acidity and gastric ulcer healing rates after 2, 4 and 8 weeks of treatment. There was a lesser correlation between gastric ulcer healing and the suppression of nocturnal acidity than was seen for duodenal ulcer. However, gastric ulcer healing was related to the same parameters of antisecretory therapy as was seen in duodenal ulcer, which implies that the two conditions are not

materially different in their response to antisecretory treatment despite
some differences in the initial and untreated levels of acid secretion.

   Thus, these several studies suggested that the extent of antisecretory
therapy could be defined in terms of three parameters: degree of effect,
duration of effect, and length of therapy. An increase in any one or all of
these parameters results in an increase in the proportion of ulcers healed at
any arbitrary time point.

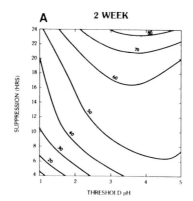

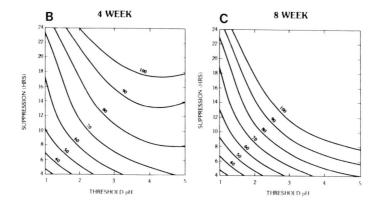

FIGURE 1   Contour plots calculated for fixed, predefined durations of
duodenal ulcer therapy at 2 weeks(A), 4 weeks(B), and 8 weeks(C).
Each contour plot shows the predicted healing rate as "isolines" which
connect points of equal healing as indicated by the numerical proportions
on each line.   (From Burget DW, Chiverton SG and Hunt RH.
Gastroenterol 1990;99:345-351 with acknowledgement)

A further model was therefore constructed to define the relationship between duodenal ulcer healing and antisecretory therapy that would be able to address fully these three parameters [10]. Acid suppression data was obtained directly from the investigators whose pharmacodynamic studies had already been subjected to meta-analysis [9]. The raw data from 24h studies of intragastric pH from seven investigators provided 490 24-hour studies using 19 different treatment regimens. Healing data was collected from a meta-analysis of published clinical trials of duodenal ulcer healing. A total of 144 published trials in 14,208 patients provided the data for healing at several endoscopic endpoints for the 19 drug regimens for which intragastric acidity data was available. A weighted least squares polynomial regression analysis was used to define the parameters of antisecretory treatment which contributed most to duodenal ulcer healing, and to define the shape of the response surface. The analysis demonstrated a highly significant correlation (r=0.9814,p<0.0001) between the degree of acid suppression, the duration of acid suppression and the length of therapy, and ulcer healing. By evaluating the degree of acid suppression in 0.2 incremental steps in pH the analysis defined pH as the critical threshold. The shape of the contours representing this relationship demonstrates clearly that healing continues to increase as the duration of acid suppression increases and as intragastric pH increases (Figure 1). However, increasing this suppression above pH 3.0 does not increase further the proportion of ulcers healed.

In Figure 1 it can be seen that there is very little increase in the proportion of ulcers healed with an increase in pH above pH3 and that the total duration of suppression during the 24 hour period is of much greater importance.

The results confirmed the highly significant and predictable relationship between the defined parameters of antisecretory therapy and ulcer healing, namely the degree and duration of suppression of intragastric acidity and the length of treatment. Furthermore, a longer duration of antisecretory effect and/or a longer duration of treatment are of greater importance than potency of acid suppression for duodenal ulcer healing.

CONCLUSION

Thus, it is clear that there is a marked discrepancy between the intraluminal pH at which mucosal damage occurs in experimental animal systems and that required to optimize the environment to initiate healing of peptic ulcer in humans. The importance of pepsin in relation to ulceration and healing remains to be explored, but residual peptic activity in gastric juice after ulceration has occurred may require a high pH for effective inactivation of peptic activity and to achieve optimal ulcer healing.

REFERENCES

1. Schiffrin and Warren (1942). Some factors concerning the production of experimental ulceration of the gastrointestinal tract in cats. Am J Dig Dis 9(6):205-209.

2. Wallace JL (1989). Gastric resistance to acid: is the "mucus bicarbonate barrier" functionally redundant? Am J Physiol 256:G31-G38.

3. Morris GP, Wallace JL (1981). The roles of ethanol and of acid in the production of gastric mucosal erosions in rats. Virchows Arch 38:23-38.

4. Kiviluoto, Voipio & Kivilaakso (1988). Subeipthelial tissue pH of rate gastric mucosa exposed to luminal acid, barrier breaking agents, and hemorrhagic shock. Gastroenterol 94:695-702.

5. Schwarz K (1910). Ueber penetriende Magen-Und Jejunalgeschwure. Beitr Z Klin Chir 67:96-128.

6. Chiverton SG, Hunt RH. Medical regimens in short and longterm ulcer management. In: Eds Piper DW, Peptic Ulcer. Ballieres Clinics in Gastroenterol 1988;2(3);655-676.

7. Hunt RH (1988). The protective role of acid. Scand J Gastroenterol 23(suppl);146:34-39.

8. Baron JH (1973). The clinical application of gastric secretion measurements. Clin Gastroenterol 2:293-314.

9. Jones DB, Howden CW, Burget DW, Kerr GD, Hunt RH (1987). Acid suppression in duodenal ulcer: A meta-analysis to define optimal dosing with antisecretory drugs. Gut 28:1120-1127.

10. Burget DW, Chiverton SG, Hunt RH (1990). Is there an optimal degree of acid suppression in healing duodenal ulcer? A model of the relationship between ulcer healing and acid suppression. Gastroenterol 99:345-351.

11. Howden CW, Jones DB, Peace K, Burget DW, Hunt RH (1988). The treatment of gastric ulcer with antisecretory drugs: relationship of pharmacological effect to healing rates. Dig Dis Sci 33(5):619-624.

12. Howden CW and Hunt RH (1990). The relationship between suppression of acidity and gastric ulcer healing. Aliment Pharmacol Therap 4:25-34.

13. Prichard PJ, Yeomans ND, Mihaly GW et al. Omeprazole: A study of its inhibition of gastric pH and oral pharmacokinetics after morning and evening dosage. Gastroenterol 1985;88:64-69.

PEPSIN INDUCED MUCOSAL DAMAGE COMPARED TO THAT WITH ETHANOL OR HYPERTONIC SALINE: THE ROLE OF THE ADHERENT MUCUS BARRIER

Adrian Allen, Andrea J. Leonard, J.P. Pearson, Lynda A. Sellers and *Mark K. Bennett

*Department of Physiological Sciences, Medical School, Framlington Place, Newcastle upon Tyne, UK. and *Department of Histopathology, Freeman Hospital, Newcastle upon Tyne, UK.*

ABSTRACT

An *in vivo* pepsin damage model has been developed using the pylorus ligated stomach of an anaesthetized rat. Instillation of pepsin (2 mg ml-1:0.1M HCl) over 2 hours resulted in progressive disruption of the adherent mucus layer; a large significant increase in soluble degraded mucin; small focal, haemorrhagic mucosal lesions and significant bleeding into the lumen. Histologically, localised, punctate ulcers were observed with the rest of the epithelium remaining intact and there was no evidence of re-epithelialisation. Instillation of 0.1M HCl alone did not affect the adherent mucus layer or cause any discernable histological damage. Pepsin damage differed markedly from that following ethanol (70%, 45 sec) or 2M NaCl (30 min) where rapid penetration of the adherent mucus barrier results in exfoliation of the epithelium, a large drop in mucosal P.D., increased permeability to i.v. radioactive inulin, but no haemorrhagic lesions. A thick mucoid coat, absent with pepsin damage, was observed with recovery and re-epithelialisation after ethanol or 2M NaCl damage. Pepsin potentiated damage by 70% ethanol or 2M NaCl, producing deep seated mucosal lesions and significant mucosal bleeding. It is concluded (1) pepsin will cause mucosal damage under conditions where 0.1M acid is ineffective, (2) the mucosal response to pepsin damage is significantly different from that following ethanol or hypertonic NaCl, (3) the adherent gastric mucus gel is normally a barrier to pepsin but not ethanol or 2M NaCl aggression *in vivo*.

INTRODUCTION

Luminal pepsin can potentiate gastroduodenal mucosal damage in animal models. An increased incidence of gastric ulceration in rats has been observed when pepsin 1 mg ml^{-1} was added to acid (pH 1.3) perfusates under pressure [1] while addition of pepsin to gastric juice perfusates increased mucosal lesions in both rat stomach and duodenum [2]. Pepsin but not acid pH 2.2 has been shown to cause a collapse in the resistance of frog gastric and oesophageal mucosa *in vitro* [3,4].

It has been postulated that the adherent gastroduodenal mucus gel is an important protective barrier against pepsin attack of the underlying epithelium [5,6]. This is based firstly, on the demonstration that gastric mucus gel effectively acts as a diffusion barrier to large sized proteins such

7

as pepsin [7]. Secondly there is a substantial body of evidence to support a continuous adherent mucus-gel layer covering the surface of the undamaged mucosa [8-15] although the continuity of the gastric mucus layer has been disputed by some workers [16,17]. The adherent gastric mucus layer on unfixed mucosal sections is continuous with a median thickness of 80um in the rat and 180um in man with minimum thickness values of 10um and 50$\underline{u}$m respectively [18,19].

While luminal pepsin does not penetrate into the mucus gel by diffusion, evidence from detailed structural studies *in vitro* [7], and in man *in vivo* [20] show the surface mucus gel layer is progressively solubilised at its surface by pepsin. Since an adherent and continuous gastric mucus gel layer is observed *in vivo*, mucus secretion must be normally sufficient to replenish that lost by peptic erosion. Here we describe a gastric damage model in the anaesthetized rat where an excess of pepsin (2 mg ml^{-1}, five times maximal secretion) is instilled in order to increase the rate of degradation of the adherent mucus barrier.

METHODS

Fasted, male Wistar rats 180g-220g were anaesthetized with 25% urethane; 1.5g Kg^{-1} intramuscularly and maintained at 35°C. Laparotomy was performed, the pylorus was ligated and a double lumen cannula was passed through a transverse incision in the oesophagus, fed distally into the stomach and the top and bottom of the oesophagus were ligated around the cannula.

Each experiment comprised five successive 30 min periods. 4 ml of fresh solution was instilled into the stomach at the start of each period and aspirated after 30 min. 4 ml volumes were used to ensure complete contact of the entire mucosal surface area with the instilled solution [21].

After an initial control period of 4 ml 0.1M HCl made isotonic with 0.05M NaCl (30 min), the following solutions were instilled in 4 ml volumes for four further 30 min periods.

Group I: 0.1M HCl/0.05M NaCl (4 x 30 min).

Group II: 0.1M HCl/0.05M NaCl/pepsin 2 mg ml^{-1} (4 x 30 min).

Group III: 70% v/v ethanol for 45 sec followed by 0.1M HCl/0.05M NaCl (4 x 30 min).

Group IV: 2M NaCl for 30 min followed by 0.1M HCl/0.05M NaCl (3 x 30 min).

Group V: 70% ethanol for 45 seconds followed by 0.1M HCl/0.05M NaCl/pepsin 2 mg ml^{-1} (4 x 30 min).

Group VI: 2M NaCl for 30 min followed by 0.1M HCl/0.05M NaCl/pepsin 2 mg ml^{-1} (3 x 30 min).

The mean pH of the 0.1M HCl instillates for all groups remained between pH 1 - 1.3 (4 x 30 min) during instillation.

Pepsin was assayed using succinyl albumin substrate and trinitrobenzene chromagen [6]. Following instillation of pepsin (2 mg ml^{-1}) the concentration of active pepsin in the collected instillates was always 2 $\pm$ 0.4 mg ml^{-1}.

Mucin glycoprotein in the instillates was assayed by digesting samples with papain (75ug ml^{-1} per instillate) and exhaustively dialysing for three days to remove digested protein which otherwise interferes with the assay. Digested mucin glycopeptides remain within the dialysis sac during this procedure. Mucin glycoprotein was assayed by the periodic acid-Schiff method [22] using pig gastric mucin as standard.

Adherent mucus gel thickness was measured by direct observation of unfixed sections of mucosa [9]. Mucosal sections continually bathed in saline were mounted transversely on a glass slide and viewed under an inverse microscope using an eyepiece graticule to measure gel thickness.

Mucosal permeability was assessed by leakage into the instillate of tritiated inulin (100 uCi ml^{-1}) given in saline as a 0.2 ml bolus dose via a jugular vein cannula, 15 min beforehand to allow equilibrium of the marker across the mucosa. Transmucosal potential difference was monitored continuously using idential Ag/AgCl electrodes.

Mucosal bleeding in instillates was quantified as a total iron content measured by atomic absorption at 248.3 nm.

Histology was monitored after formalin fixation by staining 5 um sections with haemotoxylin and eosin, periodic acid Schiffs and using an indirect immunoperoxidase technique for fibrinogen/fibrin.

RESULTS AND DISCUSSION

PEPSIN INDUCED MUCOSAL DAMAGE

Following instillation of 0.1M HCl for 2.5 hours (includes 30 min washout) (Group I), the rat gastric mucosa showed no blood in the instillates, no visible mucosal damage and histology was that of a normal epithelium.

Instillation of pepsin (2 mg ml^{-1}) pH 1 for 2 hr (Group II), in contrast to acid alone, consistently produced pin point focal haemorrhagic lesions and blood in the instillates. Estimation of blood content as haemoglobin iron measured by atomic absorption proved a rapid and simple way of quantitating bleeding in the instillates. The iron content of instillates only increased above basal values when blood was visible and there was a qualitative correlation between the extent of visible bleeding (assessed on a scale of 1-3) and iron content of instillate. Control values of iron in instillates in the absence of mucosal bleeding (e.g. Group I, HCl only) ranged from 0.01-2.14 ug ml^{-1} (mean 0.49 ug ml^{-1}) (Figure 1). The blood in the instillates following pepsin:HCl over 2 hours (Group II) was matched by a progressive and significantly increased iron content over that from 0.1M

HCl alone where no bleeding occurred (Figure 1). Mucosal scrapings from the surface of individual rat stomachs contained a mean of 0.35 ug ml^{-1} of iron, less than the mean control values. This showed that contamination by mucosal tissue did not contribute to observed increases in iron associated with bleeding following pepsin:HCl.

Histological examination of gastric mucosa following instillation of pepsin (Group II) for 2 hours showed focal areas of mucosal disruption, which were quite severe in places and affected up to 20% of the mucosal surface area. Sites of damage showed desquamation of the surface foveolar cells and deeper necrosis of the pit epithelium with the resultant exposure of the lamina propria. The specialised glands beneath this were normal. There was no evidence of fibrin exudation or re-epithelialisation. The epithelium, away from the sites of damage, appeared relatively normal. Although regenerative changes were visible (with mitotic activity extending to the upper portions of the crypts), many cells showed mucin loss, having presumably discharged their intracellular stores.

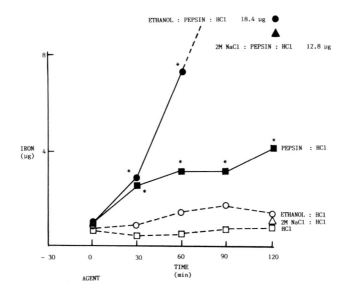

FIGURE 1: *Gastric mucosal permeability to i.v. [³H]-inulin measured as dpm in instillates. 30 min instillation of 0.1M HCl followed by 4 x 30 min instillates each of 4 ml. Instillations were 0.1M HCl alone [□] or 70% ethanol (45 sec) followed by instillation of 0.1M HCl [O]; or 2M NaCl (30 min) followed by instillation of 0.1M HCl [Δ]; with pepsin, closed symbols and solid line; without pepsin, open symbols and dotted line; (n = 5 or 6 in each group). Values are mean ± SEM.*
* *significantly different (p<0.05) to 0.1M HCl by Student's t-test.*

These results show pepsin has the potential to cause mucosal damage under conditions where acid alone is ineffective and points to the epithelial layer *per se* being susceptible to pepsin hydrolysis. The amount of instilled pepsin, 2 mg ml^{-1}, while deliberately made high in order to overwhelm the mucosal barrier, was the minimum that consistently produced mucosal haemorrhage. This concentration of pepsin was five-fold the maximum pepsin output (0.37 mg ml^{-1} for 30 min) in the rat, measured in these studies following maximal stimulation with insulin (125 units kg^{-1}). The maximum stimulated dose in man is reported as 0.7 mg ml^{-1} [23]. Pig pepsin was used in these studies because of its ready availability and its equivalent electrophoretic mobility, proteolytic and mucolytic activity to human pepsin 3 [6].

ETHANOL (70) AND HYPERTONIC NaCl (2M) INDUCED DAMAGE: POTENTIATION BY PEPSIN

Ethanol induced gastric damage was similar to that previously reported in the rat stomach [16,21,24,25]. No mucosal bleeding occurred following acute ethanol damage with basal iron values in the subsequent instillates of 0.1M HCl (Group III) (Figure 1). However, in contrast to pepsin, histology showed complete exfoliation of the epithelium had occurred. At the surface there was a mucoid coat which was formed from fibrin (positively stained by immunoperoxidase), contained large numbers of necrotic cells and was associated with the PAS positive staining of epithelial mucus. There was evidence for extensive re-epithelialisation after 2 hours of acid instillation, although punctate full mucosal thickness ulcers were present on up to 10% of the mucosa. Such ulcers were not seen if subsequent recovery was in isotonic NaCl.

2M NaCl (30 min) caused extensive exfoliation of cells across the whole gastric mucosa with some evidence of re-epithelialisation after 90 min. subsequent exposure to 0.1M HCl (Group IV). A fluffy mucoid coat of necrotic cells and mucin formed over the mucosa but this coat did not stain for fibrin, suggesting it is not the same composition as that formed following acute ethanol damage.

The contrast between the focal haemorrhagic damage by pepsin and the complete exfoliation of the epithelium by ethanol was further emphasised by studies with the transmucosal potential difference and leakage of i.v. [^{3}H]-inulin into the instillates. The gastric transmucosal P.D. was unchanged during instillation of 0.1M HCl (Group I) or pepsin, pH 1 (Group II) over 2 hours, mean P.D. for each stomach ranged from -29mV - 35.5mV. Following ethanol for 45 seconds (Group III) the mucosal P.D. immediately dropped to -5mV and there was no recovery during subsequent acid instillation. Leakage into the instillates of i.v. [^{3}H]-inulin gave low values during instillation of acid or pepsin (Figure 2). Following ethanol (45 sec) damage there was an immediate three-fold increase in [^{3}H]-inulin in the subsequent acid instillates and a five-fold increase with 2M NaCl for 30 min (Figure 2). Because of the difficulties of interpreting the passage of the large molecular weight [^{3}H]-inulin through the mucoid coat, it was not possible to say how much of the fall in [^{3}H]-inulin levels in the later instillations following ethanol and 2M NaCl was due to recovery of mucosal integrity rather than trapping of inulin at the surface.

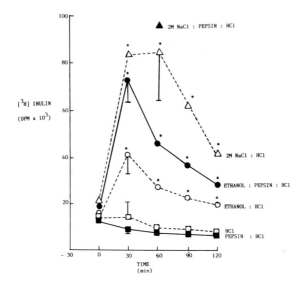

FIGURE 2: *Pepsin induced gastric mucosal bleeding measured as total iron content in instillates: 30 min instillation of 0.1M HCl followed by 4 x 30 min instillations each of 4 ml. Instillations were 0.1M HCl alone [□] or 70% ethanol (45 sec) followed by instillation of 0.1M HCl [O]; or 2M NaCl (30 min) followed by instillation of 0.1M HCl [△]; with pepsin, closed symbols and solid line; without pepsin, open symbols and dotted line; (n = 9-12 in each group). Values are medians. * significantly different to 0.1M HCl, p<0.05 by Mann Whitney U test.*

        Instillation of pepsin:0.1M HCl following acute 70% ethanol or 2M NaCl enhanced mucosal damage considerably over that seen following instillation of 0.1M HCl alone after these agents. In both groups there was extensive haemorrhage of the mucosa and blood (iron) in the instillates, greatest with instillation of pepsin following acute ethanol damage (Figure 1). This contrasted markedly with the controls of 70% ethanol (45 sec) or 2M NaCl (30 min) followed by 0.1M HCl alone, where no bleeding was observed and only basal iron levels were in the instillates. Histology following instillation of pepsin:0.2M HCl after ethanol damage (Group V) showed between 10-50% of the mucosal surface area was ulcerated with lesions extending through 30-50% of the mucosal thickness. There was extensive necrosis of the foveolar, cryptal and specialised glandular epithelium, within the lamina propria, the capillaries were dilated but there was little evidence of an 'inflammatory' response to the insulates. In areas where ulceration was absent, tissue regeneration and re-epithelialisation were present under a surface gelatinous coat of fibrin and necrotic cells.

In summary, the depth and severity of observed histological damage was in the order HCl (Group I - no damage) << ethanol/HCl,NaCl/HCl (Groups III and IV) < pepsin/HCl (Group II) << ethanol/pepsin/HCl, NaCl/pepsin/HCl (Groups V and VI). Superimposed on this was a qualitative difference between the localised damage seen following exposure to pepsin and total exfoliation of the epithelium, with re-epithelialisation and formation of a mucoid coat following acute ethanol or 2M NaCl damage. Furthermore only when pepsin was included in the instillate with 0.1M HCl did mucosal bleeding occur and this was enhanced by prior acute damage from 70% ethanol or 2M NaCl.

THE ADHERENT MUCUS BARRIER AND PEPSIN MUCOLYSIS

Pepsin mucolysis of the adherent mucus layer was followed by (1) measurement of degraded mucus in the instillates, and (2) observation of unfixed gastric mucosal sections and measurement of mucus thickness (Table 1).

There was clear evidence of mucolysis of the adherent mucus layer following instillation of pepsin:HCl for 2 hours (Group II), with a sharp and significant increase in the content of degraded mucin in the instillates compared to that from the 0.1M HCl control (Group I). The maximum release of degraded mucin following pepsin (280ug) was reached in the instillate period 30-60 min, representing a threefold increase over the corresponding 0.1M HCl control (82ug) and this rate of release was maintained throughout the remainder of the time course. Gel filtration on Sepharose 2B confirmed the PAS positive material was mucin [22].

The most apparent change in the adherent mucus layer following pepsin:HCl instillation for 2 hours was that the gel became noticeably disrupted and granular with discontinuities, 12% of the total number of readings. Discontinuities were never seen following exposure for 2.5 hr to HCl or in the fasted animal. Median mucus thickness following pepsin was not significantly lower than control values after exposure to 0.1M HCl alone (Table 1), although demarcation between the mucus gel and the mucosa was indistinct and only an approximation of mucus thickness could be obtained. The absence of a significant decrease in mucus thickness following pepsin mucolysis and with only 12% of the readings showing discontinuities indicates a relatively slow rate of penetration of the mucus barrier by this concentration of pepsin (2 mg ml^{-1}). Adherent gastric mucus is a 5% by weight mucin gel [7] and relatively large amounts of degraded mucin will be released on mucolysis for only a small decrease in adherent mucus gel thickness (as observed). Higher concentrations of pepsin (e.g. 5 mg ml^{-1}) in this model do produce significant decreases (30%) in mucus thickness over 2 hours *in vivo*.

TABLE 1.

ADHERENT AND SOLUBLE MUCUS FOLLOWING PERFUSION OF ANAESTHETIZED RAT
STOMACH WITH PEPSIN, ETHANOL OR HYPERTONIC NaCl

| Agent | Mucus thickness (um) | | | Soluble mucus |
	Medial	Range	% zero readings	(ug 2 hr^{-1}) (mean ± SEM)
0.1M HCl (Group I)	120	20-400	0	405 ± 45
pepsin (2mg/ml) HCl (Group II)	100	0-800	12%	925 ± 58*
70% ethanol (45 secs)-HCl (Group III)	210*	20=1100	0	988 ± 146
70% ethanol (45 sec)-pepsin:HCl (Group IV)	160	0-1000	6%	2942 ± 280*
2M NaCl (30 min)-HCl (Group IV)	200*	10-860	0	2790 ± 300*
2m NaCl (30 min)-pepsin:HCl (Group VI)	195*	0-1000	0.8%	3092 ± 310*

Experiments in vitro show pepsin only penetrates the mucus gel by progressive mucolysis at the surface and not by diffusion through the gel matrix [7]. Therefore it is deduced that the continuous adherent mucus layer in vivo is a protective barrier to luminal pepsin [5,15]. The experiments in this study give strong support for the adherent mucus layer providing a major protective barrier against pepsin. The results demonstrate that excess pepsin activity in the lumen can swing the dynamic balance across the mucus layer between erosion and secretion in favour of the former and once the mucus barrier is breached, epithelial digestion results. The limited focal nature of pepsin damage is in keeping with only 12% of the mucus thickness readings being zero. These are presumably the sites where pepsin has penetrated the thinnest points of the mucus gel while the rest of the epithelium remains intact, protected by a continuous mucus layer. Under normal levels of pepsin, new mucus secretion presumably balances that lost by pepsin mucolysis and mechanical erosion to maintain the continuous layer of adherent mucus gel. It should be noted that the protective role of the mucus layer depends on it being continuous over the undamaged mucosa and that evidence strongly supporting this now exists from many quite different experimental sources [8-15].

MUCOID COAT FORMATION FOLLOWING ETHANOL AND 2M NaCl DAMAGE

Previous studies have demonstrated that the adherent mucus barrier is rapidly permeated by 70% ethanol and 2M NaCl to cause extensive epithelial exfoliation [5,24,25]. The thick gelatinous or mucoid surface coat associated with subsequent gastric epithelial repair in rat is substantially thicker (median thickness 680um compared to 80um), and visibly less rigid than the adherent mucus layer of the undamaged mucosa. Also it is quite different in composition, consisting of fibrin gel with overlying necrotic cells and some mucus [25]. The formation of a fibrin based mucoid coat was observed in these studies following recovery from acute ethanol damage (Group III). However the thickness of the mucoid coat (210um), while representing a significant two-fold increase compared to that with 0.1M HCl alone (120um), was substantially thinner than that previously observed for the fully developed fibrin based mucoid coat (mean 680um) [25]. A possible explanation for this observation is that, in the present studies, some of the mucoid coat was removed from the mucosal surface by successive instillations and aspirations (four 4 x 4 ml) over the 2 hour period. Evidence for this is seen by the 1.5-fold rise in mucin glycoprotein content of washouts following acute damage with ethanol compared with the 0.1M HCl control alone (Table 1).

A similar mucoid coat was observed to form following recovery in HCl after 2M NaCl for 30 min. However this coat was not as stable as that formed following ethanol damage in that it was thinner and accompanied by a three-fold rise in soluble mucin in the instillates (Table 1). This together with the absence of a fibrin staining already noted suggests that the mucoid coat associated with repair following 2M NaCl damage may be substantially different from that following ethanol damage.

The mucoid coat associated with ethanol damage and subsequent recovery in HCl was significantly thinner and severely disrupted following pepsin instillation. Some fibrin was present at the surface following pepsin but clearly hydrolysis of the mucoid coat had occurred as shown by the large increase in soluble mucin in the instillates (Table 1). Other studies have shown higher concentrations of pepsin (5 mg ml^{-1}) will hydrolyse the mucoid coat following acute ethanol damage [26].

SUMMARY

These studies show the response of the mucosa to pepsin induced mucosal damage is quite different in important aspects to that caused by ethanol or 2M NaCl. Damage with ethanol or 2M NaCl results from the agent rapidly penetrating the mucus barrier and causing gross epithelial exfoliation and increased mucosal permeability. This is followed by epithelial repair associated with the formation of a mucoid coat over the re-epithelialising surface. The absence of bleeding following instillation of 70% ethanol or 2M NaCl in the present studies shows that under the conditions used, deeper seated vascular damage had not occurred. In contrast, pepsin damage was not associated with epithelial exfoliation or increased mucosal permeability but with focal haemorrhagic damage and bleeding. Furthermore, pepsin damage is not associated with any of the histological features of epithelial repair or the formation of a gelatinous coat. These differences between mucosal damage with pepsin and that with ethanol or hypertonic NaCl can be explained at least in part by the flow of interstitial fluid associated with the latter which will dilute and neutralise the acid and damaging agent at the surface, as well as facilitate epithelial repair and formation of the mucoid coat. The pepsin damage model described here thus offers an alternative animal model to the well documented ethanol damage model for investigation of potential mucosal protective agents. Particularly since pepsin is a natural endogenous aggressor while ethanol is an exogenous damaging agent.

This work provides evidence that a major mucosal barrier to luminal pepsin damage *in vivo* is the adherent mucus gel which when penetrated by pepsin reveals an underlying epithelia which is not resistant to digestion Studies have shown that gastric juice from peptic ulcer patients has increased mucolytic activity associated with a rise in the proportion of pepsin type 1 [6] and this can be correlated with an observed defect in the structure of the gastric mucus barrier in peptic ulcer disease [19,27]. It is possible that such increased pepsin aggression will progressively weaken the mucus barrier in a chronic situation and is one of the factors associated with the aetiology of peptic ulcer disease.

REFERENCES

1.   Alphin RS, Vokac VA, Gregory RL et al.   Role of intragastric pressure, pH and pepsin in gastric ulceration in the rat. Gastroenterology 1977; 73: 495-500.

2.   Joffe SN, Roberts NB, Taylor WH, Baron JH.   Exogenous and endogenous acid and pepsins in the pathogenesis of duodenal ulcers in the rat.   Dig Dis Sci 1980; 25: 837-841.

3.   Kivilaakso E, Fromm D, Silen W.   Effect of bile salts and related compounds on isolated oesophageal mucosa.   Surgery 1980; 87: 280-285.

4.   Kivilaakso E, Barzilai A,m Schiessel R, Craff R, Silen W.   Ulceration of isolated amphibian gastric mucosa. Gastroenterology 1979; 77: 31-37.

5.   Allen A, Hunter AC, Leonard AJ, Pearson JP, Sellers LA.   Peptic activity and the mucus-bicarbonate barrier.   In: Garner A, Whittle BJR eds.   Advances in drug therapy of gastrointestinal ulceration. John Wiley, 1989; 139-155.

6.   Pearson JP, Ward R, Allen A, Roberts NB, Taylor WH.   Mucus degradation by pepsin: comparison of mucolytic activity of human pepsin 1 and pepsin 3: implications in peptic ulceration.   Gut 1986; 27: 243-248.

7.   Bell AE, Sellers LA, Allen A, Cunliffe WJ, Morris ER, Ross-Murphy SB. Properties of gastric and duodenal mucus: effect of proteolysis, disulphide reduction, bile, acid, ethanol and hypertonicity on mucus gel structure. Gastroenterology 1985; 88: 269-280.

8.   Bickel M, Kauffman GL.   Gastric mucus gel thickness: effects of distension, 16,16-dimethyl prostaglandin E2 and carbenoxolone. Gastroenterology 1981; 80: 770-775.

9.   Kerss S, Allen A, Garner A.   A simple method for measuring the thickness of the mucus gel layer adherent to rat, frog and human mucosa: influence of feeding, prostaglandin, N-acetylcysteine and other agents. Clin Sci 1982; 63: 187-195.

10   McQueen S, Allen A, Garner A.   Measurements of gastric and duodenal mucus gel thickness.   In: Allen A, Flemstrom G, Garner A, Silen W, Turnberg LA, eds.   Mechanism of mucosal protection in the upper gastrointestinal tract.   New York: Raven, 1984; 215-221.

11.   Tobin M, Turnberg LA.   Gastric mucus thickness measured by scanning electron microscopy. Gut 1989; 30: A740-741.

12.   Sturrock N, Hopwood D.   The effects of mucus on the binding of cationized ferritin by human and animal gastrointestinal epithelium. Histochemistry 1986; 85: 255-258.

13.   Bollard JE, Vanderwee MA, Smith GW, Tasman-Jones C, Gavin JB, Lee SP.   Preservation of mucus in situ in rat colon.   Dig Dis Sci 1986; 31: 1338-1344.

14.   Holm L, Flemstrom G.   Microscopy of acid transport at the gastric surface in vivo. J Int Med 1990; 228: in press.

15.   Allen A.   Pre-epithelial factors in resistance to acid and pepsin. Eur J Gastroenterol Heptaol 1990; 2: 168-171.

16.   Morris GP, Harding RJ, Wallace JL.   A functional model for extracellular gastric mucus in the rat.   Virchows Arch (Cell Pathol) 1984; 46: 239-251.

17.   Wallace JL.   Gastric resistance to acid: is the "mucus-bicarbonate barrier" functionally redundant? Am J Physiol 1989; 256: G31-G38.

18.   Sellers LA, Carroll NJH, Allen A.   Misoprostil-induced increases in adherent gastric mucus thickness and luminal mucus output. Dig Dis Sci 1986; 31: 91S-95S.

19.   Allen A, Cunliffe WJ, Pearson JP, Venables CW.   The adherent gastric mucus gel barrier in man and changes in peptic ulceration. J Int Med 1990; 228: in press.

20.   Younan F. Pearson JP, Allen A. Gastric mucus degradation in vivo
       in peptic ulcer patients and the effects of vagotomy. In: Chantler
       EN, Elder JB, Elstein M. eds. Mucus in health and disease II. New
       York/London, Plenum, 1982; 253-273.

21.   Lacy ER, Ito S. Rapid restitution of the rat gastric mucosa after
       ethanol injury. Lab Invest. 1984; 52: 573-;1583.

22.   Mantle M, Allen A. A colorimetric assay for glycoproteins based on
       the periodic acid/Schiff stain. Biochem Soc Trans 1978; 6: 607-9.

23.   Venables CW. An assessment of the value of measuring uncollected
       gastric secretion during routine secretion studies in man. Brit J Surg
       1972; 59: 473-477.

24.   Silen W, Ito S.   Mechanisms for rapid re-epithelialisation of the
       gastric mucosal surface. Ann Rev Physiol 1985; 47: 217-229.

25.   Sellers LA, Allen A, Bennett MK.   Formation of a fibrin based
       gelatinous coat over repairing rat gastric epithelium following acute
       ethanol damage: interaction with adherent mucus. Gut 1987; 28: 835-
       843.

26.   Wallace JL, Whittle BJR. Role of mucus in the repair of gastric
       epithelial damage in the rat. Gastroenterology 1986; 91: 603-611.

27.   Younan F, Pearson JP, Allen A, Venables CW. Changes in the
       structure of the mucus gel on the mucosal surface of the stomach in
       association with peptic ulcer disease.   Gastroenterology 1982; 82:
       827-831.

HELICOBACTER PYLORI

Dr J R Lambert, Dr S K Lin, Mr M Schembri

*Monash University Department of Medicine,
Prince Henry's Hospital, Melbourne, Australia*

ABSTRACT

Helicobacter pylori (H. pylori) is the commonest infectious disease with the frequency of infection varying in different populations. This bacterium colonizes the gastric mucosa and causes nonspecific, antral chronic active gastritis (so called Type B). H. pylori is most likely transmitted via the fecal-oral or oral-oral route between humans.

H. pylori is found in subjects with chronic duodenal ulcer (97%), gastric ulcer (75%), non ulcer dyspepsia (65%) and gastric carcinoma (32%). Its role in these diseases is unclear. In chronic duodenal ulcer disease antimicrobials including colloidal bismuth subcitrate (DeNol), metronidazole and furazolidone are effective in ulcer healing. The relapse of ulcer disease is diminished after CBS therapy when compared with H2 receptor antagonists. More recently, eradication of H. pylori in subjects with chronic duodenal ulcer disease has resulted in a marked decrease in ulcer relapse with up to 3 year follow-up studies reported suggesting an important pathogenic role.

A plausible hypothesis exists to link H. pylori, gastric acid and ulcer disease. Acquired gastric metaplasia of the proximal duodenum occurs in >85% of subjects with duodenal ulcer disease. This occurs as a result of high (probably hereditary) gastric acid output. Colonization of the metaplastic mucosa with H. pylori, resulting in duodenitis, makes the mucosa more susceptible to ulceration. The pathogenesis of the inflammatory response induced by H. pylori is unclear with the role of bacterial cytotoxins, adhesions, chemotactic factors, ureases and proteases currently being evaluated.

The effects of H. pylori associated gastroduodenitis on the mucosa are multiple and include impaired mucus structure and function, surface epithelial cell damage, altered mucosal blood flow and increased prostaglandin levels. The expected increase in inflammatory mediators such as tumour necrosis factor, leukotrienes and interleukins has been identified.

Helicobacter pylori thus plays an important role in upper gastrointestinal disease, particularly duodenal ulcer disease. Because it provides stable, long-term colonization associated with inflammation it is an ideal model for studying bacterial host interactions.

INTRODUCTION

Helicobacter pylori (H. pylori) are gram-negative, microaerophilic, spiral organisms isolated from the inflamed human gastric mucosa [1]. This motile curved bacillus possesses a unipolar flagellum and is highly adapted to its environment which is close to gastric epithelial cells in the stomach and duodenum. Protection is provided from the hostile luminal environment by overlying mucus. The bacteria produces a number of products which are summarised in Table 1.

TABLE I

PRODUCTS SYNTHESIZED BY HELICOBACTER PYLORI
1. Enzymes — urease — oxidase — catalase — lipase — phospholipase — protease
2. Chemotactic factor - monocytes, neutrophils
3. Cytotoxin
4. Adherence factors - adhesins
5. Gastric acid inhibitory protein

Diagnosis of H. pylori can most readily be made using fresh antral biopsies by culture under microaerophilic and humid conditions [2] or histology of stained biopsies using Giemsa, or other specific stains. Detection of the large concentrations of urease produced by the organism provides a further rapid, simple and accurate diagnostic method of identification using commercial or standard laboratory techniques [3]. Phase contrast microscopy is another rapid and reliable technique for diagnosing H. pylori infection [4].

Non-invasive tests requiring no endoscopy and antral biopsy include the ^{13}C or ^{14}C urea breath test and serology. The urea breath test is highly sensitive and specific for H. pylori. Subjects are given a dose of carbon labelled urea orally and, if H. pylori is present, the urea is metabolized and isotopic carbon is detected in the breath. The ^{13}C-urea breath test is expensive, complex to measure and non-radioactive. In contrast, the ^{14}C-urea breath test is a cheap and simple alternative, with its only disadvantage being the ingestion of a small radioactive dose. Breath tests are an accurate and safe diagnostic tool suitable for the long term follow up of subjects [5].

Antibodies to H. pylori have been assessed by various methods the best of which is probably the enzyme-linked immunosorbent assay (ELISA) to detect elevated IgG and IgA concentrations in the serum of colonised patients [6]. The various reported assays have high sensitivity and specificity and are particularly useful in epidemiological studies. The slow fall in titre after eradication of the organisms makes serology less useful in following subjects.

This review of H. pylori relates particularly to the epidemiology of the organism and its association with disease. In addition, its possible pathogenic mechanisms and mucosal effects will be reviewed.

EPIDEMIOLOGY AND MODE OF TRANSMISSION

H. pylori has a worldwide distribution with the frequency of infection increasing with age at a rate of ~1%/year in Western countries. The onset and rate of acquisition of H. pylori in many underdeveloped countries is much more rapid. Ethnic and race differences in the frequency of H. pylori have been identified. These differences in part may reflect the higher frequency in lower socioeconomic groups and certain geographic areas.

H. pylori infection causes histological Type B antral gastritis [7]. All diseases associated with antral gastritis are also associated with H. pylori infections including duodenal ulcer, gastric ulcer, and gastric carcinoma (Table II). The frequency of essential non-ulcer dyspepsia appears to be similar to that of the asymptomatic population.

TABLE II

PREVALENCE OF DISEASES ASSOCIATED WITH HELICOBACTER PYLORI	
Duodenal ulcer	97%*(85-100%)+
Gastric ulcer	75% (58-96%)
Gastric carcinoma	32% (21-80%)
Non-ulcer dyspepsia	65% (40-90%)
Histological antral gastritis	85% (70-100%)
Pernicious anaemia	30% (21-36%)
* Melbourne experience + Literature range	

H. pylori has a predilection for the surface of human gastric mucosal cells. Colonization of gastric mucosa includes heterotopic and metaplastic gastric tissue wherever it exists in the gastrointestinal tract. Current data would suggest oral-oral or fecal-oral human to human transmission. No non-human reservoirs of H. pylori have been detected in any animals, the water supply or food substances. In humans, H. pylori has not been isolated from stool, saliva or the oral cavity, a result which may reflect inadequate methodology.

A higher prevalence of H. pylori in institutionalized mentally handicapped patients and third world countries parallels the rates of acquisition of other enteric pathogens transmitted by the fecal-oral route, including hepatitis A. Further support comes from a higher prevalence amongst gastroenterologists and gastrointestinal nursing staff. Transmission of H. pylori via contaminated endoscopes and pH probes supports oral-oral transmission.

Transmission within families has been suggested in several small studies, however, these have been limited by inadequate control groups for comparison. No evidence of sexual transmission has been identified.

PATHOGENIC MECHANISMS

Heterogeneity of the species H. pylori has been postulated to account for pathogenic and non-pathogenic strains of the bacteria.

It is thus important to understand the mechanisms whereby H. pylori can cause damage to the gastric and duodenal epithelium. Currently, this is unknown, however, there are several putative virulence factors for H. pylori. Two of these are structural parts of the bacterium - flagella and adhesins, while the other factors are extracellular products, namely, urease, cytotoxins, mucin degrading proteases, gastric acid inhibitory protein and chemotactic factor.

The H. pylori urease enzyme is a 500-600Kda protein with a high substrate affinity and is probably localized in the outer membrane and periplasmic space of the bacteria. Urease negative strains of H. pylori are non-virulent in a pig model. The ammonia produced by the urease activity may account for the organisms' survival in gastric juice. Ammonia is toxic to eukaryotic mammalian cell lines. Urease production is almost invariable in H. pylori isolates, however the amount seems to differ.

Lysates or culture filtrates of H. pylori have cytotoxic effects on different cell lines. The cytotoxin is a large molecule of greater than >50Kda and is inactivated at 60^0C. In the gnotobiotic piglet model strains of H. pylori differing in motility and cytotoxin production were tested. A good correlation between motility and virulence was observed with a questionable correlation between cytotoxin production and virulence. About 55% of H. pylori strains produce cytotoxins. In a recent study 100% of subjects with a duodenal ulcer had serum anti-cytotoxin antibodies compared with 48% of subjects with H. pylori who had infection and no ulcers.

H. PYLORI – MEDIATORS OF INFLAMMATORY RESPONSE

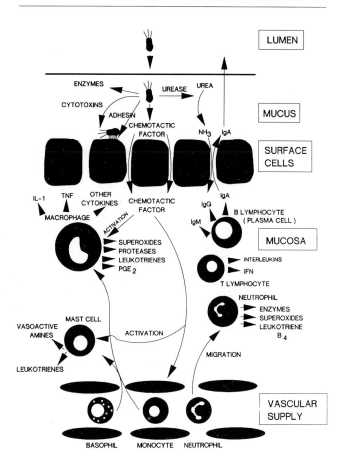

FIGURE 1.   *Hypothesis to link Helicobacter pylori in the pathophysiology of chronic duodenal ulcer disease.*

Mucus degradation occurs by the action of proteases, lipases and phospholipase A produced by H. pylori. H. pylori may also inhibit acid secretion from gastric parietal cells by a protein termed gastric acid inhibitory protein.

Chemotactic factors for monocytes and neutrophils have been recently identified which are heat sensitive, protease resistant and less than 3Kd in size. These most likely are N-formyl-methonyl-oligopeptides similar to those produced by other gut pathogens.

Adherence of H. pylori to the surface epithelial cells by adhesion pedestals has been identified by electron microscopy. These "adhesins" or "colonization factor antigens" are fibrillar glycosubstances most likely N-acetylneuramenyl lactose-binding haemagglutinin which react with sialic acid and/or a glycolipid of gastric epithelial cells.

The importance and prevalence of these virulence factors is still largely unknown. It is likely that strains of H. pylori may differ in virulence and in the future initiation of therapy may be guided by both the clinical imformation as well as the presence of virulence and other bacterial factors.

DUODENAL ULCER

A strong association exists between chronic duodenal ulcer disease and H. pylori associated gastro-duodenitis reaching 100% in some studies (Table II). A plausible hypothesis exists to link H. pylori with duodenal ulcers (Figure 1). Acquired gastric metaplasia within the duodenum occurs probably as a result of higher gastric acid output. This metaplastic mucosa becomes infected with H. pylori leading to duodenitis and an increased susceptibility to ulceration. The factors initiating the ulcer formation are unknown. Support for this hypothesis relates to the pathological findings within the duodenum in duodenal ulcer disease [8] and the lower relapse rate of ulcers in subjects eradicated of H. pylori [9]. More recently, H. pylori associated gastritis has been shown to be accompanied by an elevation of stimulated gastrin release from G cells of the antrum. Preliminary studies suggest the increased release of gastrin returns to normal following bacterial eradication.

GASTRIC ULCER AND NON-ULCER DYSPEPSIA

The role of H. pylori in gastric ulcer and essential non-ulcer dyspepsia is still unclear. The heterogeneous aetiology of these conditions makes study of the relationship to H. pylori difficult.

GASTRIC CANCER

Gastric atrophy is considered the final stage of H. pylori induced gastritis. Gastric atrophy with intestinal metaplasia is thought to be the precursor lesion for gastric carcinoma. The sequence of events which leads to intestinal metaplasia in the stomach is one of progression from superficial H. pylori gastritis through atrophic gastritis to gastric atrophy. The factors causing progression to gastric atrophy are unknown and may reflect early acquisition of infection, genetic predisposition and environmental agents such as foods, alcohol and smoking. In countries with a high incidence of gastric carcinoma (eg Japan, Colombia) the populations have a high prevalence of H. pylori infection and have acquired the infection at an early age. The relationship between H. pylori and cancer requires further investigation.

MUCOSAL EFFECTS OF H. PYLORI

H. pylori gastritis has a number of effects on the gastroduodenal mucosa. These include damage to surface epithelial cells, altered physicochemical properties of mucus, changed mucosal blood flow and elaboration of inflammatory mediators and components (Table III). Many of these effects are the result of the pathogenic mechanisms as discussed above.

TABLE III

EFFECT OF HELICOBACTER PYLORI INDUCED GASTRITIS ON GASTRODUODENAL MUCOSA

Mucus   -   degradation of protein/lipids
           -    physical properties
             .   viscosity
             . H^+ diffusion
 	
Surface epithelial cells
           -    vacuolization
           -    surface damage
 	
Mucosal blood flow - increased in antrum
 	
Inflammatory mediators/components
           -    prostaglandins
           -    leukotrienes
           -    cytokines - interleukin 1
                             - tumor necrosis factor
           -    reactive oxygen intermediates
 	
Endocrine cells - increased gastrin release

Mucus degradation by protease, lipase and phospholipases results in impaired viscosity, increased H^+ diffusion and reduced hydrophobicity has been reported [10,11]. Recent investigations have disputed the suggested proteolytic activity of H. pylori on gastric mucus.

Human gastric mucosal blood flow has recently been studied in vivo using endoscopic laser Doppler methods. Despite methodological problems, an increased mucosal flow has been observed in the antrum with eradication of H. pylori resulting in restoration to normal flow [12].

   The inflammatory response, directed against H. pylori produced antigenic material (including urease, cytotoxins and chemotactic factor), results in the rapid local recruitment of antigen presenting cells and antigen-specific T helper lymphocytes to stimulate the proliferation and differentiation of antibody-producing B cells.   This marked immune response requires down regulation by antigen-specific T suppressor/cytotoxic cells. The mucosal surface then becomes a reservoir of immunocompetent cells elaborating a number of defined agents including immunoglobulins, prostaglandins (PGE$_2$), leukotrienes, cytokines (interleukins, tumour necrosis factor) and reactive oxygen intermediates.   A schematic representation of some of the interaction between H. pylori virulence factors and the inflammatory response is shown in Figure 2.

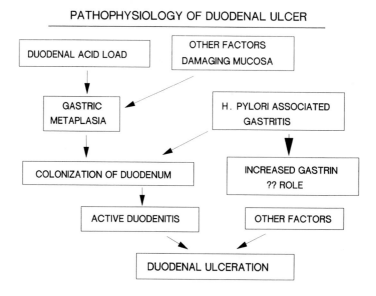

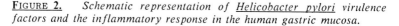

FIGURE 2.   *Schematic representation of Helicobacter pylori virulence factors and the inflammatory response in the human gastric mucosa.*

THE FUTURE

   A number of important questions remain to be answered in relation to H. pylori. The most intriguing question is why H. pylori can colonize the mucosa long-term in a stable response in an apparently immunologically hostile environment. Despite the host mobilizing both humoral and cellular immunity at the infected site the bacteria still remains viable.   The mechanisms to avoid these host responses have not yet been adequately studied.

The relationship between H. pylori and gastric carcinoma, gastric ulcer and non-ulcer dyspepsia requires further study. Long-term epidemiological studies along with well conducted placebo controlled trials of H. pylori eradication are required to define the aetiologic role in these diseases. A cheap, reliable animal model with stable long-term H. pylori colonization may be required to observe mucosal-progression to gastric atrophy, intestinal metaplasia and carcinoma formation.

Finally, the important question of the most effective and safest method of H. pylori eradication remains. Despite being sensitive to a wide range of antimicrobial agents in vitro, most single agents are ineffective in eradicating H. pylori. The most effective regimen combines colloidal bismuth subcitrate with metronidazole and tetracycline or amoxicillin. This triple therapy is capable of eradicating H. pylori from over 85% of subjects, however, side effects occur in up to one third [13,14]. Further studies in improving antimicrobial delivery to the site of colonization as well as increasing the organisms susceptibility to these agents will be required to minimize toxicity.

The initial skepticism in accepting H. pylori as an important gastrointestinal pathogen thus appears to be ill founded. The stable inflammatory gastric mucosal response induced by H. pylori has now provided an important model for evaluating host/bacterial interrelationships. Moreover, as with other new areas of research it has resulted in successful collaboration of many disciplines including gastroenterology, pathology, immunology, biochemistry, genetics and molecular biology.

REFERENCES

1.   Marshall B J, Warren J R. Unidentified curved bacilli in the stomach of patients with gastritis and peptic ulceration. Lancet 1984; 1:1311-1315.

2.   Goodwin C S, Blincow E, Warren J R, Waters T E, Sanderson C R, Easton L. Evaluation of cultural techniques for isolating Campylobacter pyloridis from endoscopic biopsies of gastric mucosa. J Clin Path 1985; 138:1127-1131.

3.   Lambert J R, Borromeo M, Pinkard K J. Evaluation of cultural techniques for isolating Campylobacter pyloridis. J Clin Path 1987; 40:462-464.

4.   Pinkard K J, Harrison B, Lambert J R. Detection of pyloric CLO by phase contrast microscopy. J Clin Path 1986; 39:112-115.

5.   Graham D Y, Klein P D, Evans D J Jr, Alpert L C, Opekun P R, Boutton T W. Campylobacter pylori detected non-invasively by the ^{13}C-urea breath test. Lancet 1987; 1:1174-1177.

6.   Goodwin C S, Blincow E, Peterson G. Enzyme-linked immunosorbent assay for Campylobacter pyloridis: correlation with presence of C. pyloridis in gastric mucosa. J Inf Dis 1987; 155:488-494.

7.   Lambert J R, Yeomans N D. Campylobacter pylori-gastroduodenal pathogen or opportunistic bystander. Aust NZ J Med 1988; 18:555-556.

8.   Wyatt J I , Rathbone B J, Dixon M F, Heatley R V. Campylobacter pyloridis and acid induced gastric metaphasia in the pathogenesis of duodenitis. J Clin Path 1987; 40:841-848.

9.   Marshall B J, Goodwin C S, Warren J R. Prospective double-blind trial of duodenal ulcer relapse after eradication of Campylobacter pylori. Lancet 1988; 2:1437-1442.

10.   Slomiary B L, Bilski J, Sarosiek J. Campylobacter pyloridis degrades mucin and undermines gastric mucosal integrity. Biochem Biophys Res Commun 1987; 144:307-314.

11.   Coggin P M, Marrero J M, Jazrawi R P, Corbishley C M, Yu C W, Northfield T C. Effect of Helicobacter pylori infection on gastric mucosal hydrophobicity in man. Gastroenterology 1990; 98:A49.

12.   Murakami A, Tada M, Yanai H, Karita M. Effect of Helicobacter pylori on gastric mucosal blood flow. Proceedings of World Congresses of Gastroenterology, Sydney 1990.

13.   Borody T, Cole P, Noonan A, Morgan G. Long-term Campylobacter pylori recurrence part eradication. Gastroenterology 1988; 94:A43.

14.   Lambert J R, Lin S K, Borromeo M, Nicholson L, Korman M G, Hansky J. Eradication of Helicobacter pylori with colloidal bismuth subcitrate/antibiotic combinations. Gastroenterology 1990; 98:A74.

INHIBITION OF GASTRIC BICARBONATE SECRETION BY NSAIDs: IMPORTANCE OF LUMINAL EXPOSURE

John Crampton, Linda Gibbons, Wynne Rees

Hope Hospital, University of Manchester
School of Medicine, Salford, U.K.

ABSTRACT

Non-steroidal anti-inflammatory drugs are capable of disrupting the pH gradient on the surface of gastric epithelium by inhibiting active bicarbonate secretion and this may be an important mechanism by which mucosal damage occurs. This study has examined the effect of a pro-drug, fenbufen on gastric bicarbonate secretion by isolated mucosa *in vitro*, and also in man using a perfusion technique. Neither fenbufen nor its main metabolite, biphenylacetic acid, significantly affected bicarbonate secretion *in vitro* from either fundic or antral mucosa in concentrations ranging from 10^{-7} to 10^{-5}M. Indomethacin 10^{-6}M produced significant inhibition of bicarbonate secretion in both fundic and antral mucosa. Perfusion of the stomach of healthy volunteers with fenbufen 600 mg/hr resulted in no significant change in bicarbonate secretion (mean change - 2%). Indomethacin perfusion (25mg/hr inhibited gastric bicarbonate secretion (mean change - 45%). These results suggest that direct exposure of the epithelium to NSAIDs is necessary to impair gastric mucosal defence mechanisms.

INTRODUCTION

Gastric damage due to NSAIDs poses considerable clinical problems [1]. Oral administration of NSAIDs can be shown to cause acute gastric mucosal erosions and petechiae [2]. Furthermore the increasing incidence of peptic ulcer disease in elderly women has been linked to increasing use of NSAIDs by this group [3] and there is evidence that the drugs may play a role in ulcer complications, such as haemorrhage [4] and perforation [5]. Their injurious properties may be due to a number of factors including reduction in mucus synthesis [6], mucus gel thickness [7], bicarbonate secretion [8], epithelial hydrophobicity [9] and mucosal blood flow [10]. Prostaglandins are thought to play a major regulatory role in all of these mucosal functions and the impairment produced by NSAIDs may be due to their common property of cyclooxygenase inhibition. The inhibitory effect of NSAIDs on bicarbonate secretion is particularly interesting since this is likely to impair the functional integrity of the mucus-bicarbonate barrier which is thought to constitute a physiological defence mechanism against endogenous acid [11].

29

Since NSAIDs play an important role in the treatment of inflammatory joint disease there have been recent attempts at producing drugs which have less ulcerogenic potential. Prodrugs, such as Fenbufen, have the theoretical advantage of having little capacity for topical damage to gastric mucosa. Circulating metabolites, such as biphenylacetic acid (BPAA) from Fenbufen, may however impair mucosal defence mechanisms either directly or through inhibition or prostaglandin synthesis. In the current study we have examined the capacity of Fenbufen and BPAA to inhibit gastric bicarbonate secretion, a component of the mucus-bicarbonate barrier, using isolated amphibian gastric mucosa and in the intact human stomach.

MATERIALS AND METHODS

IN VITRO STUDIES

These studies on gastric bicarbonate secretion were performed on isolated gastric mucosa obtained from the bullfrog *Rana Catesbeiana* using methods previously described [13]. Briefly the mucosa was dissected free of all muscularis externa and mounted as a membrane (surface area 1.8cm) between two halves of a perspex chamber so that serosal and luminal surfaces could be separately bathed by circulating solutions. The unbuffered luminal solution was gassed with 100% oxygen and the buffered serosal side solution with a mixture of 95% oxygen and 5% carbon dioxide. The serosal solution bathing gastric mucosae contained Na^+ 102.4mM; K^+ 4.0 mM; Ca^{2+} 1.8mM; Mg^{2+} 0.8mM; Cl^- 91.4mM; HCO_3 17.8mM; H_2PO_4 0.8mM; SO_4^{2-} 0.8Mm and glucose 5mM (osmolarity 220m0sm). The luminal solution differed in that HCO_3 and H_2PO_4 was replaced by mannitol 11.3mM to maintain osmolarity. The pH of the luminal solution was maintained at pH 7.4 by the continual automatic titration of 5mM hydrochloric acid from a pH stat system (ABU13 and TT2, Radiometer, Copenhagen, Denmark). Luminal alkalinisation rate could thus be measured. Antral mucosa spontaneously secreted alkali but in the case of fundic mucosa acid secretion was first inhibited by addition of cimetidine 10^{-3} M to the serosal side solution. In all preparations transmucosal potential difference could be continuously measured by means of paired calomel electrodes. The mucosal and serosal solutions were maintained at $20^{\circ}C$ by water jackets perfused by a Haak G circulator.

IN VIVO STUDIES

These studies examined the effect of fenbufen on gastric bicarbonate secretion using a perfusion method in healthy volunteers [14]. The experiments had been approved by Salford District Ethical Committee and all volunteers provided written informed consent. Subjects swallowed a multilumen polyethylene tube positioned by fluroscopy so that its tip lay in the distal duodenum. This allowed perfusion of the stomach with ^{3}H-polyethylene glycol (PEG) from a perfusion port in the proximal stomach and an aspiration port in the antrum. Similarly the duodenum could be perfused with a separate non-absorbable marker, ^{14}C-PEG. Perfusion rates were at 2ml/minute and the markers dissolved in N/saline. Subjects received ranitidine 150mg orally one hour before commencement of the study and 25mg/hour i.v. during the study to inhibit acid secretion. They were instructed to aspirate all saliva during the study with a dental sucker. After stable basal aspiration rates had been established the experiments consisted of collecting aspiration specimens from both stomach and duodenum into 10 minute aliquots. Half way through each time period a separate 1ml specimen was removed in a closed syringe for the immediate determination of pH and pCO2 using a Corning 170 blood gas analyser. Marker concentrations were determined by liquid scintillation counting for dual isotopes using a Wallace 4000 liquid scintillation counter. Bicarbonate concentration in the aspirates was calculated from the Henderson-Hasselbach equation and secretory volumes from non-absorbable marker dilution with correction for duodenogastric reflux.

DRUGS AND CHEMICALS

Fenbufen and BPAA were obtained as amorphous powders from Lederle Laboratories, Hampshire, England. These were dissolved in small volumes of bathing solution so that addition of 100ul aliquot of stock solutions produced the concentration range $10^{-7}M$ to $10^{-5}M$ for experiments on isolated mucosa. For the human studies 600mg fenbufen was dissolved in 120ml of 0.15M saline, containing ^{3}H-PEG as the non-absorbable marker. Indomethacin was obtained from Sigma Chemicals Limited and prepared likewise, being added at a concentration of $10^{-6}M$ in the *in vitro* experiments and 25mg/120ml in the human gastric perfusate.

STATISTICAL ANALYSIS

For each *in vitro* experiment the mean values for bicarbonate secretion and transmucosal potential difference per 15 minutes were calculated from the 5 minute recordings and drugs added after a minimum period of 30 minutes stable basal secretory rate. Differences between values obtained before and after administration of fenbufen, BPAA or indomethacin were evaluated using a Student's paired t-test. In the human experiments, 30 minute samples and differences were also evaluated with a paired t-test.

RESULTS

IN VITRO STUDIES

Mucosal side application of fenbufen ($10^{-7}M$ to $10^{-5}M$) to fundic and antral mucosa resulted in no change in luminal alkalinisation or transmucosal potential difference (Table 1). Further experiments examined the effect of serosal application of fenbufen metabolite, biphenylacetic acid, on gastric alkalinisation.

TABLE 1.

EFFECT OF FENBUFEN ON HCO_3^- SECRETION BY
ISOLATED GASTRIC MUCOSA

Tissue	Concentration (M)	Potential difference (mV)		HCO_3^- secretion ($umol.cm^{-2}.hr^{-1}$)	
		Control	Test	Control	Test
a. Fundus	10^{-7}	10.8±2.2	10.9±2.3	0.33±.06	0.34±.07
n = 4	10^{-6}	11.1±2.3	11.2±2.5	0.25±.05	0.24±.07
	10^{-5}	9.0±1.7	8.8±1.6	0.51±.12	0.49±.12
b. Antrum	10^{-7}	13.5±1.9	13.2±2.1	0.36±.05	0.28±.05
n = 4	10^{-6}	14.0±2.0	13.9±2.0	0.32±.05	0.35±.04
	10^{-5}	14.3±2.7	14.3±2.7	0.31±.02	0.26±.03

This also failed to produce any significant change in either bicarbonate
secretion or transmucosal potential difference in the range of
concentrations that may be achieved in vivo (Table 2).

TABLE 2.

EFFECT OF FENBUFEN METABOLITE ON HCO_3^- SECRETION BY
ISOLATED GASTRIC MUCOSA

Tissue	Concentration (M)	Potential difference (mV)		HCO_3^- secretion ($umol.cm^{-2}.hr^{-1}$)	
		Control	Test	Control	Test
a. Fundus	10^{-7}	12.3±1.9	11.9±1.7	0.32±.11	0.31±.15
n = 4	10^{-6}	11.1±1.0	10.9±0.8	0.36±.02	0.33±.03
	10^{-5}	10.3±1.4	10.2±1.4	0.44±.05	0.38±.08
b. Antrum	10^{-7}	8.6±1.2	8.5±1.1	0.37±.08	0.32±.07
n = 4	10^{-6}	8.5±0.9	8.6±0.9	0.29±.08	0.21±.07
	10^{-5}	8.5±1.3	8.5±1.3	0.17±.06	0.19±.05

In contrast, mucosal application of indomethacin ($10^{-6}M$) produced
significant inhibition of bicarbonate secretion from 0.49±0.09 to
0.36±0.08 $umol/cm^{-2}/hr^{-1}$ in fundic mucosa (p<0.05; n=6) and 0.45±0.08 to
0.36±0.07 $umol/cm^{-2}/hr^{-1}$ in antral mucosa (p<0.05; n=6).

IN VIVO STUDIES

In six healthy volunteers basal gastric bicarbonate secretion was 297±112 umol/30min (mean ± SD). During fenbufen perfusion (600 mg/hr) this was not changed at 291±93 umol/30min and also not significantly altered in the hour after fenbufen at 230±86 umol/30 min (Figure 1). There was no effect on gastric volumes or duodenogastric reflux.

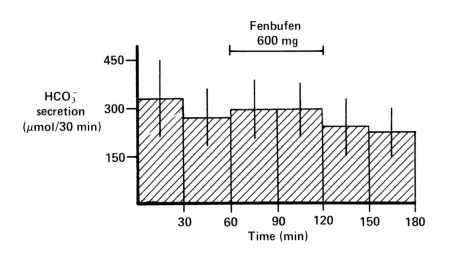

FIGURE 1: *The effect of fenbufen on gastric bicarbonate secretion in 6 healthy volunteers: basal secretion measured in the first hour with fenbufen added to the perfusate during the second hour.*

Serum drug levels indicated rapid absorption of the perfused drug, with fenbufen levels of 5.1±2.3 mg/L (mean + SD) within 30 minutes of commencing the perfusion and 10.3±8.6 mg/L at 60 minutes after which levels slowly fell. Serum drug levels of the main metabolite, biphenylacetic acid, also rose to 13.3±10 mg/L at 60 minutes and to 28.8±16 mg/L at 90 minutes indicating that the parent drug was being actively metabolised. Perfusion of fenbufen into the distal duodenum in 4 volunteers produced no change in gastric bicarbonate secretion (124±70 umol/30 min to 241±50 umol/30 min) although the drug was equally rapidly absorbed. In a group of 7 subjects, indomethacin (25 mg) was perfused over one hour and gastric bicarbonate secretion was reduced from 464±142 umol/hr to 225±60 umol/30 min (p<0.05) and this inhibition was maintained into the third hour (284±67 umol/30 min, Figure 2).

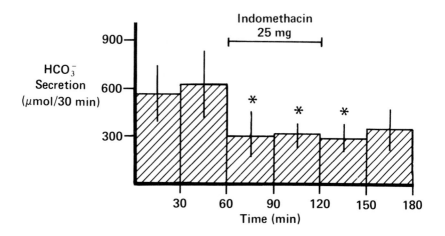

FIGURE 2:   *The effect of indomethacin on gastric bicarbonate secretion in 7 healthy volunteers: indomethacin added to the perfusate during the second hour.*

DISCUSSION

These studies demonstrate that fenbufen does not cause direct inhibition of gastric bicarbonate secretion *in vitro* or *in vivo*. Indomethacin, in contrast, inhibits bicarbonate secretion in both experimental models confirming earlier observations [15]. These findings are of potential importance in view of the role which bicarbonate secretion plays in sustaining a pH gradient across the mucus gel layer of gastroduodenal mucosa [16]. The effect of indomethacin and non-steroidal anti-inflammatory drugs in general on bicarbonate secretion has been widely held to occur via inhibition of prostaglandin synthesis [15]. Thus fenbufen, as a pro-drug devoid of intrinsic prostaglandin synthetase inhibition, may not be expected to affect alkalinisation. However, our observations have somewhat broader implications when evaluating the effect of the active metabolite BPAA. Surprisingly, this also did not affect gastric bicarbonate secretion by isolated mucosa using concentrations encountered in plasma after a standard oral dose. In the human studies the concentrations of BPAA recorded from serum samples were also within the range expected following oral therapy so that it may be implied that neither fenbufen nor its active metabolite reduced gastric bicarbonate output. Since BPA has been shown to inhibit cyclooxygenase activity the observation may suggest that NSAIDs inhibit gastric bicarbonate secretion by a direct cellular action rather than through inhibition of local prostaglandin metabolism.

According to these findings therefore, fenbufen would not be expected to influence the "mucus-bicarbonate barrier" overlying gastric mucosa which prevents exposure of the surface epithelial cells to luminal acid. However, this study does not exclude other injurious actions of fenbufen or BPAA on mucosal defence mechanisms which may be equally important such as blood flow, epithelial hydrophobicity and restitution.

ACKNOWLEDGEMENTS

The authors with to thank Valerie Harrison for preparing the manuscript, Lederle Laboratories for sponsoring the project and the Department of Medical Illustration, Hope Hospital, Salford, for producing the figures.

Dr. Crampton was in receipt of a North West Authority Grant.

REFERENCES

1. Cockell R. NSAIDs - should every prescription carry a government health warning? Gut 1987; 28:515-518.

2. Lanza FL, Umbenhauer ER, Nelson RS, Rack MF, Daurio CP, White LA. A double-blind randomised placebo controlled gastroscopic study to compare the effects of indomethacin capsules and indomethacin suppositories on the gastric mucosa of human volunteers. J. Rheumatol. 1982; 9:415-419.

3. Walt R. Logan R, Katschinski B, Ashley J, Langman M. Rising frequency of ulcer perforation in elderly people in the United Kingdom. Lancet 1986; i:489-492.

4. Somerville K, Faulkner G, Langman M. Non-steroidal anti-inflammatory drugs and bleeding peptic ulcer. Lancet 1986; i:462-464.

5. Collier D St.J, Pain JA. Non-steroidal anti-inflammatory drugs and peptic perforation. Gut 1985; 26:359-363.

6. Kent PW, Allen A. The biosynthesis of intestinal mucins. The effect of salicylate on glycoprotein biosynthesis by sheep colonic and human gastric mucosal tissues in vivo. Biochem J. 1968; 108;645-658.

7. Bickell M. Kaufman GL. Gastric mucus gel thickness: effect of distension, 16,16-dimethyl prostaglandin E2 and carbenoxolone. Gastroenterology 1981; 80:770-775.

8.   Garner A, Flemstrom G, Heylings JR.   Effects of anti-inflammatory agents and prostaglandins on acid and bicarbonate secretions in the amphibian isolated gastric mucosa. Gastroenterology 1979; 77:457-461.

9.   Lichtenberger LM, Richards JE, Hills BA.   Effect of 16,16-dimethyl prostaglandin E2 on surface hydrophobicity of aspirin treated canine gastric mucosa. Gastroenterology 1985; 88:308-314.

10.   Main IHM, Whittle BJR.   Investigation of the vasodilator and antisecretory role of prostaglandins in the rat gastric mucosa by use of non-steroidal anti-inflammatory drugs.   Br J Pharmacol. 1975; 53:217-224.

11.   Rees WDW, Turnberg LA.   Mechanisms of gastric mucosal protection: a role for the mucus bicarbonate barrier. Clin. Sci. 1982; 62:343-348.

12.   Birnhaum JE, Tolman EL, Sloboda AE, Sparano BM, McClintock DK.   Effects on gastric prostaglandin synthesis produced by fenbufen, a new non-steroidal anti-inflammatory agent with low gastrointestinal toxicity. Pharmacology 1982; 25(Suppl.1):27-38.

13.   Flemstrom G. Active alkalinisation by amphibian gastric fundic mucosa in vitro. Am J Physiol. 1977; 233:E1-E12.

14.   Rees WDW, Botham D, Turnberg LA.   A demonstration of bicarbonate production by the normal human stomach in vitro. Dig Dis Sci. 1982; 27:961-966.

15.   Smeaton LA, Hirst BA, Allen A, Garner A.   Gastric duodenal HCO^- transport in vivo: influence of prostaglandins.   Am J Physiol 1983; 245:G751-G795.

16.   Ross IN, Bahari HMM, Turnberg LA.   The pH gradient across mucus adherent to rat fundic mucosa in vivo and the effect of potential damaging agents. Gastroenterology 1981; 24:784-789.

17.   Rees WDW, Gibbons LC. Turnberg LA.   Effects of non-steroidal anti-inflammatory drugs and prostaglandins on alkali secretion by rabbit gastric fundus in vitro. Gut 1983, 24, 784-789.

ACID SECRETORY AND MUCOSAL ULCEROGENIC RESPONSES INDUCED BY LOWERING BODY TEMPERATURE - A PATHOGENIC IMPORTANCE OF BODY TEMPERATURE

K. Takeuchi, H. Niida, K. Ueshima and S. Okabe

Department of Applied Pharmacology, Kyoto Pharmaceutical University, Misasagi, Yamashina, Kyoto, Japan

ABSTRACT

We examined the relation of body temperature to acid secretory and mucosal ulcerogenic responses induced by cold exposure and investigated the role of thyrotropin-releasing hormone (TRH) in these responses in the anaesthetized rat. Lowering of body temperature ($< 32^{\circ}C$) induced acid hypersecretion and damage in the gastric mucosa. These responses reached the maximum at body temperature of $28^{\circ}C$ and were significantly blocked by vagotomy or various antisecretory agents such as atropine. Microinjection of TRH-antiserum (i.c.v.) also inhibited these responses induced by hypothermia. In contrast, TRH given i.c.v. caused an increase of acid secretion, in pattern similar to that observed during hypothermia, resulting in mucosal damage. The blood levels of thyroid-stimulating hormone elevated significantly during hypothermia, and this response preceded to the onset of acid hypersecretion and lesion formation. Hypothermia did not affect the acid secretory and mucosal ulcerogenic responses induced by carbachol in the vagotomized rat. Thus, lowering of body temperature induced vagally-dependent acid hypersecretion, mediated in part by TRH released in response to cold exposure, and may be involved in the aetiology of stress ulceration.

INTRODUCTION

Ulceration induced by stress is an important clinical cause of upper gastrointestinal bleeding in man, but the aetiology of such ulceration has not been fully understood [1]. Exposure of animals to cold-restraint stress also induces ulceration in the stomach with lowering of body temperature (BT) [2,3]. Since lowering of BT alone modifies the acid secretory and motility responses of the stomach in the rat [4-6], BT may be an important element in the pathogenesis of stress ulceration. Recent studies showed that cold stimulus releases thyrotropin-releasing hormone (TRH) [7] and that this peptide given intracisternally causes acid hypersecretion and gastric lesioins in the rat [8,9]. However, the role of TRH in gastric functional alterations induced by hypothermia remains undefined.

In the present study, we demonstrated that lowering of BT caused acid hypersecretion and lesions in the stomach and investigated the possible involvement of TRH in these responses observed during hypothermia.

37

MATERIALS AND METHODS

Male SD rats (250-300 g), kept in individual cages with wide mesh bottoms, were deprived of food but allowed free access to tap water for 18 h prior to the experiments.

GENERAL PROCEDURES:

Since the purpose of this study is to examine the effect of hypothermia on gastric function under unrestrained conditions, the experiments were performed in the rats anaesthetized with urethane (1.25 g/kg, i.p.). The animals were placed in a styrene foam box, and the BT was varied between 36 and $24^{\circ}C$ by raising it with a heat lamp and lowering it with a refrigerant pack.   The rectal temperature was continuously monitored using the rectal thermometer.   Under these conditions, gastric acid secretion and blood levels of thyroid-stimulating hormone (TSH) were measured for 4 h, and at the end of the experiments the stomachs examined for lesions under a dissecting microscope (x 10).   Acid secretion was determined in the acute fistula rat according to the modified method originally described by Tache et al [8].   Briefly, the stomach was washed with 2 ml of saline through the fistula every 15 min, and the gastric samples were titrated to pH 7.0 against 0.1 N NaOH using an autoburette.   In some animals a 22-gauge stainless steel cannula was implanted for intracerebroventricular (i.c.v.) administration of TRH and rabbit TRH-antiserum, so that its tip was inside the right lateral cerebral ventricule [10]. Correct placement of the cerebral cannula was verified after each experiment using a dye (Evans blue). In another group of animals the blood was sampled from the cervical vein at various time points during hypothermia ($28^{\circ}C$), and the TSH levels were determined by radioimmunoassay using (I^{125})TSH and rat TSH-antiserum [11].   In another group of rats, carbachol (20 ug/kg/h) was infused intravenously for 4 h in the vagotomized rats, and the acid secretory and mucosal ulcerogenic responses were compared under normal ($36^{\circ}C$) and hypothermic ($28^{\circ}C$) conditions.

STATISTICS

Data are presented as the mean $\pm$ SE from 4-8 rats. The statistical analysis was performed using a two-tailed Dunnett's multiple comparison test [12], and the values of $P < 0.05$ were regarded as significant.   A regression analysis was used to determine a correlation coefficient between two different variates.

RESULTS

Lowering of BT ($< 32^{\circ}C$) produced a marked increase of acid output, followed by damage in the stomach (Figure 1A).   Although the maximal output obtained was not significantly different between BT at $30^{\circ}C$ to $24^{\circ}C$, this response persisted for 4 h only at $28^{\circ}C$, total acid output being 211.5 $\pm$ 29.5 uEq/4 h, 461.0 $\pm$ 39.6 uEq/4 h and 365.2 $\pm$ 44.3 uEq/4 h, respectively, at $30^{\circ}C$, $28^{\circ}C$ and $26^{\circ}C$.   Even in the group of BT at $24^{\circ}C$, the increased acid secretory response was noted when BT was lowered at around $32^{\circ}C$, reached the maximum at 28°C, but followed by a decrease when BT was further reduced and maintained at 24°C. The severity of gastric lesions also reached the maximum (25.8 ± 6.1 mm^2) at 28°C; a significant relationship was found between the lesion score and acid output (r = 0.936)(Figure 1B). During hypothermia (<32°C) the animals showed characteristic body movements such as head turning, shivering and rearing.

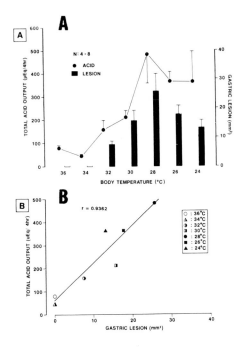

FIGURE 1 *Gastric acid secretion and lesion formation in anaesthetized rats under various body temperature (36-24°C)(A) and the relationship between acid output and lesion score under various body temperatures (B)> Body temperature was lowered by varying ambient temperature using a refrigerant pack and a heat lamp. Data represent the mean ± SE from 4 to 8 rats per group.*

The increased acid secretion caused by hypothermia (28°C) was completely blocked by bilateral cervical vagotomy and significantly inhibited by s.c. injection of atropine (1 mg/kg), hexamethonium (10 mg/kg), clonidine (1 mg/kg) or cimetidine (100 mg/kg) (Table 1 & Figure 2A). These secretory responses were also significantly inhibited by i.c.v. injection of TRH-antiserum (10 ul/rat) (Figure 2A). Although acid output in the animals treated with TRH-antiserum was gradually increased in response to

TABLE 1

EFFECTS OF VARIOUS AGENTS ON ACID SECRETORY AND MUCOSAL
ULCEROGENIC RESPONSES INDUCED BY HYPOTHERMIA IN
ANAESTHETIZED RATS (28°C)

Treatment	Dose mg/kg	No. of rats	Acid Output (μEq/4h)	Inhibition (%)	Mucosal Lesion (mm^2)	Inhibition (%)
Control	-	8	461.0 ± 39.6	-	25.8 ± 6.1	-
Atropine	1	6	65.0 ± 7.4*	85.9	0*	100.0
Hexamethonium	10	6	215.9 ± 57.7*	53.2	6.2 ± 2.2*	76.0
Cimetidine	100	6	100.0 ± 18.3*	78.3	2.5 ± 1.5*	90.3
Clonidine	1	6	137.4 ± 31.2*	70.2	2.8 ± 1.9*	89.1

Values are presented as the mean ± SE from 6-8 rats per group.
Each agent was given subcutaneously 10 min before cold exposure.
Acid output was calculated as the total output for 4 h under hypothermic conditions (28°C).
Gastric lesions were examined at the end of 4 h experiment.
*Statistically significant from controls, at $P < 0.05$.

hypothermia, the maximal value reached was 19.3 ± 4.2 *u*Eq/15 min which was significantly lower than that (46.6 ± 6.2 *u*Eq/15 min) observed in the control group given normal rabbit serum.

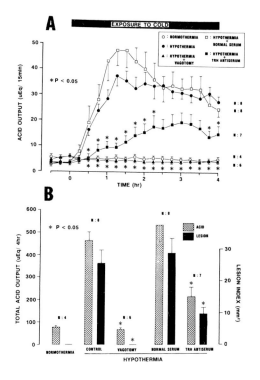

<u>FIGURE 2</u> *Effects of vagotomy and TRH-antiserum on acid hyper-secretion (A) and gastric lesions (B) induced by hypothermia (28°C) in anaesthetized rats. Vagotomy was performed bilaterally at cervical portion 1 h before cold exposure. TRH-antiserum was injected intracerebroventricularly (i.c.v.) in a dose of 10 ul/rat 5 min before cold exposure. Control animals received rabbit normal serum i.c.v. Data represent the mean ± SE from 4-8 rats. * Statistically significant from the corresponding controls, at P < 0.05.*

Total acid output in this group was 183.4 ± 35.1 *u*Eq/4 h, which was about 1/3 of that in the control group (533.4 ± 75.7 *u*Eq/4 h). Gastric lesions induced by hypothermia were also completely blocked by vagotomy and significantly prevented by the above agents or TRH-antiserum (Table 1 & Figure 2B). In contrast, i.c.v. administration of TRH (10 *u*g/rat) produced a marked stimulation of acid secretion in the rat stomach at normothermia (36°C), in pattern similar to that observed during hypothermia (not shown).

Although these responses persisted for a relatively short period and ceased within 1 h, the lesions were induced in the stomach 2 h after i.c.v. microinjection of TRH, the lesion score being 6.1 ± 2.3 mm^2.

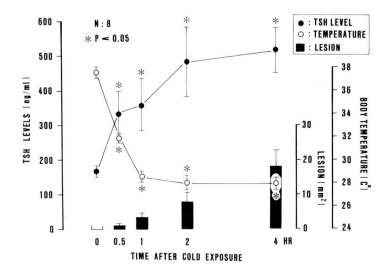

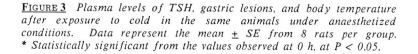

FIGURE 3 *Plasma levels of TSH, gastric lesions, and body temperature after exposure to cold in the same animals under anaesthetized conditions. Data represent the mean ± SE from 8 rats per group. * Statistically significant from the values observed at 0 h, at P < 0.05.*

Since it is known that TRH releases TSH from the anterior pituitary, we also measured blood TSH levels at different time periods during hypothermia (28°C). As evidenced in Figure 3, exposure of the animals to cold produced a lowering of BT with a mirror-image increase of blood TSH levels; they were elevated significantly from 171.7 ± 8.9 ng/ml to 334.2 ± 68.8 ng/ml 30 min after exposure to cold when BT was lowered to 32°C, progressively increased during hypothermia at 28°C, reached the plateau values of 478.7 ± 111.3 ng/ml at 2 h, and remained elevated 4 h later. At 1 h after cold exposure half the animals already showed haemorrhagic lesions in the stomach (2.3 ± 1.2 mm^2), and both the incidence and the severity of lesions were increased with time.

In the vagotomized rats, carbachol (20 ug/kg/h, i.v.) stimulated acid secretion and caused haemorrhagic damage in the mucosa 4 h later. However, the magnitude of these responses induced by carbachol was not significantly affected by lowering of BT; the lesion score was 12.8 ± 2.1 mm^2 and 11.8 ± 4.2 mm^2 at 36°C and 28°C, respectively.

DISCUSSION

Previous studies have shown that exposure of the animals to cold worsens gastric lesions induced by restraint stress [2,3] or noxious agents [5]. Several functional alterations have been reported in association with cold exposure [4-6], yet the relation of body temperature to these changes remains to be still unclear. The present study clearly demonstrated that lowering of BT ($< 32^\circ$C) induced vagally-mediated acid hypersecretion and damage in the gastric mucosa, and suggested an importance of hypothermia in the genesis of stress ulceration.

As expected, the acid secretory and mucosal ulcerogenic responses were significantly prevented by vagotomy, atropine or hexamethonium, suggesting involvement of the vagus nerves and the cholinergic system in the mechanism. Of interest, these phenomena induced by hypothermia (28°C) were significantly attenuated by pretreatment of the animals with i.c.v. administration of TRH-antiserum as well as atropine and hexamethonium. TRH which is found in high amounts in the medulla (dorsal motor nucleus of vagus, etc) is believed to serve as a central regulator of peripheral autonomic function [13]. In agreement with the findings by Jobin et al [7] and Tache et al [8], i.c.v. injection of TRH markedly increased acid secretion and motility, similar to hypothermia, and the levels of TSH were elevated in response to cold exposure. These observations strongly suggest that lowering of BT activates the thermogenic system in the brain, releases TRH which in turn induces acid secretion and motility via the vagus nerves. The finding that clonidine significantly antagonized the functional changes induced by hypothermia supports the involvement of TRH in these responses, since this agent is known to inhibit the acid stimulatory action of TRH by its central mechanism [14]. It should be noted that during hypothermia the animals exhibited the characteristic movements such as head turning and body shakes which are known as typical behavioural effects of TRH [15].

The acid secretory response reached the maximum at BT of 28°C and rather diminished when BT was above or below 28°C. This may indicate that 28°C is the optimal BT for eliciting the vagal-cholinergic excitation of the stomach function. Lower BT may reduce the cell response to vagal excitation, while TRH may not be liberated sufficiently to elicit the vagal activation at higher BT. Acid secretion was rather decreased at BT of 34°C as compared to the control group (36°C). It is known that the thermogenic response to hypothermia in the brain involves other substances such as prostaglandin and GABA as well as TRH. In contrast to TRH and GABA [6,8,16], prostaglandin causes a decrease of acid secretion in various species of the animals [17]. Thus, it may be assumed that the biphasic response of acid secretion induced by hypothermia is attributable to the interaction of the above substances released in response to cold stimulation.

Yano et al [18] showed that the gastric contractile response to acetylcholine in the vagotomized rat was augmented by lowering of ambient temperature, suggesting the presence of local mechanism (suppression of the inhibitory nerves) for functional alteration induced by hypothermia.

However, since both acid secretory and ulcerogenic responses to carbachol in the vagotomised rat were similarly observed under normal and hypothermic conditions, it is unlikely that the present findings are caused by peripheral events other than central ones in association with hypothermia.

The haemorrhagic lesions were induced in the stomach by lowering of BT below $32^{o}C$ for 4 h, and a close relationship was found between lesion score and acid output. These results suggest that acid hypersecretion may be important in the pathogenesis of the lesions induced by hypothermia. The finding with TRH-antiserum is consistent with recent observation that immunization of endogenous TRH leads to total blockade of cold restraint-induced gastric lesions [19,20]. Since exposure of the animals to stress induces a profound hypothermia in addition to several functional alterations in the stomach [4-6], TRH may serve as a possible mediator in the pathophysiology of stress ulceration.

Taken together, the present study clearly showed that lowering of BT induced vagally-mediated acid hypersecretion and mucosal lesions, mediated in part by TRH released in response to cold stimulation, and suggested an importance of the thermogenic-brain-gut axis in the pathophysiology of stress ulceration.

REFERENCES

1.   Grossman MI. Peptic Ulcer; A guide for the practicing physician. Year Book Medical Publishers, INC. Chicago. 1981.

2.   Brodie DA, and Valotski LS. Production of gastric haemorrhage in rats by multiple stresses. Proc Soc Expo Biol Med 1963; 1134: 998-1001.

3.   Senay EC and Levine RJ. Synergism between cold and restraint for rapid production of stress ulcers in rats. Proc Soc Exp Biol Med 1967; 124: 1221-1223.

4.   Mersereau WA and Hinchey EJ. Hypothermia-induced gastric hypercontractility in the genesis of the restraint ulcer. Can J Surg 1981; 24: 622-625.

5.   Robert A, Lancaster C, Kolbasa KP, Olafsson A and Lum J. Potentiation of aspirin-induced gastric lesions by exposure to cold in rats. Gastroenterology 1989; 97: 1147-1158.

6.   Takeuchi K, Nishiwaki H, Niida H and Okabe S. Body temperature-dependent action of baclofen in rat stomach: Relation to acid secretion and ulcerogenicity. Dig Dis Sci 1990; 35: 458-466.

7.   Jobin M, Ferland L, Cote J and Labrie F. Effect of exposure to cold on hypothalamic TRH activity and plasma levels of TSH and prolactin in the rat. Neuroendocrinology 1975; 18: 204-212.

8. Tache Y, Vale W and Brown M. Thyrotropin-releasing hormone: CNS action to stimulate gastric acid secretion. Nature 1980; 287: 149-151.

9. Goto Y and Tache Y. Gastric erosions induced by intracisternal thyrotropin-releasing hormone in rats. Peptides 1985; 6: 153-156.

10. Noble EP, Wurtman RJ annd Axelrod J. A simple and rapid method for injecting H^3-norepinephrine into the lateral ventricule of the rat brain. Life Sci 1967; 6: 281-291.

11. Mori M, Kobayashi I and Wakabayashi K. Suppression of serum thyroptropin (TSH) concentration following thyroidectomy and cold exposure by passive immunization with antiserum to thyrotropin-releasing hormone (TRH). Metabolism 1978; 27: 1485-1490.

12. Dunnett CW. A multiple comparison procedure for comparing several treatments with a control. Am J Stat Assoc 1955; 50: 1096-1121.

13. Kubek MJ, Rea MA, Hodes ZI and Aprison MH. Quantitation and characterization of thyrotropin-releasing hormone in vagal nuclei and other regions of the medulla oblongata of the rat. J Neurochem 1983; 40: 1307-1313.

14. Horita A, Carino MA and Lai H. Pharmacology of thyrotropin-releasing hormone (TRH). Ann Rev Pharmacol & Toxicol 1986; 26: 311-332.

15. Maeda-Hagiwara M, Watanabe H and Watanabe K. Inhibition by central alpha2-adrenergic mechanism of thyrotropin-releasing hormone-induced gastric acid secretion in the rat. Japan J Pharmacol 1984; 36: 131-136.

16. Goto Y and Debas HT. GABA-mimetic effect on gastric acid secretion: Possible significance in central mechanism. Dig Dis Sci 1983; 28: 56-60.

17. Robert A. Prostaglandins and the gastrointestinal tract. In "Physiology of the gastrointestinal tract", Johnson LR, et al (Eds), Raven Press, New York, pp 1407-1434, 1981.

18. Yano S, Matsukura H, Shibata M and Harada M. Stress procedures lowering body temperature augment gastric motility by increasing the sensitivity to acetylcholine in rats. J Pharm Dyn 1982; 5: 582-592.

19. Hernandez DE, Hennes L and Emerick SG. Inhibition of gastric acid secretion by immunoneutralization of endogenous brain thyrotropin-releasing hormone. Brain Research 1987; 401: 381-384.

20. Basso N, Nagarani M, Pekary AE, Genco A and Materia A. Role of thyrotropin-releasing hormone in stress ulcer formation in the rat. Dig Dis Sci 1988; 33: 819-823.

ASSESSMENT OF CELL DEATH IN HYPOXIC CELL INJURY

Anna-Liisa Nieminen, Gregory J. Gores, Roberto Imberti, Brian Herman and John J. Lemasters

Department of Cell Biology & Anatomy, School of Medicine, University of North Carolina at Chapel Hill, Chapel Hill, North Carolina, U.S.A.

ABSTRACT

The critical events which underlie the transition from reversible to irreversible injury remain unclear. Here, we review recent studies with rat hepatocytes where we have focused on lethal cell injury following anoxia and chemical hypoxia. The latter is a model of metabolic inhibition with cyanide and iodoacetate which mimics the ATP depletion and reductive stress of anoxia. We observed three stages of cell injury during anoxia and chemical hypoxia. Stage I consisted of the formation of numerous bleb-like evaginations of plasma membrane. Subsequently in Stage II of injury, the blebs grew and coalesced by fusion to form one to a few large terminal blebs. Ultimately, one of the terminal blebs lysed causing fluorescent probes trapped in the cytosol to be lost and normally impermeant dyes such as propidium iodide to label cell nuclei. These changes mark the onset of cell death and the beginning of Stage III of injury. Because labelling of nuclei of non-viable cells by propidium iodide resulted in an enhancement of fluorescence, a new fluorometric assay using propidium iodide fluorescence was developed to monitor cell viability continuously and nondestructively in cell suspensions and cultured cells. Employing this cytotoxicity screening assay, protection by numerous agents against lethal injury was evaluated during chemical hypoxia. Acidosis was shown to protect strongly against the onset of cell death during ATP depletion from chemical hypoxia. The efficient glycolytic substrate, fructose, but not glucose, also gave strong protection against cyanide toxicity provided that iodoacetate, a glycolytic inhibitor, was not present. Antioxidants and certain inhibitors of phospholipases and proteases protected implicating a role for oxygen radicals, phospholipases and proteases in lethal hypoxic injury. Osmotic agents which prevent cell swelling and miscellaneous other putative protective agents were without effect. The results show the utility of the propidium iodide cytotoxicity screening assay for characterizing hypoxic cell injury.

INTRODUCTION

Hypoxic injury is commonly involved in the pathophysiology of human disease. Oxygen deprivation leads to primary inhibition of mitochondrial oxidative phosphorylation and ensuing hydrolysis of ATP. Glycolysis may temporarily prevent complete loss of ATP but, in general, cannot maintain ATP levels for very long since glycolytic substrates quickly become exhausted.

The critical events which underlie the transition from reversible to irreversible injury after ATP depletion remain unclear. A number of hypotheses have been proposed to explain hypoxic cell death, including activation of autolytic enzymes, plasma membrane phospholipid degradation, free radical formation and mitochondrial dysfunction [1-3]. Here, we present recent work investigating the critical events marking the transition from reversible to irreversible injury during anoxic and hypoxic stress. We describe how cell death in hypoxic and anoxic injury occurs as the consequence of a sudden loss of plasma membrane integrity. Subsequent labelling of cell nuclei with normally impermeant fluorescent dyes forms the basis for monitoring cell viability continuously in cell suspensions and cultures. Using this new assay, we present evidence that proteases, phospholipases and oxygen free radicals can contribute to the onset of irreversible injury in a pH-dependent fashion.

METHODS

HEPATOCYTE ISOLATION AND CULTURE

Hepatocytes were isolated from overnight-fasted Sprague-Dawley rats (200-300 g) by collagenase perfusion [4]. Viability of hepatocytes was greater than 90% as determined by trypan blue exclusion. Freshly isolated cells were suspended in Krebs-Ringers-Hepes buffer containing 0.2% bovine serum albumin or cultured in Waymouth's medium MB-752/1 supplemented with 26.7 mM $NaHCO_3$, 5% fetal calf serum, 10 nM dexamethasone, and 100 nM insulin on glass coverslips coated with rat tail collagen or in 96-well microtiter plates in 5% CO_2, 95% air at $37^\circ C$.

FLUORESCENCE SPECTRA OF PROPIDIUM IODIDE

Fluorescence emission and excitation spectra were collected with a Perkin-Elmer Model 850-40 fluorescence spectrophotometer equipped with a magnetic stirrer and warmed with recirculating water at $37^\circ C$.

LACTATE DEHYDROGENASE (LDH)

At desired time intervals LDH was measured in the medium of cultured cells. LDH activity after exposure of cells to 375 uM digitonin was taken as 100% release.

CYTOTOXICITY SCREENING ASSAY

Cell viability in suspended and cultured cells was monitored using propidium iodide fluorescence. For cells in suspension, freshly isolated hepatocytes (100,000/ml) were incubated in Krebs-Ringers-Hepes buffer containing 1 uM propidium iodide and 0.2% bovine serum albumin at $37^\circ C$ [5]. Fluorescence was monitored with a filter fluorometer (Sequoia-Turner Model 450) using 520 nm (8 nm band pass) excitation and 605 nm (long pass) emission filters. Hepatocytes cultured on microtiter plates (50,000/well) were incubated in Krebs-Ringers-Hepes buffer containing 50 uM propidium iodide. Fluorescence was measured using a microtiter plate fluorescence reader (Model VIP Fluorescence Concentration Analyzer, Baxter Health Care) with 545 nm excitation and 575 nm emission interference filters. In both assays, fluorescence was measured every 15 to 30 minutes. At the end of each experiment, 375 uM digitonin was added to permeabilize all cells and obtain a maximal fluorescence reading corresponding to 100% cell death. Percent viability was calculated using the formula: $V = 100(B - X)$ $(B - A)$ where V is viability in percent, B is fluorescence after digitonin treatment, X is fluorescence at any given time point, and A is baseline fluorescence. Assays were routinely performed in triplicate.

RESULTS AND DISCUSSION

BLEB FORMATION DURING ANOXIA AND CHEMICAL HYPOXIA

Previously, we characterized changes of cell morphology in single cultured hepatocytes by phase contrast microscopy and scanning electron microscopy during anoxia and chemical hypoxia [4,6,7]. The earliest structural change occurred in as little as 5 minutes and was the formation of numerous bleb-like evaginations of the plasma membrane (Stage I of injury). Subsequently, the blebs grew and coalesced by fusion to form one to a few large blebs called terminal blebs. This phase constituted Stage II of injury. Bleb growth in Stage II continued until one of the blebs ruptured. This abrupt event was indicated by 1) loss of trapped cytosolic dyes such as bis-carboxyethylcarboxyfluorescein and Fura-2, 2) onset of nuclear labelling with trypan blue and its fluorescent counterpart, propidium iodide, and 3) lysis and disappearance of a bleb in many instances. Scanning electron microscopy of cells immediately following bleb rupture demonstrated a discontinuity, literally a hole, in the plasma membrane at the place of rupture. These changes signified the onset of cell death which we have termed Stage III of injury. In anoxic hepatocytes, bleb rupture also marked the transition from reversible to irreversible injury, namely the point at which reoxygenation could no longer rescue the cells [4].

Our findings demonstrated that death of cells, like death of organisms, is a singular all or nothing event. After bleb rupture, life of cells cannot be sustained because ion and electrical gradients across the plasma membrane have collapsed, and soluble enzymes and metabolic intermediates of the cytosol have been lost. Indeed, commonly used indicators of loss of cell viability monitor the loss of integrity of the plasma membrane: nuclear staining by membrane-impermeant dyes (e.g., trypan blue, ethidium bromide, propidium iodide), release of trapped cytosolic probes (e.g. fluorescein diacetate), and leakage of intracellular enzymes and proteins (e.g. lactate dehydrogenase, transaminase, creatine kinase, ^{51}Cr-label).

NONDESTRUCTIVE ASSAY OF VIABILITY OF HEPATOCYTE SUSPENSIONS AND CULTURES USING PROPIDIUM IODIDE FLUORESCENCE

Single cell studies are time-consuming, and many cells must be studied in order to characterize a population. Accordingly, we sought to develop an assay for monitoring cell viability of entire populations of cells which was nondestructive and continuous, i.e., suitable for making serial measurements of the same cells. We developed such an assay by exploiting the observation that an enhancement and spectral shift of propidium iodide fluorescence occurred when it bound to chromatin. In the absence of cells, propidium iodide had excitation and emission maxima near 500 nm and

625 nm, respectively (Figure 1, no cells). When digitonin-permeabilized hepatocytes (10,000 - 100,000/ml) were added, an increase of fluorescence and a red shift of the excitation spectra of propidium iodide occurred (Figure 1). A similar fluorescence enhancement occurred for the emission spectrum with a slight blue shift. These spectral changes were maximal at excitation and emission wavelengths of 540 and 610 nm, respectively. In the absence of digitonin, the changes to propidium iodide fluorescence caused by addition of viable hepatocytes were greatly diminished.

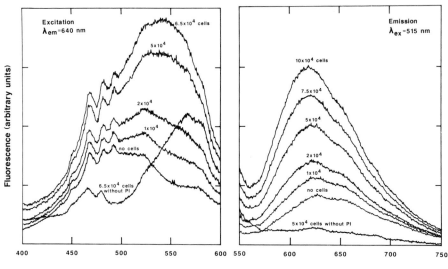

Wavelength (nm)

FIGURE 1.   *Fluorescence excitation and emission spectra of propidium iodide in the presence of digitonin-permeabilized hepatocytes - Fluorescence excitation and emission spectra were recorded from hepatocytes suspended in Krebs-Henseleit-Hepes buffer containing 10 mM glucose, 1.0 uM propidium iodide and 500 uM digitonin. Minor peaks are lamp artifacts.*

Fluorescence microscopy of digitonin-permeabilized cells revealed uniform nuclear labelling of all cells by propidium iodide. Also, we observed a 100% correspondence between labelling by trypan blue and propidium iodide of cell nuclei in our models of lethal injury. Thus, the changes of propidium iodide fluorescence appeared to be specific for nonviable cells.

Propidium iodide concentration and cell number were varied to determine optimal conditions for measuring loss of cell viability. In digitonin-permeabilized cell suspensions, the percent increase of fluorescence over baseline was greatest with 1 and 3 uM propidium iodide and was linear with cell number up to 150,000 cells/ml [5]. Accordingly, a propidium iodide concentration of 1 uM and a cell number of 100,000 cells/ml were selected for experiments with cell suspensions. For hepatocytes cultured in microtiter plates, the increase of fluorescence was greatest with 20-100 uM propidium iodide and was linear up to 75,000 cells/well. Thus, 50 uM propidium iodide and a cell concentration of 50,000 cells/well were employed in experiments with cultured cells. Evidently, the microtiter plate fluorescence reader used with cultured cells was less sensitive to propidium iodide fluorescence than the filter fluorometer. The poorer sensitivity of the fluorescence reader was due, in part, to the use of a narrow band-pass emission filter.

<u>CORRELATION BETWEEN PROPIDIUM IODIDE FLUORESCENCE, PROPIDIUM IODIDE NUCLEAR LABELLING, AND LACTATE DEHYDROGENASE RELEASE</u>

In hepatocyte suspensions treated with cyanide, the percent increase of propidium iodide fluorescence was identical to percent nuclear staining with propidium iodide and percent lactate dehydrogenase release into the extracellular medium [5]. Similarly, in cultured hepatocytes exposed to cyanide plus iodoacetate, the increase of propidium iodide fluorescence was linearly proportional to lactate dehydrogenase release into the medium (Figure 2).

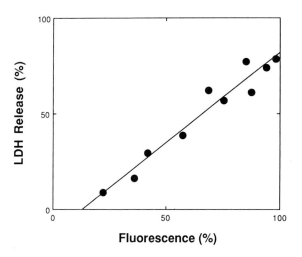

FIGURE 2. *Propidium iodide fluorescence and lactate dehydrogenase release by cultured hepatocytes during chemical hypoxia - Hepatocytes (50,000/well) were cultured overnight on 96-well microtiter plates as described in METHODS. Culture media was changed to Krebs-Ringers-Hepes buffer containing 50 uM propidium iodide, and 2.5 mM KCN plus 0.5 mM iodoacetate were added. Fluorescence was measured every 15 minutes with a microtiter plate fluorescence scanner. Simultaneously, aliquots of supernatant were removed from the wells and analyzed for LDH. A 100% response of fluorescence and LDH release was taken as that after addition of 375 uM digitonin at the end of the experiment.*

Propidium iodide fluorescence increased slightly before LDH began to appear in the incubation medium. This delay of LDH release reflects the time required for the enzyme to diffuse from nonviable cells into the bulk medium in this unstirred system.

MODEL OF CHEMICAL HYPOXIA

Using the propidium iodide assay, we developed a model of "chemical hypoxia" in order to screen potential protective agents in hypoxic and ischemic injury. Chemical hypoxia employs the metabolic inhibitors, cyanide and iodoacetate, to mimic the ATP depletion and reductive stress of anoxia. Cyanide inhibits mitochondrial respiration at cytochrome c oxidase, the site at which respiration is inhibited during anoxia. As in anoxia, cyanide causes reduction of pyridine nucleotides, quinones, cytochromes and other electron carriers which feed into cytochrome oxidase. Inhibition of respiration also inhibits completely ATP formation by oxidative phosphorylation, whereas iodoacetate inhibits ATP formation by glycolysis. Thus after chemical hypoxia, ATP is 95% depleted within 5 minutes [5].

Chemical hypoxia provides a reproducible model of the ATP depletion and reductive stress of anoxia which avoids the technical difficulties and paraphernalia associated with removal of oxygen from biological systems. Typically, hepatocyte killing after chemical hypoxia begins after a characteristic latency of about 30 minutes, is 50% complete after 60 minutes, and is more than 90% complete after 120 minutes. The propidium iodide assay of cell killing after chemical hypoxia has proven to be sensitive, inexpensive and easy to use. It has afforded us the opportunity to screen a wide variety of compounds for cytoprotection during chemical hypoxia, and we have been able to measure reliably even small amounts of cytoprotection. In Tables I and II, we summarize our experience to date.

ACIDOTIC pH

Acidosis is a characteristic feature of ischemia and systemic hypoxia. Early reports suggested that acidotic pH was protective in ischemia and hypoxia [8,9], but prevailing opinion has been that acidosis is harmful [10,11]. During chemical hypoxia, however, acidotic pH exerted a powerful protective effect, and cell killing was delayed by 2 hours or more at values of pH between 5.5 and 6.5 [5]. Decreases of as little as 0.2 pH units below a physiologic pH of 7.4 provided a delay of cell killing. Protection by acidotic extracellular pH was mediated by intracellular acidification, and in general the greater the intracellular acidification, the greater the protection [12]. Acidosis also protected against lethal injury from several toxic chemicals [13]. However, when normal pH was restored, cell killing rapidly accelerated. This phenomenon may contribute to the worsening of ischemic injury after reperfusion [5,14].

ANTIOXIDANTS

In the model of chemical hypoxia, oxygen is nevertheless present, and formation of toxic oxygen species such as superoxide and hydroxy radical may contribute to cell killing. The antioxidants, mannitol, desferrioxamine, and cyanidanol, as well as anoxia itself provided a reproducible 15 to 30 minutes delay in cell killing after chemical hypoxia [15]. The membrane-impermeant antioxidants, superoxide dismutase and catalase, were without effect, presumably because they did not gain access to the cells. Protection by anoxia correlated with a reduction of formation of hydroperoxides as detected by dichlorofluorescein fluorescence [15]. Although xanthine oxidase has been implicated as a source of oxygen radicals in hypoxia/reperfusion injury [3], allopurinol was not protective (Table I), and mitochondria appear to be a more likely source of the toxic oxygen species [16]. The "reductive stress" caused by respiratory inhibition appears to favour formation of toxic oxygen species by mitochondria which may contribute to lethal cell injury during intermittent or incomplete oxygen deprivation.

OSMOTIC AGENTS

Hepatocytes swell during chemical hypoxia, and we tested the hypothesis that swelling precipitates bleb rupture and cell death [15]. Sucrose, an effective osmotic agent, prevented cell swelling but had no effect on cell viability. Other osmotic agents including polyethyleneglycol, polyvinylpyrolidone, glycerol, and albumin also did not protect (Table I). Although mannitol did protect, mannitol passed readily through the plasma membranes of hepatocytes and did not prevent cell swelling [15,17]. Thus, protection by mannitol was not exerted through an osmotic mechanism.

CYTOSKELETAL ANTAGONISTS

The ability of eukaryotic cells to adopt different cell shapes depends on cytoskeleton-associated proteins. In cell injury, bleb formation has been postulated to occur as the result of disruption of cytoskeletal attachments to the plasma membrane [18,19]. Disappearance of vinculin, a protein involved in cytoskeleton-membrane attachment, has been described in ischemic heart [20]. Okayasu et al [21] reported that cytochalasin which depolymerizes actin microfilaments delays the onset of anoxic cell death in cultured hepatocytes. Colchicine which causes microtubule depolymerization was without effect. In our model of chemical hypoxia, however, neither cytochalasin nor phalloidin, which stabilizes microfilaments, delayed the onset of cell death (Table I). Taxol which stabilizes microtubule was also without effect.

Our data indicate that cytoskeletal agents, in general, do not influence the progression of lethal cell injury during chemical hypoxia. Although nocodazole had some protective effect, colchicine had none. Thus, protection by nocodazole may not be related to its action on microtubules, or it may be due to more efficient transport of nocodazole into the cells. In contrast to Okayasu et al [21], cytochalasin also did not protect. Cytochalasin inhibits sugar transport across plasma membranes in addition to depolymerizing actin microfilaments [22]. Anoxia stimulates glycogenolysis, and in the experiments by Okayasu et al., cytochalasin may have prevented the loss of glycogen-derived glucose from the cells. Such glucose could extend cell viability by serving as a substrate for glycolytic ATP formation. This protective mechanism would not be operative in chemical hypoxia where glycolysis is strongly inhibited with iodacetate.

TABLE 1.

SURVEY OF POTENTIAL PROTECTIVE AGENTS DURING CHEMICAL HYPOXIA IN
HEPATOCYTE SUSPENSIONS - SUSPENSIONS OF FRESHLY ISOLATED HEPATOCYTES
(100,000 cells/ml) WERE EXPOSED TO 2.5 mM KCN AND 0.5 mM
IODOACETATE (EXCEPT AS NOTED) AFTER 30 MINS OF PREINCUBATION WITH
AGENTS TO BE TESTED. CELL VIABILITY WAS ASSESSED BY PROPIDIUM IODIDE
(1uM) FLUOROMETRY AS DESCRIBED IN METHODS. AGENTS WHICH DELAYED
CELL KILLING WERE CONSIDERED PROTECTIVE.

NO BENEFIT OR TOXIC	PROTECTIVE
HYDROGEN ION	
Alkaline pH (>7.4)	Mildly acidic pH (5.5-7.2)
Very acidic pH (<5.0)	
ANTIOXIDANTS	
Allopurinol (50uM-1mM)	Mannitol (300-500mM)
Superoxide dismutase (25U/ml)	Desferrioxamine (300uM-1mM)
Catalase (500U/ml)	Cyanidanol (100-500uM)
Superoxide dismutase + catalase	Anoxia
OSMOTIC AGENTS	
Polyethyleneglycol (2.5-20%)	
Polyvinylpyrolidone (5-20%)	
Albumin (2.5-5%)	
Glycerol (10%)	
Sucrose (100-500 mM)	
CYTOSKELETAL AGENTS	
Taxol (10uM)	Nocodazole (10-50uM)
Colchicine (10uM)	
Phalloidin (10-50uM)	
Cytochalasin B (10-50uM)	
PHOSPHOLIPASE INHIBITORS	
Mepacrine (25-100ug/ml)	
Quinacrine (25-100uM)	
Chlorpromazine (100uM)	
Dibucaine (80-250uM)	
PROTEASE INHIBITORS	
Leupeptin (100 - 150ug/ml)	
Antipain (50-100uM)	
E-64 (50-100uM)	
PMSF (50-100uM)	
Iminodiacetic acid (50-100uM)	
1,10-Phenanthroline (50-300uM)	
CALCIUM ANTAGONISTS	
Verapamil (1-100uM)	Nisoldipine (1-10uM)
Flunarizine (1-50uM)	Nitrendipine (1-10uM)
Lidoflazine (1-50uM)	Nicardipine (1-10uM)
MISCELLANEOUS AGENTS	
H-7 (1-100uM)	
Tetradecanoylphorbol acetate (0.1-2uM)	
Glucose (20mM)*	Fructose (20mM)*

*In presence of cyanide only.

TABLE 2.

SURVEY OF POTENTIAL PROTECTIVE AGENTS DURING CHEMICAL HYPOXIA IN
CULTURED HEPATOCYTES - HEPATOCYTES CULTURED OVERNIGHT ON 95-WELL
MICROTITER PLATES (50,000 cells/ml) WERE EXPOSED TO 2.5 mM KCN AND
0.5 mM IODOACETATE AFTER 30 MINUTES OF PREINCUBATION WITH AGENTS
TO BE TESTED. CELL VIABILITY WAS ASSESSED BY PROPIDIUM IODIDE ($50u$M)
FLUOROMETRY AS DESCRIBED IN METHODS. AGENTS WHICH DELAYED CELL
KILLING WERE CONSIDERED PROTECTIVE.

NO BENEFIT OR TOXIC	PROTECTIVE
PHOSPHOLIPASE INHIBITORS	
	Dibucaine (100-$500u$M)
PROTEASE INHIBITORS	
Antipain (50-$100u$M)	$1,10$-Phenanthroline(100-$500u$M)
Leupeptin (5-$10u$g/ml)	Pepstatin A ($500u$M)
E-64 (50-$500u$M)	
PMSF (10-$50u$M)	
Iminodiacetic acid (100-$500u$M)	

PHOSPHOLIPASE AND PROTEASE INHIBITORS

Several studies have shown that alterations in the content and
composition of phospholipids in cellular membranes occur in ischemic and
hypoxic injury [2,23,24]. An increase in phospholipase A_2 activity may be
responsible. Similarly, accelerated proteolysis may contribute to cell killing
[25]. Thus, we evaluated protection by inhibitors of phospholipases and
proteases. None showed any protection in freshly isolated hepatocyte
suspensions (Table I). However, the phospholipase inhibitor, dibucaine, and
the protease inhibitors, 1,10-phenanthroline and pepstatin, delayed cell
killing in cultured hepatocytes (Table II). The basis for these differences
between freshly isolated and cultured hepatocytes has not been identified,
but the results suggest that both proteolysis and phospholipid hydrolysis can
contribute to lethal cell injury after ATP depletion in some situations.

In glomerular mesangial cells, Bonventre et al [26] recently
demonstrated that protein kinase C in the presence of Ca^{2+} can modulate
the activation of phospholipase A_2, possibly by phosphorylating
phospholipase A_2 modulatory proteins or phospholipase A_2 itself. With this
in mind, we evaluated the effects of H-7, a protein kinase C inhibitor, and
tetradecanoylphorbol acetate, a protein kinase C agonist, on lethal cell
injury during chemical hypoxia (Table I). However, neither agent changed
the rate of cell killing.

CALCIUM ANTAGONISTS

Previously we determined the relationship between cell surface blebbing, cytosolic free Ca^{2+}, and the onset of cell death in hepatocytes during chemical hypoxia [6,27]. An increase of free Ca^{2+} did not precede cell surface blebbing or the onset of cell death. Thus, an increase of cytosolic free Ca^{2+} was not required for cell death to occur. However, calcium channel blockers have been described to protect against hypoxic and toxic injury in intact liver [28,29]. To determine whether this was a direct effect on hepatocytes, we evaluated different calcium antagonists for protection against lethal hypoxic injury during chemical hypoxia. Verapamil, flunarizine and lidoflazine did not protect, but the dihydropyridine-type blockers, nitrendipine, nisoldipine and nicardipine, provided a small but reproducible delay of 10 to 20 minutes in cell killing during chemical hypoxia (Table I). This protection occurs despite reports that hepatocytes do not have voltage-gated calcium channels [30].

MISCELLANEOUS AGENTS

Fructose is an efficient substrate for glycolytic ATP formation in liver. In glycogen-depleted livers from fasted rats, fructose protected against lethal cell injury from anoxia [31]. Similarly, fructose protected isolated hepatocytes against cell killing after respiratory inhibition with cyanide [5]. Glucose, which is not effectively taken up and metabolized by ATP-depleted hepatocytes, did not protect. Fructose also protected in models of toxic cell injury with ionophores and oxidative chemicals suggesting that disruption of mitochondrial ATP synthesis contributes to toxicity in these settings [13]. However, in the model of chemical hypoxia, iodoacetate inhibits glycolysis, and fructose no longer protects against the onset of cell death. These experiments illustrate the critical importance of ATP availability in toxic and hypoxic injury.

CONCLUSION

The results we review here demonstrate that the transition from reversible to irreversible hypoxic injury occurs as a consequence of an abrupt breakdown of the plasma membrane permeability barrier. By screening several potential protective agents with a new fluorescent cytotoxicity assay, this strongly pH-dependent terminal event was shown to be accelerated by the action of proteases, phospholipases and oxygen free radicals.

ACKNOWLEDGEMENT

*This work was supported in part by Grants AG07218
and DK30874 from the National Institutes of Health
and by Grant J-1433 from the Office of Naval Research*

REFERENCES

1.   Farber JL, Chien KR, Mittnacht S. The pathogenesis of irreversible
      cell injury in ischemia. Am J Pathol 1981; 102: 171-178.

2.   Chien KR, Abrams J, Serroni A, Martin JT, Farber JL. Accelerated
      phospholipid degradation and associated membrane dysfunction in
      irreversible, ischemic liver cell injury. J Biol Chem 1978; 253: 4809-
      4817.

3.   Adkison D, Hollwarth ME, Benoit JN, Parks DA, McCord JM,
      Granger DN. Role of free radicals in ischemia-reperfusion injury to
      the liver. Acta Physiol Scand 1986; Suppl 548: 101-107.

4.   Herman B, Nieminen A-L, Gores GJ, Lemasters JJ. Irreversible
      injury in anoxic hepatocytes precipitated by an abrupt increase in
      plasma membrane permeability. FASEB J 1988; 2: 146-151.

5.   Gores JG, Nieminen A-L, Fleishman KE, Dawson TL, Herman B,
      Lemasters JJ. Extracellular acidosis delays onset of cell death in
      ATP-depleted hepatocytes. Am J Physiol 1988; 255: C315-322.

6.   Lemasters JJ, DiGuiseppi J, Nieminen A-L, Herman B. Blebbing, free
      Ca^{2+} and mitochondrial membrane potential preceding cell death in
      hepatocytes. Nature 1987; 325: 78-81.

7.   Nieminen A-L, Gores GJ, Wray BE, Tanaka Y, Herman B, Lemasters
      JJ. Calcium dependence of bleb formation and cell death in
      hepatocytes. Cell Calcium 1988; 9: 237-246.

8.   Bing OHL, Brooks WW, Messer JV. Heart muscle viability following
      hypoxia: protective effect of acidosis. Science 1973; 180: 1297-1298.

9.   Penttila A, Trump BF. Extracellular acidosis protects Erlich ascites
      tumor cells and rat renal cortex against anoxic injury. Science 1974;
      185: 277-278.

10.   Rouslin W, Erickson JL. Factors affecting the loss of mitochondrial
      function in autolyzing cardiac muscle. J Mol Cell Cardiol 1986; 18:
      1187-1195.

11.   Belzer FO, Southard JH. Principles of solid-organ preservation by
      cold storage. Transplantation 1988; 45: 673-676.

12.   Gores GJ, Nieminen A-L, Wray BE, Herman B, Lemasters JJ.
      Intracellular pH during 'chemical hypoxia' in cultured rat
      hepatocytes. J Clin Invest 1989; 83: 386-396.

13.   Nieminen A-L, Dawson TL, Gores GJ, Kawanishi T, Herman B,
      Lemasters JJ. Protection by acidotic pH and fructose against lethal
      injury to rat hepatocytes from mitochondrial inhibitors, ionophores
      and oxidant chemicals. Biochem Biophys Res Commun. 1990; 167:
      600-606.

14.   Currin RT, Gores GJ, Thurman RG, Lemasters JJ. Protection by
       acidic pH against anoxic injury in perfused rat liver: evidence for a
       'pH paradox'. FASEB J 1989; 3: A626.

15.   Gores GJ, Flarsheim CE, Dawson TL, Nieminen A-L, Herman B,
       Lemasters JJ. Swelling, reductive stress, and cell death during
       chemical hypoxia in hepatocytes. Am J Physiol 1989; 257: C347-354.

16.   Gores GJ, Dawson TL, Herman B, Lemasters JJ. Subcellular sites
       producing reactive oxygen species during reductive stress of chemical
       hypoxia. J Cell Biol 1989; 107: 349a.

17.   Alpini G, Garrick RA, Jones MJT, Nunes R, Tavoloni N. Water and
       nonelectrolyte permeability of isolated rat hepatocytes. Am J Physiol
       1986; 251: C872-882.

18.   Lemasters JJ, Stemkowski CJ, Ji S, Thurman RG. Cell surface
       changes and enzyme release during hypoxia and reoxygenation in the
       isolated, perfused rat liver. J Cell Biol. 1983; 97: 778-786.

19.   Thor H, Mirabelli F, Salis A, Cohen GM, Bellomo G, Orrenius S.
       Alterations in hepatocyte cytoskeleton caused by redox cycling and
       alkylating quinones. Arch Biochem Biophys. 1988; 266: 397-407.

20.   Steenbergen C, Hill ML, Jennings RB. Cytoskeletal damage during
       myocardial ischemia: Changes in vinculin immunofluorescence
       staining during total in vitro ischemia in canine heart. Circ Res.
       1987; 60: 478-486.

21.   Okayasu T, Curtis MT, Farber JL. Cytochalasin delays but not
       prevent cell death from anoxia. Am J Pathol 1984; 117: 163-166.

22.   Kasanicki MA, Cairns MT, Davies A, Gardiner RM, Baldwin SA.
       Identification and characterization of the glucose-transport protein
       of the bovine blood/brain barrier. Biochem J 1987; 247: 101-108.

23.   Chien KR, Sen A, Reynolds R, Chang A, Kim Y, Gunn MD, Buja LM,
       Willerson JT. Release of arachidonate from membrane phospholipids
       in cultured neonatal rat myocardial cells during adenosine
       triphosphate depletion. J Clin Invest 1985; 75: 1770-1780.

24.   Buja LM, Hagler HK, Willerson JT. Altered calcium homeostasis in
       the pathogenesis of myocardial ischemic and hypoxic injury. Cell
       Calcium 1988; 9: 205-217.

25.   Nicotera P, Hartzell P, Baldi C, Svensson S-A, Bellomo G, Orrenius S.,
       Cystamine induces toxicity in hepatocytes through the elevation of
       cytosolic Ca^{2+} and the stimulation of a nonlysosomal proteolytic
       system. J Biol Chem 1986; 261: 14628-14635.

26.   Bonventre JV, Swidler M.   Calcium dependency of prostaglandin E_2 production in rat glomerular mesangial cells.   J Clin Invest   1988; 82: 168-176.

27.   Nieminen A-L, Gores GJ, Wray BE, Tanaka Y, Herman B, Lemasters JJ.   Calcium dependence of bleb formation and cell death in hepatocytes. Cell Calcium   1988; 9: 237-246.

28.   Landon EJ, Naukam RJ, Sastry BVR.   Effects of calcium channel blocking agents on calcium and centrilobular necrosis in the liver of rats treated with hepatotoxic agents.   Biochem Pharmacol   1986; 35: 697-705.

29.   Thurman RG, King JN, Lemasters JJ.   Nitrendipine protects the liver against hypoxia-induced damage at submicromolar concentrations in the perfused rat liver.   J Cardiovasc Pharmacol   1987; 9(Suppl.4): 571-576.

30.   Grollman EF.   Calcium signals in the liver.   In: Arias IM, Jakoby WB, Popper H, Schachter D, Shafritz DA, eds.   The Liver: Biology and Pathobiology. 2nd ed. New York: Raven Press, 1988; 777-783.

31.   Anundi I, King J, Owen DA, Schneider H, Lemasters JJ, Thurman RG.   Fructose prevents hypoxic cell death in liver.   Am J Physiol 1987; 253: G390-396.

ROLE OF 16,16 dmPGE$_2$ IN GASTRIC CELL PROTECTION AGAINST BILE SALTS

Adam J. Dziki, John W. Harmon, Shmuel Batzri,
Barbara L. Bass and Richard M. Ugarte

*Department of Surgery, V.A. Medical Center, Washington, D.C., and
Uniformed Services University of the Health Sciences, Bethesda, Maryland*

INTRODUCTION

Prostaglandins have been termed to be cytoprotective [1,2]. This implies that they protect cells from injury directly on the cellular level. This is in contradistinction to the mechanisms of protection which occur at a tissue level acting by controlling the external environment of the cells. These would include reducing acid secretion or increasing bicarbonate secretion to maintain neutral pH and prevent cellular acidity. Another non-cellular mechanism would be protection mediated by increased blood flow clearing toxic agents and providing oxygen and bicarbonate. Still another would be the mucus gel which coats the mucosa and which, with the unstirred water layer, has the potential to protect mucosal cells. Prostaglandins are known to affect all of the above tissue-mediated mechanisms of protection. And yet these mechanisms do not seem to fully explain their protective effects. Therefore the concept of cytoprotection has been proposed.

In the current experiments we explored the possibility that prostaglandins could protect gastric mucosal cells from bile salt-induced injury. Our cellular system utilizes dispersed rabbit gastric mucosal cells. The cell types are present as in the intact mucosa with no enrichment of any fraction. This system has been utilized extensively for the study of parietal cell secretion [3,4,5]. In the current experiments we characterized the effects of deoxycholate-induced cellular injury. Trypan Blue exclusion was used as a measure of cellular viability. Oxygen consumption was also assessed. Intracellular free calcium levels were measured with the fluorescent dye FURA 2/AM. Changes in these parameters were characterized after exposure to the bile salt deoxycholate for various time periods and at various concentrations. Having characterized deoxycholate injury to the mucosal cells, we then searched for evidence of possible protective effects of the long- acting E type prostaglandin analogue 16,16 di-methyl PGE$_2$. We also assessed the effect of reducing endogenous prostaglandins in these cells by pretreating the donor rabbits with indomethacin. These studies had the dual aims of characterizing bile salt injury to the gastric mucosa on a cellular basis and identifying a cytoprotective effect of prostaglandin E$_2$.

METHODS

PREPARATION OF GASTRIC CELLS

Dispersed rabbit gastric cells were prepared from rabbit gastric glands as described in detail elsewhere [6]. In short, gastric glands were harvested from rabbit gastric mucosa, which was excised after a high pressure aortic injection. After the glands were prepared they were washed once with Ca^{2+}-free buffer (pH 7) and incubated with 12 mM EDTA for 10 minutes at $37^{o}C$. They were then washed twice with buffer (pH 7) containing 0.1 mM Ca^{2+} and resuspended in buffer (pH 7) containing 0.1% collagenase and 0.2% bovine serum albumin. After a 20 minute incubation period at $37^{o}C$ with gentle stirring, an equal volume of fresh buffer (pH 7) was added and the suspension, containing mostly single cells, was passed through a nylon mesh to remove cell clumps. The cells were collected by centrifugation (100 x g for 5 minutes) and resuspended in the appropriate buffer containing 1 mM Ca^{2+}. Cell concentration was determined by two independent individuals using a hemocytometer.

TREATMENT OF THE CELLS WITH PROSTAGLANDINS

To test the potential protective effect of prostaglandins on bile-induced injury, a cell suspension (1×10^6 cells/ml) previously loaded with FURA 2/AM was preincubated for 15 minutes at $37^{o}C$ alone or with $1 u$M dmPGE$_2$ prior to exposure to the bile salt-induced injury. In other experiments to inhibit synthesis of the endogenous prostaglandins, the rabbit was injected intramuscularly with indomethacin (10mg/kg) 1 hour prior to harvesting the gastric mucosal cells. To validate the effect of the indomethacin, platelet aggregation was assessed. Platelet aggregation was inhibited by 80% in indomethacin treated rabbits compared to controls.

MEASUREMENT OF INTRACELLULAR FREE CALCIUM

Gastric cells were preincubated with $1 u$M FURA 2/AM for 20 minutes at $37^{o}C$. The cells were then washed three times, diluted to obtain 10^6 cells/ml and resuspended in media containing 1 mM Ca^{2+}. Intracellular free calcium was measured utilizing a spectrofluorometer (Perkin-Elmer, LS 5) set at emission wavelength of 510nm, with the excitation wavelength setting oscillating rapidly between 340nm and 380nm to obtain a fluorescence intensity ratio (340/380). The amount of intracellular free calcium was calculated according to the method described by Grynkiewicz et al [7] as follows:

$$[Ca^{2+}]_i = K_d \quad * \quad \frac{R - R_{min}}{R_{max} - R} \quad * \quad \frac{S_{f2}}{S_{b2}}$$

Where K_d is the dissociation constant of the calcium-FURA complex equal to 224 nM, R is the fluorescence intensity ratio (340/380) of the measured sample, R_{max} is the fluorescence intensity ratio (340/380) obtained after the cells have been lysed by 0.1% Triton, thereby allowing entry of Ca^{2+} into the cells, and R_{min} is the fluorescence intensity ratio (340/380) with no extracellular calcium, which is bound by 25 mM EDTA. S_{f2} is the fluorescence intensity at 380 nm of the dye with no extracellular calcium and S_{b2} the fluorescence intensity at 380 nm of the dye under maximum intracellular free calcium. The process was repeated for cells with no FURA to measure tissue autofluorescence. All ratios were calculated following subtraction of tissue autofluorescence. To eliminate the contribution of dye leak (about 5% after one hour of incubation at room temperature) the time between washing the FURA-loaded cells and measuring $[Ca^{2+}]_i$ never extended beyond 30 minutes.

We validated our cellular system for measuring $[Ca^{2+}]_i$ in a number of ways. First we assessed whether $[Ca^{2+}]_i$ remained stable in resting, unperturbed cells. To demonstrate this the fluorescence intensity ratio of the cell sample was recorded at 0, 2, 5, 10, and 20 minutes.

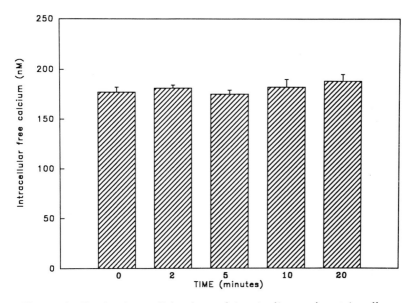

FIGURE 1   Resting intracellular free calcium in dispersed gastric cells.

Figure 1 displays the results of these measurements. $[Ca^{2+}]_i$ measured at all time intervals remained the same. In other experiments $[Ca^{2+}]_i$ remained stable for up to 3 hours.

Next we performed an experiment to examine potential deoxycholic acid (DC) interference with the FURA 2/AM calcium measurement. DC was added to a cuvette containing FURA 2/AM and a known amount of free calcium and the fluorescence intensity ratio (340/380) was registered prior to and after adding DC. Deoxycholic acid did not change the fluorescence intensity ratio.

Finally, to verify that the range of cell concentration used has no influence on the determination of $[Ca^{2+}]_i$, the cells loaded with FURA 2/AM and those used to measure tissue autofluorescence were diluted from 10^6 to 5 x 10^5 cells/ml [1:2] and 3 x 10^5 cells/ml [1:3]. The fluorescence intensity ratio (340/380) was then measured and $[Ca^{2+}]_i$ calculated by the Grynkiewicz equation. The measurement of $[Ca^{2+}]_i$ did not vary in this cell concentration range.

MEASUREMENT OF RESPIRATION

Gastric cell oxygen consumption was measured with a differential respirometer (Gilson), using air as the gas phase [8,9]. Aliquots of cells were suspended in respiratory media. Deoxycholic acid was added to separate flasks containing 2 ml of the cell suspension to final concentrations of 0.2 mM, 0.5 mM and 1 mM. Three or four flasks served as controls without DC. All flasks were equilibrated for 20 minutes at $37^{\circ}C$. Oxygen consumption was then recorded at 10 minute intervals for 40 - 60 minutes, and the rate of oxygen consumption calculated from the slope of the graph of oxygen disappearance versus time. The results were normalized for the dry weight of the cells in each preparation and expressed as ul/mg dry weight/h.

TRYPAN BLUE EXCLUSION TEST

The Trypan Blue exclusion test is a test of cellular viability, based on the fact that viable cells exclude the dye. The test was conducted in experiments by 2 individuals who counted the percentage of cells stained by 0.1 - 0.3% (w/v) Trypan Blue. Cells were treated with different concentrations of DC (0.2 mM, 0.5 mM or 1 mM) for 10 minutes and washed. Trypan Blue was then added. The percentage of cells that excluded Trypan Blue from their cytoplasm was recorded. At least 200 cells were evaluated in each test.

STATISTICAL ANALYSIS

Each experiment was performed at least three times. Significant differences at the 95% confidence level were computed using analysis of variance or the Student's t-test. Results are expressed as the mean $\pm$ one standard error of the mean (SEM).

RESULTS

$[Ca^{2+}]_i$ IN GASTRIC CELLS

The basal $[Ca^{2+}]_i$ measured in dispersed rabbit gastric cells was 177 $\pm$ 5nM and $[Ca^{2+}]_i$ maintained a range between 175nM and 188nM during measurements taken at 2, 5, 10 and 20 minutes.

The basal $[Ca^{2+}]_i$ in gastric cells treated with $dmPGE_2$ was 231 $\pm$ 11 nM and also did not change during measurements taken over the same time period. The gastric cells obtained from rabbits injected with indomethacin yielded measurements similar to the former measurements (213 $\pm$ 12nM) and these were also stable over time.

To determine the effect of the deoxycholic acid on $[Ca^{2+}]_i$, the fluorescence intensity ratio (340/380) was measured prior to the addition of DC (time 0), and then again at 2, 5, 10, and 20 minutes after the addition of various concentrations of DC (0.2 mM, 0.5 mM, or 1 mM). Deoxycholate increased $[Ca^{2+}]_i$ by 1.6 to 32-fold. The minimal concentration of DC which caused this increase was 0.2 mM. These increases occurred within 2 minutes and did not rise significantly at subsequent time intervals up to 20 minutes. The maximal $[Ca^{2+}]_i$ in the dispersed gastric cells following treatment with 0.2 mM DC reached 285 ± 24 nM, while the maximal levels were 639 ± 49 nM with 0.5 mM DC, and 5649 ± 1002 nM with 1 mM DC.

The $[Ca^{2+}]_i$ in those cells treated with prostaglandins reached 356 ± 6 nM following incubation with 0.2 mM DC, 550 ± 42 with 0.5 mM DC and 2440 ± 757 nM with 1 mM DC. Similarly dispersed gastric cells from indomethacin treated rabbits reached $[Ca^{2+}]_i$ levels of 354 ± 64 nM following treatment with 0.2 mM DC, 571 ± 48 nM with 0.5 mM DC and 4080 ± 262 nM with 1 mM DC. These results are shown in Figure 2.

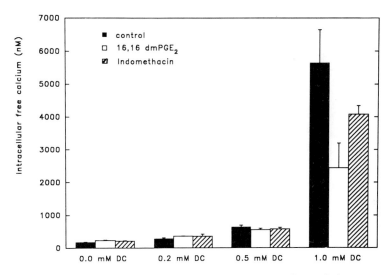

FIGURE 2   *Effect of PGE_2 and indomethacin on deoxycholate induced increase in intracellular free calcium.*

Effect of Prostaglandins on Oxygen Consumption During Deoxycholate Injury

Resting cells used 20 ± 0 ul of oxygen/mg dry weight/h. Incubation of the cells with 0.2 mM deoxycholic acid increased respiration to 24 ± 3 ul O_2/mg dry weight/h. However, incubation with higher concentrations of DC diminished the rate of respiration to 15 ± 2 ul/mg dry weight/h (0.5 mM DC) or nearly ablated it to 2 ± 1 ul/mg dry weight/h (1 mM DC). Cells pretreated with dmPGE$_2$ utilized a similar quantity of oxygen as control cells: 20 ± 1 ul/mg dry wt/h in resting conditions, 31 ± 1 after incubation with 0.2 mM DC, 15 ± 0 with 0.5 mM DC, and 8 ± 1 ul/mg dry wt/h with 1 mM DC. Gastric cells from indomethacin treated rabbits and thereby with lower levels of prostaglandins showed a similar pattern in oxygen consumption: 21 ± 2 ul/mg dry wt/h in resting conditions, 32 ± 3 ul/mg dry wt/h after incubation with 0.2 mM DC, 12 ± 3 with 0.5 mM DC and 6 ± 0 ul/mg dry wt/h with 1.0 mM DC. These results are shown in Figure 3.

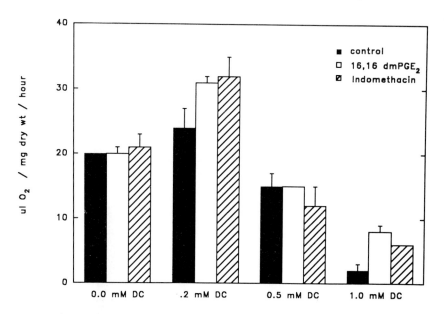

FIGURE 3   *Effect of PGE$_2$ and indomethacin on Trypan Blue exclusion in deoxycholate injured cells.*

EFFECT OF PROSTAGLANDINS ON THE TRYPAN BLUE EXCLUSION TEST AFTER DEOXYCHOLATE INJURY

This test determined that at time zero prior to exposure to deoxycholate 98% of the cells used as controls, as well as those treated with prostaglandins or obtained from rabbits injected with indomethacin, were able to exclude Trypan Blue and were thus deemed "viable" by this test. Incubation of the cells with 0.2 mM deoxycholate was not injurious to the cells in that the same percentage of cells were "viable" as in the control trial. Incubation with 0.5 mM DC diminished the percentage of "viable" cells to $91\% \pm 3$. The percentage of "viable" cells was equivalent for the prostaglandin treated cells ($90\% \pm 3$) and for the indomethacin treated cells ($91\% \pm 3$). Exposure to 1 mM DC diminished the "viability" of the control cells to $38\% \pm 15$ and similarly reduced the "viability" of the prostaglandin ($35\% \pm 19$) and indomethacin treated ($37\% \pm 21$) cells. These results are shown in Figure 4.

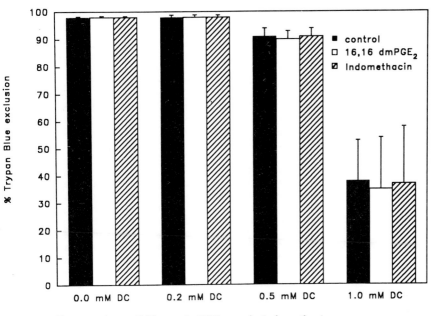

FIGURE 4   *Effect of PGE_2 and indomethacin on oxygen consumption in deoxycholate injured cells.*

DISCUSSION

Neither reducing endogenous prostaglandins with indomethacin nor supplementing exogenous prostaglandins with 16,16 di-methyl prostaglandin E_2 dramatically modulated the degree of injury produced in dispersed gastric mucosal cells by a range of concentrations of the bile salt deoxycholate.

There were two exceptions to the overall lack of effect. First, both $dmPGE_2$ and indomethacin tended to reduce the rise in $[Ca^{2+}]_i$ produced by deoxycholate. Because neither $dmPGE_2$ nor indomethacin affected the $[Ca^{2+}]_i$ of resting cells, it appears that their effect on the deoxycholate injury could be specific. The second exception was a trend towards the preservation of oxygen consumption, again in both the $dmPGE_2$ and the indomethacin treated groups. As neither of these effects was statistically significant, and because the effects were seen in both the $dmPGE_2$ and indomethacin groups, it does not appear likely that the effects seen were biologically significant evidence of a cytoprotective effect of $dmPGE_2$.

Most of the studies demonstrating a protective effect of prostaglandins in the gastric mucosa have used ethanol as the injurious agent. It is apparently easier to demonstrate this effect in alcohol injury than in other forms of injury. One of the few examples of an *in vivo* study demonstrating protection against bile acid-induced injury is Tepperman's report in which 16,16 $dmPGE_2$ protected against histamine release and permeability alterations in the canine oxyntic mucosa [10]. The protective

effect reported in Tepperman's paper provides a rationale for searching for
a protective effect of dmPGE$_2$ against bile salt-induced damage on a cellular
level.

Our failure to find a direct cytoprotective effect of dmPGE$_2$ is in
contrast to a report by Terano et al which describes the protection of
cultured rat gastric cells from taurocholate injury [11]. The analogue,
dosage, and pretreatment regimen were similar in the two studies. The bile
salt and species were different. Most of the experiments demonstrating
cytoprotection have been carried out in rats so the species difference may be
important.

When results are negative as in this study it is important to assess the
quality of the techniques. We cannot rule out the possibility that our study
failed to reveal a protective effect of dmPGE$_2$, but we did assess injury over
a range of concentrations of deoxycholate including the minimally injurious
0.2 mM up to the rather severe 1.0 mM to see if effects could be seen at
either end of the range. We used a variety of indices of injury that assess
very different functions of the cell. We also assessed the removal of
dmPGE$_2$ in the indomethacin experiments. We have shown that the dosing
regimen of indomethacin used reduces arachidonic-stimulated platelet
aggregation by 80% in our rabbit model.

Regarding our measurements of $[Ca^{2+}]_i$ with the FURA 2/AM we
performed significant validation experiments. We demonstrated that neither
deoxycholate nor dmPGE$_2$ in the concentrations used here interfered with
FURA's ability to measure free calcium in calibration experiments without
cells.

Our study is not unique in failing to identify a protective effect of
dmPGE$_2$ in dispersed gastric cells. While Cherner et al showed a protective
effect of 16,16 dmPGE$_2$ against ethanol injury to dispersed chief cells from
the guinea pig stomach [12], Szabo et al reported that neither PGE$_2$ (1 uM -
10mM) nor its analogue 16,16 dmPGE$_2$ protected dispersed rat gastric cells.
In his study, PGE$_2$ failed to protect against ethanol and 16,16 dmPGE$_2$
against HCl- induced injury [13].

The ability of prostaglandins to protect the gastric mucosa of the rat
against ethanol-induced injury is well documented and dramatic. The precise
mechanism of the protection has thus far eluded detection. Our studies fail
to support the contention that PGE$_2$ protects cells by a universal
cytoprotective mechanism and directs attention back towards other
possibilites such as alterations in the microcirculation.

REFERENCES

1.   Robert, A., Nezamis, J.E., Lancaster, C. and Hanchar, A.J.   (1979):
      Gastroenterology, 77:433-443.

2.   Miller, T.A. (1983): Am. J. Physiol., 245:G601-623.

3.   Batzri, S., Harmon, J.W., Walker, M.D., Thompson, W.F. and Toles, R. (1982): Biochim. Biophys. Acta, 720:217-221.

4.   Batzri, S., Harmon, J.W., Dyer, J. and Thompson, W.F. (1982): Mol. Pharmacol., 22:41-47.

5.   Batzri, S., Harmon, J.W. and Thompson, W.F. (1982): Mol. Pharmacol., 22:33-40.

6.   Batzri, S. and Gardner, J.D. (1978): Biochim. Biophys. Acta, 508:328-338.

7.   Grynkiewicz, G., Poenie, M. and Tsien, R.Y. (1985): J. Biol. Chem., 260:3440-3450.

8.   Batzri, S. (1985): Am. J. Physiol., 248:G360-368.

9.   Chew, C.S. and Hersey, S.J. (1982): Am. J. Physiol., 242:G505-512

10. Tepperman, B.L. (1979): Can. J. Physiol. Pharmacol., 57:251-256.

11. Terano, A., Shinichi, O., Mach, T., Hiraishi, H., Stachura, J., Tarnawski, A. and Ivey, K.J. (1986): Gastroenterology, 92:669-677.

12. Cherner, J.A., Naik, L., Tarnawski, A., Brzozowski, T., Stachura, J. and Singh, G. (1989): Am. J. Physiol., 256:G704-714.

13. Szabo, S., Pihan, G., Spill, W.F., Zetter, B.R. (1988):Gastroenterology, 94:A451.

ROLE OF GASTRIC MICROVASCULAR PERFUSION IN MUCOSAL PROTECTION AGAINST ETHANOL INJURY

Gary M. Frydman, Angela G. Penney, Cathy Malcontenti, Paul E. O'Brien

Monash University Department of Surgery, Alfred Hospital, Melbourne, Australia

INTRODUCTION

Virchow first proposed that ischaemia played a central role in the pathogenesis of gastric mucosal disease in 1853 [1]. Recent studies have shown that vascular injury plays a critical role in the pathogenesis of ethanol induced gastric mucosal damage [2-5]. Although both microvascular injury and epithelial cell necrosis occurs rapidly after ethanol injury it appears likely that endothelial cell damage precedes epithelial necrosis. Stasis of blood flow was noted by 49 seconds after exposure to ethanol yet the earliest histological evidence of epithelial cell necrosis was at 2.5 minutes [6]. Szabo et al [4] showed an increase in endothelial leakage and increased monastral blue staining to the damaged endothelium 1 minute after ethanol exposure. Ultrastructural studies have also shown that endothelial damage is evident prior to epithelial cell necrosis [7-9].

Prior administration of various agents, including prostaglandin E_2 (PGE_2) sucralfate (SUC), or colloidal bismuth subcitrate (CBS) have been shown to reduce the extent of deep mucosal necrosis caused by ethanol(10). Despite extensive investigation, the nature of their protective effects still remains unclear. It has been proposed that these agents may protect the gastric microcirculation and preserve gastric mucosal blood flow, thereby significantly limiting epithelial injury. Maintenance of gastric mucosal blood flow permits ongoing delivery of oxygen and nutrients, the clearance of mucosal toxic agents and the stabilization of mucosal acid-base balance [11].

In this study we examine the effects of different concentrations of ethanol (100%, 50%, and 25%) on the rats gastric microvascular structure and we explore the influence of pretreatment by PG, SUC and CBS on the gastric microvascular effects of 100% ethanol.

MATERIALS AND METHODS

Adult male Long Evans rats (weight 200-250 g) were fasted for 24 hours prior to each experiment but allowed free access to water. Each animal was briefly anaesthetized with immersion in 100% CO_2 to allow for instillation of the test or control agent.

PREPARATION OF TEST AGENTS

PGE$_2$ was purchased from Sigma (St. Louis) as a crystalline powder, which was dissolved in absolute ethanol to give a stock solution containing 1 mg/ml PGE$_2$, which was stored at -4°C. Immediately prior to use, the stock solution was diluted with normal saline to a final concentration of 25 ug/ml. Colloidal bismuth subcitrate (CBS) (De-Nol, Parke Davis) was obtained as tablets containing 107.7 mg of bismuth. Each tablet was crushed and dissolved in normal saline to a concentration of 4 mg/ml. Sucralfate (DuPont) was obtained as tablets containing 1g sucralfate. Each tablet was crushed and dissolved in saline to prepare a test solution of 10 mg/ml. All drug solutions were prepared on the day of experiment.

MICROVASCULAR CASTING

Fifteen minutes after instillation of the test agent absolute ethanol was instilled into the rat's stomach in a dose of 0.5 ml/100g rat body weight. Ten minutes later each animal was anaesthetized with methohexitone sodium (Lilly) at a dose of 75 ug/kg by intraperitoneal injection, and the thoracic aorta exposed and cannulated. The casting medium consisted of Mercox CL (Vilene Hospital Inc. & Co. Tokyo), methylmethacrylate (BDH, Poole Inc.) and Mercox NA catalyst was perfused into the animal according to the technique previously described [12]. After the cast had set, the stomach was removed and the tissues dissolved away by immersion in 20% NaOH solution. The casts were then examined under scanning and electron microscope by an observer unaware of the experimental group. At least ten casts were examined for each experimental group.

RESULTS

NORMAL MICROVASCULAR STRUCTURE

The normal microvascular architecture of the rat gastric mucosa has been described previously [12]. In brief, it consists of a capillary network which arises from submucosal arterioles and passes between the gastric glands towards the lumen of the stomach to form a network of capillaries around the necks of the glands beneath the surface epithelial layer (Figure 1). These vessels then drain into infrequent venules which traverse the mucosa without further tributaries, to the submucosal veins.

Study of the microvascular structure of the control group of rats which were not exposed to ethanol consistently showed a generally intact microvascular network with only occasional areas where there was failure to completely fill the superficial capillary loops (Figure 1). No areas of deep loss of patency of the capillaries or of extravasation of the casting material were seen in any of the specimens.

EFFECTS OF 100% ETHANOL

Damage of the gastric microvasculature at 15 minutes after absolute ethanol administration is characterised by the presence of patchy areas of loss of patency of the capillary network, generally extending almost to the submucosal vessels (Figure 2). Extravasation of casting material is frequently seen on the surface of the cast and is commonly seen at the interface between areas of deep loss of patency of the capillaries and areas of relatively normal microvascular cast.

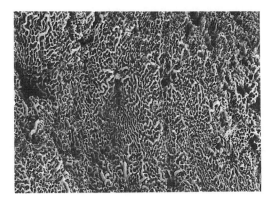

FIGURE 1: *A view of the intact surface capillary network in control rats given saline. Almost all areas show an intact filling of the cast up to the honeycomb capillary loops which surround the gastric glands. Note the presence of some incomplete loops .*

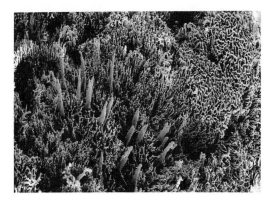

FIGURE 2: *An overview of the luminal aspect of a cast after 100% ethanol damage. Note the patchy appearance of the cast with areas of gross disruption of the normal microvascular architecture. In one area there is deep microvascular damage with complete loss of patency of the mucosal microvessels to the level of the submucosa. Only venules can be seen. However immediately above and to the right of this area there is an area of the cast which shows the normal microvascular structure.*

In the areas which demonstrate deep loss of patency of the capillary network the tufts of capillaries can be seen to arise from submucosal arterioles but no filling occurs beyond these tufts. The submucosal venules do fill presumably by retrograde flow at the level of the submucosa, thus indicating that the abnormality as demonstrated by the cast is confined to the capillary loop between the initial site of origin from the arteriole and the point of drainage into the venule (Figure 2).

MODIFICATION OF ETHANOL DAMAGE BY PGE_2, SUC AND CBS

Pretreatment of the stomach by each of these agents prior to ethanol exposure resulted in virtual absence of areas of deep loss of patency of the capillary network (Figure 3). No difference in the effectiveness was noted between the three agents. Areas of loss of patency of the more superficial capillary loops were again noted as was extravasation of casting material onto the surface of the cast (Figure 4). However, the characteristic focal areas of deep loss of patency of the capillaries seen after exposure to ethanol alone was virtually absent from these casts.

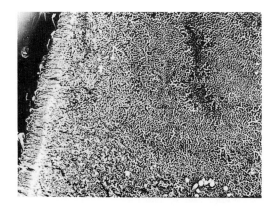

FIGURE 3: *A microvascular cast of the rat mucosa which had been pretreated with PGE_2 followed by exposure to 100% ethanol. The lower right aspect of the cast shows some areas where the surface capillary network is incomplete. There are some small spherical extravastions in the upper field. The remainder of the cast shows an intact appearance. A similar appearance is noted in rats pretreated with CBS or sucralfate prior to ethanol administration.*

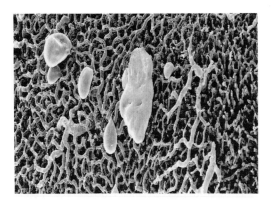

FIGURE 4 *The luminal aspect of the stomach following pretreatment with CBS prior to 100% ethanol. In the centre of the picture leakage of casting material can be seen to be coming from intact superficial capillaries. On the left hand side of the cast an area of loss of patency of the superficial capillary network is noted.*

DISCUSSION

The results of these studies indicate that major changes occur in the gastric microvasculature following ethanol application. The findings of deep deficits in the filling of the microvascular casts as well as extravasation of cast material may correlate with the necrotic lesions seen on histological examination and the obvious mucosal haemorrhage seen macroscopically after ethanol exposure. The presence of cast extravasations appearing at the junction of intact with damaged microvasculature along with the fact that they were noticed only on the surface of an intact capillary network suggests that these changes occur prior to loss of patency of the surface mucosal capillaries. This loss of patency of capillaries may indicate loss of these vessels in association with adjacent tissue loss, closure of the vessels due to thrombosis or loss of flow, compression of the capillary by surrounding tissue or fluid, or constriction of proximal or distal blood vessels. Our technique does not allow us to differentiate between these possible mechanisms. Studies utilising *in-vivo* microscopy have suggested that ethanol causes blood flow stasis due to possible intracapillary thrombosis [3,5,13].

Pretreatment with PGE_2, SUC and CBS clearly protected the microvasculature from ethanol damage. Damage that was present was confined to the more superficial levels of the microvaculature and was less extensive. These findings support the proposal that these agents protect the gastric mucosa by maintaining the integrity of the gastric microvessels thereby preserving mucosal blood flow.

Despite extensive investigation the mechanism by which these agents protect the gastric mucosa is still poorly understood. Robert initially proposed that the primary effect of prostaglandin was to increase the ability of the gastric mucosal cells to withstand toxic injury [14]. Reports that suggest that PGE_2 can protect isolated cell suspensions or isolated mucosa from the damaging effects of ethanol [15-20] would support Robert's initial proposal [14]. It should be noted that in these studies the concentration of ethanol utilized was in the ordder of 10% or less. This concentration of ethanol in other stuudies on the intact animal or on isolated sheets of gastric mucosa has failed to show any toxic properties [21-22]. The relevance of these *in vitro* studies which show protection from prostaglandin to this low concentration of ethanol, to the intact animal studies in which PGE_2 is seen to protect against high concentrations of ethanol remains to be established.

More recently there has been extensive investigation on the role of the gastric microvasculature as a central element in the protective effects of these agents. Many studies have focussed on the potential of various prostaglandins to alter the rate of gastric mucosal blood flow as the most likely measure of their protective effect with the expectation that the greater the increase in gastric mucosal blood flow, the greater the protective effect. This correlation has not been obtained.

The focus on an increase in gastric mucosal blood flow may be inappropriate. Increasing evidence suggests that these protective agents may mediate a protective effect on the gastric mucosa by maintaining normal rates of gastric mucosal blood flow in the face of toxic irritants rather than causing an increase in the rate of gastric mucosal blood flow.

Application of ethanol and aspirin to the stomach have been shown to cause cessation of gastric mucosal blood flow [2-3,5-6]. This microcirculatory stasis can be seen to precede cellular necrosis [6]. Utilising both in-vivo microscopy and laser doppler flowmetry, pretreatment with PGE_2, prior to ethanol injury, caused preservation of gastric mucosal perfusion [5]. Using microspheres [23] and hydrogen gas clearance [24], others support these findings of maintenance of gastric mucosal blood flow in the face of luminal irritants.

Similarly, Chen et al [25] demonstrated that SUC was able to maintain integrity of the gastric mucosal perfusion following ethanol insult using both laser doppler flowmetry and hydrogen gas clearance. In other studies, SUC pretreatment has been shown to be associated with a marked reduction in loss of albumin [26] and haemoglobin [27] in association with ethanol injury. Similar findings have been described for CBS [28].

In the present studies we have shown that the gastric microvasculature suffers patchy severe damage with deep loss of patency of the capillary network down to the level of the submucosa. Pretreatment with the protective agents PGE_2, CBS, and SUC was able to protect the gastric microvasculature from deep capillary loss, with loss of patency of superficial capillaries only. These studies therefore give further support to the proposal that, in the absence of PGE_2 or other protective agents, exposure of the gastric mucosa to an irritant leads to endothelial cell damage, followed by cessation of microvascular perfusion and as a consequence a reduction in the capacity of the gastric epithelial cells to resist direct toxic damage. Although PGE_2, SUC and CBS are capable of augmenting other components of gastric mucosal defence, we propose that the primary action of the protective agent is the prevention of endothelial cell damage. The preservation of microvascular flow allows ongoing delivery of oxygen and nutrients as well as a conduit for the removal of intra-gastric toxins thereby providing a relative increase in the capacity of the epithelium to resist damage.

ACKNOWLEDGEMENT

This study was supported by a Grant from the
National Health and Medical Research Council of Australia

REFERENCES

1.   Virchow, R, Historiches, kritisches und positives Lehre der Unterleibsaffektionen. Archiv fur pathologische Anatomie, 1853; 5: 281-387.

2.   Trier JS, Szabo S, Allan CH. Ethanol-induced damage to mucosal capillaries of rat stomach. Gastroenterology 1987; 92: 13-22.

3.   Guth PH, Paulsen G, Nagata H. Histologic and microcirculatory changes in alcohol-induced gastric lesions in the rat: effect of prostaglandin cytoprotection. Gastroenterology 1984; 87: 1083-1091.

4.   Szabo S, Trier JS, Brown A, Schnoor J. Early vascular injury and increased vascular permeability in gastric mucosal injury caused by ethanol in the rat. Gastroenterology 1985; 88: 228-36.

5.   Pihan G, Majzoubi D, Haudenschild C, Trier J, Szabo S. Early microcirculatory stasis in acute gastric mucosal injury in the rat and prevention by 16,16-dimethyl prostaglandin E_2 or sodium thiosulfate. Gastroenterology 1986; 91: 1415-1426.

6.   Bou-abboud C, Wayland H, Paulsen G, Guth P. Microcirculatory stasis precedes tissue necrosis in ethanol induced gastric mucosal injury in the rat. Dig Dis Sci 1988;33:872-877.

7.   Tarnawski A, Hollander D, Stachura J. Ultrastructural changes in the gastric mucosal microvessels after ethanol. Gastoenterol Clin Biol 1985; 9: 93-97.

8.   Tarnawski A, Stachura J, Hollander D, Sareh IJ, Bogdal J. Cellular aspects of alcohol-induced injury and protection of the human gastric mucosa. Focus on mucosal microvessels. J Clin Gastroenterol 1988; 10: S35-S45.

9.   Tarnawski A, Stachura J, Gergely H, Hollander D. Microvascular
Endothelium - A major target for alcohol injury of the human gastric
mucosa. Histochemical and ultrastructural study. J Clin Gastroenterol
1988; 10: S53-S64.

10.   O'Brien PE, Frydman GM, Holmes R, Malcontenti C, Phelan D.
Evaluation of putative cytoprotective properties of anti-ulcer drugs
using quantitative histological techniques. Dig Dis Sci 95: In Press,
1990.

11.   Frykland J, Helander HF, Elander B, Wallmark B. Function and
structure of parietal cells after H+-K+ ATP-ase blockade. Am J
Physiol 1988;254:G399-G407.

12.   Gannon B, Browning J, O'Brien P. The microvascular architecture of
the glandular mucosa of the stomach. J Anat 1982; 135: 667-683.

13.   Oates PJ, Hakkinen JP. Studies on the mechanism of ethanol-induced
gastric damage in rats. Gastroenterology 1988; 94: 10-21.

14.   Robert A, Nezamis JE, Lancaster C, Hanchar AJ. Cytoprotection by
Prostaglandins in Rats. Prevention of gastric necrosis produced by
alcohol, HCl, NaOH, hypertonic NaCl, and thermal injury.
Gastroenterology 1979; 77: 433-443.

15.   Sewell RB, Ling TS, Yeomans ND. Ethanol-induced cell damage in
cultured rat antral mucosa assessed by chromium-51 release. Dig Dis
Sci 1986; 31: 853-858.

16.   Terano A, Mach T, Stachura J, Tarnawski A, Ivey KJ. Effect of 16,16
dimethyl prostaglandin E_2 on aspirin induced damage to rat gastric
epithelial cells in tissue culture. Gut 1984; 25: 19-25.

17.   Cherner JA, Naik L, Tarnawski A, Brzozowski T, Stachura J, Singh
G. Ability of prostaglandin to reduce ethanol injury to dispersed
chief cells from guinea pig stomach. Am J Physiol 1989;256: G704-
G714.

18.   Tarnawski A, Brzozowski T, Sarfeh IJ, Krause WJ, Ulich TR, Gergely
H, Hollander D. Prostaglandin protection of human isolated gastric
glands against indomethacin and ethanol injury. J Clin Invest 1988;
81: 1081-1089.

19.   Terano A, Shiga J, Hiraishi H, Ota S, Sugimoto T. Protective action
of tetraprenylacetone against ethanol-induced damage in rat gastric
mucosa. Digestion 1986; 35: 182-188.

20.   Arakawa T, Fukuda T, Kobayashi K. Protection of isolated rat
gastric cells by prostaglandins from damage caused by ethanol. J Clin
Gastroenterol 1988;10: 528-534.

21.   Eastwood GL, Kirchner JP. Changes in the fine structure of mouse
      gastric epithelium produced by ethanol and urea. Gastroenterology
      1974; 67: 71-84.

22.   Dinoso VP, Ming SC, McNiff J. Ultrastructural changes of the the
      canine gastric mucosa after topical application of graded
      concentrations of ethanol. Am J Dig Dis 1976; 21: 626-632.

23.   Gaskill HV, Sirinek KR, Levine BA. Prostacyclin-mediated gastric
      cytoprotection is dependent on mucosal blood flow. Surgery 1982; 92:
      220-225.

24.   Arakawa T, Nakamura H, Chono S, Satoh H, Fukuda T, Saeki Y,
      Kobayashi K. Absence of effect of 16,16-dimethyl prostaglandin E_2
      on reduction of gastric mucosal blood flow caused by indomethacin
      in rats. Dig Dis Sci 1989; 34: 1369-1373.

25.   Chen BW, Hiu WM, Lam SK, Cho CH, Ng MMT, Luk CT. Effect of
      sucralfate on gastric mucosal blood flow in rats. Gut 1989; 30: 1544-
      1551.

26.   Nagashima S, Hoshino E, Hinohara Y, Sakai K, Hata S, Nakano H.
      Effect of sucralfate on ethanol induced gastric mucosal damage in
      the rat. Scand J Gastroenterol 1983; 18 Suppl 83: 17-20.

27.   Tarnawski A, Hollander D, Gergely H, Stachura J. Comparison of
      antacid, sucralfate, cimetidine, and ranitidine in protection of the
      gastric mucosa against ethanol injury. Am J Med 1985; 79 Suppl2C:
      19-23.

28.   Konturek SJ, Kwiecien N, Obtulowicz W, Hebzda Z. Olesky J. Effects
      of colloidal bismuth subcitrate on aspirin-induced gastric
      microbleeding, DNA loss, and prostaglandin formation in humans.
      Scand J Gastroenterol 1988; 23: 861-866.

ROLE OF AMBIENT Cl⁻ IN THE ELECTROPHYSIOLOGIC RESPONSE OF AMPHIBIAN GASTRIC MUCOSA TO INJURY

J.B. Matthews and A. Garner

Department of Surgery, Beth Israel Hospital, Boston, USA.
Department of Biochemistry, University College of Wales, Aberystwyth, U.K.

ABSTRACT

The gastric mucosa appears to have minimal H^+ conduction pathways in either Cl^- containing or Cl^- free solutions when observed electrical changes are corrected for liquid junction potentials. The electrophysiologic response to anoxia plus acidosis differs from the response to anoxia alone; anoxia plus acidosis results in a striking discontinuity in both the PD and R traces termed the sudden potential drop (SPD). This event depends on the presence of Cl^- in the bathing media and is independent of luminal pH. The absence of Cl^- in the bathing media appeared to extend the tolerance of the mucosa to 90% N_2-10% CO_2 gassing, as measured by the degree of recovery of the electrical parameters. Complex effects on Cl^- permeability and Cl^- transport largely account for the observed electrophysiological response of amphibian gastric mucosa to anoxia and acidosis, and the absence of ambient Cl^- under these conditions may protect the epithelial cells by preventing the development of cell edema.

INTRODUCTION

Vertebrate gastric mucosa possesses a remarkable but still incompletely understood ability to withstand the corrosive actions of its own digestive secretions and maintain a million-fold proton gradient in the steady-state. Unlike gallbladder or small intestine, the gastric mucosa is a relatively tight epithelium, with an electrical resistance (R) of approximately 100-600 ohms-cm² depending on the acid secretory state [1]. The paracellular shunt pathway contributes approximately 20% to the total conductance of fundic mucosa [2]. Active transport, particularly of Cl^-, generates a sizeable potential difference (PD) with the luminal side negative with respect to the serosal side. In mammals there is a small but significant contribution of active Na^+ absorption to the PD [3].

Conditions which disrupt the gastric mucosal "barrier" to H^+ back-diffusion typically result in a marked decrease or elimination of the transmucosal PD. However, a fall in PD may also be observed under a variety of conditions which do not appear to damage the surface epithelial cells, and therefore the use of the PD as a measure of the function or integrity of the barrier must be discouraged [4,5]. Extensive damage to the

81

epithelial cells and tight junction complexes (such as by 1 M NaCl or absolute ethanol) causes a loss of ionic permselectivity and an increase in shunt conductance, which manifests as a precipitous fall in R in addition to a sharp drop in PD [6,7].   While the combined use of both PD and R to assess barrier function is probably preferable than the use of either parameter alone, interpretation of results is not always straightforward. For example, stimulation of amphibian gastric mucosa by histamine or forskolin is in no way injurious to the tissue, yet causes a fall in PD and a prominent decrease in R to the range characteristic of leaky epithelia [4].   This effect is related to the large increase in apical membrane area of oxynticopeptic cells that accompanies the transition from resting to stimulated state [8].

Cl⁻ is the central ionic moiety in the generation of the gastric mucosal PD. We have recently re-examined the role of ambient Cl⁻ in the electrophysiologic response to luminal acidification and anoxia.

METHODS

Stomachs from doubly-pithed bullfrogs (*Rana catesbeiana*) were removed, opened along the lesser curvature, stripped of their external muscle layers, and mounted as mucosal sheets in conventional lucite Ussing-style chambers.   Luminal (L) and nutrient (N) bathing solutions were circulated in a gas-lift apparatus with 95% O_2-5% CO_2.   The compositions of standard and Cl⁻ free L and N appear in Table 1.   Cimetidine 10^{-3} M was added to N. Paired halves of fundic tissue were used unless otherwise noted; antrum was distinguished by its generally paler appearance and lack of mucosal folds.

Transmucosal PD was continuously monitored via 4M KCl agar electrodes connected to a voltage/current clamp and chart recorder. Transepithelial R was calculated from the change in PD after a 1 second pulse of 25 uA delivered across the tissue by an additional two electrodes. Correction was made for the fluid resistance (approximately 45 ohms-cm^2) measured for each experiment.

Luminal acidification was accomplished by manually adding a small aliquot of either 1N HCl for Cl⁻ containing solutions or 1N H_2SO_4 for Cl⁻ free conditions.   A saturated KCl glass electrode was used for pH measurements. The liquid junctional potential which developed when the luminal solution was rapidly acidified from pH 5 to pH 2 was estimated by the change in PD after acidification of the luminal-side compartment using a porous paraffin membrane rather than tissue separating the chamber halves.

RESULTS AND DISCUSSION

Traditional models of gastric mucosal injury depict H⁺ back-diffusion as an initiating or at least a damage-promoting process [5]. Since the conditions which cause an increased loss of luminal H⁺ into the tissue are often accompanied by deterioration of electrical parameters, an interrelationship between the electrophysiologic properties of the stomach and the ability to withstand autodigestion has long been postulated.

TABLE 1

COMPOSITION OF SOLUTIONS

	Nutrient, mM		Luminal, mM	
	Standard	Isethionate	Standard	Isethionate
Na^+	102.4	102.4	102.4	102.4
K^+	4.0	4.0	4.0	4.0
Mg^{2+}	0.8	0.8	0.8	0.8
Ca^{2+}	1.8	1.0	1.8	1.0
Cl^-	91.4		91.4	
Isethionate		83.3		100.4
HCO_3^-	17.8	17.8		
$H_2PO_4^-$	0.8	0.8		
SO_4^{2-}	0.8	3.8	10.1	3.8
TES				
Mannitol		5.4	19.3	17.4
Glucose	10.0	10.0		
Osmolarity (mosM)	229.8	229.8	229.8	229.8

However, the mechanism of H^+ movement across the normal and damaged gastric epithelium remains obscure; in fact, the details of proton flux across simple lipid bilayers are controversial [9]. Net H^+ movement across artificial membranes may be influenced in part by the permeability of the counter-ion species, since bulk electroneutrality must be maintained; for example, in one study, it was observed that dissipation of pH gradients in a lipid vesicle model was enhanced by the K^+ ionophore valinomycin and retarded by the presence of an impermeant anion [10].

As measured by luminal ion substitution, Cl⁻ appears to be the major conductive species across the apical aspect of gastric mucosa. Changes in luminal (Na^+) and (K^+) are without effect on the transmucosal PD, whereas, in our experiments, luminal anion substitution showed the selectivity pattern $Br^- > Cl^- > NO_3^- >$ isethionate = HCO_3^-. In Cl⁻ containing media buffered by HCO_3^-/CO_2 in the nutrient bath, changes in luminal pH from 5 to 2 resulted in minimal change in PD, similar in magnitude to the liquid junction potential for these conditions [11]. Since H^+ back diffusion has been postulated to be coupled in some fashion to Cl⁻ flux in the direction L to N [12], we tested whether an H^+ conductance could be uncovered in Cl⁻ free media. In cimetidine-treated fundic tissue, rapid titration of luminal pH from 5 to 2 with H_2SO_4 in isethionate media caused a marked hyperpolarization of the PD by 8.3 ± 0.7 mV (n=5), in the direction consistent with an H^+ diffusion potential. However, the liquid junction potential measured in isethionate media was approximately 8mV and therefore completely accounted for the observed change in PD. No major proton conductive pathways were therefore detectable. This observation is consistent with data from chief cell monolayers which suggest that apical membrane permeability to H^+ is low [13]. In our experiments, at higher luminal acidity (pH < 1) many tissues showed an irreversible decrease in PD after an initial hyperpolarization accompanied by a fall in R, implying tissue damage.

Stress ulceration in critically ill patients is often associated with gastric mucosal ischemia and systemic acidosis and is usually preventable if gastric acidity is controlled [14]. The effects of ischemia on the *in vitro* amphibian gastric mucosa are complex and appear to be influenced by the presence of tissue acidosis. Kidder observed that the electrophysiologic response of chambered amphibian gastric mucosa to anoxia differed strikingly if induced with 90% N_2-10% CO_2 rather than 95% N_2-5% CO_2 or 100% N_2 [15]. Under the latter gassing conditions the PD was observed to decline steadily toward zero as R increased, whereas with 90% N_2-10% CO_2 the slowly declining PD trace was interrupted at approximately -10 mV by a sudden, precipitous fall to near-zero accompanied by a rapid decrease in R.

This event has been termed the "sudden potential drop" (SPD) and generally occurred 10-20 minutes into the anoxic period.

We further explored this unusual electrical response and found it could be produced with either 95% N_2-5% CO_2 or 100% N_2 gassing provided that the nutrient pH was made less than approximately 7.2 by lowering nutrient (HCO_3^-)[16]. We and others [12] have also observed an "aerobic" SPD response with TES or HEPES as the nutrient buffer species and nutrient pH was titrated to less than 7.0. The SPD response did not occur in antrum, suggesting a requirement for oxynticopeptic cells. One of the more interesting aspects of the SPD was that, although the event was characterized by a rapid fall in PD and R, there appeared to be no obvious accompanying tissue damage at either the light or electron microscopic level, and the electrical parameters were rapidly reversible upon restoration of control conditions [17]. This reversibility distinguishes the SPD from conditions which cause a rapid decrease in PD and R by virtue of epithelial damage [7].

In the present study, the SPD response to 90% N_2-10% CO_2 appeared similar in tissues exposed to either luminal pH 2 or luminal pH 5, and, immediately following the SPD, reoxygenation of tissue at both luminal pH values resulted in a return to near-baseline levels of PD and R (n=4). After a longer period of anoxia (30 minutes), PD and R only partially recovered, and after 60 minutes the PD remained zero and R remained low despite 2 hours of reoxygenation (n=5). At luminal pH 1, the SPD response was irreversible, and a permanent absence of acid secretory capacity has been measured [18]. Kidder has measured an augmented voltage response to changes in luminal pH following the SPD [18], but when correction was made for liquid junction potentials, we could not confirm this in our experiments.

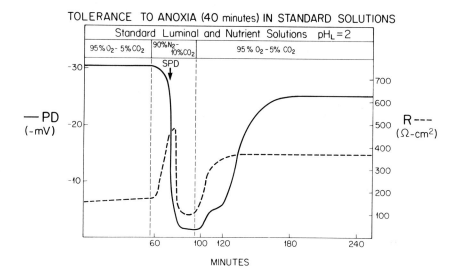

TOLERANCE TO ANOXIA (40 minutes) IN STANDARD SOLUTIONS

Figure 1: *Sudden potential drop (SPD) produced in cimetidine treated fundus exposed to 90% N2-10% CO₂. After 40 minutes of anoxia, the PD and R changes are partially reversible.*

    Although the SPD occurs when either Na^+ or K^+ are absent from the bathing media, the response is prevented by replacement of Cl^- with SO_4^{-2} [19], acetate, or isethionate but not NO_3^- [16]. In fact, the SPD will not occur with substitution for luminal Cl- alone.

    The voltage change produced by luminal Cl^- substitution was found to be markedly increased following the SPD, leading us to speculate that the response reflected an increased Cl^- permeability across the apical membrane. However, the transmucosal flux of ^{36}Cl was noted to be markedly <u>decreased</u> after the SPD response and the voltage change produced by <u>nutrient</u> Cl^- substitution was nearly eliminated after the SPD [15], suggesting that movement of Cl^- across the basolateral membrane was somehow restricted despite the apparent increased apical anion permeability. These observations are similar to those seen in inhibited tissues bathed in HCO_3^- free media [20]. An increased permeability to Cl^- across the apical membrane alone does not entirely explain the electrical phenomenon, since the transmucosal PD and R response requires charge to be carried across the basolateral membrane as well. The identity of the charge-carrying species for the basolateral membrane is unknown, and an effect on shunt conductance has not been conclusively excluded.

Preservation solutions used clinically for organ transplantation are designed to extend the tolerance of a harvested organ to prolonged periods of ischemia. A notable characteristic of the composition of University of Wisconsin preservation solution is the substitution of lactobionate for Cl^-; theoretically, the use of this large impermeant anionic species retards the development of intracellular edema which follows the inhibition of active ion pumps [21]. By analogy, we wondered if the use of Cl^- free solutions would extend the tolerance of *in vitro* fundus to ischemia, as measured by the reversibility of the electrophysiologic parameters. Indeed, the electrical parameters were completely reversible after 60 minutes exposure to 90% N_2 10% CO_2 for tissues bathed in Cl^- free media (n=4) but were irreversible in Cl^- containing media (n=6) (Figures 2 and 3).

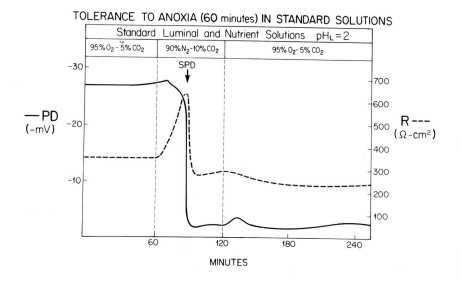

FIGURE 2:   *Sixty-minute exposure to 90% N_2-10% CO_2 in Cl^- containing media with luminal pH = 2. An SPD response is observed. After reoxygenation, there is no recovery of PD or R despite 2 hours of observation.*

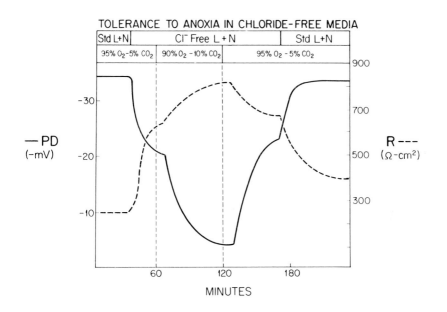

FIGURE 3: *Sixty-minute exposure to 90% N_2-10% CO_2 in Cl⁻ free media with luminal pH = 2. No SPD is observed. After reoxygenation, there is a rapid recovery of electrical parameters, and return to Cl⁻ containing solutions restores baseline PD and R.*

These results held for tissues exposed to either luminal pH 2 or pH 5. The tissues bathed in Cl⁻ containing solutions demonstrated the SPD response, which was always absent under Cl⁻ free conditions. There is, however, insufficient data as yet to relate the occurrence of the SPD itself to the ability of the mucosa to tolerate anoxia and acidosis. Removal of ambient Cl⁻ significantly altered the electrophysiologic response to anoxia and acidosis and appeared to prolong the tolerance of the epithelium to these conditions. One may speculate that ischemia causes a loss of volume regulatory capacity which leads, in the presence of a permeant anionic species, to the development of intracellular edema, followed ultimately by cell death.

REFERENCES

1.   Fromter E, Diamond JM.   Route of passive ion permeation in
      epithelia. Nature. 1972; 235: 9-12.

2.   Spenney JG, Shoemaker RL, Sachs G.   Microelectrode studies in
      fundic mucosa. J Membrane Biol. 1974; 19: 105-128.

3.   Machen TE, Silen W, Forte JG.   Na$^+$ transport by mammalian
      stomach. Am J Physiol. 1978; 234: E228-W235.

4.   Silen W. Gastric mucosal defense and repair.   In: Physiology of the
      Gastrointestinal Tract. 2nd Ed.   Johnson LR (ed).   Raven Press, New
      York 1987; 1055-1069.

5.   Thjodleifsson B, Wormsley KG.   Back-diffusion - fact or fiction?
      Digestion 1977; 15: 53-72.

6.   Dawson DC, Cooke AR.   Parallel pathways for ion transport across
      rat gastric mucosa: effect of ethanol. Am J Physiol 1978; 235:E7-E15.

7.   Svanes K, Ito S, Takeuchi K, Silen W.   Restitution of the surface
      epithelium of the *in vitro* frog gastric mucosa after damage with
      hyperosmolar sodium chloride. Gastroenterology 1982; 82: 1409-26.

8.   Clausen C, Machen TE, Diamond JM.   Use of AC impedance analysis
      to study membrane changes related to acid secretion in amphibian
      gastric mucosa. Biophys J. 1983; 41: 167-178.

9.   Gutknecht J.   Proton/hydroxide conductance through lipid bilayer
      membranes. J Membrane Biol. 1984; 82: 105-112.

10.   Barreto JC, Lichtenberger LM.   The gastric mucosal barrier need not
      be impermeable to protons. Gastroenterology 1988; 94: 610.

11.   Barry PH, Diamond JM.   Junction potentials, electrode standard
      potentials, and other problems of interpreting electrical properties of
      membranes. J Membrane Biol. 1970; 3: 93-122.

12.   Durbin RP.   Back-diffusion of H$^+$ in isolated frog gastric mucosa.
      Am J Physiol. 1984; 246: G114-119.

13.   Sanders MJ, Ayalon A, Roll M, Soll AH.   The apical surface of
      canine chief cell monolayers resists H$^+$ back-diffusion. Nature 1985;
      313: 52-54.

14.   Priebe JH, Skillman JJ. Bushell LS, et al.   Antacid versus cimetidine
      in preventing acute gastrointestinal bleeding. N Engl J Med. 1980;
      302: 426-430.

15.   Kidder GW, Montgomery CW.   The sudden potential drop in frog
      gastric mucosa.   Am J Physiol. 1976; 230: 61-66.

16.   Matthews JB, Rangachari PK, Rowe PH, et al.   Characteristics of sudden potential drop in bullfrog gastric mucosa.   Am. J Physiol. 1985; 248: G587-593.

17.   Matthews JB, Ito S, Silen W.   Further studies on the mechanisms of the sudden potential drop in frog gastric mucosa. In: Hydrogen Ion Transport in Epithelia. Forte J (ed). John Wiley & Sons 1984:379-87.

18.   Kidder FW.   Further studies on the sudden potential drop, and a model for stress ulcer etiology.   In: Hydrogen Ion Transport in Epithelia. Schulz I, et al. (eds).   Elsevier Press. 1980; 217-224.

19.   Kidder GW.   Ionic conditions for the sudden potential drop in frog gastric mucosa. In: Gastric Hydrogen Ion Secretion. Kasebekar DK, et al (eds).   Dekkar, New York 1976; 54-74.

20.   Manning EC, Machen TE.   Effects of bicarbonate and pH on chloride transport by gastric mucosa.   Am J Physiol. 1983; 243: G60-68.

21.   Belzer FO, Southard JH.   Principles of solid organ preservation by cold storage.   Transplantation   1988; 45: 673-676.

THE RELATIONSHIP BETWEEN ALKALINE SECRETION AND MUCOSAL PERMEABILITY IN DUODENUM

Olof Nylander and Manaf Sababi

*Department of Physiology and Medical Biophysics,
Biomedical Center, Uppsala University, Sweden*

ABSTRACT

A 3cm segment of proximal duodenum was perfused with saline and the relationship between alkaline secretion and mucosal permeability studied under various experimental conditions in anaesthetized rats. Mucosal permeability was assessed by measuring the clearance of ^{51}Cr-EDTA from blood to lumen and the rate of luminal alkalinization was determined by back titration. Intravenous infusion of vasoactive intestinal peptide (13.5ug/kg/h for 60 min) induced a 2.7-fold increase in luminal alkalinization and a 50% decrease in mucosal permeability. Indomethacin induced a marked increase (160%) in alkalinization and 60 min after the injection, alkalinization was still 50% above basal. Perfusion of duodenum with either 50 or 100 mM hydrochloric acid for 5 min increased mucosal permeability threefold and fourfold, respectively. 50 min after cessation of perfusion with 100 mM hydrochloric acid, mucosal permeability was 2.6-fold higher than the pre-acid control. Hydrochloric acid increased luminal alkalinization by about 30-50%. It is concluded that no causal relationship exists between luminal alkalinization and mucosal permeability indicating that the transepithelial movement of ^{51}Cr-EDTA and HCO_3^- does not necessarily occur through the same "pore". The hydrochloric acid-induced stimulation of luminal alkalinization may, however, be due to an increased paracellular permeability of HCO_3^-. Brief exposure of rat duodenum to hydrochloric acid at a concentration of 50 mM or higher affects mucosal integrity.

INTRODUCTION

Ovesen et al [1] have recently shown that patients with pancreatic insufficiency have about the same capability to neutralize hydrochloric acid emptied from the stomach as healthy volunteers. This indicates that the duodenal mucosa possesses a remarkable capability to neutralize excessive amounts of H+ in the luminal fluid. It has been suggested that HCO_3^-, secreted by the surface epithelial cell, together with the mucus layer constitute an acid-neutralizing layer that protects the duodenal mucosa against H^+ attack [2]. A growing body of evidence indicates that the rate of alkaline secretion is under the influence of several physiological control mechanisms [2-8]. In a recent study [9] it was shown that basal luminal alkalinization was 4 to 5 times higher in duodenum than in jejunum.

A similar difference was noted between the segments with regard to basal mucosal permeability, duodenum being higher. It is thus possible that the difference in the rate of alkalinization between the segments simply reflects differences in mucosal permeability. The objective of the present investigation was to study the relationship between alkaline secretion and mucosal permeability in duodenum during various experimental conditions. This was accomplished by modifying the rate of luminal alkalinization by using agents that increase (vasoactive intestinal peptide and hydrochloric acid) or inhibit (indomethacin) alkaline secretion. The rate of luminal alkalinization was determined by back titration of the effluent and mucosal permeability was assessed by measuring the clearance of ^{51}Cr-EDTA from blood to duodenal lumen.

MATERIALS AND METHODS

SURGICAL PROCEDURE.

The surgical procedure for perfusion of rat duodenum was the same as previously described by Nylander et al. [9]　Briefly, Sprague Dawley male rats (ALAB, Sollentuna, Sweden) weighing 250 to 400 grams were used. The rats were fasted for 16-18 hours before anaesthesia but had free access to drinking water.　The animals were anaesthetized with 120 mg/kg bodyweight Na-5-ethyl-1-(1'-methyl-propyl)-2-thiobarbituric acid (Inactin^R) injected intraperitoneally.　A tracheotomy was performed and the right femoral vein and femoral artery were catheterized with PE-50 polyethylene tubing.　The vein was used for infusion of drugs and the arterial catheter was connected to a pressure transducer and a Grass Polyrecorder to monitor arterial blood pressure and for blood withdrawals during the experiment.　A laparotomy was performed and both renal pedicles ligated to prevent excretion of ^{51}Cr-EDTA in the urine.　The common bile duct was catheterized with a PE 10 polyethylene tubing close to its entrance into duodenum to avoid pancreaticobiliary secretions from entering the duodenal segment under study.　A soft plastic tubing was introduced into the mouth and pushed along the esophagus into the stomach and through the pylorus. The cannula was secured by two ligatures 2-4 mm distal to the pylorus. Another cannula (PE 320) was inserted into duodenum about 3 cm distal to the pylorus and secured by ligatures.　The proximal duodenal cannula was connected to a peristaltic pump (Gilson minipuls) and the segment continuously perfused with isotonic sodium chloride (saline).

MEASUREMENT OF LUMINAL ALKALINIZATION

The rate of luminal alkalinization was determined by titration of the effluent to pH 6.00 with 50 mM HCl under continuous gassing (100% N_2) using a Radiometer pH-stat equipment (Autoburette ABU 12, TTT 80 Titrator and PHM 64 pH meter, Radiometer, Copenhagen, Denmark).　The pH electrode (Gk 2321C) was routinely calibrated with standard buffers (pH 6.00 and 1.00) before the start of the titration.　The rate of luminal alkalinization was expressed as the amount (microequivalents) of base secreted per cm intestine per hour.

MEASUREMENT OF MUCOSAL PERMEABILITY

Immediately following surgery, 75 uCi of ^{51}Cr-EDTA diluted in saline was injected intravenously. After a one hour equilibration period, the first blood sample was taken (0.25 ml) and 5 min later the experiment started. The duodenal segment was perfused with either saline (150 mM NaCl) or two different concentrations of hydrochloric acid at a rate of 0.5 ml/min. The effluent was collected in vials and these were exchanged every 5 or 10 minutes. The second blood sample was taken immediately after termination of the experiment. The blood volume loss due to blood sampling was compensated for by injection of 0.3 ml of a Ficoll solution (5%). After centrifugation of the blood samples, a volume of 50-100 ul of plasma was taken. A 1 ml sample of the luminal perfusate and the plasma samples were analysed for ^{51}Cr-EDTA activity in a gamma counter. The clearance of ^{51}Cr-EDTA from blood to lumen was calculated according to the following formula:

^{51}Cr-EDTA clearance =

$$\frac{\text{perfusate cpm/ml x perfusion rate ml/min x 100}}{\text{Plasma cpm/ml x tissue weight}}$$

The ^{51}Cr-EDTA clearance is expressed as ml/min/100gm wet tissue weight.

EXPERIMENTAL PROTOCOL

In the first series of experiments the effects of intravenous infusion of vasoactive intestinal peptide (VIP) on ^{51}Cr-EDTA clearance and luminal alkalinization were examined. After a 30 min control period VIP was continuously infused at a dose of 13.5 ug/kg/h for 1 hour. The experiment was terminated 60 min after cessation of the VIP-infusion. In another series of experiments the duodenum was perfused with saline for a total time of 80 min. Indomethacin was injected intravenously as a bolus dose of 1.6 mg/kg 20 min after the onset of saline perfusion. The effects on ^{51}Cr-EDTA clearance and luminal alkalinization were determined.

In the third and fourth series of experiments, the duodenum was perfused with saline for 40 min and then by either 50 mM or 100 mM hydrochloric acid for 5 min. This was followed by another saline perfusion period of 50 min. ^{51}Cr-EDTA clearance and the rate of luminal alkalinization were determined.

CHEMICALS

Na-5-ethyl-1-(1'-methyl-propyl)-2-thiobarbituric acid (Inactin^R) was obtained from Byk-Gulden, Konstantz, FRG. Bovine albumin, vasoactive intestinal peptide, Ficoll (type 400) and NaCl were all purchased from Sigma Chemical Co., St. Louis, MO, USA. Indomethacin (Confortid^R for injection) was obtained from Dumex Co., Copenhagen, Denmark, and heparin from KabiVitrum, Stockholm, Sweden. ^{51}Cr-EDTA was purchased from Du Pont, Wilmington, LE, US. Saline solution was made fresh every day with Millipore water. The HCl containing solutions (50 and 100mM) were made from a stock solution of 1 M HCl (Titrisol^R, E. Merck, FRG) and adjusted to isotonicity by the addition of NaCl.

<u>STATISTICS</u>

Values are expressed as means $\pm$ SE. The statistical significance of data was tested by using Student's t-test for paired samples comparing results obtained during the saline perfusion (control) period with those during or after the infusion of VIP, injection of indomethacin or luminal perfusion of HCl. Comparison of differences between groups of animals was performed by using Student's t-test for unpaired samples. A P value of < 0.05 was considered significant (two-tailed test).

RESULTS

<u>EFFECTS OF VASOACTIVE INTESTINAL PEPTIDE</u>

Spontaneous luminal alkalinization was about $9u$Eq/cm/h. Continuous intravenous infusion of VIP increased the rate of luminal alkalinization markedly (2.7-fold) and a steady state rate of secretion was attained 40 min after the onset of infusion (Figure 1). After cessation of the VIP-infusion the rate of luminal alkalinization decreased to the basal level. ^{51}Cr-EDTA clearance remained fairly stable during the control period preceding the VIP-infusion. A gradual decrease in ^{51}Cr-EDTA clearance occurred in response to the VIP-infusion and one hour after the onset of infusion the decrease in mucosal permeability was 50% (P<0.01).

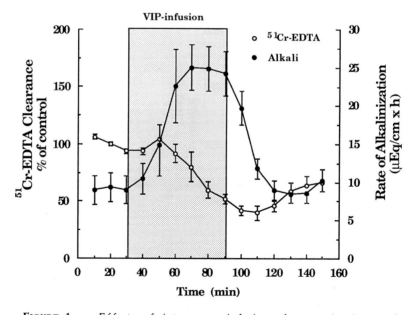

<u>FIGURE 1.</u>   *Effects of intravenous infusion of vasoactive intestinal peptide (VIP) on* ^{51}Cr-EDTA *clearance (o) and luminal alkalinization (o). VIP; was infused at a rate of 13.5ug/kg/h for 60 min. Values are means $\pm$ SE, n = 6-8.*

<u>EFFECTS OF INDOMETHACIN</u>

A bolus injection of indomethacin at a dose of 1.6 mg/kg induced an immediate increase in ^{51}Cr-EDTA clearance (Figure 2). This increase was followed by a gradual decrease and 60 min after the injection ^{51}Cr-EDTA clearance was about 45% below that in the preceding control (P<0.05). Unexpectedly, indomethacin induced a marked increase in the rate of luminal alkalinization. The rate of luminal alkalinization attained its maximal value (160% above basal, P<0.02) 20 min after the bolus injection. One hour after the administration of indomethacin the rate of luminal alkalinization was still 50% higher (P<0.05) than before the injection of the drug.

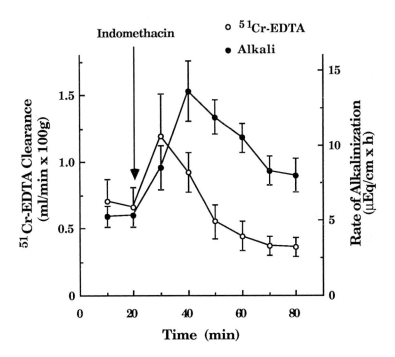

<u>FIGURE 2.</u> *Effects of indomethacin on* ^{51}Cr-EDTA *clearance (o) and luminal alkalinization (o). Indomethacin was administered as a bolus dose of 1.6 mg/kg. Values are means ± SE, n = 6.*

EFFECTS OF LUMINAL PERFUSION WITH HYDROCHLORIC ACID

Luminal perfusion of duodenum with 50 mM HCl for 5 min increased ^{51}Cr-EDTA clearance in all six experiments (Figure 3). 50 min after cessation of the acid perfusion the ^{51}Cr-EDTA clearance was not statistically different from pre-acid control.

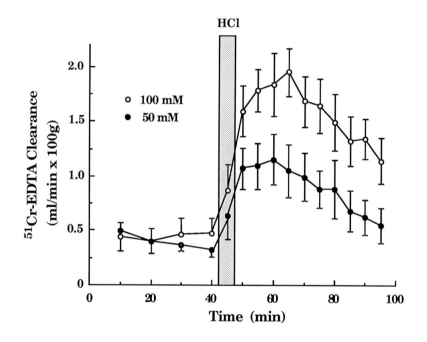

FIGURE 3. *Effects of luminal perfusion of duodenum for 5 min with 50 mM (o) or 100 mM (i) hydrochloric acid (HCl) on* ^{51}Cr-EDTA *clearance. Values are means ± SE, n = 6-8.*

Perfusion of duodenum with 100 mM HCl for 5 min induced a 4-fold increase in ^{51}Cr-EDTA clearance (Figure 3) and 50 min after cessation of the acid perfusion ^{51}Cr-EDTA clearance was still 2.6-fold higher than the pre-acid control (P<0.01). Spontaneous luminal alkalinization was stable in both groups. Luminal perfusion with either 50 or 100 mM hydrochloric acid for 5 min increased the rate of alkalinization by about 50% (P<0.05) and 30% (P<0.05) respectively (Figure 4).

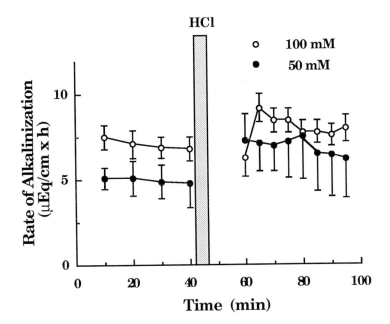

FIGURE 4. *Effects of luminal perfusion of duodenum for 5 min with 50 mM (o) or 100 mM (o) hydrochloric acid (HCl) on luminal alkalinization. The rate of luminal alkalinization could not be accurately determined in the two effluents subsequent to the HCl-perfusion period. These effluents had a pH<6.0 and were therefore excluded in figure. Values are means ± SE, n = 7-9.*

DISCUSSION

The aim of the present investigation was to elucidate the relationship between duodenal alkaline secretion and mucosal permeability. The latter was assessed by measuring the clearance of ^{51}Cr-EDTA from blood-to-duodenal lumen. Previous studies have shown that intestinal clearance of water soluble molecules greater than approximately 150 dalton, including EDTA, is blood flow-independent indicating that the rate limiting barrier for the diffusion of EDTA from blood to intestinal lumen is the intestinal epithelium [9,10]. Recent investigations have demonstrated that intestinal perfusion with various agents including hydrochloric acid [9,11], ethanol [12] or the chemotactic peptide N-formyl methioyl-leucyl-phenylalanine [13], all increase mucosal permeability in a dose-related fashion. Of interest in this context is that mucosal permeability is higher in patients with intestinal disorders than in healthy individuals [14]. Thus, the ^{51}Cr-EDTA clearance technique allows for detection of subtle and large changes in mucosal integrity [15].

Brief exposure of duodenum to hydrochloric acid increases alkaline secretion and the release of VIP [4,7,16,17]. Considering that VIP is an effective stimulant of duodenal alkaline secretion [2,6] and that the increase in luminal alkalinizaion in response to HCl is inhibited by an VIP-antagonist [18], VIP is a probable mediator of the HCl-induced rise in alkaline secretion. It is thus possible that the HCl-induced stimulation of bicarbonate transport, mediated via VIP, also increases ^{51}Cr-EDTA clearance. However, the 2.7-fold increase in luminal alkalinization in response to VIP was associated with a 50% decrease in basal ^{51}Cr-EDTA clearance. This suggests that the HCl-induced increase in ^{51}Cr-EDTA clearance is not mediated via stimulation of duodenal alkaline secretion but may raher reflect disturbance of mucosal integrity. These data further suggest that VIP stimulates duodenal alkaline secretion via a direct effect on the HCO_3^- secreting cell.

Intravenous administration of the cyclooxygenase inhibitor indomethacin induced a large increase in the rate of luminal alkalinization. This is an unexpected finding since previous investigations have shown that indomethacin inhibits rather than stimulates basal duodenal alkaline secretion [4,5,7,8]. The rise in luminal alkalinization in response to indomethacin does probably not reflect an increase in paracellular conductance for HCO_3^-. There was thus no relationship between the changes in ^{51}Cr-EDTA clearance and the rate of luminal alkalinization. The latter was still increased above basal one hour after the injection of the drug while ^{51}Cr-EDTA clearance was reduced by 45%. The mechanism of action of indomethacin in stimulating duodenal alkaline secretion is not known and remains to be elucidated.

In the present study, the rise in luminal alkalinization in response to either 50 mM or 100 mM HCl was small (30 to 50%). Recently, it was shown that perfusion of jejunum with 10 mM HCl for 40 min increased the rate of luminal alkalinization threefold. This increase in alkalinization was correlated to the increase in ^{51}Cr-EDTA clearance suggesting passive movement of bicarbonate into the luminal solution [9]. Similarly, there is strong reason to believe that the increase in duodenal alkalinization in response to 100 mM HCl is due to an increased passive flux of HCO_3^- rather than stimulation of active transport of this ion. The ^{51}Cr-EDTA clearance increased 4-fold in response to luminal perfusion with 100 mM HCl, indicating a marked increase in paracellular permeability, and 50 min after cessation of the HCl perfusion the clearance was still 2.6-fold higher than basal. These results together with the morphological data recently reported by Leung et al [19] strongly suggests that luminal perfusion with 100 mM HCl for 5 min causes mucosal damage in duodenum of the rat. Furthermore, previous investigations suggest that a large portion of alkaline secretion by the intact duodenal mucosa is due to a metabolic dependent secretory process and that passive movement of HCO_3^- is a minor part of alkalinization [2,20,21]. Assuming that the passive movement accounts for 10-30% of basal alkaline secretion and provided that active secretion of HCO_3^- does not change (due to mucosal damage), a threefold increase of passive flux of HCO_3^- (as for ^{51}Cr-EDTA) would increase total alkalinization by 20 to 60%. These figures are in the same range as those obtained in response to hydrochloric acid (50 or 100 mM) in the present investigation.

In conclusion, the results of the present study indicate absence of a causal relationship between luminal alkalinization and mucosal permeability. This in turn suggests that the transepithelial movement of ^{51}Cr-EDTA and base (HCO_3^-) does not necessarily occur through the same "pore" and that luminal alkalinization seems to be due to transcellular rather than paracellular movement of base. During pathophysiological conditions as when the duodenum is exposed to excessive amounts of H+, the intercellular tight junction structure may be disrupted resulting in a higher paracellular permeability of both ^{51}Cr-EDTA and HCO_3^-. With the use of the ^{51}Cr-EDTA clearance technique, it may be possible to detect and quantify early mucosal damage and thus gain new knowledge about the pathophysiological mechanisms that enhance the susceptibility of the duodenal mucosa to HCl and other noxious agents.

ACKNOWLEDGEMENTS

This work was supported by Grants from the Swedish Medical Research Council, Stockholm, Sweden, and from Hassle AB, Molndal, Sweden

The authors thank Mrs Hjordis Andersson for excellent technical assistance.

REFERENCES

1. Ovesen L, Bendtsen T, Tage-Jensen U, Pedersen NT, Gram BR, Rune SJ. Intraluminal pH in the stomach, duodenum and proximal jejunum in normal subjects and patients with exocrine pancreatic insufficiency. Gastroenterology 1986; 90: 958-962.

2. Flemstrom G. Gastric and duodenal mucosal bicarbonate secretion. In: Johnson LR, ed (2nd ed.). Physiology of the Gastrointestinal Tract. New York: Raven, 1987: 1011-1030.

3. Fandriks L, Jonson C, Nylander O, Flemstrom G. Neural influences on gastroduodenal secretion. In: Szabo S, Pfeiffer CJ, eds. Ulcer Disease: new aspects of pathogenesis and pharmacology. Boc Raton: CRC Press, 1989: 193-205.

4. Flemstrom G, Garner A, Nylander O, Hurst BC, Heylings JR. Surface epithelial HCO_3^- transport by mammalian duodenum in vivo. Am J Physiol. 1982; 243: G348-G358.

5. Granstam S-O, Flemstrom G, Nylander O. Bicarbonate secretion by the rabbit duodenum in vivo: effects of prostaglandins, vagal nerve stimulation and some drugs. Acta Physiol Scand 1987; 131: 377-384.

6.   Isenberg JI, Wallin B, Johansson C, Smedfors B, Mutt V, Tatemoto K, Emas S. Secretin, VIP and PHI stimulate rat proximal duodenal surface epithelial bicarbonate secretion *in vivo*. Regul Pept 1984; 8: 315-320.

7.   Konturek SJ, Bilski J, Tasler J, Laskiewicz J. Gastroduodenal alkaline response to acid and taurocholate in conscious dogs. Am J Physiol 1984; 247: G149-154.

8.   Smeaton LA, Hirst BH, Allen A, Garner A. Gastric and duodenal HCO_3^- transport in vivo: Influence of prostaglandins. Am J Physiol. 1983; 245: G751-G759.

9.   Nylander O, Kvietys P, Granger DN. Effects of hydrochloric acid on duodenal and jejunal mucosal permeability in the rat. Am J Physiol. 1989; 257: G653-G660.

10.   Winne D. Blood flow in intestinal absorption models. J Pharmacokin Biophar 1978; 6: 55-78.

11.   Wilkes JM, Garner A, Peters TJ. Mechanisms of acid disposal and acid-stimulated alkaline secretion by gasroduodenal mucosa. Dig Dis Sci 1988; 33: 361-367.

12.   Kvietys PR, Twohig B, Dansell J, Specian RD. Ethanol-induced injury to the rat gastric mucosa. Role of neutrophils and xanthine oxidase-derived radicals. Gastroenterology 1990; 98: 909-920.

13.   Von Ritter C, Sekizuka E, Grisham MB, Granger DN. The chemotactic peptide N-formyl methioyl-leucyl-phenylalanine increases mucosal permeability in the distal ilium of the rat. Gastroenterology 1988; 95: 651-659.

14.   Menzies IS. Transmucosal passage or inert molecules in health and disease. In: Skadhauge E, Heintze K, eds. Intestinal absorption and secretion London: MTP Press, 1983: 527-543.

15.   Crissinger KD, Kvietys PR, Granger DN. Pathophysiology of gastrointestinal mucosal permeability. J Internal Medicine 1990; 228: Suppl 1 (in press).

16.   Isenberg JI, Smedfors B, Johansson C. Effect of graded doses of intraluminal H+, prostaglandin E_2 and inhibition of endogenous prostaglandin synthesis on proximal duodenal bicarbonate secretion in unanaesthetized rats. Gastroenterology 1985; 88: 303-307.

17.   Smedfors B, Theodorsson E, Aly A, Musat A, Panja AB, Johansson C. HCl-induced duodenal HCO_3^- secretion is associated with concentration related release of local prostaglandin E_2, vasoactive intestinal peptide, neurokinin A and substance P in the rat. Eur J Gastroenterol and Hept 1989; 1: 193-199.

18.   Algazi MC, Pandol SJ, Rivier, Isenberg JI. Effect of VIP antagonist
       on VIP-, PGE_2-, and acid-stimulated duodenal bicarbonate secretion.
       Am J Physiol 1989; 256: G833-G836.

19.   Leung FW, Miller JC, Reedy TJ, Guth PH. Exogenous prostaglandins
       protects against acid-induced deep mucosal injury by stimulating
       alkaline secretion in rat duodenum. Dig Dis Sci 1989; 34: 1686-1691.

20.   Heylings JT, Feldman M.   Basal and PGE_2-stimulated duodenal
       bicarbonate secretion in the rat in vivo. Am J Physiol 1988; 255:
       G470-G475.

21.   Simson JNL, Merhav A, Silen W. Alkaline secretion by amphibian
       duodenum. I. General characteristics. Am J Physiol 1981; 240: G410-
       G408.

ROLE OF SENSORY NEUROPEPTIDES IN GASTRIC MUCOSAL DAMAGE AND PROTECTION

P. Holzer[1,2], H.E. Raybould[2], I.Th. Lippe[1,] R. Amann[1],
E.H. Livingston[2], B.M. Peskar[3], B.A. Peskar[4], Y. Tache[2] & P.H. Guth[2]

[1]Dept. of Experimental & Clinical Pharmacology, University of Graz, Austria,
[2]Center for Ulcer Research & Education, University of California at Los Angeles
and Veterans Admin. Wadsworth Medical Center, Los Angeles, [3]Dept. of
Experimental Clinical Medicine, University of Bochum, FRG, and [4]Dept of
Pharmacology & Toxicology, University of Bochum, FRG

ABSTRACT

The gastric mucosa and particularly the submucosal blood vessels are densely innervated by primary afferent neurons containing peptides such as substance P (SP) and calcitonin gene-related peptide (CGRP). (i) Stimulation of these sensory neurons by acute intragastric administration of capsaicin (10-640 uM) increases gastric mucosal blood flow (GMBF) and protects the gastric mucosa from experimental injury. (ii) Acute administration of capsaicin is able to augment the release of CGRP into the gastric circulation. (iii) Close arterial infusion of CGRP, but not SP, to the rat stomach facilitates GMBF and prevents experimental damage of the mucosa. (iv) GMBF also increases in response to acid back-diffusion through a disrupted gastric mucosal barrier. This rise in GMBF is inhibited after ablation of CGRP-containing afferent neurons of spinal but not vagal origin. Concomitantly, injury to the mucosa is aggravated by sensory neuron ablation. These findings indicate that peptidergic afferent neurons play a physiological role in the regulation of GMBF and gastric mucosal integrity.

INTRODUCTION

Apart from autonomic and enteric neurons, the gastric mucosa and submucosa is innervated by primary afferent neurons which arise from cell bodies in either the dorsal root (spinal afferents) or nodose ganglia (vagal afferents) [1,2]. The nerve endings of these afferent nerve fibres form a particularly dense plexus around submucosal blood vessels, which suggests that they are involved in the regulation of mucosal blood flow. The functional implications of some of these afferent neurons can be examined by virtue of their sensitivity to capsaicin. This drug enables selective manipulation of the state of activity of certain primary afferent neurons with unmyelinated (C-) or thinly meylinated (Aδ-) nerve fibres [3,4], and it is two actions of capsaicin which can be taken use of. Acute administration of low nontoxic doses of the drug can be employed to stimulate capsaicin-sensitive afferent neurons whereas systemic administration of high neurotoxic doses of capsaicin is used to produce a long-lasting defunctionalization of the neurons sensitive to the drug.

In addition to their afferent function, capsaicin-sensitive sensory neurons play a local effector function by way of the release of neuropeptide transmitters from their peripheral nerve endings [4]. Sensory neuropeptides such as substance P (SP) and calcitonin gene-related peptide (CGRP) are involved in inflammatory reactions of many tissues which are interpreted as protecting or as promoting repair of damaged tissue [4]. There also is twofold evidence for a physiological role of peptidergic sensory neurons in controlling protective mechanisms of the gastric mucosa. (i) Ablation of capsaicin-sensitive afferent neurons has been found to exacerbate gastric lesion formation in response to a variety of endogenous and exogenous factors including acid [5,6], platelet-activating factor [7], indomethacin [8,9] and ethanol [8,10,11]. (ii) Stimulation of sensory nerve endings by intragastric administration of capsaicin protects from gastric mucosal damage induced by acid [5], ethanol [12,13] or aspirin [14]. Analysis of the pathways and mechanisms of the protective action of sensory nerve stimulation has suggested that sensory neurons strengthen gastric mucosal defence against injury by local vasodilator reflexes within the gastric wall [12,15]. The aims of the present study were (i) to confirm that sensory neurons are involved in the control of gastric mucosal circulation and (ii) to examine which neuropeptides mediate the vasodilator and protective role of sensory neurons. Considering that capsaicin-sensitive afferent neurons are sensitive to hydrogen ions [16,17] we also investigated whether these neurons were to monitor acid influx into the mucosa and to signal the increase in mucosal blood flow which is a well-known sequel of acid back-diffusion [18,19].

METHODS

All experiments were performed on adult Sprague-Dawley rats which were fasted overnight and anaesthetized with urethane (1.5 mg/kg subcutaneously). Functional ablation of capsaicin-sensitive neurons was achieved by two different methods of capsaicin treatment. Subcutaneous injection of a total dose of 125 mg/kg capsaicin 10-14 days before the experiments was used to defunctionalise all afferent neurons sensitive to the drug [3,4]. Administration of a 1% solution of capsaicin to the cervical vagus nerve trunks or to the coeliac ganglion for 30 min was used to selectively ablate vagal or spinal sensory neurons, respectively, supplying the stomach [20]. Also in this instance a period of 10-14 days was allowed to elapse until the rats were used for experiments. The animals were fitted with a tracheal cannula, a cannula in a carotid artery for recording of the blood pressure and a cannula in a jugular vein for constant infusion of saline (1 ml/h) [6,8,13,14,15]. The body temperature of the animals was kept at 36-37°C. The stomach was constantly perfused at a rate of 0.75 ml/min via catheters inserted in the forestomach and pylorus. For close arterial administration of substances to the stomach, a catheter (PE-10) was inserted retrogradely in the splenic artery close to the coeliac artery. Gastric mucosal blood flow (GMBF) was measured by the hydrogen gas clearance technique, the recording needle-type elecrode being inserted at the interface between muscularis mucosae and submucosa [13]. Acid output or acid loss from the lumen was determined by titration of the gastric perfusate fractions to pH 7. Gross damage of the gastric mucosa was evaluated by either a semiquantitative scoring method [12,13] or computerized image analysis [13]. In addition, the mucosae were also examined by routine histology techniques to quantitate the depth of injury [13]. The data are presented as means ± SEM. Statistical analysis of the results was performed with the nonparametric U or H tests, values of P<0.05 being regarded as significant.

RESULTS AND DISCUSSION

<u>Stimulation of sensory neurons increases gastric mucosal blood flow and resistance against injury.</u>

Perfusion of the stomach with capsaicin (1-640 uM) in saline led to a prompt and sustained increase in GMBF as measured by the hydrogen gas clearance technique [13,21]. The effect of capsaicin was dose-dependent and most likely related to mucosal vasodilatation since systemic blood pressure was not changed [21]. This observation confirms previous findings obtained with the gastric clearance of aniline, an indirect measure of GMBF [15]. The increase in GMBF was also seen when capsaicin was administered together with an injurious concentration of 25% ethanol [13,21]. The gastric mucosal vasodilatation caused by 10-640 uM capsaicin closely correlated (P <0.01) with a reduction of gross lesion formation [21]. This result can be taken to hypothesize that the protective effect of capsaicin is due to augmented blood flow through the mucosa. The protective effect of capsaicin manifested itself not only in a reduction of macroscopically visible damage but also in prevention of histologically deep injury. Superficial injury to the mucosa, however, was not prevented by capsaicin as shown by both light and scanning electron microscopy [13].

Separate experiments established that both the capsaicin-induced mucosal vasodilatation and protection from ethanol injury were mediated by sensory neurons [12,21]. Ablation of sensory neurons by pretreatment of the experimental animals with subcutaneous capsaicin abolished the capsaicin-induced increase in GMBF and protection from ethanol injury [12,21]. This observation indicates that both the vasodilator and protective effects of intragastric capsaicin arise from stimulation of sensory neurons. Other experiments revealed that the protective effect of capsaicin does not involve the autonomic nervous system and hence is most likely due to a local neural mechanism within the stomach [12]. However, both the vasodilator and protective effects of intragastric capsaicin were inhibited by tetrodotoxin (60 ng/min), a blocker of nerve conduction [21]. This finding shows that the gastric effects of capsaicin involve nerve conduction and hence are brought about by a neural reflex within the gastric wall.

<u>Calcitonin gene-related peptide as a mediator of sensory nerve-mediated gastric mucosal vasodilatation and protection.</u>

Inherent in the assumption that capsaicin-induced mucosal vasodilatation results from a local reflex within the stomach is the question as to what transmitter substances of capsaicin-sensitive nerve endings mediate the increase in GMBF. CGRP and SP whose presence in sensory nerve endings of the stomach is well established [1,2] are likely candidates because they exhibit vasodilator activity in other vascular beds [4]. Using a preparation of the vascularly perfused rat stomach we found that intraarterial infusion of capsaicin (10 uM) induced a large increase in the release of immunoreactive CGRP into the venous effluent (Figure 1)[22]. High performance liquid chromatography of the released material indicated that the majority of the immunoreactivity corresponded to authentic CGRP [22]. Other work has shown that SP also is released by capsaicin in the rat and guinea-pig stomach [23].

Vascularly perfused rat stomach

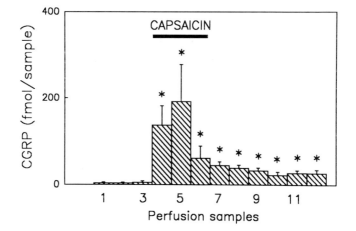

FIGURE 1. *Effect of capsaicin (10 uM, added to the vascular perfusion medium as indicated) on the release of immunoreactive calcitonin gene-related peptide (CGRP) into the venous effluent of the vascularly perfused stomach of the rat. Each perfusion sample consisted of 60 drops. Means ± S.E.M., n = 4. *P<0.05 (Quade test) versus pre-capsaicin values. Data taken from reference 24.*

If CGRP and/or SP were to be mediators of capsaicin-sensitive nerve endings in the stomach they also should be able to mimick the vasodilator and protective effects of capsaicin on the gastric mucosa. This hypothesis was tested by investigating whether close arterial infusion of the peptides to the rat stomach is able to increase GMBF and to protect from experimental injury. Using the hydrogen gas clearance technique we observed that infusion of rat α-CGRP, the prevalent form of CGRP in primary afferent neurons of the rat [24], increased GMBF at doses (15 pmol/min) which were too low to cause systemic hypotension (Figure 2)[25]. Higher doses of the peptide (75 pmol/min) facilitated blood flow to a larger extent but also lowered blood pressure. In contrast, SP (125 or 625 pmol/min) failed to alter GMBF although the higher dose of the peptide caused significant hypotension [25]. These findings show that CGRP is a very potent vasodilator and thus is a likely candidate mediator of the sensory nerve-induced increase in GMBF.

Further experiments corroborated the hypothesis that CGRP is a mediator of sensory nerve-mediated gastric mucosal protection. Close arterial administration of CGRP to the rat stomach, at the same dose (15 pmol/min) that stimulated gastric mucosal blood flow [25], reduced gross injury produced by 25% ethanol (Figure 2) or acidified aspirin [26], the two injury models in which capsaicin previously had been found to be protective [12,13,14].

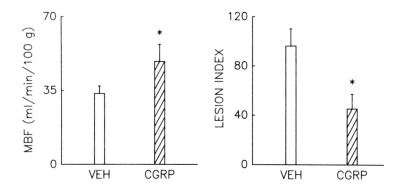

FIGURE 2. *Effect of close arterial infusion of calcitonin gene-related peptide (rat alpha-CGRP, 15 pmol/min) into the rat stomach on gastric mucosal blood flow (MBF; left panel) and gross lesion formation in response to ethanol (right panel). In the latter case, the stomach of urethane-anaesthetized rats was perfused with 25% ethanol for a period of 30 min after which gross injury was estimated semiquantitatively by calculating a lesion index (26). MBF was measured by the hydrogen gas clearance technique (13). The infusion of CGRP was started 5 min before measurement of MBF or the start of the ethanol perfusion. Means ± S.E.M., n = 6. *P<0.05 (U test) versus infusion of vehicle (VEH). Data taken from references 25 and 26.*

Thus CGRP is able to strengthen the resistance of the rat gastric mucosa against injurious factors, an effect which is very likely related to its potent vasodilator action. In view of the inactivity of SP in affecting GMBF we did not examine its effect on gastric mucosal lesion formation. There is information, however, that subcutaneous administration of SP fails to reduce experimental injury [27].

Prostaglandins and other eicosanoids which play a role in maintaining mucosal integrity have been ruled out as mediators of sensory nerve-mediated gastric mucosal protection. This conclusion is derived from the finding that indomethacin administered at doses shown to inhibit gastric prostaglandin synthesis failed to alter the protective action of intragastric capsaicin against ethanol injury [13]. Furthermore, capsaicin given intragastrically at a dose known to prevent ethanol-induced injury did not affect the *ex vivo* formation of prostaglandin E_2, 6-oxo-prostaglandin $F_{1\alpha}$ and leukotriene C_4 [13].

PHYSIOLOGICAL ROLE OF CGRP-CONTAINING SENSORY NEURONS IN THE GASTRIC VASODILATOR RESPONSE TO ACID BACK-DIFFUSION.

Given that stimulation of sensory neurons in the stomach strengthens the resistance of the gastric mucosa against injury by way of an increase in GMBF, the question arises as to the physiological or pathophysiological conditions under which capsaicin-sensitive sensory neurons are called into effect to facilitate GMBF. Since these neurons are sensitive to acid [16,17] we examined whether augmented back-diffusion of acid into the gastric mucosa is a condition which stimulates sensory neurons and thereby leads to an increase in GMBF, a phenomenon that has been well documented [18,19]. In our experimental model, acid back-diffusion into the gastric mucosa was induced by disrupting the gastric mucosal barrier with 15% ethanol in the presence of exogenous acid (0.15 N HCl). This procedure caused a marked and sustained increase in GMBF and enhanced acid loss from the gastric perfusion medium [6]. Since systemic blood pressure was not altered it seems likely that the rise of GMBF resulted from mucosal vasodilatation. Sensory denervation by subcutaneous pretreatment of rats with a neurotoxic dose of capsaicin inhibited the blood flow increase caused by barrier disruption in the presence of exogenous acid [6]. Associated with this inhibition of the blood flow response was a signficant exacerbation of gross lesion formation and a significant increase in the mucosal depth of the lesions [6]. Mean arterial blood pressure, basal GMBF and acid loss from the gastric perfusion medium were not altered by ablation of capsaicin-sensitive sensory neurons [6].

Additional evidence that the vasodilator response to acid back-diffusion is mediated by neurons came from experiments in which tetrodotoxin, a blocker of nerve conduction, was infused close arterially to the stomach (60 ng/min)[6]. This drug suppressed the blood flow increase evoked by acid back-diffusion and aggravated gross damage in the gastric mucosa [6]. As reported previously [19], atropine failed to change the gastric blood flow response to acid back-diffusion indicating that postganglionic parasympathetic neurons or cholinergic vasodilator neurons of the enteric nervous system are not implicated [6]. Also unlikely is an involvement of the sympathetic nervous system since stimulation of sympathetic efferent neurons causes mucosal vasoconstriction [28]. However, the data obtained with tetrodotoxin indicate that the rise in GMBF due to acid back-diffusion is brought about by a neural reflex. In analogy with the local effector function of sensory nerve endings in other tissues [4] it is hypothesized that vasodilatation involves only sensory neurons and is the result of an axon reflex between different branches of sensory nerve fibres in the stomach. This explanation, however, does not take account of a possible implication of the enteric nervous system, which also needs to be considered.

To investigate the origin of the sensory neurons which mediate gastric mucosal vasodilatation in response to acid back-diffusion, vagal or spinal sensory neurons were selectively ablated by local capsaicin pretreatment of the vagus nerve trunks or coeliac ganglion, respectively [20]. Perivagal capsaicin treatment failed to change the rise in blood flow evoked by barrier disruption in the presence of exogenous acid, and gross damage of the mucosa was likewise unaltered. In contrast, pericoeliac treatment with capsaicin significantly inhibited the mucosal vasodilator response to acid back-diffusion and significantly exacerbated mucosal lesion formation (Table 1)[20].

TABLE 1

EFFECT OF PERICOELIAC CAPSAICIN TREATMENT (selective ablation of spinal afferent neurons supplying the stomach) ON THE CONSEQUENCES OF ACID BACK-DIFFUSION AND PEPTIDE CONCENTRATIONS IN THE RAT STOMACH.

Parameter	Control	Sensory neuron ablation
Blood flow rise [A]	43 ± 11	20 ± 5*
Gross injury [B]	7 ± 1	16 ± 3*
Substance P content [C]	40 ± 4	38 ± 5
CGRP [C]	38 ± 8	10 ± 5*

Means ± SEM, n = 7-10. *P<0.05 (U test).
[A] Blood flow rise given in ml/min/100g.
[B] Gross injury expressed as a percentage of the area of the corpus mucosa.
[C] Peptide levels given in pmol/g wet tissue.

Neither perivagal nor pericoeliac (Table 1) capsaicin treatment had any effect on the SP content of the gastric wall as measured by radio-immunoassay. The CGRP content was unchanged after perivagal but significantly reduced after pericoeliac capsaicin treatment (Table 1)[20]. These data confirm previous reports that most of the gastric CGRP originates from spinal ganglion neurons [1,2,24] whereas SP derives primarily from enteric neurons. Furthermore, the present results indicate that gastric mucosal vasodilatation in response to acid back-diffusion is mediated, at least in part, by primary afferent neurons that arise from dorsal root ganglia and contain CGRP. It would appear, therefore, that CGRP is an important candidate mediator of gastric mucosal vasodilatation evoked by sensory nerve stimulation.

CONCLUSIONS

The present findings reveal an hitherto unknown pathway by which mechanisms of gastric mucosal resistance to injury are called into effect and co-ordinated by the nervous system. Capsaicin-sensitive sensory neurons in the stomach monitor acid influx into the superficial mucosa and in turn signal for an increase in GMBF to strengthen gastric mucosal defense against deep acid injury. This hypothesis is in keeping with the concept that maintenance or facilitation of GMBF is an important mechanism of gastric mucosal protection [18,19,28,29]. A new perspective in the physiology and pathophysiology of the gastric mucosa opens up if one considers that the long-term integrity of the gastric mucosa may be under the subtle control of acid-sensitive sensory neurons and that, vice versa, improper functioning of these neural control mechanisms may predispose to gastric ulcer disease. The present data demonstrate that some of the peptides contained in gastric sensory nerve endings might fulfill a transmitter or mediator role in controlling GMBF and gastric mucosal integrity. CGRP, which in the rat gastric mucosa originates exclusively from spinal sensory neurons [1,2,24], appears to be important in this respect. This peptide is released following sensory nerve stimulation and is extremely potent in facilitating GMBF and protecting the mucosa from injurious factors. To the contrary, selective ablation of spinal sensory neurons containing CGRP weakens the resistance of the gastric mucosa against acid injury.

ACKNOWLEDGEMENTS

Work performed in the authors' laboratories was supported by the Austrian Scientific Research Funds (grants 5552 and 7845), the Max Kade Foundation, the National Institute of Health, Veterans Administration Research Funds and the Franz Lanyar Foundation of the Medical Faculty of the University of Graz.

REFERENCES

1.   Sternini C, Reeve JR and Brecha N. Distribution and characterization of calcitonin gene-related peptide immunoreactivity in the digestive system of normal and capsaicin-treated rats. Gastroenterology 1987; 93: 852-862.

2.   Green T and Dockray GJ. Characterization of the peptidergic afferent innervation of the stomach in the rat, mouse and guinea-pig. Neuroscience 1988; 25: 181-193.

3.   Buck SH and Burks TF. The neuropharmacology of capsaicin: review of some recent observations. Pharmacol. Rev. 1986; 38: 179-226.

4.   Holzer P.   Local effector functions of capsaicin-sensitive sensory nerve endings: involvement of tachykinins, calcitonin gene-related peptide and other neuropeptides. Neuroscience 1988; 24: 739-768.

5.   Szolcsanyi J and Bartho L.   Impaired defense mechanism to peptic ulcer in the capsaicin-desensitized rat.   In: Gastrointestinal Defense Mechanisms. G. Mozsik, O. Hanninen and T. Javor, Eds. Pergamon Press and Akademiai Kiado.   Oxford and Budapest, U.K. and Hungary. 1981; pp 39-51.

6.   Holzer P, Livingston EH and Guth PH.   Sensory neurons signal for an increase in rat gastric mucosal blood flow in response to acid back-diffusion. Gastroenterology 1990; 98: A175.

7.   Esplugues JV, Whittle BJR and Moncada S.   Local opioid-sensitive afferent sensory neurons in the modulation of gastric damage induced by Paf. Br J Pharmacol. 1989; 97: 579-585.

8.   Holzer P and Sametz W.   Gastric mucosal protection against ulcerogenic factors in the rat mediated by capsaicin-sensitive afferent neurons. Gastroenterology 1986; 91: 975-981.

9.   Evangelista S, Maggi CA and Meli A.   Evidence for a role of adrenals in the capsaicin-sensitive "gastric defence mechanism" in rats. Proc Soc Exp Biol Med 1986; 182: 568-569.

10.   Evangelista S, Maggi CA and Meli A.   Influence of peripherally-administered peptides on ethanol-induced gastric ulcers in the rat. Gen Pharmacol 1987; 18: 647-649.

11.   Esplugues JV and Whittle BJR.   Morphine potentiation of ethanol-induced gastric mucosal damage in the rat.   Role of local sensory afferent neurons. Gastroenterology 1990; 98: 82-89.

12.   Holzer P and Lippe IT.   Stimulation of afferent nerve endings by intragastric capsaicin protects against ethanol-induced damage of gastric mucosa. Neuroscience 1988; 27: 981-987.

13.   Holzer P, Pabst MA, Lippe IT, Peskar BM, Peskar BA, Livingston EH and Guth PH.   Afferent nerve-mediated protection against deep mucosal damage in the rat stomach. Gastroenterology 1990; 98: 838-848.

14.   Holzer P, Pabst MA and Lippe IT.   Intragastric capsaicin protects against aspirin-induced lesion formation and bleeding in the rat gastric mucosa. Gastroenterology 1989; 96: 1425-1433.

15.   Lippe IT, Pabst MA and Holzer P.   Intragastric capsaicin enhances rat gastric acid elimination and mucosal blood flow by afferent nerve stimulation. Br J Pharmacol 1989; 96: 91-100.

16.   Clarke GD and Davison JS. Mucosal receptors in the gastric antrum and small intestine of the rat with afferent fibres in the cervical vagus. J Physiol (London) 1978; 248:55-67.

17.   Bevan S and Yeats JC. Protons activate a sustained inward current in a sub-population of rat isolated dorsal root ganglion (DRG) neurones. J Physiol (London) 1989; 417:81P.

18.   Whittle BJR. Mechanisms underlying gastric mucosal damage induced by indomethacin and bile salts, and the actions of prostglandins. Br. J. Pharmacol. 1977; 60: 455-460.

19.   Bruggeman TM, Wood JG, and Davenport HW. Local control of blood flow in the dog's stomach: vasodilatation caused by acid back-diffusion following topical application of salicylic acid. Gastroenterology 1979; 77: 736-744.

20.   Raybould HE, Holzer P, Sternini C and Eysselein VE. Selective ablation of spinal sensory neurons containing CGRP inhibits the increase in rat gastric mucosal blood flow due to acid back-diffusion. Gasrtroenterology 1990; 98: A198.

21.   Holzer P, Livingston EH and Guth PH. Close correlation between sensory nerve-induced increase in rat gastric mucosal blood flow and prevention of ethanol injury. Gastroenterology 1990; 98: A60.

22.   Holzer P, Peskar BM, Peskar BA, and Amann R. Release of calcitonin gene-related peptide induced by capsaicin in the vascularly perfused rat stomach. Neurosci Lett 1990; 108: 195-200.

23.   Renzi D, Santicioli P, Maggi CA, Surrenti C, Pradelles P and Meli A. Capsaicin-induced release of substance P-like immunoreactivity from the guinea pig stomach in vitro and in vivo. Neurosci Lett 1988; 92: 254-258.

24.   Varro A, Green T, Holmes S and Dockray GJ. Calcitonin gene-related peptide in visceral afferent nerve fibres: quantification by radioimmunoassay and determination of axonal transport rates. Neuroscience 1988; 26: 927-932.

25.   Holzer P, Tache Y and Guth PH. The vasodilator peptides alpha-CGRP and VIP, but not substance P and neurokinin A, increase rat gastric mucosal blood flow. Gastroenterology 1990; 98: A175.

26.   Lippe IT, Lorbach M and Holzer P. Close arterial infusion of calcitonin gene-related peptide into the rat stomach inhibits aspirin- and ethanol-induced hemorrhagic damage. Regul Pept 1989; 26: 35-46.

27.   Evangelista S, Lippe IT, Rovero P, Maggi CA and Meli A. Tachykinins protect against ethanol-induced gastric lesions in rats. Peptides 1989; 10: 79-81.

28.   Guth PH and Leung FW. Physiology of the gastric circulation. In: Physiology of the Gastrointestinal Tract. Johnson LR. Ed. Raven Press. New York. NY. 1987; pp.1031-1053.

29.   Gannon B, Browning J and O'Brien P.   The microvascular architecture of the glandular mucosa of rat stomach.   J Anat 1982; 135: 667-683.

PERIPHERAL OPIOID-SENSITIVE MECHANISMS OF MUCOSAL INJURY AND PROTECTION.

J.V. Esplugues and B.J.R. Whittle*

*Departments of Pharmacology, University of Valencia, Valencia, Spain and
Wellcome Research Laboratories, Beckenham, Kent, U.K.

ABSTRACT

The existence of perpheral opioid-sensitive mechanisms that could influence the ability of the gastric mucosa to withstand damage has been investigated in the rat. Morphine (9 mg kg^{-1}, i.v.) significantly potentiated the level of macroscopic damage induced by 5-min intragastric challenge with ethanol (25% - 100%). These effects of morphine were inhibited by the opioid antagonists naloxone and the peripherally acting N-methylnalorphine. Pretreatment of rats with capsaicin, 2 weeks before the study to induce functional ablation of primary afferent neurons, likewise augmented the damage induced by ethanol, to an extent similar to that observed following treatment with morphine. The area of gastric damage induced by ethanol (50% and 100%) was substantially reduced by prior administration (10 min) of PGE$_2$ (25-100 ug kg^{-1}, p.o.). However, pretreatment with morphine led to significant reduction in the protective effects of PGE$_2$ against ethanol-induced gastric mucosal damage. These observations thus indicate the involvement of opioid-sensitive processes in the mechanisms contributing to the protection of the gastric mucosa against damage, and suggest that interaction with such processes may contribute to the protective effects of prostaglandins.

INTRODUCTION

Local sensory afferent neurons, particularly those that are capsaicin-sensitive, are considered to regulate protective mechanisms of the gastric mucosa against damage. Ablation of capsaicin-sensitive afferent neurons increases the degree of macroscopically apparent mucosal damage induced by several pro-ulcerogenic or irritant agents [1,2,3]. Furthermore, acute stimulation with capsaicin of afferent nerve endings in the gastric mucosa protects against different ulcerogenic procedures [1,4,5].

Morphine and other opioids potentiate gastric mucosal injury in various experimental models [6,7,8], although the mechanisms underlying such action remain unclear. Following observations on the regulatory effects of opioids and enkephalins on neuropeptide-release by sensory nerve endings [9,10], studies on vascular permeability and blood flow in the skin have suggested that opioids can inhibit the activity of primary afferent neurons [11,12,13,14]. Furthermore, studies in analgesia have indicated that morphine-like opioids modulate afferent sensory neurons by an action at peripheral sites [15,16].

In the present paper, we have analyzed the possibility that opioids could influence the ability of the mucosa to withstand mucosal damage by exerting a peripheral action on local capsaicin-sensitive neuronal mechanims. To evaluate this concept, we have investigated the effects of primary afferent neuronal desensitization that follows systemic capsaicin pretreatment, on the gastric damage elicited by intragastric ethanol and have compared this with the actions of morphine. Furthermore, since opiates can also inhibit the stimulatory effects of E-type prostaglandins on certain sensory neurones [17], the effects of morphine on the protection of the rat gastric mucosa against ethanol-induced damage elicited by PGE_2 were also studied.

METHODS

Male Wistar rats (220-260g body weight) were deprived of food, but not water, for 18-20 h before the experiment. One ml of ethanol (25%, 50% or 100%, v/v in saline) or vehicle was administered orally by gavage, and the rats killed by cervical dislocation 5 min later. The stomachs were opened, pinned to a wax block immersed in neutral buffered formalin and photographed on colour transparency film. The extent of damage was calculated via computerized planimetry, and expressed as the percent of the total gastric mucosa showing macroscopically visible damage. In one group of experiments, morphine (9 mg kg^{-1}) or saline was injected (1 ml kg^{-1}) into the tail vein 15 min before the administration of ethanol. To investigate the effects of opioid antagonists, rats were pretreated (i.v.) 5 min before the administration of morphine with naloxone (1 mg kg^{-1}) or N-methylnalorphine (6 mg kg^{-1}). In a second group of experiments, adult rats were treated with capsaicin, under halothane anaesthesia, for three consecutive days (20, 30 and 50 mg kg^{-1}, s.c.) as described previously in detail [3]. Control animals received a similar regimen of treatment with the capsaicin vehicle (10% ethanol, 10% Tween 80, 80% saline). Two weeks after completion of the capsaicin treatment the gastric mucosa was challenged with ethanol. In a third group of experiments, rats were treated with PGE_2 (25, 50 and 100 μg kg^{-1}, p.o.) 10 min before morphine (9 mg kg^{-1}, i.v.), and intragastric ethanol administered 15 min later. PGE_2 (Upjohn) was stored in absolute ethanol and an aliquot (20 μl) was diluted in saline prior to use. All results are shown as mean $\pm$ s.e. mean. Student's t-test was used for evaluating statistical significance, and probability values p<0.05 were taken as significant.

RESULTS

EFFECTS OF MORPHINE-PRETREATMENT ON ETHANOL-INDUCED MUCOSAL DAMAGE.

The intragastric administration of 1 ml of ethanol 25%, 50% or 100% resulted in macroscopically detectable damage involving 8% $\pm$ 1% (n=16), 20 $\pm$ 2% (n=28) and 43% $\pm$ 5% (n=27) respectively of the total area of the rat gastric mucosa (Figure 1). Gastric mucosal damage was not observed in any

animal, either treated or control that received only saline. As shown in
Figure 1, the pretreatment with morphine (9 mg kg^{-1}, i.v.) 15 min before
challenge significantly increased the extent of gastric mucosal damage
elicited by the administration of 1 ml of ethanol (25% - 100%).
Macroscopically, the potentiation by morphine of ethanol-induced mucosal
damage was characterised as a significant increase in the area of the lesions
affecting the corpus region.   Furthermore, morphine induced the
appearance of hemorrhagic lesions in the antral mucosa, an area not
exhibiting distinct macroscopic damage following challenge with ethanol
alone.   When analyzed histologically, pretreatment with morphine also
augmented the degree of ethanol-induced damage that was observed in the
mucosa of both the corpus and the antrum of the rat stomach [18]. The
nature of the damage was characterised by the same histological features
that were observed with ethanol alone, but with a significantly greater
degree of deep hemorrhagic damage.

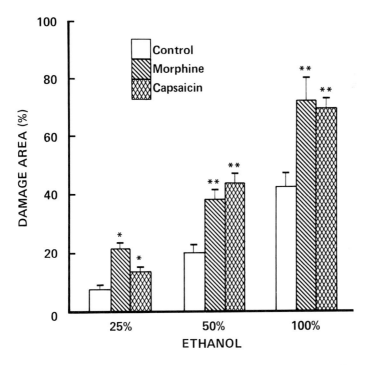

FIGURE 1 *Potentiation by pretreatment with morphine (9 mg kg^{-1} i.v., 15
min) or capsaicin (2 weeks earlier) of the rat gastric mucosal damage
induced by various intragastric concentrations of ethanol (25% - 100%).
Results, shown as the percent of the total mucosal area that exhibited
macroscopically assessed damage 5 min after challenge, are the mean ±
s.e. mean of 6 to 28 experiments in each group. Significant difference
from the respective control ethanol-alone groups is given as *p<0.05, and
**p<0.01. Results are adapted from Esplugues and Whittle [18].*

The potentiating effect of morphine on ethanol-induced gastric damage cannot be attributed to variations in the rate of gastric emptying, since intragastric volume determined after challenge with ethanol was not different in control or morphine pretreated rats. Furthermore, intragastric concentrations of the non absorbable marker phenol red, administered simultaneously with ethanol to control and morphine pretreated rats, was likewise not significantly different between the two groups, indicating no difference in the rate of gastric emptying [18].

The enhancing effect of morphine on gastric damage induced by ethanol appeared to be mediated through a specific interaction with classical opiate receptors since low doses of the classical opioid antagonist naloxone, which can act on both central and peripheral opioid receptors, abolished such potentiation.

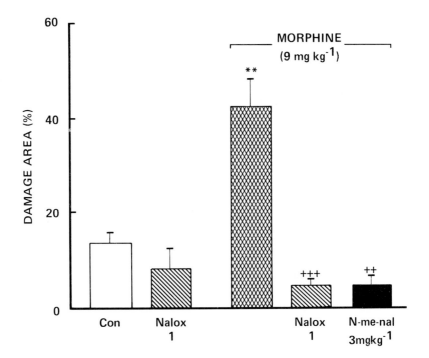

FIGURE 2   *Effects of the opiate antagonists naloxone (1 mg kg^{-1}, i.v.) and N-methyl nalorphine (6 mg kg^{-1}, i.v.) on the potentiation by morphine (9 mg kg^{-1}, i.v.) of the gastric damage induced by the intragastric administration of ethanol 50% (1 ml). Results, shown as the % of the total mucosal area that exhibited macroscopically assessed damage, are the mean ± s.e. mean of 4 to 12 experiments in each group. Significant difference from the ethanol control is given as **p<0.01, and from the combination of morphine and ethanol by ++p<0.01 and +++p<0.001. Results are adapted from Esplugues & Whittle [18].*

Furthermore, the opioid receptors involved appear to be located peripherally since N-methyl nalorphine, a peripherally acting quaternary opioid receptor antagonist which does not penetrate the blood brain barrier [12] equally inhibited the potentiating action of morphine (Figure 2). In the absence of morphine pretreatment, neither naloxone nor N-methylnalorphine significantly modified the level of mucosal damage induced by ethanol alone. Although the opioid receptors involved in this potentiating effect have not been fully characterized, the specificity of morphine, naloxone and N-methylnalorphine seems to indicate the involvement of u receptors in this mechanism.

EFFECTS OF CAPSAICIN-PRETREATMENT ON ETHANOL-INDUCED GASTRIC MUCOSAL DAMAGE.

As with morphine, capsaicin-pretreatment itself did not induce any macroscopic damage to the rat gastric mucosa when analysed two weeks later. However, animals systemically pretreated with capsaicin showed a significant enhancement in the extent of macroscopically apparent gastric mucosal damage observed after the intragastric administration (1 ml) of the three different ethanol concentrations (25%, 50% and 100%) as shown in Figure 1. Macroscopically, there was an increase in the area of haemorrhagic damage to the corpus mucosa, with the appearance of distinct hemorrhagic lesions in the antral mucosa to an extent comparable to that observed following treatment with morphine.

EFFECTS OF PRETREATMENT WITH PGE$_2$ ON MORPHINE POTENTIATION OF ETHANOL-INDUCED GASTRIC DAMAGE.

Intragastric pretreatment with PGE$_2$ (25 and 200 ug kg^{-1}) substantially reduced by 67% and 95% respectively ($p<0.01$ for both) the level of damage induced by 100% ethanol (Figure 3). Administration of PGE$_2$ (100 ug kg^{-1}) alone did not cause any macroscopically detectable changes to the rat gastric mucosa.

The area of damage induced by 100% ethanol was significantly increased ($p<0.01$) following 15 min intravenous pretreatment with morphine (9 mg kg^{-1}). Under those conditions of morphine and ethanol (100%) challenge, prior administration (10 min) of PGE$_2$ (25 ug kg^{-1}, p.o.) did not significantly modify the degree of mucosal damage. Furthermore, although with the highest dose of PGE$_2$ (100 ug kg^{-1}, p.o.) there was a significant ($p<0.05$) reduction in the extent of damage, 41 $\pm$ 7% (n=5) of the total area of the gastric mucosa still exhibited distinct macroscopic damage (Figure 3).

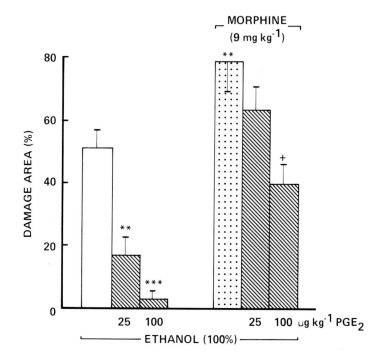

FIGURE 3   *Effects of pretreatment with PGE$_2$ (25 and 100 ug kg^{-1}, p.o.) on the gastric mucosal damage induced by the intragastric administration of 100% ethanol (1 ml) alone or after morphine pretreatment (9 mg kg^{-1}, i.v.). Results, shown as the % of the total mucosal area that exhibited macroscopically assessed damage 5 min after challenge, are the mean ± s.e. mean of 4 to 10 experiments in each group. Significant difference from the control ethanol-alone group is given as **p<0.01, *** p<0.001 and from the ethanol + morphine group as + p<0.05.*

    Since the failure of PGE$_2$, at the dose employed in our study, to inhibit the damage induced by the combination of 100% ethanol and morphine could possibly have reflected the increased extent of damage, further studies with a lower ethanol concentration under these conditions were conducted.

As shown in Figure 4, pretreatment with morphine (9 mg kg^{-1}, i.v.) augmented the area of damage induced by 50% ethanol to a level not significantly different from that observed with 100% ethanol alone. However, even under these conditions, pretreatment with PGE$_2$ (50 ug kg^{-1}, p.o.) did not significantly inhibit damage caused by this combination of 50% ethanol and morphine, although gastric mucosal damage induced by 50% and 100% ethanol alone was decreased by 79 $\pm$ 6% and 86 $\pm$ 10% (p<0.01 and p<0.001 respectively), as shown in Figure 4.

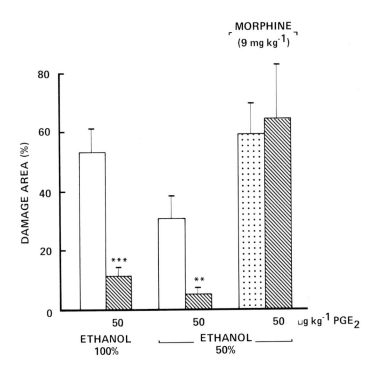

FIGURE 4 *Effects of pretreatment with PGE$_2$ (50 ug kg^{-1}, p.o.) on the gastric mucosal damage induced by the intragastric administration of 50 or 100% ethanol (1 ml) alone and on the potentiation by morphine pretreatment (9 mg kg^{-1}, i.v.) of the damaging effects of 50% ethanol. Results, shown as the % of the total mucosal area that exhibited macroscopically assessed damage 5 min after challenge, are the mean $\pm$ s.e. mean of 4 to 12 experiments in each group. Significant difference from the respective ethanol-alone group is given as **p<0.01 or ***p<0.001.*

DISCUSSION

This study has shown that opioids can enhance the degree of gastric mucosal damage induced by intragastric challenge with different concentrations of ethanol. This effect appears to be brought about by interaction at classical opiate receptors located in the periphery, as demonstrated by the effects of the peripherally acting antagonist. Opioids, acting peripherally, have been shown to inhibit the activity of sensory neurons [11, 12, 13 14]. It is therefore relevant that ablation of primary afferent neurons, following capsaicin-pretreatment in adult rats, also augmented the damaging effects of ethanol on the gastric mucosa to a similar extent to that observed after morphine administration. When compared, both macroscopically and histologically, the major features of the increased damage appearing after both treatments were also similar [18] providing, therefore, good evidence to suggest a common mechanism of action.

Microcirculatory disturbances have been proposed to mediate the initial stages in the pathogenesis of gastric lesions induced by ethanol [19,20]. Recent studies have demonstrated that both capsaicin-pretreatment and the administration of morphine, equally potentiate the changes in gastric mucosal blood flow induced by certain ulcerogens such as Paf [21]. These findings would suggest that opioid-sensitive primary afferent neurones may modulate blood flow in the gastric microcirculation, perhaps by the release of vasodilator sensory neuropeptides, and that such endogenous neuropeptides may thus protect against mucosal injury by a local vascular mechanism.

Treatment with morphine or capsaicin did not induce any detectable mucosal damage when administered alone to non-challenged stomachs. These observations imply that peripheral sensory neurons play a protective modulatory role in the gastric mucosa only under pathological situations such as those following challenge by a noxious stimuli. The lack of effect of the opioid-antagonists used in our experiments to influence the degree of ethanol-mucosal damage when administered alone, underlies that in this model of acute gastric damage, endogenous enkephalins do not appear to modulate the activity of peripheral sensory neurons. However, this finding does not exclude the possibility that, during certain stress situations, the endogenous release of high levels of enkephalins could inhibit the activity of such neurons and, therefore, aggravate gastric mucosal damage.

Since the early description of the protection elicited by prostaglandins against ethanol-induced gastric damage [22], exogenously administered prostaglandins have been reported to decrease gastric mucosal injury in a wide variety of models of experimental ulceration, but as yet the mechanisms responsible for such action are not clearly understood [23]. Acute stimulation with capsaicin of peripheral afferent sensory fibres located in the gastric mucosa has been shown to prevent deep mucosal injury induced by ethanol, and other ulcerogens [4,5], a protective effect similar to that induced by prostaglandins. Furthermore, prostaglandins, particularly the E-type, have been shown to stimulate sensory neurons, an effect inhibited by opioids [17]. However, gastric mucosal protection mediated by afferent nerves does not depend on prostanoid formation [2]. In the present study, administration of morphine, at doses that exert comparable effects on ethanol damage as those induced by capsaicin desensitization, led to a significant reduction in the protective effects of PGE_2 against ethanol-induced gastric mucosal damage. Although high doses of PGE_2 still exerted some protection, lower doses were ineffective. Similar findings on the effects of morphine pretreatments have been previously observed with the potent prostaglandins analogue 16, 16 dimethyl PGE_2 [24]. These observations thus indicate the involvement of opioid-sensitive processes in the mechanisms contributing to protection of the gastric mucosa by prostaglandins against challenge. Opioids, acting on peripheral sites, thus appear to mimic the actions of capsaicin-pretreatment in enhancing gastric mucosal damage induced by ulcerogenic agents. Such effect may be brought about by prevention of the release of protective neuropeptides such as calcitonin-gene related peptide (CGRP) from local sensory neurons. Not only do such sensory neurons and their mediators appear to modulate the ability of the mucosa to withstand challenge, the present studies also suggest that the protective mechanisms of other endogenous mediators such as PGE_2 may also involve interactions with opioid-sensitive sensory processes.

ACKNOWLEDGEMENT

*The preparation of this manuscript has been supported by grants
(FAR No. 89-0432) from
"Programa Nacional de Investigacion y Desarrollo Farmaceutico"
and (FIS No. 88/1947) from
"Fondo de Investigaciones Sanitarias" (Spain).*

REFERENCES

1.   Szolcsanyi J. Bartho L. Impaired defense mechanisms to peptic ulcer in the capsaicin-desensitized rat. In: Gastrointestinal defense mechanisms. Mozsik Gy. Hanninen O. Javor T. (eds) Oxford and Budapest: Pergamon Press and Akademiai Kiado: 1981; pp 39-51

2.   Holzer P. Sametz W. Gastric mucosal protection against ulcerogenic factors in the rat mediated by capsaicin-sensitive afferent neurons. Gastroenterology 1986; 91: 975-81.

3.   Esplugues JV. Whittle BJR. Moncada S. Local opioid-sensitive afferent sensory neurones in the modulation of gastric damage induced by Paf. Br J Pharmacol. 1989; 97: 579-85.

4.   Holzer P. Lippe ITh. Stimulation of afferent nerve endings by intragastric capsaicin protects against ethanol-induced damage of the gastric mucosa. Neuroscience 1988; 27: 981-87.

5.   Holzer P. Pabst MA. Lippe ITh. Intragastric capsaicin protects against aspirin-induced lesion formation and bleeding in the rat gastric mucosa. Gastroenterology 1989; 96: 1425-33.

6.   Selye M. A syndrome produced by diverse nocuous agents. Nature 1935; 138: 32-40.

7.   Gyires K. Furst S. Farczadi E. Marton A. Morphine potentiates the gastroulcerogenic effect of indomethacin. Pharmacology 1985; 30: 25-31.

8.   Till M. Gati T. Rabai K. Szombath D. Szekeley JI. Effect of [D-Met^2-Pro^5] enkephalinamide on gastric ulceration and transmucosal potential difference. Eur J Pharmacol 1988; 150: 325-30.

9.   Konishi S. Tsunoo A. Yanaihara N. Otsuka M. Peptidergic excitatory and inhibitory synapses in mammalian sympathetic ganglia: roles of substance P and enkephalin. Biomed Res 1980; 1: 528-35.

10.   Brodin E. Gazelius B. Panopoulos P. Olgart L. Morphine inhibits substance P release from peripheral sensory nerve endings. Acta Physiol Scand 1983; 117: 567-72.

11.   Bartho L. Szolcsanyi J. Opiate agonists inhibit neurogenic plasma extravasation in the rat. Eur J Pharmacol. 1981; 73: 101-4.

12.   Smith TW, Buchan P, Parsons DN, Wilkinson S. Peripheral antinoceptive effects of N-methylmorphine. Life Sci 1982; 31: 1205-8.

13.   Lembeck F. Donnerer J. Opioid control of the function of primary afferent substance P fibres. Eur J Pharmacol. 1985; 114: 241-6.

14.   Gamse R, Saria A. Antidromic vasodilatation in the rat hindpaw measured by laser Doppler flowmetry: pharmacological modulation. J Auton Nerv Syst 1987; 19: 105-11.

15.   Ferreira SH, Nakamura M. II-Prostaglandin hyperalgesia. The peripheral analgesic activity of morphine, enkephalins and opioid antagonists. Prostaglandins 1979; 18: 191-200.

16.   Russell NJW. Schaible H-G, Schmidt RF. Opiates inhibit the discharges of fine afferent units from inflamed knee joint of the cat. Neurosci Lett 1987; 76: 107-12.

17.   Coleridge HM. Coleridge JCG. Ginzel KH. Baker DG, Banzett RB. Morrison MA. Stimulation by "irritant" receptors and afferent C-fibres in the lung by prostaglandins. Nature (Lond) 1976; 264: 451-453.

18.   Esplugues JV. Whittle BJR. Morphine potentiation of ethanol-induced gastric mucosal damage in the rat: Role of local sensory afferent neurons. Gastroenterology 1990; 98: 82-89.

19. Guth PH. Paulsen G. Nagata H. Histologic and microcirculatory changes in alcohol-induced gastric lesions in the rat: effect of prostaglandin cytoprotection. Gastroenterology 1984; 87: 1083-90.

20. Szabo S, Trier JS, Brown A, Schnoor J. Early vascular injury and increased vascular permeability in gastric mucosal injury caused by ethanol in the rat. Gastroenterology 1985; 88: 228-36.

21. Pique JM, Esplugues JV. Whittle BJR. Influence of morphine or capsaicin pretreatment on rat gastric microcirculatory response to PAF. Am J Physiol 1990; 258: G352-57.

22. Robert A. Cytoprotection by prostaglandins in rats. Prevention of gastric necrosis produced by alcohol, HCl, NaOH, Hypertonic NaCl, and thermal injury. Gastroenterology 1979; 77: 433-443.

23. Whittle BJR. Vane JR. Prostanoids as regulators of gastrointestinal function. In: Physiology of the gastrointestinal tract. Jonhson LR. Christensen J. Jackson MJ. Jacobson ED. Walsh JH. (Eds) New York: Raven Press (2nd Edition): 1987; 143-80.

24. Esplugues JV. Whittle BJR. Prostaglandin protection of the rat gastric mucosa is attenuated by opioids. Gastroenterology 1990; 98:A-42.

ROLE OF THE ENDOGENOUS VASOACTIVE MEDIATORS, NITRIC OXIDE, PROSTANOIDS AND SENSORY NEUROPEPTIDES IN THE REGULATION OF GASTRIC BLOOD FLOW AND MUCOSAL INTEGRITY

Brendon J.R. Whittle and Barry L. Tepperman

*Department of Pharmacology, Wellcome Research Laboratories,
Langley Court, Beckenham, Kent, U.K.*

ABSTRACT

The interactions between the endothelium-derived relaxing factor, nitric oxide (NO), the sensory neuropeptides released from primary afferent neurones, and the endogenous prostanoids, in the regulation of gastric mucosal blood flow and integrity has been investigated. The inhibitor of NO biosynthesis, N^G-monomethyl-L-arginine (L-NMMA, 0.8 - 50mg kg^{-1} i.v.) induced a dose-dependent fall in resting gastric mucosal blood flow as determined by laser Doppler flowmetry (LDF) in the anaesthetised rat. In rats pretreated with capsaicin, two weeks prior to study to deplete sensory neuropeptides from primary afferent neurones, the fall in LDF induced by sub-threshold doses of L-NMMA was substantially augmented. This indicates an interaction between sensory neuropeptides and NO in the modulation of microvascular perfusion. Treatment with indomethacin (5mg kg^{-1} i.v.), to inhibit endogenous prostanoids, did not significantly enhance the fall in LDF induced by L-NMMA in either control or capsaicin-pretreated rats. This suggests a minimal role of endogenous prostanoids in the regulation of mucosal blood flow under these conditions. Whereas L-NMMA alone did not induce acute mucosal damage, extensive haemorrhagic necrosis was observed in capsaicin-pretreated rats, which was further augmented by indomethacin administration. These findings thus suggest that the interactions between endogenous vasoactive mediators NO, sensory neuropeptides and prostanoids play a crucial role in the regulation of mucosal integrity, which may involve effects on both mucosal blood flow and the continuity of the microvasculature.

INTRODUCTION

The integrity of the gastric mucosa is critically dependent on adequate microvascular perfusion. Thus, agents that cause direct vasoconstriction, can induce acute gastric mucosal injury. Such endogenous local vasoconstrictor mediators exerting pro-ulcerogenic actions on the gastric mucosa include thromboxane A_2 [1,2], endothelin-1 [3,4] noradrenaline and neuropeptide Y [5].

A reduction in the release or activity of local vasodilator mediators in the gastric microcirculation can also compromise mucosal integrity. Thus, inhibition of vasodilator prostanoid synthesis by non-steroid anti-inflammatory agents is considered to be one mechanism by which treatment with such agents can lead to gastric injury and make the mucosa more susceptible to damage [6]. Furthermore, the mechanism by which pretreatment with capsaicin augments damage induced by pro-ulcerogenic agents is likely to involve the destruction of primary afferent neurones, resulting in depletion of their vasodilator sensory neuropeptides such as calcitonin gene-related peptide (CGRP), in the gastric mucosa [7,8,9].

A further vasodilator mediator that may play a crucial role in the microcirculation is the endothelium-derived relaxing factor, nitric oxide [10,11,12], formed from L-arginine [13]. The biosynthesis of nitric oxide (NO) can be inhibited by the L-arginine analogue, N^G-monomethyl-L-arginine (L-NMMA) both *in vitro* and *in vivo* [14,15]. Furthermore, in doses that also elevate systemic arterial blood pressure in the rat [16], L-NMMA can reduce resting gastric mucosal blood flow, as estimated by hydrogen gas clearance [17].

These endogenous vasodilator mediators may interact in the regulation of the gastric microcirculation and mucosal integrity [18]. In the present study, therefore, the mechanisms by which depletion of sensory neuropeptides or inhibition of cyclo-oxygenase can greatly potentiate the mucosal injury by L-NMMA [18], has been investigated. Thus, the effects of intravenous administration of L-NMMA on gastric mucosal blood flow, as measured by laser Doppler flowmetry, has now been determined following capsaicin-pretreatment or indomethacin administration in the rat.

METHODS

MEASUREMENT OF GASTRIC MUCOSAL BLOOD FLOW

Male Wistar rats (230-260g body weight) were deprived of food but not water for 18-20 hours before the experiment. Animals were anaesthetised with sodium pentobarbitone (60 mg kg^{-1} i.p.) and the stomach exposed by a mid-line incision. A short small bore (8.5 mm OD) plastic cannula was then inserted via a small incision in the forestomach and tied in place, to allow free access to the gastric lumen. Any gastric contents were gently aspirated and gastric blood flow was recorded continuously using a laser Doppler blood flow monitor (Moor Instruments Model MBF3D).

The principles and use of laser Doppler flowmetry for assessment of gastric mucosal blood flow in the rat has previously been described [19]. In the present study, a stainless steel laser optic probe (1.65mm OD; Moor Instruments) was inserted into the gastric lumen via the plastic cannula and was allowed to rest gently on the upper regions of the gastric fundic mucosa. Changes in laser Doppler flow (LDF) were assessed in response to intravenous bolus injection (0.1-0.5 ml) of isotonic saline or the compounds under investigation, L-NMMA (Figure 1; Wellcome Research Laboratories) or indomethacin (Sigma Chemical Company). Average LDF values were determined for the 3 min period just prior to drug administration. Similarly the average LDF was calculated for a subsequent 3 min period when values of LDF had stabilised, usually 5 min after drug administration.

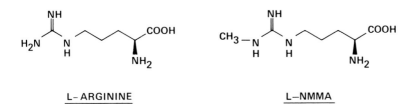

L–ARGININE   L–NMMA

FIGURE 1   *Chemical structure of the substrate for nitric oxide (NO) synthesis, L-arginine, and of the NO-synthase inhibitor, N^G-monomethyl-L-arginine (L-NMMA).*

Compounds were administered via the intravenous route using a 25G hypodermic needle and 0.3 mm polyethelene cannula inserted into a tail vein. The mean systemic arterial blood pressure (BP) was also measured from a cannula inserted into a carotid artery and connected to a pressure transducer (Bell and Howell, Ashford, U.K.) and a chart recorder (Grass model 7D polygraph).

ASSESSMENT OF GASTRIC MUCOSAL DAMAGE

Male Wistar rats (230-260g), were anaesthetized with sodium pentobarbitone (60 mg kg^{-1}, i.p.), the stomach exposed by a mid-line incision and 2 ml of acid saline (100mM HCl) was instilled into the gastric lumen via a needle inserted through the forestomach, followed by bolus intravenous administration of L-NMMA through a tail vein. Forty-five minutes later, the stomachs were opened along the greater curvature, pinned to a wax block, immersed in neutral buffered formalin and photographed. The percentage of the total gastric mucosa showing macroscopically visible damage was determined via computerized planimetry in a randomized manner.

CAPSAICIN-PRETREATMENT

To deplete sensory neuropeptides, adult rats (190-210g) were treated under halothane anaesthesia with capsaicin in increasing doses (20, 30 and 50 mg kg^{-1}, s.c.) over three consecutive days and the animals were used 2 weeks later, as described previously in detail [18].

STATISTICAL ANALYSIS

All data are expressed as mean ± s.e. mean. Comparisons between groups of parametric data were made by Student's t-test for unpaired data, or analysis of variance and Duncan's multiple range test, where P values of less than 0.05 were taken as significant.

RESULTS

EFFECTS OF L-NMMA ON GASTRIC BLOOD FLOW

In control studies, resting laser Doppler flow (LDF), the index of gastric mucosal blood flow, remained stable over a 1h period. Intravenous bolus injection of L-NMMA (0.8-50 mg kg^{-1}) induced a dose-dependent fall in LDF, as shown in Figure 2. The fall in LDF began within 1 min of administration of L-NMMA, and reached its maximal fall within 3 min. The maximal reduction in LDF achieved with L-NMMA (50 mg kg^{-1}), was 28 $\pm$ 9% (n = 5; P<0.05).

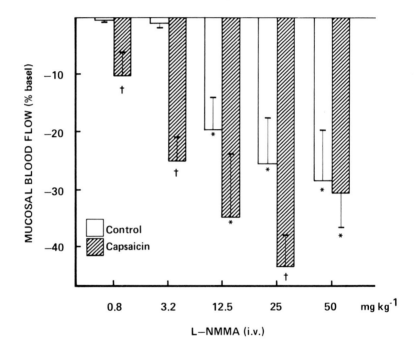

FIGURE 2.   Effects of capsaicin-pretreatment (2 weeks earlier) on the fall in gastric mucosal blood flow induced by L-NMMA (0.8 - 5 mg kg^{-1} i.v.), as assessed by laser Doppler flowmetry in the anaesthetised rat. Results, expressed as the reduction, % of basal, are the mean $\pm$ s.e. mean of 5 experiments for each group, where significant change from basal is shown as *P<0.05 and from L-NMMA alone as $^{+}$P<0.05.

EFFECTS OF CAPSAICIN

In rats pretreated 2 weeks earlier with capsaicin, intravenous administration of sub-threshold doses of L-NMMA (0.8 and 3.2 mg kg^{-1}), now induced substantial (P<0.05) dose-dependent reductions in LDF (Figure 2).

Likewise, the effects of the higher dose of L-NMMA (25 mg kg^{-1}) was significantly greater than in vehicle-pretreated rats, with a maximal reduction in LDF of 43 ± 6% (n = 4, P<0.05). Capsaicin administration did not, however, increase the reduction in the LDF induced by the maximal dose of L-NMMA (Figure 2).

EFFECTS OF INDOMETHACIN

Intravenous administration of indomethacin (5 mg kg^{-1}) did not significantly augment the reduction in LDF induced by L-NMMA (0.8 - 50 mg kg^{-1} i.v.,), as shown in Figure 3. Furthermore, indomethacin administration did not further enhance the augmented reduction in LDF induced by L-NMMA in capsaicin-pretreated rats (Figure 3). This dose of indomethacin alone did not significantly reduce resting LDF over this observation period (n = 4).

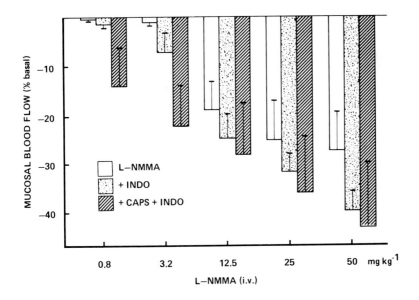

FIGURE 3. *Effects of pretreatment (15 min) with indomethacin (5 mg kg^{-1} i.v.) on the fall in gastric mucosal blood flow induced by L-NMMA (0.8 - 50 mg kg^{-1} i.v.) in vehicle or capsaicin-pretreated rats. Results, expressed as the reduction, % of basal, are the mean ± s.e. mean of 5 experiments for each group. Indomethacin did not significantly (P<0.05) augment the changes in either control or capsaicin-pretreated rats.*

EFFECTS ON SYSTEMIC ARTERIAL BLOOD PRESSURE.

Intravenous administration of L-NMMA (0.8 - 50 mg kg^{-1}) induced a dose-dependent rise in systemic arterial blood pressure, reaching a maximal value of 48 ± 3 mmHg (n = 5; P<0.01) above its resting value (101 ± 3 mmHg: n = 24). Administration of indomethacin (5 mg kg^{-1} i.v.) did not significantly alter this hypertensive response to L-NMMA (Figure 4). Furthermore, the apparent depression of the dose-response relationship with L-NMMA, or with L-NMMA in combination with indomethacin, in animals pretreated with capsaicin, did not reach significance (Figure 4).

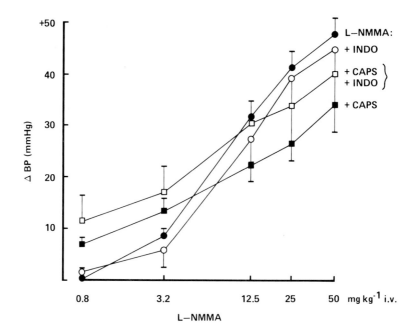

FIGURE 4.   Effects of L-NMMA (0.8 mg kg^{-1} i.v.) on systemic arterial blood pressure (BP) in the rat, in control experiments and following pretreatment with capsaicin (CAPS) or administration of indomethacin (INDO: 5 mg kg^{-1} i.v.). Results shown as BP (mmHg), are the mean ± s.e. mean of 4-5 experiments for each group.

MUCOSAL DAMAGE AND L-NMMA

Intravenous administration of L-NMMA (12.5 and 100 mg kg^{-1}) alone did not lead to macroscopically detectable mucosal damage, when assessed 45 min after administration.   However, significant areas of mucoal injury could be observed following L-NMMA administration in capsaicin-pretreated rats (Figure 5). This mucosal injury was apparent macroscopically as surface cell damage, vasocongestion and haemorrhage. Capsaicin-pretreatment alone did not induce detectable damage to the mucosa (Figure 5).

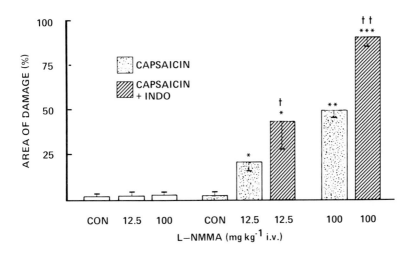

FIGURE 5. *Potentiation of the gastric mucosal damage induced by L-NMMA (12.5 and 50 mg kg^{-1} i.v.) by capsaicin-pretreatment and indomethacin (5 mg kg^{-1} i.v.) administration. Results, given as the % of the total mucosal area that exhibited macroscopic mucosal damage, are the mean ± s.e. mean of 4-5 experiments in each group, where significant difference from the corresponding control is shown as *P<0.05, **P<0.01, ***P<0.001 and the increase by indomethacin in the corresponding group as +P<0.05, ++P<0.01. This data is derived in part from the study of Whittle et al [18].*

The dose-dependent mucosal injury induced by L-NMMA (12.5 and 100 mg kg^{-1} i.v.) over the 45 min period in capsaicin-pretreated rats was further significantly augmented by the administration of indomethacin (5mg kg^{-1} i.v.) as shown in Figure 5. At the higher dose of L-NMMA under these conditions, this damage involved the total area of the mucosa including both corpus and antral regions and was macroscopically apparent as wide-spread epithelial sloughing, vasocongestion, with distinct haemorrhagic and necrotic lesions.

DISCUSSION

The present study demonstrates that the inhibitor of NO synthase, L-NMMA, reduces resting gastric mucosal blood flow in the rat, as assessed by laser Doppler flowmetry. These findings, which confirm our previous observations using hydrogen-gas clearance to measure mucosal blood flow

[17], thus implicate endogenous NO, synthesized from L-arginine by the vascular endothelial cells, in the modulation of the gastric microcirculation.

Pretreatment with capsaicin substantially augmented the reduction in mucosal blood flow following L-NMMA administration, particularly those induced by sub-threshold doses. Such effects suggest significant interactions between sensory neuropeptides and NO in the regulation of blood flow. Indeed, the anatomical close-proximity of the capsaicin-sensitive primary afferent neurones to the submucosal microvasculature [20] would provide adequate opportunity for such vascular actions to occur.

It was not possible to assess whether such capsaicin-pretreatment itself reduced resting mucosal blood flow in the current study, since the laser Doppler technique used can only determine relative changes in the same animal. However, present studies using hydrogen gas clearance have demonstrated that treatment of neonates with capsaicin, which permanently destroys primary afferent neurones, did not subsequently affect resting mucosal blood flow in the adult rat [21]. These findings suggest that depletion of sensory neuropeptides alone is not sufficient to affect resting blood flow when adequate endogenous NO is available to the microcirculation. However, under conditions of partial reduction in NO synthesis, such as those following administration of L-NMMA, the demands of the microcirculation may be met at least in part, by the local release of sensory neuropeptides. The occurrence of such interactive mechanisms in the regulation of vascular tone and blood flow would seem appropriate in view of its importance for tissue integrity.

Administration of indomethacin, in a dose sufficient to inhibit near-maximally gastric mucosal cyclo-oxygenase [6], did not significantly augment the fall in mucosal blood flow induced by L-NMMA, nor did it further enhance the L-NMMA-induced fall in mucosal blood flow in capsaicin-pretreated rats. These findings thus suggest that under the present experimental conditions, endogenous prostanoids do not make a significant contribution to the regulation of blood flow in the mucosa under conditions of reduced NO formation and depletion of sensory neuropeptides.

Acute administration of L-NMMA induced dose-related mucosal injury in capsaicin-pretreated rats, but not in vehicle-pretreated rats [18]. Like the effects on mucosal blood flow, the entantiomer D-NMMA which does not inhibit NO synthesis [14], had no such damaging effect, while the actions of L-NMMA on both mucosal blood flow and injury could be reversed by concurrent administration of L-arginine [17,18]. The injurious actions of L-NMMA under these conditions could be related to the enhanced reduction in mucosal blood flow seen clearly with the lower doses of L-NMMA in capsaicin-pretreated rats, leading to levels of microvascular perfusion inadequate for tissue survival. However, the findings that the mucosal injury induced by high doses of L-NMMA was also augmented in capsaicin-pretreated rats, yet the fall in blood flow was not further enhanced, could suggest that sensory neuropeptides may also exert additional protective actions, such as by enhancing the integrity of the microvasculature. It has been proposed that damage to the endothelium and capillary network is a primary event in the pathogenesis of mucosal injury and necrosis induced by topical irritants [22,23] and such local intravascular events are also likely to operate with other pro-ulcerogenic mediators [24]. Indeed, the vasocongestion and haemorrhagic necrosis induced by L-NMMA in capsaicin-pretreated rats further suggests that these pathological events are initiated at the level of the microcirculation. In addition, endogenous NO could also contribute to the maintenance of endothelial continuity and hence protect the mucosa from injury, both by blood-borne mediators or by topical challenge.

The findings of a substantial increase in mucosal damage induced by L-NMMA in capsaicin-pretreated rats following indomethacin administration, but with no additional reduction in mucosal blood flow, suggests a pro-ulcerogenic mechanism following prostanoid inhibition, not related directly to a further compromised microvascular perfusion. It is relevant therefore that the protective effects of exogenous prostanoids against topical challenge in the gastric mucosa has been attributed to the prevention of microvascular stasis, rather than to direct vasodilatation [22,25], an effect that may reflect actions on the integrity of the microvascular endothelium. Thus, inhibition of endogenous mucosal prostanoids, including endothelium-derived prostacyclin, along with depletion of sensory neuropeptides, may make the microvasculature more susceptible to the detrimental effects of reduced blood flow following L-NMMA, leading to the extensive mucosal damage observed.

The present study thus provides further evidence of the importance of blood flow and vasoactive mediators in the modulation of mucosal injury. The findings suggest that NO, prostanoids and sensory neuropeptides interact not only in the maintenance of adequate blood flow, but in the preservation of microvascular and tissue integrity. Such interactions between diverse physiological mediators appear essential for the provision of mucosal stability and protection against damage.

ACKNOWLEDGEMENT

*Barry L. Tepperman is a recipient of a
Commonwealth Medical Fellowship.*

REFERENCES

1. Whittle BJR, Kauffman GL, Moncada S. Vasoconstriction with thromboxane A2 induces ulceration of the gastric mucosa. Nature 1981; 292: 472-474.

2. Esplugues JV, Whittle BJR. Close-arterial administration of the thromboxane mimetic U-46619 induces damage to the rat gastric mucosa. Prostaglandins 1988; 35: 137-148.

3. Whittle BJR, Esplugues JV. Induction of rat gastric damage by the endothelium-derived peptide, endothelin. Br J Pharmacol 1988; 95: 1011-1013.

4.   Wallace JL, Cirino G, de Nucci G, McKnight W, MacNaughton WK.
      Endothelin has potent ulcerogenic and vasoconstrictor actions in the
      stomach. Am J Physiol 1989; 256: G661-666.

5.   Tepperman BL, Whittle BJR.   Actions of noradrenaline and
      neuropeptide Y on gastric mucosal blood flow and integrity in the
      anaesthetized rat. J Physiol 1990; 426: 87P.

6.   Whittle BJR. The mechanisms of gastric damage by non-steroid anti-
      inflammatory drugs. In: Cohen M (ed) Biological Protection with
      Prostaglandins, Florida: CRC Press 1986; 1-27.

7.   Holzer P, Sametz W. Gastric mucosal protection against ulcerogenic
      factors in the rat mediated by capsaicin-sensitive afferent neurones.
      Gastroenterology. 1986; 91: 975-981.

8.   Szolcsany J, Bartho L. Impaired defense mechanism in peptic ulcer
      in the capsaicin-desensitized rat. In: Mozsik GH, Hanninen O, Javor
      T (eds). Gastrointestinal defense mechanisms. Oxford and Budapest:
      Pergamon Press and Akademiai Kiaod, 1981; 39-51.

9.   Holzer P. Local effector functions of capsaicin-sensitive sensory
      nerve endings: involvement of tachykinins, calcitonin gene-related
      peptide and other neuropeptides. Neuroscience 1988; 24: 739-768.

10.   Palmer RMJ, Ferridge AG, Moncada S. Nitric oxide release accounts
      for the biological activity of endothelium-derived relaxing factor.
      Nature 1987; 327: 524-526.

11.   Khan MT, Furchgott RF. Additional evidence that endothelium-
      derived relaxing factor is nitric oxide. In: Rand MJ, Raper C. (eds).
      Pharmacology, New York, Elsevier. 1987; 341-344.

12.   Ignarro LJ, Buga GM, Wood KS, Byrns RE, Chaudhuri G.
      Endothelium-derived relaxing factor produced and released from
      artery and vein is nitric oxide. Proc Natl Acad Sci USA 1987; 84:
      9265-9269.

13.   Palmer RMJ, Ashton DS, Moncada S. Vascular endothelial cells
      synthesize nitric oxide from L-arginine. Nature 1988; 333: 664-666.

14.   Rees DD, Palmer RMJ, Hodson HF, Moncada S. A specific inhibitor
      of nitric oxide formation from L-arginine attenuates endothelium-
      dependent relaxation. Br J Pharmacol 1989; 96: 418-424.

15.   Rees DD, Palmer RMJ, Moncada S. Role of endothelium-derived
      oxide in the regulation of blood pressure. Proc Natl Acad Sci USA
      1989; 86: 3375-3378.

16.   Whittle BJR, Lopez-Belmonte J, Rees DD. Modulation of the
      vasodepressor actions of acetylcholine, bradykinin, substance P and
      endothelin in the rat by a specific inhibitor of nitric oxide
      formation. Br J Pharmacol 1989; 98: 646-652.

17. Pique JM, Whittle BJR, Esplugues JV. The vasodilator role of endogenous nitric oxide in the rat gastric microcirculation. Eur J Pharmacol 1989; 171: 293-296.

18. Whittle BJR, Lopez-Belmonte J, Moncada S. Regulation of gastric mucosal integrity by endogenous nitric oxide: interactions with prostanoids and sensory neuropeptides in the rat. Br J Pharmacol 1990; 99: 607-611.

19. Holm-Rutili L, Berglindh T. Pentagastrin and gastric mucosal blood flow. Am J Physiol. 1988; 250: G525-580.

20. Green T, Dockray GJ. Characterization of the peptidergic afferent innervation of the stomach in the rat, mouse, and guinea-pig. Neuroscience 1988; 25: 181-193.

21. Pique JM, Esplugues JV, Whittle BJR. Influence of morphine or capsaicin pretreatment on rat gastric microcirculatory response to PAF. Am J Physiol 1990; 258: G352-357.

22. Guth PH, Paulsen G, Nagata H. Histological and microcirculatory changes in alcohol-induced gastric lesions in the rat: effect of prostaglandin cytoprotection. Gastroenterology 1984; 87: 1083-1090.

23. Szabo Sj, Trier JS, Brown A, Schnoor J. Early vascular injury and increased vascular permeability in gastric mucosal injury caused by ethanol in the rat. Gastroenterology 1985; 88: 228-236.

24. Whittle BJR, Esplugues JV. Pro-ulcerogenic eicosanoids and related lipid mediators in gastro-intestinal damage. In: Garner A, Whittle BJR. (eds) Advances in Drug Therapy of Gastrointestinal Ulceration, Chichester, England. John Wiley & Sons 1989; 165-188.

25. Pihan G, Majzoubi D, Haudenschild C, Trier JS, Szabo S. Early microcirculatory stasis in acute gastric mucosal injury in the rat and prevention by 16, 16-dimethyl prostaglandin E2 or sodium thiosulfate. Gastroenterology 1986; 91: 1415-1426.

MEDIATION OF NSAID-INDUCED GASTROPATHY BY LEUKOCYTES AND LEUKOCYTE-DERIVED PRODUCTS

John Wallace, Catherine Keenan, Webb McKnight, and Paula Vaananen

Gastrointestinal Research Group, University of Calgary, Calgary, Alberta, Canada

ABSTRACT

The role of neutrophils in the pathogenesis of ulceration induced by non-steroidal anti-inflammatory drugs was investigated. Neutrophil adherence to the vascular endothelium may be involved in producing the reduction of mucosal blood flow which precedes the onset of ulceration. In addition, neutrophil-derived products could contribute to the tissue necrosis which follows the administration of this class of drugs. These hypotheses were tested by examining the effects of: 1. depletion of circulating neutrophils by pretreatment with an anti-neutrophil serum; 2. depletion of tissue-associated granulocytes in the gastric mucosa; 3. increasing the number of tissue-associated granulocytes in the gastric mucosa; 4. prevention of the adherence of circulating leukocytes to the vascular endothelium; 5. treatment with an enzyme which is capable of scavenging oxygen-derived free radicals. Reduction of circulating neutrophil numbers by >95% by treatment with anti-neutrophil serum was accompanied by a significant decrease (~85%) in the extent of injury induced in the rat stomach by indomethacin. Decreasing or increasing the levels of mucosal tissue-associated granulocytes did not modify the susceptibility to indomethacin-induced damage. Prevention of leukocyte adherence to the vascular endothelium resulted in complete prevention of indomethacin-induced gastric damage in the rabbit. Intravenous administration of the hydrogen peroxide scavenging enzyme, catalase, resulted in a significant reduction of indomethacin-induced gastric damage in the rat. These results support a role for the circulating leukocyte, especially the neutrophil, in the pathogenesis of gastric injury induced by non-steroidal anti-inflammatory drugs.

INTRODUCTION

Leukocytes, particularly neutrophils, have been implicated in the pathogenesis of several types of gastrointestinal ulceration. For example, neutrophils have been shown to play an important role in experimental models of ischemia-reperfusion injury in the intestine [1] and hemorrhagic shock-induced damage in the stomach [2]. More recently, neutrophils have been suggested to be involved in ethanol-induced gastric damage [3].

139

Neutrophils might contribute to ulceration by adhering to the vascular endothelium of mucosal vessels, thereby occluding the vessels and reducing mucosal blood flow.   Neutrophils also can release a number of substances which can cause tissue necrosis, including oxygen-derived free radicals, myeloperoxidase, hypochlorous acid and proteases.   These products are capable of producing damage to the vascular endothelium, a characteristic of NSAID-induced gastropathy seen within minutes of administration of these drugs to experimental animals [4,5].

In the present study, we have investigated the possible contribution of leukocytes to the pathogenesis of ulceration induced by non-steroidal anti-inflammatory drugs (NSAIDs).   While it is clear that the ulcerogenic properties of NSAIDs correlate well with their ability to inhibit gastric prostaglandin synthesis, it is not clear how such inhibition contributes to the development of ulcers.   NSAIDs cause a reduction of mucosal blood flow in the regions which eventually ulcerate [6-8], and this has been shown to be preceded by the formation of "white thrombi" in mucosal microvessels [7]. It is therefore possible that leukocyte adherence to the vascular endothelium is a precipitating event in the pathogenesis of NSAID-induced ulceration, and that the subsequent release of various products, such as free radicals, may contribute to the production of tissue necrosis.

METHODS

Male, Wistar rats (175-225 g), or male New Zealand white rabbits (500-700 g), were deprived of food, but not water, for 18-24 hours prior to an experiment.   In the rat experiments, gastric damage was induced by oral administration of indomethacin at a dose of 20 mg/kg.   Control rats received an equivalent volume of the vehicle (1.25% sodium bicarbonate). The rats were killed 3 hours later and the extent of macroscopically visible hemorrhagic damage scored by an observer unaware of the treatment.   The lesions were counted and their lengths measured.   The gastric damage score for each stomach was the sum of the lengths of all lesions, in mm.

Effects of Depletion of Circulating Neutrophils

In order to determine the contribution of neutrophils to the ulceration induced in the rat stomach by indomethacin, the effects of prior depletion of circulating neutrophils was assessed.   One group of rats was treated intraperitoneally with an anti-neutrophil serum (ANS) raised in goats against rat neutrophils [2] 18 hours prior to administration of indomethacin.   A blood sample was taken from each rat and differential counts were performed to confirm that neutropenia had been induced.   In all rats treated with ANS, the circulating neutrophil count was reduced by >95% [5].   Control rats did not receive any treatment prior to indomethacin administration.   A second control group were treated with normal goat serum in place of ANS.

EFFECTS OF INCREASING OR DECREASING THE NUMBERS OF TISSUE-ASSOCIATED GRANULOCYTES.

In order to determine if tissue-associated granulocytes might play a role in the pathogenesis of indomethacin-induced ulceration, experiments were performed using rats in which gastric myeloperoxidase (MPO) levels had been significantly reduced or increased. MPO is an enzyme found primarily in the azurophilic granules of neutrophils, and has been used extensively as a biochemical marker of granulocyte infiltration into various tissues. Reduction of gastric MPO levels was accomplished by pretreatment with dexamethasone (4 mg/kg s.c.) 30 and 6 hours prior to administration of indomethacin. In addition to scoring the damage, tissue samples (~100 mg) were excised from the corpus region for subsequent determination of MPO activity. Enhancement of gastric MPO levels was accomplished by infecting rats with 3000 stage 3 larvae (s.c.) of *Nippostrongylus brasiliensis* 40 days prior to the experiment. Worm expulsion is virtually complete by 15 days after infection. In addition to increasing tissue MPO levels, this infection results in mast cell hyperplasia within the mucosa.

EFFECTS OF INHIBITION OF LEUKOCYTE ADHERENCE ON INDOMETHACIN-INDUCED GASTROPATHY

Rabbits were pretreated with the monoclonal antibody IB-4, which is directed against the β subunit (CD_{18}) of the leukocyte adhesion glycoprotein [9], 2 hours prior to intragastric instillation of indomethacin (5 mg/ml). The indomethacin solution was left in the stomach for 30 minutes, after which 100 mM HCl was instilled for one hour. At the end of this period the stomach was excised and the area of hemorrhagic damage measured by an observer unaware of the treatment, using micrometer calipers. Tissue samples were taken from the corpus for subsequent histological examination. Rabbits were used in these experiments because the antibody, which is directed against human CD_{18}, does not cross-react with rat CD_{18}.

EFFECTS OF A FREE RADICAL SCAVENGING ENZYME ON INDOMETHACIN-INDUCED GASTROPATHY

A perfused rat stomach preparation was used, similar to that described previously by Smith et al. [2]. Damage was assessed by measurement of blood to lumen clearance of ^{51}Cr-EDTA. ^{51}Cr-EDTA (87 uCi) was injected i.v. at the beginning of the experiment. After a 20 minute stabilization period, the stomach was perfused for 30 minutes with normal saline, followed by indomethacin (10 mg/ml for 30 min) and hydrochloric acid (100 mM for 60 min). The gastric perfusate was collected into tubes on a fraction collector, and blood samples were taken from the carotid artery every 15 minutes so that the blood level of ^{51}Cr-EDTA could be determined. In the experimental group, an intravenous infusion of catalase (25,000 U/kg/hour) was started at the time when the intragastric perfusion with saline was started, and was continued until the end of the experiment. Control rats received an intravenous infusion of the vehicle

(phosphate-buffered saline).   Catalase is an enzyme which catalyses the
conversion of hydrogen peroxide to water and molecular oxygen, and has
been shown to prevent the adherence of neutrophils to vascular endothelial
cells in vitro in response to hydrogen peroxide [10].

RESULTS

EFFECTS OF DEPLETION OF CIRCULATING NEUTROPHILS

Depletion of circulating neutrophils by administration of ANS
resulted in a significant change in the susceptibility of the gastric mucosa to
injury induced by indomethacin (Figure 1).   Neutropenic rats were virtually
spared of damage induced by a high dose of indomethacin.   This reduction
of damage was not due to effects of the ANS on gastric acid secretion, nor
to effects of the ANS on the inhibition of gastric cyclo-oxygenase by
indomethacin [5].   The effect of ANS also did not appear to be a non-
specific response to the foreign serum, since treatment of rats with normal
goat serum did not significantly affect the susceptibility to indomethacin-
induced gastric damage.

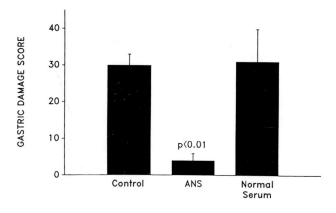

FIGURE 1. *Effects   of   depletion   of   circulating   neutrophils   on
susceptibility to indomethacin-induced gastric damage.   Rats were
pretreated with an anti-neutrophil serum (ANS), the vehicle or with
normal goat serum 18 hours prior to oral administration of indomethacin
(20 mg/kg).   Damage was scored three hours later by an observer
unaware of the treatment.   The ANS reduced circulating neutrophil
numbers by >95%. Each bar represents the mean ± SEM of at least 5
experiments. Figure adapted from data presented in reference 5.*

EFFECTS OF INCREASING OR DECREASING THE NUMBERS OF TISSUE-ASSOCIATED GRANULOCYTES.

As shown in Figure 2, treatment with dexamethasone resulted in almost complete abolition of MPO activity in the stomach   Despite the decrease in tissue-associated MPO activity, this treatment did not significantly affect the susceptibility to indomethacin-induced gastric damage.   On the other hand, a three-fold increase in gastric MPO activity, as was seen in rats previously infected with *Nippostrongylus brasiliensis*, did not significantly alter susceptibility to indomethacin-induced gastropathy.

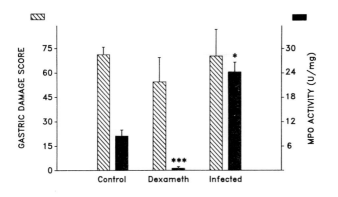

FIGURE 2: *Effects of decreasing (with dexamethasone treatment) or increasing (with N. brasiliensis infection) the numbers of tissue-associated granulocytes (as measured by myeloperoxidase (MPO) activity) on susceptibility to gastric damage induced by indomethacin (20 mg/kg p.o.). Dexamethasone was administered (4 mg/kg s.c.) 6 and 30 hours prior to indomethacin administration.   The infection with N. brasiliensis was performed 40 days prior to the experiment. While the parasite is virtually eliminated from the rat by 15 days post-infection, mastocytosis and elevated MPO levels persist for many weeks thereafter. Each bar represents the mean ± SEM of at least 5 experiments.*

EFFECTS OF INHIBITION OF LEUKOCYTE ADHERENCE ON INDOMETHACIN-INDUCED GASTROPATHY.

Intragastric administration of indomethacin to the rabbit produced numerous small hemorrhagic erosions, largely confined to the corpus.   These lesions were usually on the order of 2-3 mm long and 1 mm wide.   In rabbits pretreated with the monoclonal antibody directed against CD18 (IB-4), the extent of indomethacin-induced damage was significantly reduced

(Figure 3). Only a few lesions per stomach were observed in this group of rabbits. In fact, the extent of damage in the group pretreated with IB-4 did not differ significantly from that in rabbits which received the vehicle (1.25% sodium bicarbonate) intragastrically instead of indomethacin (data not shown).

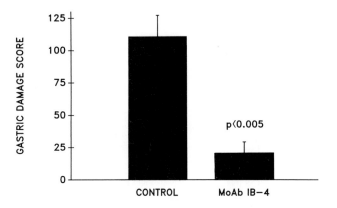

FIGURE 3: *Effects of pretreatment with a monoclonal antibody (IB-4) directed against the β subunit of the leukocyte adhesion complex on susceptibility of the rabbit to indomethacin-induced gastric damage. The rabbits were pretreated with IB-4 or the vehicle 2 hours prior to intragastric instillation of indomethacin at a concentration of 5 mg/ml. Damage was scored one hour after exposure to indomethacin by an observer unaware of the treatment. The level of damage observed in the group treated with IB-4 did not differ significantly from that observed in a control group which did not receive intragastric indomethacin. Each bar represents the mean ± SEM of 6 experiments.*

Histological examination of tissue samples from rabbits in the indomethacin control group revealed extensive vascular congestion associated with regions of leukocyte margination in mucosal and, to a lesser extent, submucosal vessels. While quantitative differentiation of the leukocytes was not performed, it was clear that the vast majority of the marginated leukocytes were neutrophils. These leukocytes were frequently observed to be occluding microvessels within the mucosa. In rabbits pretreated with IB-4, leukocyte margination and vascular congestion were much less prominent.

EFFECTS OF FREE RADICAL SCAVENGING ENZYMES ON INDOMETHACIN-INDUCED
GASTROPATHY.

Intragastric administration of indomethacin resulted in a marked
increase in the permeability of the gastric mucosa to ^{51}Cr-EDTA. As shown
in Figure 4, leakage of ^{51}Cr-EDTA into the lumen of the stomach increased
further when indomethacin was removed from the stomach and was replaced
with 100 mM HCl. When the stomachs were examined at the conclusion of
the experiment, there was extensive hemorrhagic damage (mean damage
score of 110 ± 6). Intravenous infusion of catalase resulted in a highly
significant (p<0.001) reduction of ^{51}Cr-EDTA leakage into the gastric lumen
during the period when indomethacin bathed the mucosa, and during the
subsequent two periods when the mucosa was exposed to 100 mM HCl. The
amount of ^{51}Cr-EDTA leakage in the catalase-treated group did not differ
significantly from that in a group of animals which received the vehicle for
indomethacin intragastrically (data not shown). Catalase infusion also
resulted in a significant decrease in macroscopically visible damage (mean
damage score of 60 ± 8; p<0.05).

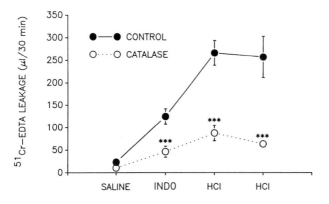

FIGURE 4: *Effects of intravenous infusion of catalase (25,000
U/kg/hour) on permeability of the gastric mucosa before, during and
after exposure to indomethacin (10mg/ml). ^{51}Cr-EDTA was injected
intravenously 20 minutes prior to the start of the experiment. The
leakage of ^{51}Cr-EDTA into the gastric lumen in rats treated with catalase
did not differ significantly from that observed in rats which did not
receive intragastric indomethacin. Asterisks denote a significant
difference between the two groups (p<0.001). Each point represents the
mean ± SEM of at least 5 experiments.*

DISCUSSION

The present results support the hypothesis that adherence of leukocytes to the vascular endothelium following administration of NSAIDs contributes significantly to the production of hemorrhagic erosions. Depletion of circulating neutrophils through treatment with an anti-neutrophil serum, or prevention of neutrophil (and other leukocyte) adherence through treatment with an antibody directed against the adhesion complex on these cells resulted in near-complete protection against indomethacin-induced gastric damage. It is not yet clear through what mechanism neutrophils or other leukocytes might contribute to ulceration. One possibility is that adherence of these cells to the endothelium results in reduced mucosal perfusion, thereby rendering the mucosa susceptible to injury by luminal acid. This hypothesis is supported by the observations of Kitahora and Guth [7] who noted the appearance of white thrombi in mucosal vessels shortly after topical application of aspirin. Mucosal blood flow subsequently slowed in the regions where the thrombi were observed, and eventually ulcers formed. The hypothesis is also supported by the histological evidence of leukocyte margination within the mucosa following administration of indomethacin to the rabbit. Neutrophil activation subsequent to adherence would also lead to the release of various products, such as free radicals and proteases, which could contribute to the ulceration process. We have previously shown that vascular endothelial damage occurs within 15 minutes of the administration of indomethacin to the rat, and that such damage does not occur in rats depleted of circulating neutrophils by pretreatment with ANS [5].

It is interesting that tissue-associate granulocytes, as detected by measurement of MPO activity, do not seem to play an important role in NSAID-induced gastric injury. Depletion of gastric MPO did not alter the susceptibility to ulceration, nor did increasing the tissue content of MPO-containing cells through infection with a nematode. It should be noted that although MPO is often measured as a biochemical marker of neutrophil numbers in a tissue, it is likely that eosinophil peroxidase might cross-react in most assays for MPO. It is not yet known to what extent tissue levels of MPO in the normal rat stomach is attributable to neutrophils versus other peroxidase containing cells. It is also not known to what extent the increase in MPO activity in the stomach of rats infected with *Nippostrongylus brasiliensis* is attributable to elevated numbers of neutrophils.

The hypothesis that neutrophil-derived free radicals might contribute to NSAID-induced ulceration is supported by the observation that catalase significantly reduced gastric injury, as determined by blood to lumen clearance of ^{51}Cr-EDTA. Although catalase did not completely prevent the formation of hemorrhagic lesions, it did reduce the changes in gastric mucosal permeability to the levels seen in control rats not receiving indomethacin. Pihan et al. [11] previously demonstrated that a higher dose of catalase (150,000 U/kg versus a total dose of 50,000 U/kg in the present study) significantly reduced the extent of macroscopically visible damage induced in the rat stomach by aspirin.   They also showed a significant reduction of damage with another free radical scavenging enzyme, superoxide dismutase.   The effects observed with catalase in the present study suggest a role for hydrogen peroxide in the pathogenesis of gastric injury induced by indomethacin.   Hydrogen peroxide might conribute to ulceration by inducing endothelial and other cellular necrosis [12].   It might also contribute to damage by promoting the adherence of circulating neutrophils to the vascular endothelium.   Lewis et al. [10] demonstrated that hydrogen peroxide increased the adherence of neutrophils to vascular endothelial cells *in vitro*, possibly through the stimulation of endothelial platelet-activating factor synthesis.   The increase in adherence could be prevented if catalase were added to the culture medium in addition to the hydrogen peroxide.

While the present study supports the hypothesis that circulating neutrophils play a critical role in the production of gastropathy following administration of NSAIDs, it remains unclear what causes the neutrophils to become activated and to adhere to the vascular endothelium.   Numerous mediators can activate neutrophils, including platelet-activating factor, leukotriene B_4 and the complement fragment C5a.   A number of cytokines, including interleukin-1 and tumour necrosis factor, can increase the expression on endothelial cells of adhesion molecules to which neutrophils bind.   On the other hand, some prostaglandins (e.g. prostacyclin) can inhibit the activation and adherence of neutrophils.   It is therefore possible that the NSAIDs might cause increased neutrophil activation by inhibiting the synthesis of factors which tonically inhibit the adherence of these cells to the vessel wall.   It is not yet clear which, if any, of these mediators are involved in the pathogenesis of NSAID-gastropathy, but it is an area that certainly warrants further investigation.

REFERENCES

1.   Grisham MB, Granger DN. Neutrophil-mediated mucosal injury: role of reactive oxygen metabolites. Dig Dis Sci 1988; 33: 6s-15s.

2.   Smith SM, Holm-Rutili L, Perry MA, Grisham MB, Arfors KE, Granger DN, Kvietys PR. Role of neutrophils in hemorrhagic shock-induced gastric mucosal injury in the rat.   Gastroenterology 1987; 93: 466-471.

3.   Kvietys PR, Twohig B, Danzell J, Specian RD.   Ethanol-induced injury to the rat gastric mucosa.   Role of neutrophils and xanthine oxidase-derived radicals. Gastroenterology 1990; 98: 909-920.

4.   Rainsford KD. Microvascular injury during gastric mucosal damage by anti-inflammatory drugs in pigs and rats.   Agents Actions 1983; 13: 457-460.

5. Wallace JL, Keenan CM, Granger DN. Gastric ulceration induced by non-steroidal anti-inflammatory drugs is a neutrophil-dependent process. Am J Physiol. (*in press*)

6. Ashley SW, Sonnenschein LA, Cheung LY, Focal gastric mucosal blood flow at the site of aspirin-induced ulceration. Am J Surg 1985; 149: 53-59.

7. Kitahora T, Guth PH. Effect of aspirin plus hydrochloric acid on the gastric mucosal microcirculation. Gastroenterology 1987; 93: 810-817.

8. Gana TJ, Huhlewych R, Koo J. Focal gastric mucosal blood flow in aspirin-induced ulceration. Ann Surg 1987; 205: 399-403.

9. Van Voorhis WC, Steinman RM, Hair LS, Luban J, Witmer MD, Koide S, Cohn SA. Specific antimononuclear phagocyte monoclonal antibodies. J Exp Med 1983; 158: 126-145.

10. Lewis MS, Whatley RE, Cain P, McIntyre TM, Prescott SM, Zimmerman GA. Hydrogen peroxide stimulates the synthesis of platelet-activating factor by endothelium and induces endothelial cell-dependent neutrophil adhesion. J Clin Invest 1988; 82: 2045-2055.

11. Pihan G, Regillo C, Szabo S. Free radicals and lipid peroxidation in ethanol- or aspirin-induced gastric mucosal injury. Dig Dis Sci 1987; 32: 1395-1401.

12. Ward PA, Till G, Kunkel S, Beauchamp C. Evidence for a role of hydroxyl radical in complement and neutrophil-dependent tissue injury. J Clin Invest 1983; 72: 789-795.

ISCHEMIA-REPERFUSION INDUCED CHANGES IN MICROVASCULAR PERMEABILITY

M.A. Perry and D.N. Granger

School of Physiology and Pharmacology, University of New South Wales, Sydney, Australia, and Department of Physiology and Biophysics, LSU Medical Centre, Shreveport, Louisiana, USA

INTRODUCTION

The first evidence that oxyradicals played a role in the microvascular injury associated with ischemia-reperfusion (I/R) of the small bowel came from a study in which the oxyradical scavenger superoxide dismutase was found to effectively prevent the increase in microvascular permeability caused by one hour of intestinal ischemia followed by reperfusion [5]. This led to the hypothesis that oxyradicals were generated during reperfusion of the ischemic tissue and were responsible for the microvascular injury. Briefly the proposed mechanism is as follows; ischemia causes the conversion of the NAD^+ reducing enzyme xanthine dehydrogenase to the oxyradical generating xanthine oxidase. At the same time catabolism of ATP results in the accumulation of hypoxanthine in the tissue. During reperfusion molecular oxygen is reintroduced and together with xanthine oxidase and hypoxanthine as the substrate, is reduced to the superoxide radical (O_2^-). Endogenous superoxide dismutase converts some of the O_2^- to H_2O_2 which, in the presence of a transition metal such as Fe^{3+} and together with O_2^- generates the hydroxyl radical (OH). These xanthine oxidase derived oxidants are cytotoxic and are capable of inflicting direct injury on the tissue by peroxidation of cell constituents.

Xanthine oxidase derived oxidants are not the only source of injury to the ischemic gut. It is obvious from histological and biochemical studies and more recently from in vivo microscopy that polymorphonuclear leukocytes are attracted to ischemic tissue. This has led to the current hypothesis (Figure 1) that xanthine oxidase derived oxidants serve to attract and activate granulocytes and that it is the oxidants and proteolytic enzymes release by these cells that mediate reperfusion induced microvascular injury [1]. This chapter will review evidence relevant to the hypothesis put forward in Figure 1 that xanthine oxidase derived oxidants and granulocytes are responsible for the changes in microvascular permeability that occur during I/R injury in the gut.

ASSESSMENT OF MICROVASCULAR PERMEABILITY

The permeability characteristics of capillaries in the gastrointestinal tract has been extensively studied, particularly in the small intestine where the permeability to plasma proteins is well documented [19, 21]. The most commonly used index of microvascular permeability is 1- δ_d, where δ_d is the osmotic reflection coefficient. The osmotic reflection coefficient for plasma protein is obtained from the lymph to plasma concentration ratio (L/P) for total protein obtained at high lymph flows. Lymph flow is increased by elevation of venous pressure which increases the convective movement of plasma proteins across the capillary wall and reduces the diffusive contribution to total exchange to a negligible level. When L/P remains constant despite further increases in filtration rate the ratio reflects the true sieving characteristics of the capillary wall [21]. δ_d is calculated as 1 - L/P (filtration rate independent). Since a reduction in the osmotic reflection coefficient reflects an increase in vascular permeability the value 1- δ_d has been used as the index of microvascular permeability.

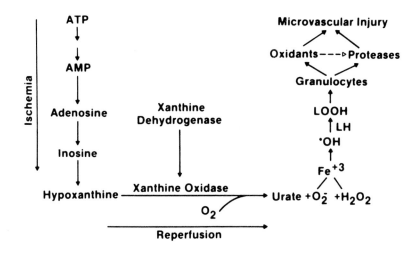

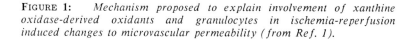

FIGURE 1:   *Mechanism proposed to explain involvement of xanthine oxidase-derived oxidants and granulocytes in ischemia-reperfusion induced changes to microvascular permeability (from Ref. 1).*

The osmotic reflection coefficient for total plasma protein in the cat small intestine is approximately 0.92. The control value for microvascular permeability is, therefore, 0.08 [6]. Osmotic reflection coefficients have also been obtained for the different molecular weight proteins found in lymph and plasma. These data have been used to describe the permeability characteristic of the microvasculature in terms of equivalent pore sizes. An example of such an analysis is shown in Figure 2, where 1- δ_d is plotted for each different sized protein. Theoretical curves relating 1- δ_d to solute radius are generated for different sized pores. The microcirculation of cat small intestine has permeability characteristic that are best described by two populations of pores; numerous small pores of 46 Å radius and far less frequent large pores of 200 Å radius.

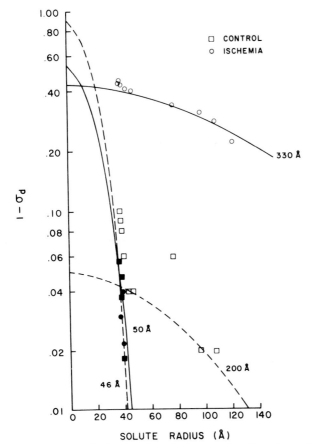

FIGURE 2: *Pore analysis for lymphatic protein flux data from small intestine under control conditions (squares) and after 1 hr of ischemia (circles). It was assumed that* $\delta_d = 1\ C_L/C_P$ *at the high capillary filtration rates studied. Note that the analysis predicts that ischemia selectively increases the size of the large pores (from Ref. 21).*

ISCHEMIA-REPERFUSION INDUCED CHANGES IN MICROVASCULAR PERMEABILITY

In the cat small intestine one hour of ischemia (local perfusion pressure of 20 mm Hg) followed by reperfusion, increased microvascular permeability (1- δ_d) from 0.08 to 0.41 (Table 1). The theoretical pore analysis indicated that this was due to an increase in the size of the large pores from 200 Å to 330 Å with little change in the size of the small pores (Figure 2). It is interesting to note that ischemia alone caused permeability to increase to only 0.15, while reperfusion caused a five-fold increase in permeability. This is consistent with the hypothesis put forward in Figure 1 suggesting that microvascular injury is most likely to occur following the reintroduction of molecular oxygen.

XANTHINE OXIDASE INHIBITORS

Many studies have shown that inhibition of oxyradical producing enzyme xanthine oxidase significantly attenuates reperfusion injury in the gastrointestinal tract [1]. Allopurinol, a competitive inhibitor of xanthine oxidase, also prevented the increase in microvascular permeability associated with one hour of ischemia followed by reperfusion (Table 1). This effect was observed at concentrations of allopurinol which effectively inhibited xanthine oxidase activity without directly scavenging free radicals [22]. Other inhibitors of xanthine oxidase including folic acid, pterin aldehyde and tungsten supplemented diets were as effective as allopurinol in preventing reperfusion induced microvascular injury.

TABLE 1.

EFFECT OF XANTHINE OXIDASE INHIBITORS ON I/R INDUCED CHANGES IN
MICROVASCULAR PERMEABILITY.

TREATMENT	MICROVASCULAR PERMEABILITY $(I- \delta_d)$	REF.
Control	0.08 ± 0.005	6
Ischemia (1 hr)	0.15 ± 0.03	1
Ischemia (1 hr) + reperfusion (I/R)	0.41 ± 0.02	6
I/R + treatment with		
allopurinol	0.18 ± 0.01	15
folic acid	0.16 ± 0.04	4
pterin aldehyde	0.15 ± 0.02	4
tungsten supplemented diet	0.20 ± 0.02	17
soybean trypsin inhibitor	0.16 ± 0.01	16

Values are mean $\pm$ SE.

The conversion of xanthine dehydrogenase to xanthine oxidase occurs by limited proteotysis, oxidation of sulfhydryl groups or both [1]. Protease inhibitors such as soybean trypsin inhibitor prevent the ischemia induced conversion of xanthine dehydrogenase to xanthine oxidase and at the same time prevent I/R induced increases in microvascular permeability (Table 1).

OXYRADICAL SCAVENGERS

The observation which implicated oxyradicals as mediators of I/R injury was that superoxide dismutase (SOD) administered intravenously following renal ligation (the enzyme is sufficiently small to be cleared by the kidneys) largely prevented I/R induced changes in microvascular permeability [5]. Similar results have been obtained with copper diisopropyl salicylate (Cu-DIPS) a lipophilic SOD-mimetic (Table 2).

Other xanthine oxidase derived oxidants generated during I/R include H_2O_2 produced by the dismutation of O_2^-, and the hydroxyl radical, generated by the iron-catalyzed Haber-Weiss reaction

$$O_2^- + Fe^{3+} \longrightarrow Fe^{2+} + O_2$$
$$Fe^{2+} + H_2O_2 \longrightarrow Fe^{3+} + OH^- + OH$$

Pretreatment with the hydroxyl radical scavenger dimethyl sulfoxide (DMSO) or the peroxidase enzyme catalase were effective in preventing the reperfusion induced increase in microvascular permeability (Table 2).

Intravascular generation of oxyradicals by infusion of hypoxanthine - xanthine oxidase into the arterial supply to the small bowel effectively increased microvascular permeability to 0.38, a value similar to that observed following I/R. This effect was not observed when the oxyradical scavengers SOD and DMSO were included in the infusion mixture (Table 2). Using a different model, the hamster cheek pouch, Ley and Arfors [13] also found that oxyradical generation caused dramatic increases in leakyness of postcapillary venules. The number of sites leaking FITC-dextran increased 10-fold following XO infusion and this was completely reversed by pretreatment with SOD conjugated to polyethylene glycol.

TABLE 2.

EFFECT OF OXYRADICAL SCAVENGERS ON I/R INDUCED
CHANGES IN MICROVASCULAR PERMEABILITY.

TREATMENT	MICROVASCULAR PERMEABILITY $(I- \delta_d^-)$	REF
Control	0.08 ± 0.05	6
Ischemia + Reperfusion (I/R)	0.41 ± 0.02	6
I/R + treatment with		
DMSO	0.19 ± 0.02	15
catalase	0.19 ± 0.01	3
Intra-arterial infusion of HX and XO	0.38 ± 0.02	18
HX-XO + SOD	0.14 ± 0.02	18
HX-XO + DMSO	0.17 ± 0.02	18

HX = hypoxanthine; XO = xanthine oxidase; DMSO = dimethylsulfoxide.

The hydroxyl radical is regarded as the most reactive and damaging of the xanthine oxidase derived oxidants. Generation of this radical is influenced by the availability of catalytically active iron. Chelation of free iron with desferoxamine or binding of iron to the protein apotransferrin presented the increase in microvascular permeability caused by reperfusion of the ischemic intestine (Figure 3). Saturation of desferoxamine and apotransferrin with iron completely negated their beneficial effects. These data indicate that hydroxyl radicals, derived from the superoxide anion by an iron catalysed Haber-Weiss reaction play a major role in I/R induced injury.

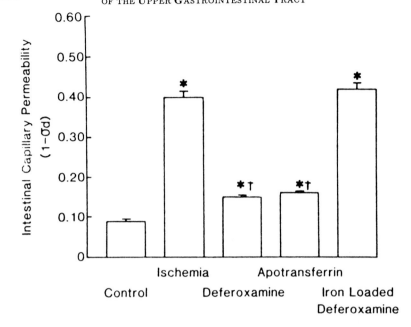

FIGURE 3: *Effect of deferoxamine, apotransferrin and iron loaded deferoxamine on intestinal vascular permeability changes induced by ischemia-reperfusion.* * $P < 0.05$ *relative to control (non-ischemic preparations).* †$P < 0.05$ *relative to untreated ischemic preparations.* σ_d = *capillary osmotic reflection coefficient of intestinal capillaries for total plasma proteins (from Ref. 9).*

GRANULOCYTES AND MICROVASCULAR PERMEABILITY

It is well recognised that granulocytes are involved in I/R injury in a variety of different tissues. When activated these cells generate superoxide radicals and release a number of destructive enzymes including myeloperoxidase (MPO) and elastase. The resulting mixture of oxidants and proteases can injure both tissue and microvasculature. The tissue concentration of MPO is commonly used as an index of neutrophil infiltration since MPO constitutes 5% of the dry weight of the neutrophil and MPO is found in only one other mammalian cell but in much lower concentration. During I/R there is a 20-fold increase in MPO activity in the small intestine indicating a dramatic increase in neutrophil adherence and extravasation [8]. In the stomach comparable conditions of I/R produced a more modest increase in MPO from 8.9 ± 2.6 to 22.7 ± 5.3 (Perry, unpublished observations). Grisham et al. [8] found that allopurinol and SOD reduced the I/R induced increased in MPO activity in the intestine. This ability of XO inhibitors and oxyradical scavengers to inhibit neutrophil infiltration suggests that XO derived oxidants play a role in attracting and possibly activating neutrophils during I/R.

TABLE 3.

EFFECT OF NEUTROPHILS ON I/R INDUCED CHANGES IN MICROVASCULAR
PERMEABILITY.

TREATMENT	MICROVASCULAR PERMEABILITY $(I-\delta_d)$	REF
Control	0.08 ± 0.005	6
Ischemia (1 hr) + reperfusion (I/R)	0.41 ± 0.02	6
(I/R) plus treatment with		
antineutrophil serum	0.13 ± 0.01	11
MoAb 60.3	0.12 ± 0.01	11
FMLP (in lumen)	0.40 ± 0.07	7
FMLP + ANS	0.19 ± 0.06	7

MoAb 60.3 = monoclonal antibody against adhesion glycoproteins;
FMLP = formyl - methionyl - leucyl - phenylalanine;
ANS = anti-neutrophil serum.

In order to determine whether neutrophils contribute towards the I/R
induced increase in microvascular permeability Hernandez et al. [11] either
depleted cats of neutrophils with anti-neutrophil serum or inhibited
neutrophil adherence to endothelium with a monoclonal antibody (MoAb 60.
3). Anti-neutrophil serum reduced the circulating neutrophil count to
between 5 and 10% of control and at the same time prevented the I/R
induced increase in permeability (Table 3). A similar result was obtained
with MoAb 60.3. This antibody not only prevents neutrophil adherence but
also neutrophil extravasation and it is as effective as the antiserum in
preventing microvascular injury during I/R.

One effect of neutrophil depletion is to reduce plugging of the
microcirculation with neutrophils and thereby improve blood flow during
ischemia. This effect has been observed in the rat where anti-neutrophil
serum protected the stomach against hemorrhagic shock induced gastric
mucosal injury, an effect which was attributed entirely to improved blood
during the ischemic period [20]. This was not the case in the study of
Hernandez et al. [11] since in their model intestinal blood flow was closely
controlled. The fact that neutrophil depletion was effective in preventing
I/R induced increases in microvascular permeability indicates that these
cells and their cytotoxic products are responsible for a major proportion of
the microvascular injury. Further support for this notion comes from a
study in which formyl - methionyl - leucyl - phenylalamine (FMLP), a
bacterial peptide known to attract and activate neutrophils, was added to
the lumen of the cat small bowel and caused a dramatic increase in
microvascular permeability. This effect was not observed when the animals
were depleted of neutrophils with anti-neutrophil serum (Figure 4). In this
study the antiserum depleted the circulating neutrophils to < 5% of control
but only reduced the MPO activity (and presumably the number of
neutrophils) in the bowel wall by 50% indicating that the circulating
neutrophils may have played the dominant role in causing microvascular
injury.

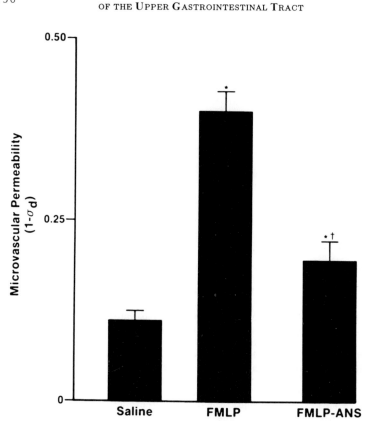

FIGURE 4:   *Effects of FMLP on intestinal microvascular permeability in control animals and ANS-treated animals. * $P < 0.05$ relative to saline †$P < 0.05$ relative to FMLP in control animals (from Ref. 7).*

POSSIBLE OXYRADICAL GENERATED CHEMOTACTIC AGENTS

The hypothesis outlined in Figure 1 suggests that oxyradicals produced during I/R cause neutrophil adherence and extravasation, and that the oxidants and proteases produced by these granulocytes exacerbate microvascular injury. Little is known, however, of the nature of the agents that are responsible for neutrophil chemotaxis and activation. Two possible mediators of leukocyte adherence are platelet activating factor (PAF) and leukotriene B_4 (LTB$_4$). Both of these substances cause dramatic increases in the adherence of neutrophils to venular endothelium in vivo. Kubes et al. [12] have recently investigated whether superoxides and leukocyte adhesion glycoproteins play a role in the leukocyte adherence and increased microvascular permeability induced by PAF. They found that SOD and a monoclonal antibody (MoAbIB$_4$ directed against the CD18 adhesion glycoprotein on the surface of the leukocyte) reduced PAF induced increase in leukocyte adherence by 30% and 66%, respectively. These agents also reduced (by 40% and 70%, respectively) the PAF induced increase in intestinal microvascular permeability. The observation that oxyradicals and leukocyte adhesion molecules are involved in PAF induced injury to the microcirculation implicates PAF as a possible mediator in I/R injury.

The relative importance of xanthine oxidase derived oxidants compared to granulocyte derived oxidants and proteins remains uncertain. It appears that both play key roles in the process of I/R, since removal of either source of injury confers protection on the tissue.

Neutrophils accumulate in the microvasculature during ischemia. This is most likely a result of the reduction in blood flow velocity and therefore a reduction in the shear force that normally opposes neutrophil adhesion to endothelium, thereby allowing the proadhesive forces to dominate. This effect is only observed on the venous side of the microvasculature, with little or no sticking of leukocytes to arterioles even at very low shear rates. The factors which regulate neutrophil-endothelial interactions during I/R and which enhance or inhibit the function of these adhesive glycoproteins, the role oxyradicals play in neutrophil-endothelial interactions and the nature of the chemical mediators produced during I/R all remain to be investigated.

REFERENCES

1. Granger DN Role of xanthine oxidase and granulocytes in ischemia-reperfusion injury. Am J Physiol 1988; 255: H1269-H1275.

2. Granger DN, Grisham MB, Hernandez LA Ischemia-reperfusion injury in the small intestine: effect of adenosine (Abstract) Federation Proc 1986; 46: 1124.

3. Granger DN, Hollwarth ME, Parks DA Ischemia-reperfusion injury: role of oxygen-derived free radicals. Acta Physiol Scand Suppl 1986; 548: 47-64.

4. Granger DN, McCord JM, Parks DA, Hollwarth ME Xanthine oxidase inhibitors attenuate ischemia-induced vascular permeability changes in the cat intestine. Gastroenterology 1986; 90: 80-84.

5. Granger DN, Rutili G, McCord JM Superoxide radicals in feline intestinal ischemia. Gastroenterology 1981; 81: 22-29.

6. Granger DN, Sennett M, McElearney P, Taylor AE Effect of local arterial hypotension on cat intestinal capillary permeability. Gastroenterology 1980; 79: 474-480.

7. Granger DN, Zimmerman BJ, Sekizuka E, Grisham MB Intestinal microvascular exchange in the rat during luminal perfusion with formyl-methionyl-leucyl-phenylalanine. Gastroenterology 1988; 94: 673-681.

8. Grisham MB, Hernandez LA, Granger DN Xanthine oxidase and neutrophil infiltration in intestinal ischemia. Am J Physiol 1986; 251 (Gastrointest Liver Physiol 14): G567-G574.

9. Hernandez LA, Grisham MB, Granger DN A role for iron in oxidant-mediated ischemic injury to intestinal microvasculature. Am J Physiol 1987; 253 (Gastrointest Liver Physiol16): G49-G53.

10.   Hernandez LA, Grisham MB, Granger DN   Effects of CU-DIPS on
ischemia-reperfusion injury. In: Biology of Copper Complexes,
Sorenson JRJ ed, Clifton NJ: Humana 1987; 201-210.

11.   Hernandez LA, Grisham MB, Twohig B, Arfors KE, Harlan JM,
Granger DN   Role of neutrophils in ischemia-reperfusion induced
microvascular injury. Am J Physiol 1987; 253 (Heart Circ Physiol
22): H699-H703.

12.   Kubes P, Suzuki M, Granger DN   Role of superoxide and CD18
adhesion proteins in PAF-induced leukocyte adherence and increased
microvascular permeability. Am J Physiol (in press).

13.   Ley K, Arfors KE   Changes in macromolecular permeability by
intravascular generation of oxygen-derived free radicals. Microvasc
Res 1982; 24: 25-33.

14.   Parks DA, Bulkley GB, Granger DN, Hamilton SR, McCord JM
Ischemic injury in the cat small intestine: role of superoxide radicals.
Gastroenterology 1982; 82; 9-15.

15.   Parks DA, Granger DN   Ischemia-induced vascular changes: role of
xanthine oxidase and hydroxyl radicals.   Am J Physiol 1983; 245
(Gastrointest Liver Physiol 8); G285-G289.

16.   Parks DA, Granger DN, Bulkley GB, Shah AK   Soybean trypsin
inhibitor attenuates ischemic injury to the feline small intestine.
Gastroenterology 1985; 89: 6-12.

17.   Parks DA, Henson JL, Granger DN   Effect of xanthine oxidase
inactivation on ischemic injury to the small intestine (Abstract).
Physiologist 1986; 29: 101.

18.   Parks DA, Shah AK, Granger DN   Oxygen radicals: effects on
intestinal vascular permeability.   Am J Physiol 1984; 247
(Gastrointest Liver Physiol 10): G167-G170.

19.   Perry MA, Granger DN   Permeability characteristics of intestinal
capillaries In "Physiology of the Intestinal Circulation" (Shepherd AP,
Granger DN eds) 1984; pp 233-247 Raven Press: New York.

20.   Smith SM, Holm-Rutili L, Perry MA, Grisham MB, Arfors KE,
Granger DN, Kvietys PR   Role of neutrophils in hemorrhagic shock-
induced gastric mucosal injury in the rat. Gastroenterology 1987; 93:
466-471.

21.   Taylor AE, Granger DN   Exchange of macromolecules across the
microcirculation. In Handbook of Physiology. The Cardiovascular
System IV (Renkin EM, Michel CC eds) 1983; Chapter 11, pp 467-520.
Am Physiol Soc: Bethesda.

22.   Zimmerman BJ, Parks DA, Grisham MB, Granger DN   Allopurinol
does not enhance antioxidant properties of extracellular fluid. Am J
Physiol 1988; 255: H202-H206.

REACTIVE OXYGEN METABOLITES: MEDIATORS OF GASTROINTESTINAL INJURY

Patrick M. Reilly, Gregory B. Bulkley

The Department of Surgery, The Johns Hopkins Medical Institutions, Baltimore, Maryland

ABSTRACT

Highly toxic metabolites of oxygen are generated normally by aerobic metabolism in most cells, which are protected from injury by multiple endogenous antioxidant mechanisms. When pathological conditions, such as ischaemia/reperfusion, increase this oxidant flux, serious tissue damage may ensue. In the small intestine, which is disproportionately susceptible to the ischemia during circulatory shock, ischemia activates xanthine oxidase, which then generates a massive burst of superoxide free radicals when oxygen is returned at reperfusion. These radicals, and their toxic oxygen metabolites, then generate much of the mucosal injury that has been previously attributed to anoxia itself, both by direct action, and by the secondary activation of circulating neutrophils. Recent evidence shows that although the mucosal epithelial cell is rich in xanthine oxidase, it is probably endothelial cell xanthine oxidase that triggers this mucosal reperfusion injury, not only in the intestine, but in the stomach and liver as well. Moreover, this superficial epithelial necrosis appears to account for a loss of the barrier function of both the stomach and intestine. This mechanism may therefore explain not only some forms of gastric and intestinal ulceration, but also explain the appearance of bacterial translocation, perhaps the basis for the "gut as the motor of multiple organ failure."

INTRODUCTION

While mucosal injury of the gastrointestinal tract in association with circulatory shock [1], and its fundamental basis in mucosal ischemia [2], have long been appreciated, we have only more recently come to appreciate that much of this injury takes place at the level of the microvasculature, and is related, at least in part, to the generation of free radicals and other toxic metabolites of oxygen at reperfusion.

A free radical is a molecule with one or more unpaired electrons in its outer orbital. Such unpaired electrons make these species quite unstable and therefore very reactive as the free radical tends to react with other molecules to pair this electron and thereby generate a more stable species (i.e. a lower energy state). The most abundant radical in biological systems is **molecular oxygen** (O_2) or **dioxygen** $(^3O_2)$[3], which has two unpaired

159

electrons. (In this ground state, the spin of both unpaired electrons is parallel, making the species relatively unreactive. When the spins are antiparallel, this species, termed **singlet oxygen** ($^1O_2$) is more reactive [4,5]) A number of other important oxygen-centered free radicals also exist. The **superoxide anion** (O_2^-) and the **hydroxyl radical** (OH·) are both species with one unpaired electron in their outer shell. The hydroxyl radical is particularly unstable and therefore much more reactive. As a result, the hydroxyl radical is short-lived ($\sim 10^{-6}$s) in biological systems [6]. Although the hydroperoxides, such as **hydrogen peroxide** (H_2O_2), are not true free radical species, they constitute an important secondary class of reactive oxygen metabolites that can also be quite toxic to tissue components.

Reactive oxygen metabolites, including free radicals, are formed continuously as a normal byproduct of cellular metabolism. The "**univalent leak**" of molecular oxygen in the mitrochondrion is one example: During oxidative phosphorylation, the mitochondrial cytochrome array couples the production of adenosine triphosphate (ATP) to the tetravalent reduction of molecular oxygen to water (Figure 1). During this process, all four electrons are effectively added at once. Because no free intermediate species containing an uneven number of electrons are formed, no free radicals are generated by this reaction. However, about 1-5% of oxygen which is reduced to water within the mitrochondrion "leaks" out from this cytochrome-catalyzed pathway and undergoes non-catalytic, stepwise, univalent reduction [7], thereby producing a continuous flux of reactive oxygen metabolites which must be "detoxified" by protective biochemical mechanisms within the cell in order to prevent injury.[8]

There are numerous other endogenous sources of free radical generation. The metabolism of arachidonic acid by **cyclooxygenase** to produce prostaglandins and **lipoxygenase** to produce leukotrienes each involves intermediate peroxy compounds as well as hydroxy radicals (Figure 2) [9,10]. A number of oxidases can, under certain circumstances and with varying degrees of efficiency, generate toxic oxygen metabolites. **Xanthine oxidoreductase** catalyzes the two step oxidation of purines, such as hypoxanthine, through xanthine, to urate [11,12]. *In vivo*, the enzyme may exist in either of two forms, a dehydrogenase (d-form), which uses NAD^+ as an electron acceptor and therefore does not generate radicals, and an oxidase (o-form) which uses molecular oxygen as an electron acceptor, and thereby produces the superoxide radical as a byproduct of purine metabolism [13]. While the superoxide radical may be a byproduct of other oxidative reactions, it is the primary product of the highly specialized **NADPH oxidase** system on the membrane surface of inflammatory cells, including neutrophils, eosinophils, monocytes, and macrophages [14,15]. This enzyme, when activated, catalyzes the sudden reduction of oxygen to hydrogen peroxide and the superoxide anion. This phenomenon, termed the "**respiratory burst**", accounts for more than 90% of oxygen consumption by a stimulated neutrophil [16]. This production of the superoxide anion is one of the major mechanisms by which phagocytes destroy micro-organisms. While this superoxide can itself be toxic, its major toxicity here is through the secondary generation of **hypochlorous acid** (HOCl, the active agent in Chlorox^R bleach) from hydrogen peroxide and chloride ions by the enzyme myeloperoxidase, which is unique to and abundant within these cells [17].

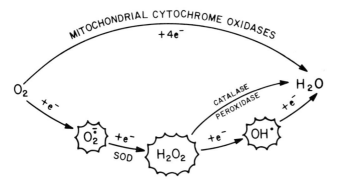

FIGURE 1:   Reduction of Molecular Oxygen.   *The mitochondrial cytochrome oxidase complex reduces molecular oxygen by the simultaneous addition of four electrons, producing water and generating ATP without the production of free toxic oxygen intermediates. However, 1-5% of oxygen "leaks" from this pathway and undergoes stepwise, univalent reduction. The one electron reduction of oxygen generates the superoxide radical (O_2^-). This can subsequently be reduced to hydrogen peroxide (H_2O_2), most commonly in a dismutation reaction catalyzed by superoxide dismutase (SOD). Hydrogen peroxide can be directly detoxified to water by a catalase or peroxidase-catalyzed reduction. Alternatively, hydrogen peroxide can be reduced, usually in an iron-catalyzed reaction, to the hydroxyl radical (OH). This highly reactive radical can subsequently abstract a hydrogen atom to reduce itself to water. While protective biochemical mechanisms are in place to detoxify the toxic intermediates generated by this "univalent leak" under normal conditions, increased concentrations of oxygen generate excessive amounts of toxic oxygen metabolites which overwhelm the protective mechanisms. (Reprinted from: Sussman MS, Buchman GB, Bulkley GB. Mechanisms of organ injury by toxic oxygen metabolites. In: Multiple Organ Failure: Pathogenesis and Management (Fry DE, ed). Chicago, Yearbook Medical Publishers, in press. With permission).*

A number of exogenous agents can also lead to the production of free radicals in biological systems.   One example is the flavoprotein-catalyzed **redox cycling** of **xenobiotics**.   A xenobiotic (e.g. the herbicide **paraquat** or the chemotherapeutic agent **doxorubicin** [Adriamycin[R]]), is reduced by NADPH, and subsequently oxidized by donating an electron to molecular oxygen, generating the superoxide anion.   Since neither the enzyme nor the xenobiotic, only oxygen, are consumed in this process, the toxic product of the reaction is produced continuously, and in great excess [18].   The acute bronchial epithelial injury and (probably) the long term carcinogenic effects of **cigarette smoke** [19], the acute hepatic injury induced by **carbon tetrachloride** (CCl4) [20,21], and the effects on any tissue (normal or neoplastic) or **ionizing radiation** (both acute [cell killing, 22,23] and chronic [mutagenesis 24,25]), are also mediated largely through free radical mechanisms.

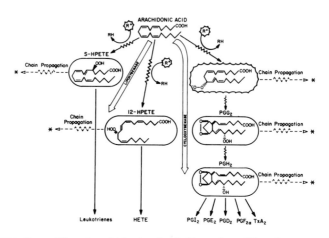

FIGURE 2:   The Arachidonic Acid Cascade. *The first step in the production of the active metabolites of arachidonic acid are lipid peroxidations (zigzag arrows), which are usually catalyzed by either cyclooxygenase or lipoxygenase. Alternatively, these reactions may be initiated by radicals (encircled by scalloped lines). The initial products of this lipid peroxidation, hydro- and endoperoxides (encircled by smooth lines), can decompose to yield radical species which can then start new chain reactions. Thus the arachidonic acid cascade can both be initiated by, and be a source of toxic oxygen metabolites. (Reprinted from: Sussman MS, Buchman GB, Bulkley GB. Mechanisms of organ injury by toxic oxygen metabolites. In: Multiple Organ Failure: Pathogenesis and Management (Fry DE, ed) Chicago, Yearbook Medical Publishers, in press. With Permission).*

Free radicals can attack any biochemical component of the cell, but lipids, proteins, and nucleic acids are particularly important targets. Because they are so highly reactive, free radicals generally react with the first structure which they encounter - most frequently the lipid component of cell or organelle membranes [26]. This mechanism of free radical-mediated lipid peroxidation is an example of a classic chain reaction. A single hydroxyl radical and molecular oxygen can react with a polyunsaturated fatty acid to generate multiple fatty acid peroxy radicals [27], which subsequently react with other lipids, proteins, or nucleic acids, thereby propagating the transfer of electrons and subsequent oxidation (destruction) of substrates. Only when two radicals react with each other, or the radicals are "scavenged" by another electron acceptor to form a less reactive species, will the chain reaction cease. Proteins, both structural and enzymatic, are also vulnerable to free radical-mediated denaturation. Toxic oxygen metabolites can also directly attack nucleic acids, causing base hydroxylation, cross-linking or scission (cutting) of DNA strands.

METHODS FOR IDENTIFYING AND QUANTITATING FREE RADICAL-MEDIATED INJURY

Direct detection of free radicals is hampered by their high reactivity and consequent short lives. As a result, free radicals rarely accumulate within tissues at concentrations high enough to allow their measurement by conventional spectrophotometric techniques. To deal with these problems, a successful alternative strategy has been employed which involves adding an indicator reagent directly to the biological system, allowing it to react with the free radical as it is formed. One then assays for the change in the indicator reagent. The most conventional approach is to use the SOD-inhibitable reduction of cytochrome C (or nitroblue tetrazolium {NBT}) as an assay of superoxide generation *in vitro*. This approach has some applications *in vivo*, but they are limited by the fact that cytochrome C does not penetrate cellular membranes and therefore cannot be used to detect superoxide generation within intact cells and organs. In addition, both cytochrome C and NBT can react with other non-free radical agents, thereby overestimating superoxide concentrations. An equivalent approach uses **electron spin resonance spectroscopy** (ESR), which is based on the absorption of microwaves by the unpaired electrons of free radicals in a magnetic field. **Electron spin trapping** involves the use of compounds (spin traps) which, when they react with free radicals, form a more stable free radical product, essentially "trapping" the unpaired electron in a spin trap adduct that can be assayed by ESR. [28]. **Nuclear magnetic resonance (NMR)** spectroscopy may enable the detection of free radicals *in vivo*. However, the steady state concentrations of free radicals in biological systems is below current imaging thresholds, and spin traps will probably be required here as well.

When free radicals return to the ground state (a lower energy level) they emit a photon, a phenomenon termed ultraweak **chemiluminescence**. The detection of this light has been used for years for the detection of free radical generation *in vitro*, for example to measure the respiratory burst of neutrophils. Recently, this has also been applied to whole organs *in vivo* [29]. Because the intensity of this photoemission is so low, it is necessary to scrupulously exclude external light sources and, often, to amplify the signal with indicator reagents such as luminol or lucigenin.

While the technological advances made in recent years are increasing the sensitivity of these direct detection techniques, they all still suffer from a theoretical limitation: they can only detect the presence of free radicals in a biologic system. They cannot establish a causal role for free radicals in a biological process. Results from studies employing these techniques alone must therefore be interpreted carefully to distinguish causes from effects and from epiphenomena.

The detection of products of free radical-mediated reactions has also been used as indirect evidence of toxic oxygen metabolite-mediated injury. The products of lipid peroxidation (hydrocarbons, conjugated dienes, malondialdehyde {MDA}) have been most widely studied. Nucleic acid products, secondary to free radical-mediated oxidative damage, have also been detected by spin trapping, again associating free radical-mediated tissue damage with the injury.

Perhaps the most common approach for the study of free radical-mediated injury is the amelioration of organ injury by various free radical inhibitors. The definitiveness of such indirect evidence, obtained with inhibitors, is directly proportional to the specificity of the inhibitor used. The enzymatic scavengers, SOD and catalase, are highly specific for the removal of superoxide [30] and hydrogen peroxide [31], respectively. Therefore, inhibition of experimental injury by these agents is highly suggestive that the pathophysiologic event is indeed mediated by one of these toxic oxygen metabolites. Allopurinol and its active metabolite, oxypurinol, specifically inhibit the enzyme, xanthine oxidase. Although allopurinol may be a hydroxyl radical scavenger at high concentrations *in vitro* [32], it has been found that this highly inefficient scavenging capability is unlikely to explain reports of classic experiments [33]. Therefore, the inhibition of experimental injury with allopurinol (at normal pharmacologic concentrations) strongly suggests a central role for a xanthine oxidase-mediated pathophysiologic mechanism. On the other hand, non-enzymatic scavengers, such as DMSO and mannitol, are relatively nonspecific. Results from experiments using these agents alone must be interpreted with great caution. The question of secondary, non-radical mechanisms of action persists whenever a nonspecific, indirect method of free radical detection is used alone in an experimental model. However, these approaches do definitively distinguish causal mechanisms from effects and epiphenomena. The obvious solution to the distinct limitations imposed by each of the above approaches is to employ combinations of techniques simultaneously. This combined approach has become the standard for evaluating proposed mechanisms of free radical-mediated tissue injury.

RESULTS OF STUDIES OF FREE RADICAL-MEDIATED GASTROINTESTINAL INJURY.

Small Intestine

The mechanisms by which toxic oxygen metabolites participate in organ injury has been most extensively studied by Granger and his colleagues in a model of post-ischemic reperfusion injury in the cat small intestine. In this model, the administration of superoxide dismutase (SOD) near the end of the ischemic period, but prior to reperfusion, largely prevented the increased capillary permeability seen after one hour of partial ischemia [34]. This was the first clear demonstration of free radical-mediated reperfusion injury in any organ.

Reperfusion injury can be defined as the damage that occurs to an organ during the resumption of blood flow following an episode of ischemia. This is distinct from the injury caused by the ischemia *per se*, although the ischemic episode is necessary to generate the conditions for free radical formation at reperfusion. One hallmark of reperfusion injury is that it may be ameliorated by interventions which are initiated at the end of the ischemic period. Therefore, injuries which were once thought to be a result of hypoperfusion, and therefore not amenable to treatment, may actually be prevented, or at least diminished by therapy initiated at the beginning of resuscitation.

In this same model, the scavenging of hydrogen peroxide with catalase [35], of hydroxyl radicals with DMSO [36], or the prevention of their formation by chelating iron with desferoxamine or transferrin [37], all ameliorated the injury. Moreover, inhibition of xanthine oxidase activity with allopurinol [38], pterin aldehyde [39], or tungsten feeding [39] provided protection equivalent to that seen with SOD. As a result, xanthine oxidase, which is in high concentration in the intestinal mucosa [40], appears to be the initial source of free radical generation at reperfusion.

In intestinal mucosal homogenates, the dehydrogenase form of xanthine oxidoreductase predominates. However, following ischaemia, irreversible limited proteolysis converts this enzyme to the oxidase form, which generates superoxide [41,42]. Serine protease inhibitors prevent this proteolytic conversion *in vitro* [43], and the consequent tissue injury *in vivo* [44], suggesting that the proteolytic activation of xanthine oxidase during ischaemia facilitates the generation of toxic oxygen metabolites when oxygen is reintroduced at reperfusion.

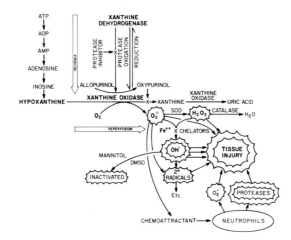

FIGURE 3: **The Generation of Toxic Oxygen Metabolites Triggered by Xanthine Oxidase at Reperfusion.** *During ischemia, the breakdown of high energy phosphate compounds (ATP) results in the accumulation of the purine metabolites hypoxanthine and xanthine. At the same time, xanthine dehydrogenase is converted to xanthine oxidase, either by reversible oxidation or irreversible limited proteolysis. At reperfusion, oxygen is reintroduced, suddenly and in excess, driving the rapid oxidation of purines, producing urate and the superoxide radical as a byproduct. This superoxide can then secondarily generate the highly toxic hydroxyl radical via an iron-catalyzed reaction. In addition to causing tissue injury themselves, these radicals may also lead to the accumulation, adherence, and activation of neutrophils. In many organs, such as the intestine, neutrophil-generated radicals and proteases contribute substantially to tissue injury, (Modified from Granger et al [34]).*

This body of work supports the hypothesis by Granger et al [34] which is summarized in Figure 3. The catabolism of ATP during ischemia leads to an increased concentration of the purine metabolites hypoxanthine and xanthine. At the same time, ischemia appears to mediate the conversion of xanthine dehydrogenase to xanthine oxidase. (While proteolysis is probably involved, the precise mechanism by which ischemia mediates this step is still unclear [45]). Oxygen, the only substrate lacking in order for superoxide to be generated, is reintroduced suddenly, and in excess, at reperfusion. The superoxide generated by xanthine oxidase then triggers a free radical chain reaction which leads to tissue injury   The fact that scavenging the hydroxyl radical, or blocking its secondary generation by iron-mediated reactions, has the same effect as blockade of the cascade more proximally suggests that some form of the hydroxyl radical, probably a perferryl radical, is the actual agent of injury [35,36].

Further studies in the cat small intestine suggest that the neutrophil plays an important role in the mediation of this reperfusion injury. The treatment of these cats with antineutrophil serum, or with a monoclonal antibody which prevents neutrophil adhesion to the microvasculature, also prevented the reperfusion-mediated capillary leak [46]. While some might interpret this finding to suggest that reperfusion injury is entirely explained by the generation of superoxide by neutrophils, it seems more likely that the neutrophil acts as an amplifier, rather than an initiator of tissue injury. Neutrophils, which generate superoxide with a NADPH oxidase (which is not inhibited by allopurinol [46] also produce a large number of toxic mediators other than oxygen metabolites, including elastase, collagenase, and other proteases [47]. The marked accumulation of neutrophils within the mucosa of the cat intestine caused by partial ischemia is prevented by xanthine oxidase inhibition with allopurinol [48]. Recent studies suggest that neutrophils accumulate and adhere to the microvascular endothelium in the post-ischemic feline small intestine in response to toxic oxygen metabolite generated by a xanthine oxidase dependent initial event [49,50], but that the capillary permeability injury itself is mediated by toxins that are then generated by the accumulated neutrophils [51].

Stomach

Following an episode of hypotension or some other form of severe physiologic stress, a mucosal lesion, characterized by hemorrhagic necrosis, is frequently seen in the stomach. Endoscopic surveillance of intensive care critically ill patients demonstrates that virtually 100% will have some evidence of mucosal ulceration. Most of these lesions disappear within 7-14 days, but these "stress ulcerations" can result in massive gastric hemorrhage and significant morbidity and mortality in the critically ill patient [52,53]. The initiating factor in this disease process is most likely an angiotensin-mediated splanchnic vasospasm causing gastric mucosal ischemia [54], followed by the generation of toxic oxygen metabolites at reperfusion. Such mucosal lesions produced in animal models of gastric injury secondary to hypotension can be prevented by either SOD or allopurinol [55,56]. In addition, the gastric ulcerations associated with the use of nonsteroidal anti-inflammatory agents may also involve a free radical-mediated mechanism.

Pancreas

The pancreas is also susceptible to a form of ischemic injury similar to that seen in the stomach and small intestine. Ischemic pancreatitis can be seen after shock, and has been noted following cardiopulmonary bypass [57]. In a canine model of ischemic pancreatitis, the administration of either allopurinol or SOD at reperfusion provided protection against this injury [58,59]. In addition, similar treatment blocks the manifestations of pancreatitis in models of gallstone and alcohol-induced hyperlipidemic pancreatitis, suggesting a possible common pathway in the development of acute pancreatitis in man [58]. However, free radicals appear to play a less important role in other models of pancreatitis, and since no currently available experimental model truly mimics the clinical situation, the exact role of toxic oxygen metabolites as mediators of human pancreatitis still remains unclear.

MULTIPLE ORGAN FAILURE

The syndrome of multisystem organ failure (MSOF) currently affects a wide variety of critically ill or injured patients. There is increasing evidence that the gastrointestinal tract may play a central role in the initial development and maintenance of the MSOF syndrome. Of all the proposed etiologies for MSOF, ischemia/reperfusion injury to the superficial gut mucosal barrier seems particularly likely. Patients subjected to circulatory shock, hypoxia, sepsis, and other initial forms of severe physiologic stress may sustain a mild, otherwise subclinical level of angiotensin-mediated nonocclusive ischemia of the (stomach and) intestine that may not progress to frank bowel necrosis. Although not recognized clinically as the classical syndrome of intestinal ischemia, it may result in the loss of the superficial mucosa, with the subsequent loss of the epithelial barrier function. Indeed, critically ill patients coming to autopsy have long been recognized to have such lesions, but they are often attributed to postmortem "autolysis" and not recognized as a premortem change.

Once the epithelial barrier function of the small intestine has been lost, the translocation of bacteria, and perhaps other luminal toxins, is facilitated. In rats subjected to hemorrhagic shock and resuscitation, this full sequence of events is seen, and is prevented by pretreatment with allopurinol, suggesting that free radicals, generated from xanthine oxidase at reperfusion, play an important role [60]. It is not known whether these agents merely trigger the release of inflammatory mediators from the gut itself, the liver, or from elsewhere. In any case, the loss of this barrier function probably provides a sound basis for the concept that the "gut is the motor of multiple organ failure" [61].

MICROVASCULAR ENDOTHELIAL CELL TRIGGER MECHANISM

The fact that allopurinol can prevent ischemia/reperfusion injury even in organs that do not contain measurable quantities of xanthine oxidase in their parenchymal cells (tissue homogenates), as well as prevent neutrophil accumulation in post-ischemic intestine, has focused attention on the endothelial cell as a possible source of xanthine oxidase generated superoxide. Immunohistochemical studies appear to localize xanthine oxidase activity in the microvascular endothelium of a number of organs, including the human heart [62,63]. We have found significant concentrations of xanthine dehydrogenase, which was rapidly converted to the oxidase, in cultured rat pulmonary artery endothelial cells subjected to relatively short periods of anoxia [64]. Moreover, 45 minutes of anoxia followed by 30 minutes of reoxygenation (simulating ischemia/reperfusion) produced endothelial cell lysis which was prevented by either allopurinol or SOD and catalase at the time of reoxygenation. These results indicate that the entire xanthine oxidase-based free radical-generating system is present and operative within the endothelial cell itself, even in the absence of neutrophils and parenchymal cells. We have proposed that this **endothelial cell trigger mechanism** is the ubiquitous initiator of free radical-mediated reperfusion injury (Figure 4).

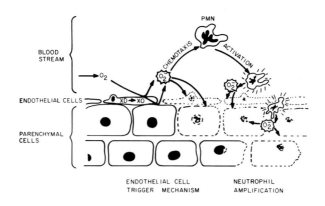

FIGURE 4: **The Endothelial Cell Trigger Mechanism of Free Radical-Mediated Reperfusion Injury.** *The entire xanthine oxidase-based free radical-generating system is present in the endothelial cell itself. Through a free radical-mediated mechanism, neutrophils accumulate, adhere, and are activated. The result is a further amplification of the initial endothelial cell injury. (Modified from Ratych, et al [64]).*

While in some organs endothelial cell injury may result in microvascular thrombosis and ultimate loss of organ function [65], in other organs (such as the intestine) this injury may only act as an initial trigger to attract and activate neurophils. How this early endothelial damage is communicated to the neutrophil, whether by non-specific injury, by a specific mediator cascade, or by up-regulation of specific endothelial or neutrophil adherence molecules, is unknown. However, the scavenging of superoxide with SOD does significantly decrease the adherence of neutrophils to the mesenteric venular endothelium following ischemia/reperfusion [66]. Once the neutrophils have adhered to the microvascular endothelium and been activated, they may cause tissue injury via toxic oxygen metabolites, proteases, or a combination of both mediators. This neutrophil amplifying system appears to be of variable quantitative importance in different organs, perhaps corresponding to the variable accumulation of neutrophils in different organs subject to ischemia [67].

SUMMARY

The generation of toxic oxygen metabolites by aerobic organisms is ubiquitous under normal circumstances, and can be greatly amplified under pathologic conditions, such that the fluxes of these highly toxic species can overwhelm the extensive endogenous antioxidant defense mechanisms. Indeed, this phenomenon is the final common pathway in a wide variety of otherwise disparate disease mechanisms. In the gastrointestinal tract, three of these mechanisms are of particular importance: 1) the generation of superoxide by microvascular endothelial cell xanthine oxidase at reperfusion following ischemia caused by angiotensin-mediated selective splanchnic vasoconstriction; 2) the generation of superoxide and hypochlorous acid by circulating neutrophils and fixed macrophages in response to the first mechanism and numerous other inflammatory stimuli; 3) the generation of, and activation by superoxide of arachidonate metabolism, via both the cyclooxygenase (prostaglandin) and lipoxygenase (leukotriene) pathways. All of these mechanisms appear to be important in the generation of mucosal injury in the gastrointestinal tract.

ACKNOWLEDGEMENT

This work was supported by NIH Grant #DK31764

REFERENCES

1.   Haglund U., Bulkley GB, Granger ND.   On the pathophysiology of intestinal ischemic injury.   Acta Chir Scand 1987; 153: 321.

2.   Bulkley BB, Kvietys PR, Parks DA, et al. Relationship of blood flow and oxygen consumption to ischemic injury in the canine small intestine. Gastroent 1985; 852-857.

3.   Fee JA and Valentine JS.   Chemical and physical properties of superoxide. In: Superoxide and Superoxide Dismutase (Michelson AM, McCord JM, Fridovich I, eds) New York, Academic Press, 1977; 19-60.

4.   Green MJ, Hill HAD.   Chemistry of dioxygen, In: Methods in Enzymology, Vol 105 (Packer L, ed.) Orlando, Academic Press, Inc., 1984; 3-22.

5.   Taube H.   Mechanisms of oxidation with oxygen.   J Gen Physiol 1965; 49: 29-50.

6.   Michelson AM. Toxic effects of active oxygen. In: Biochemical and Medical Aspects of Active Oxygen (Hayaishi O, Asada K, eds) Baltimore, University Park Press, 1977; 155-170.

7.   Boveris A, Chance B. The mitochondrial generation of hydrogen peroxide: General properties and effect of hyperbaric oxygen. Biochem J. 1973; 123: 707-716.

8.   Turrens JF, Boveris A. Generation of superoxide anion by the NADH dehydrogenase of bovine heart mitochondria. Biochem J 1980; 191: 421-427.

9.   Samuelson B. Leukotrienes: Mediators of immediate hypersensitivity reactions and inflammation. Science 1983; 220: 568-575.

10.   Kuehl FA, Humes J, Torchiana ML, et al. Oxygen-centered radicals in inflammatory processes. Adv Inflam Res 1979; 1: 419-430.

11.   McCord JM, Fridovich I. The reduction of cytochrome c by milk xanthine oxidase. J Biol Chem 1968; 243: 5753-5760.

12.   McCord JM, Fridovich I. Superoxide dismutase: An enzymatic function for erythrocuprein (Hemocuprein). J Biol Chem 1969; 244: 6049-6055.

13.   Waud WR, Rajagopalan KV. Purification and properties of the NAD-Dependent (Type D) and O_2-Dependent (Type O) forms of rat liver xanthine dehydrogenase. Arch Biochem Biophys 1976; 172: 354-364.

14.   Babior BM. Oxygen-dependent microbial killing by phagocytes. N Engl J Med 1978; 298: 659-668, 721-725.

15.   Babior BM, Peters WA. The O_2^--producing enzyme of human neutrophils: Further properties. J Biol Chem 1981; 256: 2321-2323.

16.   Klebanoff SJ. Oxygen metabolism and the toxic properties of phagocytes. Ann Intern Med 1980; 93: 480-489.

17.   Klebanoff SS. Phagocytic cells: Products of oxygen metabolism. In: Inflamation: Basic Principles and Clinical Correlates. (Gallin JI, Goldstein IM, Snyder R, eds) New York, Raven Press, 1988, 391-444.

18.   Cohen GM, Doherty M. Free radical mediated cell toxicity by redoc cycling chemicals. Br J Cancer 1987; 55, suppl VIII: 46-52.

19.   Lyons MJ, Gibson JF, Ingram DJE. Free radicals produced in cigarette smoke. Nature 1958; 181: 1003-1004.

20.   Butler TC. Reduction of carbon tetrachloride in vivo and reduction of tetrachloride and chloroform in vitro by tissues and tissue constituents. J Phar Exp Ther 1961; 134: 311-319.

21.   Reynolds ES, Ree HJ. Liver parenchymal cell injury: VII. Membrane denaturation following carbon tetrachloride. Lab Invest 1971; 25: 269-278.

22.   Hall EJ. Radiobiology for the Radiologist. Hagerstown, Harper and Row Publishers, 1973.

23.   Biaglow JE. Oxygen, hydrogen donors and radiation response. In: Hyperthermia (Bicher HI, Bruley DF, eds.). New York, Plenum Press, 1982, 147-175.

24.   Southorn PA, Powis G. Free radicals in medicine II. Involvement in human disease. Mayo Clin Proc. 1988; 63: 390-408.

25.   Oberley LW, Sierra E. Radiation sensitivity testing of cultured eukaryotic cells. In: CRC Handbook of Methods for Oxygen Radical Research (Greenwald RTA, ed). Boca Raton, CRC Press, Inc., 1985; 417-422.

26.   Mead JF. Free radical mechanisms of lipid damage and consequences for cellular membranes. In: Free Radicals in Biology (Pryor WA, ed.). New York, Academic Press, 1976; 51-56.

27.   Southorn PA, Powis G. Free radicals in medicine I. Chemical nature and biologic reactions. Mayo Clin Proc. 1988; 63: 381-389.

28.   Samuni A, Carmichael AJ, Russo JB, et al. On the spin trapping and ESR detection of oxygen-derived radicals generated inside cells. Proc Natl Acad Sci USA 1986; 83: 7593-7597.

29.   Boveris A, Cadenas E, Reiter R, et al. Organ chemiluminescence: Noninvasive assay for oxidative radical reactions. Proc Natl Acad Sci USA. 1980; 77: 347-351.

30.   Bannister JV, Bannister WH, Rotilio G. Aspects of the structure, function, and applications of superoxide dismutase. CRC Crit Rev Biochem. 1987; 22: 111-180.

31.   Forman HJ, Fisher AB. Antioxidant defenses. In: Oxygen and Living Processes and Interdisciplinary Approach (Gilbert DL, ed). New York, Springer-Verlag, 1981; 235-249.

32.   Moorhouse PC, Grootveld M, Halliwell B, et al. Allopurinol and oxypurinol are hydroxyl radical scavengers. FEBS Letters 1987; 213: 23-28.

33.   Zimmerman BJ, Parks DA, Grisham MB, et al. Allopurinol does not enhance antioxidant properties of extracellular fluid. Am J Physiol 1988; 255: H202-H206.

34.   Granger DN, Rutili G, McCord JM. Superoxide radicals in feline intestinal ischemia. Gastroenterology 1981; 81: 22-29.

35.   Granger DN, Hollwarth ME, Parks DA. Ischemia-reperfusion injury: Role of oxygen-derived free radicals. Acta Physiol Scand 1986; 548: 47-64.

36.   Parks DA, Granger DN. Ischemia-induced vascular changes: Role of xanthine oxidase and hydroxyl radicals. Am J Physiol 1983; 245 (GI 8): G285-G289.

37.   Hernandez LA, Grisham MB, Granger DN. A role for iron in oxidant-mediated ischemic injury to intestinal microvasculature. Am J Physiol 1987; 253 (GI 16): G49-G53.

38.   Parks DA, Bulkley GB, Granger DN, et al. Ischemic injury in the cat small intestine: role of superoxide radicals. Gastroenterology 1982; 82: 9-15.

39.   Granger DN. Role of xanthine oxidase and granulocytes in ischemia-reperfusion injury. Gastroenterology 1988; 255: H1269-1275.

40.   Parks DA, Granger DN. Xanthine oxidase: Biochemistry, distribution and physiology. Acta Physiol Scand 1986; 548: 97-100.

41.   McCord JM, Roy RS. The pathophysiology of superoxide: Roles in inflammation and ischemia. Can J Physiol Pharmacol 1982; 60: 1346-1352.

42.   Parks DA, Williams TK, Beckman JS: Conversion of xanthine dehydrogenase to oxidase in ischemic rat intestine: A re-evaluation. Am J Physiol 1988; 254 (GI 17): G768-G774.

43.   Batelli MG, Della Corte E, Stirpe F. Xanthine oxidase type d (dehydrogenase) in the intestine and other organs of the rat intestine. Biochem J 1972; 126: 747-749.

44.   Parks DA, Granger DN, Bulkley GB, et al. Soybean trypsin inhibitor attenuates ischemic injury to the feline intestine. Gastroenterology 1985; 89: 6-12.

45.   McKelvey TG, Hollwarth ME, Granger DN, et al. Mechanisms of conversion of xanthine dehydrogenase to xanthine oxidase in ischemic rat liver. Am J Physiol 1988; 254: G753-G760.

46.   Jones HP, Grisham MB, Bose SK, et al. Effect of allopurinol on neutrophil superoxide production, chemotaxis, or segmentation. Biochem Pharm 1985; 34: 3673-3676.

47.   Weiss SJ. Tissue destruction by neutrophils. New Engl J Med 1989; 320: 365-376.

48.   Grisham MB, Hernandez LA, Granger DN. Xanthine oxidase and neutrophil infiltration in intestinal ischemia. Am J Physiol 1986; 251 (GI 14): G567-G574.

49.   Kubes P, Suzuki M, Granger DN. The role of superoxide in platelet-activating factor-induced neutrophil adherence in cat mesentery. Gastroent 1990; 98: A457.

50.   Suzuki M, Grisham MB, Granger DN. Hydrogen peroxide promotes neutrophil adherence in cat mesenteric venules. Gastroent 1990; 98: A476.

51.   Hernandez LA, Grisham MB, Twohig B, et al. Role of neutrophils in ischemia-reperfusion induced microvascular injury. Am J Physiol 1987; 253 (Heart Circ Physiol 22): H699-H703.

52.   Peura DA, Johnson LF. Cimetidine for prevention and treatment of gastroduodenal mucosal lesions in patients in an intensive care unit. Ann Int Med 1985; 103: 173.

53.   Zinner MJ, Zuidema GS, Smith PL.   The prevention of upper gastrointestinal tract bleeding in patients in an intensive care unit. Surg Gyn Obst 1981; 153: 214.

54.   Baily RW, Bulkley GB, Hamilton SR, et al.   The fundamental hemodynamic mechanism underlying gastric "stress ulceration" in cardiogenic shock. Ann Surg 1987; 205: 597-612.

55.   Itoh M, Guth PH.   Role of oxygen-derived free radicals in hemorrhagic shock-induced gastric lesions in the rat. Gastroenterology 1985; 88: 1162-1167.

56.   Perry MA, Wadhwa S, Parks DA, et al. Role of oxygen radicals in ischemia-induced lesions in the cat stomach. Gastroenterology 1985; 90: 362-367.

57.   Warshaw A, O'Hara P. Susceptibility of the pancreas to ischemic injury in shock. Ann Surg. 1978; 188: 197-201.

58.   Sanfey H, Bulkley GB, Cameron JL.   The pathogenesis of acute pancreatitis: The source and role of oxygen-derived free radicals in three different experimental models. Ann Surg 1985; 201: 633-639.

59.   Sanfey H, Sarr MG, Bulkley GB, et al. Oxygen-derived free radicals and acute pancreatitis: A review. Acta Physiol Scand. 1986; 126: 109-118.

60.   Deitch EA, Bridges W, Baker J et al. Hemorrhagic shock-induced bacterial translocation is reduced by xanthine oxidase inhibition or inactivation. Surgery 1988; 104: 191.

61.   Meakins JL, Marshall JC. The gut as the motor of multiple system organ failure.   In: Marston A, Bulkley GB, Fiddian-Green RG, Haglund UH, eds. Splanchnic Ischemia and Multiple Organ Failure. London: Edward Arnold, 1989: 339.

62.   Jarasch ED, Bruder G, Heid HW. Significance of xanthine oxidase in capillary endothelial cells. Acta Physiol Scand 1986; 126 Suppl. 548: 39-46.

63.   Bruder G, Heid HW, Jarasch ED, et al. Immunological identification and determination of xanthine oxidase in cells and tissues. Differentiation 1983; 23: 218-225.

64.   Ratych RE, Chuknyiska RS, Bulkley GB. The primary localization of free radical generation following anoxia/reoxygenation in isolated endothelial cells. Surgery 1987; 102: 122-131.

65.   Marzella L, Jesudass RR, Manson PN, et al. Functional and structural evaluation of the vasculature of skin flaps after ischemia and reperfusion. Plast and Reconstr Surg 1988; 81: 752-750.

66.   Suzuki M. Grisham MB, Granger DN. Superoxide plays a role in reperfusion-induced leukocyte adherence to microvascular endothelium. Gastroenterology 1989; 96: A497.

67.   Grisham MB, Granger DN. Free radicals: reactive metabolites of oxygen as mediators of postischemic reperfusion injury. In: Splanchnic Ischemia and Multiple Organ Failure (Marston A, Bulkley GB, Fiddian-Green RG, Haglund UH, eds) London, Edward Arnold, 1989; 135-144.

EPITHELIAL CELL AND MEMBRANE PERMEABILITY TO PROTONS

Barry H. Hirst

*Department of Physiological Sciences, University of Newcastle upon Tyne
Medical School, Newcastle upon Tyne, England*

ABSTRACT

The net proton permeability of apical membranes from different regions of the gut is qualitatively consistent with the physiological concentrations of acid they have to resist, but have yet to be reconciled quantitatively with known properties of the cell membranes *in vivo*. The fluidity of the membranes is an important factor influencing proton permeability. Alcohols are recognised as increasing acid back-diffusion *in vivo*, and in isolated membranes increase proton permeability in parallel with increased membrane fluidity. The effects of alcohols on the isolated membranes are seen at concentrations lower than required to induce gross damage in the intact mucosa. Bile salts also perturb isolated membranes, including increasing proton permeability, at concentrations lower than that required in intact tissue. Exogenous prostaglandin E_2 is able to ameliorate the bile salt-induced increase in proton permeability, without having an effect when added alone, indicating a direct protective action on duodenal apical membranes. The studies with isolated membrane vesicles provide direct evidence that the cell membrane is likely to be a site of sensitive and early damage by barrier-breaking agents. Gastrointestinal epithelial cells in culture offer another model for studying the effect of recognized damaging agents. Growth of the cells on permeable supports allows reconstitution of a functional epithelium. Several established cell lines from the human intestine (T84 and HCT-8), and dog kidney (MDCK), grown as reconstituted epithelia form tight monolayers of high transepithelial resistance, and demonstrate substantial resistance to acidification. The resistance of these simple epithelia to acid illustrate the central role of the epithelial cell as a barrier to acid back-diffusion in the gut. The established cell lines provide a simplified epithelial system for clarifying mechanisms of the barrier to acid.

INTRODUCTION

The mucosal lining of the upper gastrointestinal tract is regularly exposed to a highly acidic environment and, in the case of the stomach, has an ability to maintain greater than one million-fold gradient of protons, termed the gastric mucosal barrier [1]. The maintenance of this barrier to acid is of explicit pathophysiological importance; breaching the barrier leads to local damage to the mucosa and is ultimately associated with ulceration. The components of this barrier to acid include the surface HCO_3^--containing mucus gel, tissue acid-base balance and mucosal blood flow ('extrinsic' factors), together with the intrinsic properties of the epithelia, including intracellular pH regulation, and the permeability of the epithelial cell apical membranes and tight junctions to protons (Figure 1).

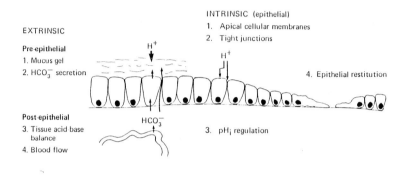

FIGURE 1:   *Components of the upper gastrointestinal barrier to acid
              [From Hirst (1)]*

The studies outlined below describe work using gastrointestinal luminal plasma membrane vesicles and cultured epithelial cells to study the resistance of epithelia to acid [2,3]. We have characterised the permeability to protons of the apical plasma membranes from various areas of the upper gastrointestinal tract [3], and the effect of damaging agents [4-6]. We have also investigated the effect of acid challenges on cultured epithelial cells grown on permeable supports to reconstitute epithelial monolayers [7].

MATERIALS AND METHODS

APICAL MEMBRANE VESICLES

Membrane vesicles were prepared from rabbit gastric, intestinal and renal membranes. Gastric vesicles were prepared from the apical membranes of parietal cells stimulated to secrete acid (stimulation-associated (SA) vesicles) [8]. Duodenal, jejunal and renal cortical brush-border membrane (BBM) vesicles were prepared by a Mg^{2+}-precipitation method [2,4,5].

Proton permeability. Proton permeability was quantified from the recovery of acridine orange fluorescence quenching [4]. Vesicles were pre-equilibrated to give an acidic (pH 6.5) intravesicular compartment, before addition to an alkaline (pH 8.0) buffer containing acridine orange. The acridine orange partitions into the intravesicular acidic environment with a rapid quenching of fluorescence. The slower leakage of protons out of the vesicles is accompanied by a recovery of fluorescence signal which may be followed with time. Figures 2 and 3 illustrate such experiments. This fluorescence recovery follows simple first-order kinetics [2,4] and enables determination of the rate constant for the recovery of the fluorescence, equivalent to proton permeation; k_{H^+}. The exponential time constant (τ) for this process is the inverse of k_{H^+}. From these values, and the radius (r) of the vesicles, the intracellular concentration of protons ($[H^+]_i$), and the intravesicular (βend) and extravesicular buffer capacities (βex), the net proton permeability coefficient (Pnet), which is the sum of the flux of protons (PH) and hydroxide (POH), may be calculated:

$$Pnet = PH + POH = \frac{r.\beta_{END} + \beta_{EX}}{3\tau[H^+]_i.\ln 10}$$

Pnet is dominated by PH under the current experimental conditions [4]. All experiments were carried out in solutions containing high K^+ and valinomycin to voltage clamp the vesicles and so prevent H^+ diffusion potentials from developing [4].

Lipid dynamics. The structural order and lipid dynamics of the hydrophobic region of the membranes were measured from the fluorescence anisotropy (r) of 1,6-diphenyl-1,3,4-hexatriene (DPH) under both steady-state and time-resolved conditions [4]. Under steady-state conditions, membrane fluidity was expressed in terms of the parameter (r_o/r)-1, where r is the observed fluorescence anisotropy, and r_o is the maximum fluorescence anisotropy. Time-resolved anisotropy decays of DPH fluorescence were analysed to yield the fluorescence lifetime (τ_f), correlation time (ϕ) and limiting anisotrophy (r∞) [4].

CULTURED EPITHELIAL CELLS

Madin-Darby canine kidney (MDCK), human ileo-caecal (HCT-8) and colonic (T84) adenocarcinoma cells were seeded onto Millicell-HA 12 mm diameter culture inserts, collagen-coated for HCT-8 and T84 cells, and used 3-7 days after seeding when a significant transepithelial resistance (Re) had developed [7]. Monolayers were then transferred to modified Ussing chambers. Each reservoir was connected by agar bridges to voltage-sensing calomel electrodes, and to Ag-AgCl electrodes used for bipolar current pulses, and Re determined from the voltage deflections. The reservoirs were filled with 4 ml of a bicarbonate-free Krebs-Ringer solution buffered with 5 mM-Tris maleate, with pH varied from 7.4 to 2.5

RESULTS

STUDIES WITH ISOLATED APICAL MEMBRANE VESICLES

Proton permeability and lipid dynamics of gastrointestinal membranes

The native proton permeability of the membranes was in the rank order gastric SA < duodenal BBM = jejunal BBM << renal BBM (Table 1). Under non-voltage clamped conditions, the rate of proton permeation was indeterminably slow, due to the development of H+ diffusion potentials [2]. Addition of bovine serum albumin (2%), to mop up any fatty acids which might act as endogenous protonophores, only resulted in a small reduction (~30%) in the rate of proton permeation [4].

The proton permeability of the membrane vesicles was not simply related to their lipid dynamics (Table 1). Under steady-state conditions, membrane fluidity $[(r_o/r)-1$; renal BBM <= deuodenal BBM < jejunal BBM <= gastric SA] tended to be inversely related to proton permeability. The fluorescence lifetimes of DPH in the different membranes were similar, and consistent with other studies [4]. The majority of the steady-state DPH anisotropy could be accounted for by the limiting anisotropy (r∞), while the membranes had rotational correlation times (ϕ) around 4 ns (Table 1).

TABLE 1

*Proton permeability and lipid dynamics of upper
gastrointestinal and renal apical plasma membrane vesicles*

Membrane	Proton Permeability Pnet (x 10^{-4}cm/s)	Membrane fluidity parameters				
		(r_o/r)-1	τf	ϕ (ns)	r∞ (ns)	Ref
Gastric SA	3.77	0.62	8.73	4.03	0.22	[4]
		0.59				[5]
Duodenal BBM	9.83	0.45	8.23	3.05	0.25	[4]
	6.30	0.50	9.14	4.26	0.25	[6]
	5.42					[9]
Jejunal BBM	5.59	0.57				[11]
Renal BBM	95.3	0.44	8.94	5.48	0.25	[4]

All variables were measured at 20^oC as described by Wilkes et al [4]. Lipid dynamic properties were characterised from 1,6-diphenyl-1,3,5-hexatriene (DPH) fluorescence anisotropy measurements. (ro/r)-1 is an indication of membrane fluidity under steady state conditions. τf is the fluorescence lifetime, ϕ correlation time, and r∞ the limiting anisotropy, determined from time-resolved fluorescence decays of DPH.

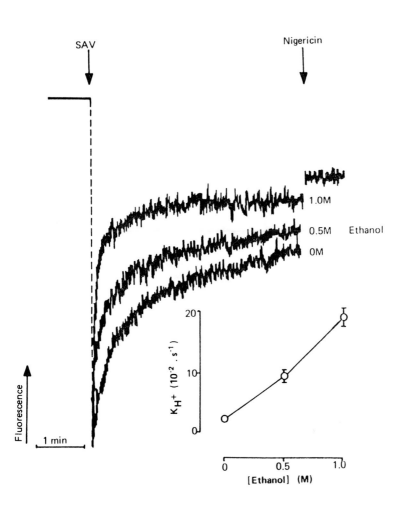

FIGURE 2   *Effects of ethanol on proton permeation in parietal cell apical membrane vesicles. Vesicles (stimulation-associated; SAV) were voltage-clamped with K^+-valinomycin, and equilibrated at pH 6.5, and then diluted into a pH 8.0 solution containing acridine orange (first arrow). Addition of vesicles leads to a quenching of the fluorescence signal as the dye accumulates in the acidic intravesicular space. Recovery of fluorescence gives the rate of H^+ permeation. Nigericin, a H^+-K^+ ionophore, was added at the second arrow and fully dissipates the proton gradient. Increasing concentrations of ethanol accelerate the rate of fluorescence recovery, i.e. increase proton permeation. Inset: apparent rate constant for the recovery of fluorescence plotted against concentration of ethanol. [From Hirst (1)]*

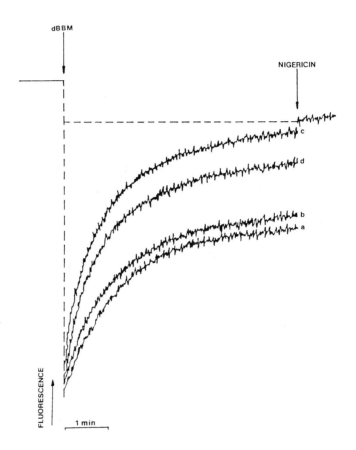

FIGURE 3   *Effect of PGE$_2$ on bile salt-induced increase in proton permeation in duodenal BBM vesicles.   On addition of vesicles equilibrated at pH 6.5 to a solution containing acridine orange, pH 8.0, fluorescence (λex 490 nm, λem 522 nm) quenching is observed. As the pH gradient is dissipated, quenching is reduced.   Addition of nigericin completely dissipates the pH gradient. The traces illustrate experiments with vesicles pre-incubated (a) under control conditions, (b) with PGE$_2$, 10^{-7} M, (c) with deoxycholate, 0.5 mM, and (d) with PGE$_2$, 10^{-7} M, plus deoxycholate, 0.5 mM. [From Zhao & Hirst (9)].*

Proton permeability in renal [4], duodenal [10] and ileal (JM Wilkes & BH Hirst, unpublished) membrane vesicles is reduced by amiloride (10^{-6}-10^{-3} M) consistent with a role for the Na^+/H^+ exchangers as a leak pathway for protons. These three membrane types have all been demonstrated to contain Na^+/H^+ exchange. In duodenal BBM, by imposing a K^+-diffusion potential, we could demonstrate the intravesicular acidification which was stimulated by addition of valinomycin, indicative of entry of protons via a conductive pathway. This mechanism was also sensitive to amiloride [10]. In gastric SA vesicles, proton permeation was insensitive to amiloride (JM Wilkes & BH Hirst, unpublished), arguably due to the absence of Na^+/H^+ exchangers in these membranes.

STUDIES WITH BARRIER-BREAKING AGENTS.

Alcohols.   Alcohols, including ethanol, increase the fluidity of gastrointestinal membranes [4,5].   These effects are observed with low concentrations of ethanol (e.g. 0.3-0.5 M). These membrane fluidising effects of alcohols are recognised as causing general increases in membrane passive permeability [3].   Proton permeability is also increased by alcohols [4]. Figure 2 illustrates the effect of increasing concentrations of ethanol on the rate of proton permeation in gastric SA vesicles.   The increase in proton permeability induced by alcohols is directly correlated with the increases in membrane fluidity [4], suggesting a causal relation.   At higher concentrations, the alcohols result in increased membrane fragility and disruption of the vesicles [5].

Bile salts.   Low concentrations of bile salts (e.g. 0.1-1.0 mM deoxycholate and its conjugates), which are below their critical micellar concentration (CMC), increase duodenal and jejunal BBM fragility and proton permeability [6,9,11].   The effect of deoxycholate, 0.5 mM, on proton permeation in duodenal BBM is illustrated in Figure 3.   In contrast to the effects of alcohols, however, the increased proton permeability was not associated with increased membrane fluidity in duodenal BBM [6].

COMPARISON OF DUODENAL AND JEJUNAL BBM

Duodenal BBM are more resistant than gastric SA membranes and jejunal BBM to increased fragility.   Thus, with alcohols as the perturbing agents higher concentrations of ethanol are required to cause significant increases in vesicle disruption [5].   Similarly, duodenal BBM are less sensitive to alcohol-induced increases in proton permeability [4]. With bile salts, duodenal BBM are again more resistant than jejunal BBM to increases in proton permeability, vesicle fragility and membrane fluidity [11].

PROTECTION WITH PROSTAGLANDINS

Addition of prostaglandin E_2 (PGE_2) *in vitro* to duodenal BBM has no effect on proton permeability.   However, PGE_2, 10^{-7}-10^{-6} M, was able to reduce the increase in proton permeability induced by bile salts (Figure 3). PGE_2 had no consistent effect on the bile salt induced increase in membrane fragility [9].

STUDIES WITH CULTURED EPITHELIAL CELLS

Acidification of the apical surface of tight monolayers (Re >700   .cm^2) of epithelial cells results in a biphasic response (Figure 4). Initially Re increases, followed by a decline as the apical pH is further reduced. In MDCK cells, the apical surface is able to withstand pH 3.0 for at least 1.5 h, whereas a decline in Re is observed upon basolateral acidification for 1.5 h (AB Chan & BH Hirst, unpublished). Neither surface is able to maintain Re with acidification down to pH 2.5 or below. Similar patterns were also observed with two other high resistance cell lines: T84 and HCT-8 [7]. Apical, but not basolateral, amiloride (10^{-3} M) reduced the ability of MDCK cell monolayers to maintain Re during apical or basolateral acidification [12], suggesting a role for apical Na^+/H^+ exchangers in the normal maintenance of epithelial integrity in the face of acidic challenges in these cells.

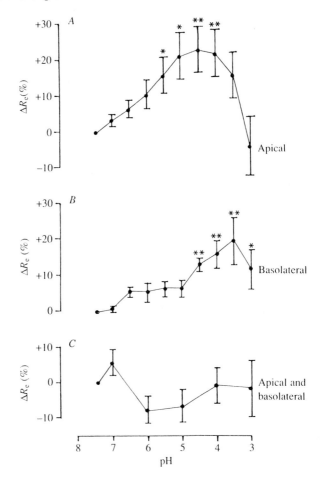

FIGURE 4. *Transepithelial electrical resistance of MDCK monolayers as a function of pH of apical or basolateral solutions. The pH of the apical (A) or basolateral (B) solution was acidified while the contralateral solution was maintained at pH 7.4. In (C), both solutions were acidified simultaneously. Even at pH 3.0, electrical resistance of the monolayers is maintained. [From Chan et al (7)].*

Aspirin (1-5 mM) alone has little effect on *Re* in either MDCK or HCT-8 cells. Similarly the cell monolayers are able to maintain *Re* during apical acidification to pH 3.0. However, addition of aspirin to the acidic solution resulted in a marked decline in *Re* [13].

DISCUSSION

The rank order for proton permeability for the four membrane types (gastric < duodenal = jejunal << renal) is in general agreement with their known physiological environments [3,4]. Quantitatively, however, these permeabilities (e.g. approximately 4×10^{-4} cm/s for gastric membranes) are one to two orders of magnitude higher than values for the intact gastric mucosa [3,4]. Only a small component of this increased proton permeability may be accounted for by contamination by endogenous protonophores. The greater pH gradient in situ might activate pH dependent factors, and cellular transmembrane potentials and the small radius of curvature of the vesicles [1,3,4] may all be factors contributing towards the differences between the in situ and vesicle estimates of proton permeability.

At least one route for the permeation of protons through the membranes is via transmembrane proteins. In the small intestine and kidney this will include permeation via amiloride-sensitive Na^+/H^+ exchangers [3,10]. The lipid membrane also constitutes a site for proton permeation, and increases in lipid dynamics by alcohols may make this route more accessible to protons [4].

Alcohols and bile salts are able to increase membrane proton permeability directly. This effect of these two recognised gastric mucosal barrier breaking agents [1] is observed at low concentrations. For example, the concentrations of ethanol required to increase proton permeability *in vitro* are equivalent to those likely to be found in the gut after moderate social drinking [5]. Similarly, the concentrations of bile salts required for this effect are similar to those found in the normal stomach [6]. The concentrations of both these agents required to perturb proton permeability in membrane vesicles are considerably lower than those required to elicit gross damage to the gastric and intestinal mucosa [1,3]. These subtle changes in proton permeability are likely to be important early events in pathophysiological damage to the mucosa in situ.

The effects of prostaglandins in the gastrointestinal tract are as diverse as they are abundant, and many are assigned to be protective in nature. Direct membrane actions have been implied from a number of studies, but the direct action of PGE_2 in reducing the bile salt increase in proton permeability [9], may be one important physiological mechanism for duodenal mucosal protection.

The ability of several cultured epithelial cell lines to maintain transepithelial electrical resistance during challenge with apical acidity, indicates that these relatively simple systems may provide a suitable model for studying epithelial resistance to acid. Acidification is initially associated with increased Re, and this is similar to that observed in isolated gastric mucosa [14]. Similarly, in both cultured cells [12] and isolated gastric mucosa [14], amiloride attenuates the acid induced increases in Re. Thus Na^+/H^+ exchangers may be involved in the normal maintenance of Re and the response to acidic challenges. The ability of these cultured cellular monolayers to withstand acid allows their use as model systems for studying gut function, including the ability to mimic local intraluminal environments which are likely to be essential features in the damaging effects of several barrier-breaking agents (e.g. pH partitioning of aspirin) [1,13]. The resistance of these simple epithelia to acid illustrate the central role of the epithelial cell as a barrier to acid back-diffusion in the gut.

ACKNOWLEDGEMENTS

The work reported from the author's laboratory was supported by grants from the Medical Research Council (G8418056CA), SmithKline Foundation, University of Newcastle upon Tyne Research Committee (563022 & 563262), and Science & Engineering Research Council CASE awards with Glaxo Group Research, Ware, Smith Kline & French Research, Welwyn, and Sterling-Winthrop Research Centre, Alnwick. The author also acknowledges the Royal Society, Biochemical Society and Pfizer Ltd. for travel awards. The author is pleased to record the scientific collaboration of Dr. J.M. Wilkes, Dr. D. Zhao, Dr. H.J. Ballard, A.B. Chan, C.N. Allen, G.E. Spencer and Dr. N.L. Simmons.

REFERENCES

1. Hirst BH. The gastric mucosal barrier. In: Forte JG (Ed). Handbook of Physiology. The Gastrointestinal System. Vol. III. Gastrointestinal Secretion. American Physiological Society: Bethesda, MD. 2nd Ed. 1989; 279-308.

2. Wilkes JM, Ballard HJ, Latham JAE, Hirst BH. Gastroduodenal epithelial cells: the role of the apical membrane in mucosal protection. In: Reid E, Cook GMW and Luzio JP (Eds). Cells, Membranes, and Disease, Including Renal. Plenum: New York. 1987; 243-254.

3. Hirst BH. Gastrointestinal epithelial barrier to acid: studies with isolated membrane vesicles and cultured epithelial cells. In: Jones CJ (Ed). Epithelia: advances in cell physiology and cell culture. Kluwer: Dordrecht. 1990: 5-27.

4. Wilkes JM, Ballard HJ, Dryden DTF, Hirst BH. Proton permeability and lipid dynamics of gastric and duodenal apical membrane vesicles. Am J Physiol 1989; 256: G553-G562.

5. Ballard HJ, Wilkes JM, Hirst BH. Effect of alcohols on gastric and small intestinal apical membrane integrity and fluidity. Gut 1988; 29: 1648-1655.

6. Zhao D, Hirst BH. Bile salt induced increases in duodenal brush-border membrane proton permeability, fluidity and fragility. Dig Dis Sci. 1990; 35: 589-595.

7. Chan AB, Allen CN, Simmons NL, Parsons ME, Hirst BH. Resistance to acid of canine kidney (MDCK) and human colonic (T84) and ileocaecal (HCT-8) adenocarcinoma epithelial cell monolayers in vitro. Qu J Exp Physiol 1989; 74: 553-556.

8. Hirst BH, Forte JG. Redistribution and characterization of (H^++K^+)-ATPase membranes from resting and stimulated gastric parietal cells. Biochem J 1985; 231: 641-649.

9. Zhao D, Hirst BH. Prostaglandin protects against bile salt-induced increases in duodenal brush-border membrane proton permeability. Gut 1991; 32: in press.

10. Briggs R, Hirst BH, Wilkes JM. Amiloride sensitivity of proton conductance in rabbit duodenal brush-border membrane vesicles in vitro. J Physiol (London) 1988; 406: 117P.

11. Zhao D, Hirst BH. Comparison of bile salt perturbation of duodenal and jejunal isolated brush-border membranes. Digestion 1991; 48: in press.

12. Chan AB, Hirst BH, Parsons ME, Simmons NL. Resistance of Medin-Darby canine kidney (MDCK) epithelial cell monolayers to acid. J Physiol (London) 1989; 409: 58P.

13. Allen CN, Eason CT, Bonner FW, Simmons NL, Hirst BH. Development of human gastrointestinal cultured cells for predictive toxicology. Human Toxicol. 1989; 8: 412.

14. Spencer GE, Spraggs CF, Stables R, Hirst BH. Effect of acid on transmucosal electrical resistance in rabbit isolated gastric mucosa. J Physiol (London) 1991; 432:22P.

SPECIALIZATION OF THE APICAL SURFACE OF PARIETAL CELLS: IDENTIFICATION AND CHARACTERIZATION OF A β-SUBUNIT OF THE GASTRIC H,K-ATPase

J.G. Forte[1], C.T. Okamoto[1], D.C.Chow[1], V.A. Canfield[2] and R. Levenson[2]

[1]Dept. of Cell & Molecular Biology, Univ. of California, Berkeley, CA and
[2]Dept. of Cell Biology, Yale Univ. School of Medicine, New Haven, CT

ABSTRACT

Histochemical studies show that a heavily glycosylated protein is present in great abundance in the parietal cell membranes that are also rich in H,K-ATPase, i.e., tubulovesicles and apical microvillar membranes. This glycoprotein has been shown to be a β-subunit of the H,K-ATPase, which we now know to function as an αβ protomer. Primary amino acid sequence of gastric β , deduced from cDNA clones, demonstrate several structural analogies between gastric β and the β-subunit isoforms of the Na,K-ATPase. Gastric β consists of 294 amino acids, with a small intracellular domain, a single transmembrane segment, and a large extracellular domain (78% of the proteic mass, as well as a high density of glycoconjugates). Six cysteine residues in the extracellular domain of gastric β may play an important role in the structural stability and functional activity of the H,K-ATPase. Strong reducing conditions lead to inhibition of enzyme activity with implications that disulfide bonds in the extracellular domain of gastric β may serve to stabilize holoenzymatic activity as well as intrinsic structure. Several interesting and characteristic features of the oligosaccharides in gastric β have been ascertained. All oligosaccharides are N-linked, complex tri- or tetra-antennary type, devoid of sialic acid, and probably containing poly-N-acetyllactosamine structure. On the basis of the high degree of glycosylation present at the extracellular membrane facing the gastric lumen, we speculate on the possibility that the oligosaccharides play a role in the cellular resistance to autodigestion.

INTRODUCTION

The question as to why the healthy stomach does not digest itself is one of great clinical and biological significance. Proteic constituents on the apical surface of parietal cells, and indeed all gastric epithelial cells, must be highly resistant to the extreme variations of pH (pH 0.8 to 7.8) and proteolytic conditions within the lumen of the stomach. Earlier work from our laboratory showed the presence of a heavy and distinctive [1], and possibly protective [2], coat of glycoprotein on the external face of parietal cell apical membranes and on the interior surface of cytoplasmic tubulovesicles. More recently [3-5] we demonstrated that this parietal cell glycoprotein is an associated β-subunit of the H,K-ATPase (gastric β). The purpose of this report is to describe additional structural and functional features of gastric β.

Histochemical studies carried out on ultrathin sections of frog [1], rat [6] and pig (unpublished) revealed that a rich coating of glycoprotein is present on parietal (or oxyntic) cell membranes. In the acid secreting cells the most intense staining was localized to the outer aspect of the apical plasma membrane, the internal surface of tubulovesicles, and within cisternae and vesicles of the Golgi complex.

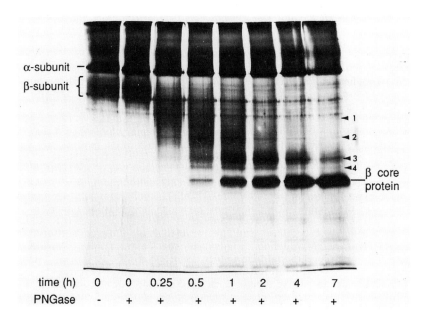

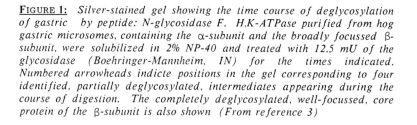

FIGURE 1: *Silver-stained gel showing the time course of deglycosylation of gastric by peptide: N-glycosidase F. H,K-ATPase purified from hog gastric microsomes, containing the α-subunit and the broadly focussed β-subunit, were solubilized in 2% NP-40 and treated with 12.5 mU of the glycosidase (Boehringer-Mannheim, IN) for the times indicated. Numbered arrowheads indicte positions in the gel corresponding to four identified, partially deglycosylated, intermediates appearing during the course of digestion. The completely deglycosylated, well-focussed, core protein of the β-subunit is also shown (From reference 3)*

IDENTFICATION OF THE β-SUBUNIT OF THE H,K-ATPASE.

Working with H,K-ATPase-rich tubulovesicles that had been purified from several species we consistently identified on SDS-PAGE a carbohydrate-staining band in the region of 60-80 kDa [2,3]. Because this glycoprotein band was so poorly focussed and rich in carbohydrate, it was poorly stained with Coomassie blue, leading others to conclude that the 94 kDa peptide(s) is the only proteic component in purified H,K-ATPase [7]. In addition to its invariant presence within gastric tubulovesicles and apical membrane fractions, the 60-80 kDa glycoprotein was found to exist in non-covalent association with the 94 kDa a-subunit [3,4]. This association was shown to be stable in several non-denaturing detergents (e.g., Nonidet-P40, Triton X100, cholate, $C_{12}E_8$), and was the initial basis for our suggestion that the gastric 60-80 kDa glycoprotein was a β-subunit of the H,K-ATPase (gastric β). Further evidence for the gastric β-subunit hypothesis came from deglycosylation studies and analyses of the α βsubunit stoichiometry.

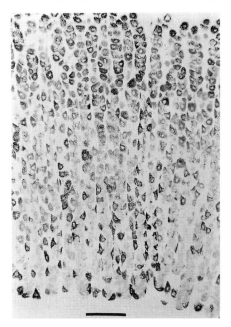

FIGURE 2: *Immunoperoxidase staining of rabbit gastric mucosa using monoclonal antibody against H,K-ATPase β-subunit (β-MAb). Rabbit fundic mucosa was fixed by freeze-substitution, embedded in paraffin and sectioned. Deparaffinized sections were probed with β-MAb, followed by anti-mouse-IgG-peroxidase. Gastric glands are shown from the neck region (top) to the lamina propria (bottom) at the base of the glands. Surface epithelial cells are completely unstained and are thus not shown. Parietal cells are the only cells that are positively stained for the gastric β-subunit antigen. Bar marker is 100 um.*

Deglycosylation of gastric β is specifically and completely effected by peptide:N-glycosidase F [3]. Figure 1 shows a time course of deglycosylation of the 60-80 kDa glycoprotein producing at least four intermediate stages of partial deglycosylation, in addition to the final deglycosylated 34 kDa core peptide of gastric β . These data reveal a well-focussed core peptide about the same molecular size as the β-subunit of the Na,K-ATPase [7], and the kinetics of deglycosylation are consistent with at least five sites of N-glycosylation on gastric β . Protein stained SDS-gels of highly purified H,K-ATPase preparations were scanned by densitometry to estimate the relative amounts of protein in the α- and β-subunits. For 14 separate gels the Coomassie blue staining of the α-subunit was 2.5 ± 1.1

times greater than the β -subunit, which is not significantly different than α β proteic mass ratio predicted from the molecular weights. Thus these data are consistent with a 1 to 1 molecular stoichiometry for α to β in the H,K-ATPase [3].

IMMUNOLOGICAL DETECTION OF GASTRIC β.

A mouse monoclonal antibody (β-MAb) was developed against gastric β for use in cytological and analytical immunodetection [9]. The pattern of gastric tissue staining with β-MAb, as shown in figure 2 , (i) is specific for parietal cells, (ii) is highly suggestive of tubulovesicular labelling, and (iii) is distributed in the same pattern as that obtained with an antibody to the α-subunit [9]. As shown by the Western blot analyses in figure 3, the antigen recognizing β-MAb is present in gastric mucosa of hog, rabbit, cow, rat, and mouse (i.e. all mammalian species thus far examined), but was not present in tissues other than stomach (i.e. colon, kidney, liver, pancreas, small intestine, brain).

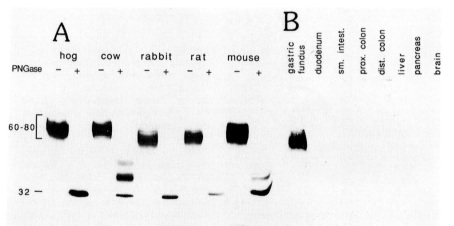

FIGURE 3: *Probing for the expression of gastric β-subunit in oxyntic mucosa of various species and in various tissues of the rabbit. A. Membrane fractions were prepared from stomachs of hog, cow, rabbit, rat and mouse, solubilized in detergent and either treated with peptide: N-glycosidase F (+) or not (-). Samples were run on SDS-PAGE, transblotted onto nitrocellulose, and probed with a monoclonal antibody against rabbit gastric (β-MAb) and a second antibody conjugated with peroxidase. Hog (10ug/lane), cow (15 ug/lane), rabbit (50 ug/lane), rat (45 ug/lane), and mouse (40 ug/lane). The apparent molecular weight of the glycosylated and deglycosylated β-subunits are indicated on the left. B. Membrane fractions prepared from various rabbit tissues, as indicated, were separated by SDS-PAGE, transblotted and probed with β-MAb as in A. Positive identification was made only in gastric tissue. Fundus (50 ug/lane), duodenum (100 ug/lane), intestine (200 ug/lane), proximal colon (97 ug/lane), distal colon (200 ug/lane), liver (136 ug/lane), pancreas (99 ug/lane) and brain (165 ug/lane).*

PEPTIDE SEQUENCING.

cDNA libraries prepared from bovine abomasum and rat gastric mucosa were screened with the β-MAb to assay protein expression, and oligonucleotides constructed from amino acid sequences obtained on fragments of gastric β. Thus, cDNA clones encoding the bovine (partial length) and rat (full length) gastric β subunits have been isolated and sequenced [10]. The open reading frame for the full length rat cDNA clone predicts that gastric β contains 294 amino acids with a molecular weight of 33,689, and a primary amino acid sequence as shown in figure 4. The hydropathy profile shown in figure 5 indicates that from the amino terminus there is a relatively short polar cytoplasmic domain, followed by a single hydrophobic transmembrane segment, and finally a rather large (228 amino acid residues) extracellular carboxy-terminal domain including seven consensus sequences of potential sites for N-linked glycosylation.

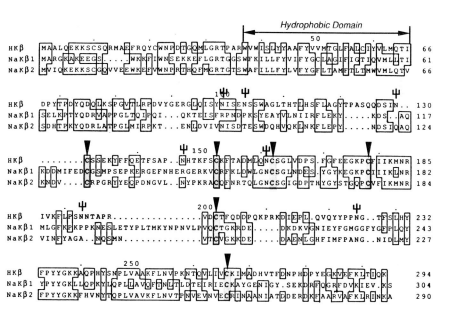

FIGURE 4: *Amino acid sequences of H,K-ATPase and Na,K-ATPase β-subunits. The deduced amino acid of the rat H,K-ATPase β-subunit (HK β , top line) was aligned with those of rat Na,K-ATPase β₁ (NaK β₁, middle line) and β₂ (NaK β₂, bottom line) subunits. Lapses in the sequence allow optimal alignment for amino acid insertions/deletions. Identical residues are enclosed. The highly conserved cysteine residues in the proposed extracellular domain of the three β-subunits are shaded (arrowheads) and consensus sequence sites for N-glycosylation are indicated by the triton symbol. The H,K-ATPase β-subunit sequence is numbered above, while amino acids for all three subunits are numbered on the right. (From reference 10). Shull has also recently cloned and sequenced the β-subunit of the rat gastric ATPase (28).*

Figure 4 also compares amino acid sequences for the β_1 and β_2 subunit isoforms of the Na,K-ATPase in a computer-aligned fit with gastric β. The sequence for rat gastric β shows 41% identity with the rat Na,K-ATPase β_2 subunit and 35% identity with the rat β_1 subunit. There are a total of nine cysteine residues within gastric β. The six cysteine residues in the putative extracellular domain of all three subunit types are very highly conserved, suggesting some fundamental role for these cysteine residues, possibly stabilizing tertiary structure through disulfide cross-linking. When analyzed either by the algorithm developed by Finer-Moore et al.[11] the predicted secondary structures for gastric β, β_1 and β_2 are quite similar. Using the 9/8/86 version of Stroud's PREDICT program [11] to suggest secondary structure we have devised the preliminary working model of gastric β depicted in figure 6. We have taken additional liberties in indicating that all seven of the potential N-linked glycosylation sites are occupied by an oligosaccharide, and have presumed three specific disulfide bonds in the extracellular domain.

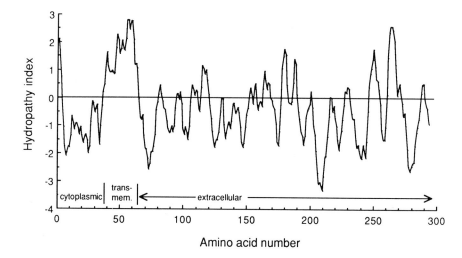

FIGURE 5: *Hydropathy profile of rat gastric H,K-ATPase β-subunit. Hydropathy plot was obtained using the algorithm and hydropathy values of Kyte and Doolittle (29). Hydrophobic regions are above the center line and hydrophilic regions are below.*

FUNCTIONAL ACTIVITY OF DISULFIDE BONDS IN THE H,K-ATPASE.

Two separate groups have presented evidence to suggest that the cysteine residues in the extracellular domain of the β-subunit of the Na,K-ATPase normally exist in the oxidized state as three disulfide bonds [12,13]. They also demonstrated that Na,K-ATPase activity was inhibited under reducing conditions where disulfides were at least partially reduced [12-15]. Because the extracellular cysteine residues of the various β-subunits are so highly conserved, we tested the sensitivity of gastric H,K-ATPase activity to

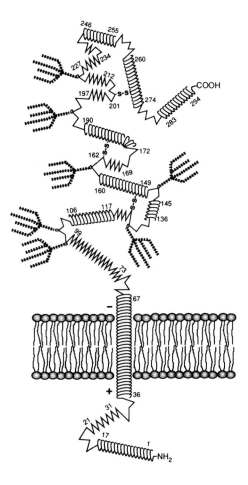

<u>FIGURE 6.</u> *Hypothetical model of H,K-ATPase β-subunit structure at the apical membrane surface. The model was constructed by combining the experimentally deduced primary sequence of rat gastric β, hydropathy data, secondary structural predictions from the 9/8/86 version of Stroud's PREDICT algorithm (11), and assumed disulfide bond arrangements. The model also assumes glycosylation of all seven predicted N-linked sites. An important missing element is the locus and nature of interaction between the β- and α-subunits.*

reducing conditions. From earlier work [16], as well as from more recent reevaluation, we concluded that relatively mild conditions of reduction (e.g., 2-10 mM 2-mercaptoethanol for 30 min, $37^{\circ}C$) had no significant effect on H,K-ATPase. However, stronger reducing conditions, using higher concentration of 2-mercaptoethanol or dithiothreitol at elevated temperatures, produced a time-dependent loss of enzyme activity. The loss of K^{+}-stimulated pNPPase activity (a marker of H,K-ATPase) produced by 400 mM 2-mercaptoethanol at $43^{\circ}C$ is shown in figure 7.

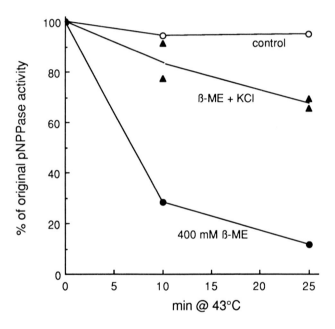

FIGURE 7: *Effect of strong reducing conditions on Gastric H,K-ATPase activity and the protective action of K+. Hog microsomal membranes were incubated at $43^{\circ}C$ with 400mM ethanol (control), or with 400 mM 2-mercaptoethanol in the absence (β-ME) or presence of 10 mM KCl (β -ME + KCl) for the times as shown. Membranes were then washed of extraneous agents by centrifugation in the cold and assayed for H,K-ATPase or K+-stimulated pNPPase (shown here) activities.*

Interestingly, the degree of inhibition was attenuated by relatively low concentrations of K^{+}, as has also been shown for Na,K-ATPase [12,15]. Among the three alkali metal cations tested for their ability to protect H,K-ATPase from disulfide reduction we found the order of effectivity to be

$Tl^+ > K^+ >> Na^+$, which is the same order for ability to catalyze the hydrolysis of ATP and pNPP [17]. These data can be taken as suggesting that external disulfide bonds on gastric β are specifically responsible for the inhibition based on (i) structural analogies with what has been shown for the Na,K-ATPase [12-15], (ii) the unlikely occurrence of stable disulfide bonds within the reducing environment of the cytoplasmic domain, and (iii) the predicted transmembrane orientation of the gastric α-subunit [18] which would allow for only one extracellular cysteine residue. Furthermore, such observations provide the first hint that the gastric β-subunit has a functional role in H,K-ATPase activity

GLYCOSYLATION OF GASTRIC β

As pointed out above there are seven potential sites of N-linked glycosylation in the exterior domain of gastric β ; there are also seven potential sites predicted on the $β_2$-subunit isoform of the Na,K-ATPase. The $β_1$-subunit isoform of Na,K-ATPase has three predicted sites of N-glycosylation, and all three have been shown to be occupied by an oligosaccharide [19]. For gastric β we have evidence that at least two of the seven consensus N-linked sites are glycosylated. Peptide fragments from gastric β which had been deglycosylated by peptide:N-glcosidase F reveal the amino acid aspartate is present in position 193 and 225 [10] instead of asparagine residues that are predicted from the cDNA sequence [10 and figure 4). Since the action of peptide:N-glycosidase F is to deamidate asparagine to aspartic acid while releasing oligosaccharide [20], we can conclude that Asn_{193} and Asn_{225} are certainly glycosylated *in situ*. It is not certain which of the remaining sites on gastric β are glycosylated (nor which sites on $β_2$), but we do know that gastric β is rich in carbohydrate. Analyses reveal that 25-30% of total mass of the gastric β glycoprotein is carbohydrate [3], with the bulk of the sugar being N-acetylglucosamine (glcNAc), galactose (gal), and mannose (man). Unlike $β_1$ and $β_2$, gastric β contains no sialic acid [2,21]. We suggest that the unique character in quality and quantity of the oligosaccharides in gastric β may serve a role in stabilizing the apical membrane of the parietal cell.

On the basis of the affinity of gastric β to various lectins, and its sensitivity to selected glycosidases, we can make some general conclusions regarding the nature of the glycosylations on the peptide. Gastric β does not bind to conconavalin A, but is very avidly bound to a number of other lectins, including ricinus communis agglutinin, wheat germ agglutinin, helix pomatia agglutinin [22,3], and to tomato and potato lectins [23]. Deglycosylation of gastric β is rapidly effected by peptide:N-glycosidase F [23], but is completely insensitive to endoglycosidase F (personal observations). In addition, the core protein produced by peptide:N-glycosidase F is the same as that produced by complete chemical deglycosylation, indicating that there is no O-linked glycosylation. Thus, all glycopeptide linkage on gastric β must occur exclusively as N-asparagine linkage, and not to serine or threonine. The nature of the oligosaccharide also appears to be fairly uniform. From the data on lectin binding and glycosidase sensitivity we conclude that gastric β oligosaccharides are not of the high mannose- nor hybrid-types, but of the complex-type, most likely in a tri- or tetra-antennary structure. On the basis of strong affinity for tomato and potato lectins it was suggested [23] that gastric β-subunit oligosaccharides are rich in poly-N-acetyllactosamine sequences (i.e., repeating glcNAc/gal sequences). This is also a characteristic for binding to wheat germ agglutinin [24], further supporting a poly-N-acetyllactosamine structure.

The functional activity of the oligosaccharides on the gastric β-subunit is unknown. For the Na,K-ATPase it is known that αβ association, processing through ER and Golgi, and plasma membrane insertion can occur in the absence of a glycosylated β-subunit [25,26]. In addition, functional activity (i.e., ATP hydrolysis and transport) can occur in completely deglycosylated forms of Na,K-ATPase [27]. However, complete inhibition of glycosylation leads to a destabilization of both the β- and α-subunits as judged by their increased sensitivity to trypsin [26]. By analogy we might propose that the oligosaccharides of the gastric β-subunit serve some stabilizing and protective function at the outer membrane surface. This issue is especially critical for the apical surface of the parietal cell where conditions of low pH and proteolysis threaten to disrupt many protein structures. Many polysaccharides are resistant to such hydrolytic conditions as would occur in the stomach lumen, and from crude structural data currently available, including the lack of sialic acid, it would seem that oligosaccharides of the gastric β-subunit may be resistant to gastric digestion. Whether and how the the glycosylated structure can afford stability and protection to the apical surface remains to be established.

REFERENCES

1. Forte TM, Forte JG. Histochemical staining and characterization of glycoproteins in acid-secreting cells of frog stomach. J Cell Biol 1970; 47: 437-52.

2. Beesley RC, Forte JG. Glycoproteins and glycolipids of oxyntic cell microsomes. I. Glyclproteins: carbohydrate composition, analytical and preparative fractionation. Biochim Biophys Acta 1973; 307: 372-385.

3. Okamoto CT, Karpilow JM, Smolka A, Forte JG, Isolation and characterization of gastric microsomal glycoproteins. Evidence for a glycosylated -subunit of the H^+, K^+-ATPase. Biochim Biophys Acta 1990; 1037: 360-372.

4. Karpilow J, Okamoto CT, Smolka A, Forte JG. Glycoprotein association with gastric H/K-ATPase. Fed Proc 1987; 46(3): 363 (Abstract #269).

5. Okamoto CT, Forte JG. Isolation and characterization of oxyntic cell microsomal membrane glycoproteins (abstract) Fed Proc 1987; 46: 365.

6. Sedar AW. Electron microscopic demonstration of polysaccharides associated with acid-secreting cells of the stomach after "inert dehydration". J Ultrastruct Res 1969; 28: 112-124.

7.   Sachs G.   The gastric proton pump: The H^+, K^+-ATPase.   In:
      Physiology of the Gastrointestinal Tract.   Second edition, edited by
      LR Johnson, NY, Raven Press, 1987 pp. 865-881.

8.   McDonough AA, Geering K, Farley RA.   The sodium pump needs
      its β-subunit. FASEB J 1990; 4: 1598-1605.

9.   Chow DC, Okamoto CT, Forte JG.   Immunological characterization of
      a 60-80 kDa glycoprotein associated with the gastric microsomal H+,
      K+-ATPase. The FASEB J 1989; 3(3): A973 (Abstract #3754).

10.   Canfield VA, Okamoto CT, Chow D, Dorfman J, Gros P, Forte JG,
      Levenson R.   Cloning of the K, K-ATPase β-subunit: Tissue-specific
      expression, chromosomal assignment, and relationship to Na,
      K-ATPase subunits. J Biol Chem 1990: In press.

11.   Feiner-Moore J, Bazan JS, Rubin J, Stroud RN.   Identity of
      membrane protein and soluble proteins secondary structural elements,
      domain structure and packing arrangement by Fourier transform
      amphipathic analysis. In: Prediction of Protein Structrure and the
      Principles of Protein Conformation.   Edited by G Fassman. NY,
      Plenum Press, 1989, pp. 719-760.

12.   Kawamura M, Nagano K.   Evidence for essential disulfide bonds in
      the β-subunit of (Na^++K^+)-ATPase.   Biochim Biophys Acta   1984;
      774: 188-192.

13.   Kirley TL.   Determination of three disulfide bonds and one free
      sulfhydryl in the β-subunit of (Na, K)-ATPase. J Biol Chem 1989;
      264(13): 7185-7192.

14.   Kawamura M, Ohmizo K, Morohashi M, Nagano K.   Protective effect
      of Na+ and K+ against inactivation of (Na^++K^+)-ATPase by high
      concentrations of 2-mercaptoethanol at high temperatures.   Biochim
      Biophys Acta   1985; 821: 115-120.

15.   Kirley TL.   Inactivation of Na^+, $K^+)$-ATPase by β-mercaptoethanol.
      J Biol Chem 1990; 265(8): 4227-4232.

16.   Forte JG, Poulter JL, Dykstra R, Rivas J, Lee HC.   Specific
      modification of gastric K^+-stimulated ATPase activity by thimerosal.
      Biochim Biophys Acta. 1981; 644: 257-265.

17.   Forte JG, Ganser AL, Ray TK.   The K^+-stimulated ATPase from
      oxyntic glands of gastric mucosa: In: Gastric Hydrogen Ion Secretion.
      Edited by DK Kasbekar, G. Sachs, and W Rehm, NY, Dekker 1976;
      pp. 302-330.

18.   Shull GE, Lingrel JB.   Molecular cloning of the rat stomach (H^++K^+)-
      ATPase. J Biol Chem 1986; 231(6): 16788-16791.

19.   Miller RP, Farley RA. All three potential N-glycosylation sites of the dog kidney (Na^++K^+)-ATPase β-subunit contain oligosaccharide. Biochim Biophys Acta 1988; 954: 50-57.

20.   Tarentino AL, Gomez CM, Plummer TH, Jr. Deglycosylation of asparagine-linked glycans by peptide: N-glycosidase G. Biochemistry 1985; 24: 4665-4671.

21.   Kyte J. Properties of 2 polypeptides of sodium-dependent and potassium-dependent adenosine-triphosphatase. J Biol Chem 1972; 247: 7642-7649.

22.   Okamoto CT, Forte JG. Distribution of lectin-binding sites in oxyntic and chief cells of isolated rabbit gastric glands. Gastroenterology 1988; 95: 334-342.

23.   Callaghan JM, Toh BH, Pettitt JM, Humphris DC, Gleeson PA. Poly-N-acetyllactosamine-specific tomato lectin interacts with gastric parietal cells. Identification of a tomato-lectin binding $60-90x10^3$ M_r membrane glycoprotein of tubulovesicles. J Cell Sci. 1990; 95: 563-576.

24.   Gallagher JT, Morris A, Dexter TM. Identification of two binding sites for wheat-germ agglutinin on polyactosamine-type oligosaccharides. Biochem J 1985; 231: 115-122.

25.   Tamkun MM, Fambrough DM. The (Na^++K^+)-ATPase of chick sensory neurons. Studies on biosynthesis and intracellular transport. J Biol Chem 1986; 261(3): 1009-1019.

26.   Zamofing D, Rossier BC, Geering K. Role of the Na, K-ATPase β-subunit in the cellular accumulation and maturation of the enzyme as assessed by glycosylation inhibitors. J Membrane Biol 1988; 104: 69-79.

27.   Zamofing D, Rossier BC, Geering K. Inhibition of N-glycosylation affects transepithelial Na^+ but not Na^+-K^+-ATPase transport. Am J Phyisol 1989; 256(Cell Physiol 25): C958-C966.

28.   Shull GE. cDNA cloning of the β-subunit of the rat gastric H,K-ATPase. J Biol Chem 1990; 265: 12123-12126.

29.   Kyte J, Doolittle RF. A simple method for displaying the hydropathic character of a protein. J. Molecular Biol. 1982; 157: 105-132.

IS THERE A ROLE FOR TRANSCELLULAR (APICAL MEMBRANE) DIFFUSION OF HYDROGEN IONS IN ACUTE ACID INJURY TO RABBIT ESOPHAGEAL EPITHELIUM?

Roy C. Orlando, Edward J. Cragoe Jr.* and Nelia A. Tobey

*University of North Carolina School of Medicine,
Department of Medicine, Chapel Hill, North Carolina.
P.O.Box 631548, Nacogdoches, Texas, U.S.A.

ABSTRACT

The initial stages of acute acid injury to esophageal epithelium involve hydrogen ion (H^+) diffusion into the epithelium and an increase in permeability across the intercellular junctions (paracellular pathway). The present investigation seeks to establish whether the major route for H^+ diffusion into the epithelium is via the apical cell membrane sodium channels and whether the potential lowering of intracellular pH (pHi) by the transcellular diffusion of luminal H^+ across the apical cell membrane could mediate the acute increase in junctional permeability. Rabbit esophageal epithelia were mounted in Ussing chambers to monitor short circuit current, Isc, (a marker of H^+ diffusion in HCl-exposed tissues) and electrical resistance, R, (a marker of epithelial permeability). Pretreatment of tissues with phenamil, an irreversible inhibitor of sodium channels, significantly reduced basal Isc but was unable to block either the HCl⁻ induced increase in Isc or the decline in R. Tissues in which pHi was lowered either by using the NH_4Cl prepulse technique, by switching from buffered Ringer to unbuffered Ringer solution, or by changing solution gassing from 5% CO_2 to 10% CO_2 - were acidified sufficiently to inhibit Isc yet R did not decline. From these results we conclude that the apical membrane Na^+ channels are not the major route for H^+ entry into the esophageal epithelium and that the transcellular (apical membrane) diffusion of H^+ even in sufficient quantities to acidify the cell is not responsible for the increase in junctional permeability associated with luminal acidification.

INTRODUCTION

Studies from our laboratory have previously described the sequential changes in epithelial structure/function leading to cell necrosis in the acid-exposed rabbit esophagus [1-3]. These studies found that acid damage could be viewed as a three stage process; stage 1, identified by increased PD, was due to H^+ diffusion into the tissue (no significant change in morphology); stage 2, identified by a decrease in PD, was due to increased permeability across the intercellular junctions (dilated intercellular spaces but no cell necrosis on electron microscopy); and stage 3, identified by abolition of PD, was due to inhibition of active transport and the development of cell necrosis.

Although it is accepted that the proximate cause of cell death from exposure to luminal acid is acidification of cells, our initial studies did not clarify whether the major route for H^+ entering and damaging the epithelium (stage 1) was via the transcellular or paracellular route or both. More recently data was obtained showing that serosal HCO_3 (and HEPES, an organic buffer impermeant to cells) protect against acid damage to esophageal epithelium by buffering H^+ within the extracellular space below the level of the junctions [4]. This finding supports the importance of the paracellular pathway as the major route for H^+ diffusion enroute to producing cell necrosis in esophageal epithelium. However, this data still does not exclude the possibility that the initial attack by H^+ was via the transcellular (apical membrane) route with the consequent lowering of pHi indirectly mediating the increase in junctional permeability. For this reason we investigated in Ussing-chambered esophageal epithelium whether lowering pHi would increase junctional permeability and, since esophageal epithelium has Na^+ channels in its apical membranes, whether these cationic channels could serve as routes for H^+ to diffuse across the apical cell membrane.

MATERIALS AND METHODS

New Zealand white rabbits weighing between 8 and 9lb were killed by administering intravenously an overdose of pentobarbital (60 mg/ml). The esophagus was excised, opened, and pinned mucosal surface down, in a paraffin tray containing ice-cold oxygenated normal Ringer's solution. The submucosa was grasped with hemostats, lifted up, and dissected free of the underlying mucosa with a scalpel. This process yielded a sheet of tissue consisting of stratified squamous epithelium and a small amount of underlying connective tissue. From this tissue, four sections were cut and mounted as flat sheets between Lucite half-chambers with an aperture of 1.13 cm^2 for measurements of potential difference (PD), short-circuit current (Isc) and resistance (R). Tissues were bathed with normal Ringer's solution (composition in mmol/L: Na^+ 140, Cl^- 120, K^+ 5, HCO_3^- 25, Ca^{2+} 1.2, Mg^{2+} 1.2, HPO_4^{-2} 2.4, $H_2PO_4^-$ 0.4, 268 mosmol/kg H_2O, pH 7.5 when gassed with 95% O_2/5% CO_2 at $37^\circ C$. Luminal and serosal solutions were connected to calomel and Ag-AgCl electrodes with Ringer-agar bridges for measurements of PD and automatic short-circuiting of the tissue with a voltage clamp (World Precision Instruments, Inc., New Haven, Conn.). Tissues were continuously short-circuited except for 5-10 second periods when the open circuit PD was read. Electrical resistance (R) was calculated using Ohm's law from the open-circuit PD and the Isc or from the current deflection to imposed voltage.

Forty-five minutes after mounting (equilibration period), one of a pair of tissues (tissues paired by R, R within 25%) was pretreated with phenamil, 10^{-4}M, for 30 min while the other served as control. Following pretreatment, tissues were acidified by the addition of 60 mM HCl to the luminal bath. After 1h of acidification, the luminal and serosal solutions were drained and replaced with normal Ringer solution (washout). PD, Isc and R were monitored before, during and after acidification.

INTRACELLULAR ACIDIFICATION.

Three manoeuvers were employed to study the effects of intracellular acidification on junctional permeability. In the first method, esophageal tissues were mounted in Ussing chambers and bathed in normal Ringer solution bubbled with 95% O_2/5% CO_2. After pairing by R as described above, one of the pair was exposed on both sides to iso-osmolar solutions containing 30 mM NH_4Cl for 30 minutes (composition mM/L: Na^+ 110, Cl^- 120, K^+ 5, HCO_3^- 25, Ca^{2+} 1.2, Mg^{2+} 1.2, HPO_4^{-2} 2.4, $H_2PO_4^-$ 0.4, NH_4^+ 30). After exposure to NH_4Cl, both bathing solutions were replaced with a Na-free Ringer solution (washout) (composition mM/L: $choline^+$ 140, Cl^- 120, K^+ 5, HCO_3^- 25, Ca^{2+} 1.2, Mg^{2+} 1.2, HPO_4^{-2} 2.4, $H_2PO_4^-$ 0.4). This manoeuver which is known to acidify cells upon washout is a modification of the "NH_4Cl prepulse technique" [5]. The use of the Na-free Ringer solution was to prolong the time of intracellular acidification by inhibition of all Na-dependent cell alkalinizing processes such as the Na^+-dependent Cl^-/HCO_3^- exchange and the previously documented Na^+/H^+ exchange [5]. Controls unexposed to NH_4Cl were also subjected to washout while monitoring R. The second manoeuver to acidify esophageal cells involved exchanging both bathing solutions of normal Ringer bubbled with 95% O_2/5% CO_2 to a bicarbonate-free (unbuffered) solution bubbled with 95% O_2/5% CO_2 (composition the same as normal Ringer except for equimolar replacements of bicarbonate by isethionate and phosphate by chloride, solution pH = 6.5 when bubbled with 95% O_2/5% CO_2). The third manoeuvre which produced an even greater reduction in pHi in this system was achieved by changing the gassing of both unbuffered bathing solutions to 10% CO_2 (and 90% O_2, unbuffered solution pH = 6.3). Each of the above methods was independently verified to acidify the cytoplasm of flourescent-dye loaded isolated esophageal cells (unpublished observations - see results).

Junction potentials were determined for all solutions used in these experiments by a modification of the method of Read and Fordtran [6]. Junction potentials for solutions with pH ≥ 2 were <1 mV and so were ignored. Junction potentials for solutions of 60 mM HCl, pH 1.5, were +5.6 mV during luminal acidification, but since they neither alter R nor alter the findings comparing changes in Isc, corrections were not required in the presentation of results.

Phenamil was synthesized for this study by the previously described method (ref 6a). This compound was dissolved in dimethyl sulfoxide and diluted to the desired concentration with the appropriate media. The final concentration of DMSO was below that which might affect test results.

RESULTS AND DISCUSSION

The possibility of a transcellular (apical membrane) route for H^+ entry into and damage to esophageal epithelium was initially considered because Powell et al [7] had shown that the major electrolyte transported across esophageal epithelium was Na^+ and Palmer [8] found that H^+ could traverse amiloride-sensitive Na^+ channels in toad bladder. To determine whether H^+ diffused primarily through Na^+ channels in esophageal epithelium we compared the rise in Isc in tissues exposed to luminal HCl in the presence or absence of phenamil, an irreversible inhibitor of Na^+

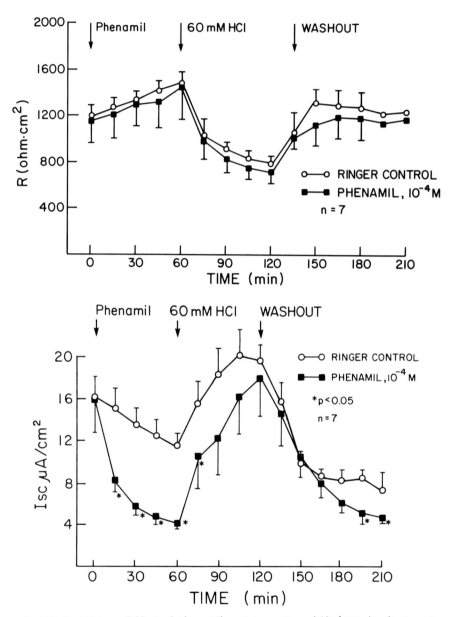

FIGURE 1A AND 1B   Effect of phenamil pretreatment on (A) short circuit current
(Isc) and (B) electrical resistance (R) in rabbit esophageal epithelia before,
during and after luminal exposure to 60 mM HCl. Phenamil, an irreversible
inhibitor of Na$^+$ channels, significantly inhibits basal Isc but does not block
either the HCl-induced increase in Isc or decline in R. Note: phenamil blockade
of Na$^+$ channels was not disrupted by acidification as evidenced by the
persistence of an inhibited Isc after washout.

channels [9]. (Note: the increase in Isc in rabbit esophagus exposed to high luminal acidity has been previously shown to primarily reflect H^+ diffusion [2]).

Figure 1a demonstrates that pretreatment with phenamil for 30 min inhibited basal Isc by 75%. Since 80% of the basal Isc in rabbit esophageal epithelium is due to active Na absorption [2,8], this degree of inhibition suggests that more than 90% of Na^+ channels were blocked by phenamil. Despite successful blockade of Na^+ channels, however, acidification of the luminal bath with HCl produced a similar increase in Isc and decline in R for phenamil and control tissues (Figures 1a and 1b respectively). This indicates that blockade of Na^+ channels neither prevents H^+ diffusion into esophageal epithelium nor does it prevent the ability of luminal HCl to injure the tissue by increasing junctional permeability. Also of note in Figure 1 - the Isc in phenamil-treated tissues remained significantly lower than in controls after washout. This indicates that the blockade of Na^+ channels by phenamil remained intact throughout the period of acidification.

Although the above experiment indicated that blockade of Na^+ channels failed to limit H^+ diffusion and its ability to increase junctional permeability, a possible role for the transcellular diffusion of H^+ through other routes could not be excluded. This was true especially since Madara et al [10] showed that junctional permeability may be under the control of cellular processes and others have documented that reductions in pHi can serve as mediator of other important cellular events [11]. One potential mechanism by which the transcellular (apical membrane) movement of H^+ may mediate the increase in junctional permeability would be through the lowering of pHi. This hypothesis was evaluated in Ussing-chambered epithelium by a series of bathing solution manouevres designed to lower pHi of esophageal cells while continuously monitoring R, a marker of tissue permeability.

Intracellular acidification was presumed to be achieved in the Ussing-chambered esophageal epithelial cells either by transient (30 min) exposure to NH_4Cl ("NH_4Cl prepulse technique"), by switching from bicarbonate-buffered to unbuffered Ringer solutions bubbled with 95% $O_2/5\% CO_2$ or by changing the gassing of the unbuffered Ringer solution from 5% CO_2 to 10% CO_2 content [6,12]. (These manouevres were verified by us to rapidly result in reductions in pHi to acidic levels in flourescent dye-loaded isolated esophageal cells. The NH_4Cl prepulse technique reduced pHi to between 6.1-6.5. The switch from buffered to unbuffered Ringer solution bubbled with 95% $O_2/5\% CO_2$ lowered pHi from 7.5 to 6.8 while the switch to gassing with 90% $O_2/10\% CO_2$ further reduced pHi to 6.3. Unpublished observations). However, as shown in figures 2 and 3, in no case did these manouevers result in a decline in R. In fact a decline in R only occurred during NH_4Cl exposure (an exposure which initially alkalinizes the cell due to the more rapid entry of NH_3 than NH_4^+) but this decline reversed and returned to baseline upon "washout" - washout precipitating intracellular acidification due to the rapid removal of NH_3 from the cell and retention of H^+ from the NH_4^+ entry).

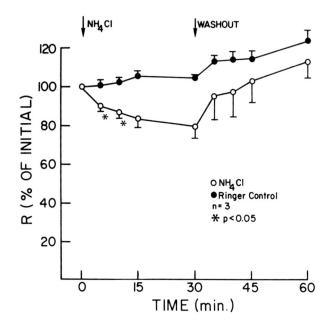

FIGURE 2.   Effect of the NH_4Cl prepulse technique on the electrical
resistance (R) of rabbit esophageal epithelium. During NH_4Cl exposure,
a period of alkalinization, R declined; however, after NH_4Cl removal and
replacement by Na-free Ringer solution (washout), manoeuvres designed
to both acidify the cell and prolong that acidification by blockage of
Na^+-dependent Cl^-/HCO_3^- exchange and/or Na^+/H^+ exchange, R
returned to normal.

    In addition, since the replacement solution was Na-free, intracellular
acidification would have been prolonged due to blockade of membrane Na-
dependent cell alkalinization processes such as the Na^+-dependent Cl^-/HCO_3^-
exchangers and Na/H exchangers the latter of which are known to be
important alkalinizers of pHi in esophageal cells [13]. Further, although the
gassing of the unbuffered Ringer solution with 5% CO_2 produced
intracellular and extracellular acidification low enough to inhibit the Isc of
esophageal epithelia (Isc reduced by 43 ± 6%, n=5), there was still no
evidence of a decline in R for any tissue (Figure 3).   These findings suggest
that the lowering of pHi even to levels that inhibit other cell functions
cannot account for the observed increase in junctonal permeability during
acute luminal acid exposure.

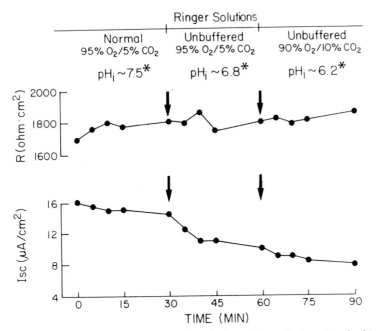

FIGURE 3. *Representative example of the effect of changing bathing solutions from normal (buffered) Ringer solution bubbled with 95% 02/5% CO_2 to unbuffered Ringer solution bubbled with 95% 02/5% CO_2 and from the latter to unbuffered Ringer solution bubbled with 90% $0_2/10\%$ CO_2 on the short-circuit current (Isc) and electrical resistance (R) of rabbit esophageal epithelium. [*Note: These manouevres cause a reduction of intracellular pH to acidic levels (values shown in figure) as documented by studies in flourescent dye-loaded isolated esophageal cells. (personal unpublished observations).] Intracellular acidification is shown to inhibit the Isc of esophageal tissue but to have no effect on R.*

In summary our 3-stage model of acute acid damage to rabbit esophagus indicates that H^+ initially diffuses across the epithelium and that this event is first followed by an increase in junctional permeability and then by cell death [1-3]. The results of the present investigation add to the evidence that the major route for H^+ entry into the epithelium enroute to producing damage is not transcellular, that is the rate of H^+ diffusion across the apical cell membrane is inconsequential from the standpoint of injury . This concept is supported by the inability of an inhibitor of Na^+ channels, the major cationic channel in the apical cell membrane of esophageal cells, to reduce lumen-to-blood diffusion of H^+ and by the observation that transcellular diffusion of H^+ even at rates that would produce intracellular acidosis could not account for the initial increase in junctional permeability. These negative results increase the likelihood that H^+ directly attacks and diffuses through the intercellular junctions enroute to producing irreversible damage (necrosis) to esophageal cells.

ACKNOWLEDGEMENT

This research was supported in part by a grant from the
National Institutes of Health #RO1DK36013-05

REFERENCES

1.   Orlando RC, Powell DW, Carney CN. Pathophysiology of acute acid injury in rabbit esophageal epithelium. J Clin Invest 1981; 68:286-293.

2.   Orlando RC, Bryson JC, Powell DW. Mechanisms of H^+ injury in rabbit esophageal epithelium. Am J Physiol 1984; 246: G718=G724.

3.   Carney CN, Orlando RC, Powell DW, Dotson MM. Morphologic alterations in early acid-induced epithelial injury of the rabbit esophagus. Lab Invest 1981; 45: 198-208.

4.   Tobey NA, Powell DW, Schreiner VJ, Orlando RC. Serosal bicarbonate protects against acid injury to rabbit esophagus. Gastroenterology 1989; 96: 1466-1477.

5.   Boron WF, Boulpaep EL. Intracellular pH regulation in the renal proximal tubule of the salamander. J Gen Physiol. 1983; 81: 29-52.

6.   Read NW, Fordtran JS. The role of intraluminal junction potentials in the generation of the gastric potential difference in man. Gastroenterology 1979; 76: 932-938.

6a.   Cragoe EJ, Woltersdorf OW, Bicking JB, Kwong SB, Jones JH. Pyrazine Diuretics: II. N-amidino-3-amino-5-substituted-6-halopyrazinecarboxamides. J Med Chem 1967; 10: 66-75.

7.   Powell DW, Morris SM, Boyd DD. Water and electrolyte transport by rabbit esophagus. Am J Physiol 1975; 229: 438-443.

8.   Palmer LG. Ion selectivity of the apical membrane Na channel in the toad urinary bladder. J Membr Biol. 1982; 67: 91-98.

9.   Garvin JL, Simon SA, Cragoe Jr EJ, Mandel LJ. Phenamil, an irreversible inhibitor of sodium channels in the toad urinary bladder. J Membrane Biol. 1985; 87: 45-54.

10.   Madara JL. Tight junction dynamics: is paracellular transport regulated? Cell; 53: 497-498.

11.   Roos A, Boron WF. Intracellular pH. Physiol Rev. 1981; 61: 296-434.

12.   Carter KJ, Saario I, Seidler U, Silen W. Effect of $PCO2$ on intracellular pH in in vitro frog gastric mucosa. Am J Physiol 1989; 256: G206-213.

13.   Agnone LM, Schmidt LN, Goldstein JL, Layden TJ. Mechanisms of regulation of intracellular pH in isolated rabbit esophageal cells. Clin Res 1989; 37: 365A.

GASTRIC MUCOSAL HYDROPHOBICITY

T.C. Northfield and P.M. Goggin

*Department of Medicine, St. George's Hospital Medical School,
Cranmer Terrace, Tooting, London, UK*

ABSTRACT

Contact angle measurements in animal studies have demonstrated that gastric mucosa has a relatively hydrophobic surface. We have developed and validated a technique for the measurement of this property on human endoscopic biopsy specimens. Mean contact angle of the gastric body (70°) and antrum (70°) was higher than duodenal bulb (62°, p<0.01) and distal duodenum (50°, p<0.001).

Subjects with duodenal ulcer and gastric ulcer had a lower contact angle than controls without ulcer (57°, n=49 and 59°, n=17 vs 66°, n=124 respectively). Helicobacter pylori infection was associated with reduced contact angle in subjects with gastritis (59° vs 70°). Contact angle was unchanged following treatment with ranitidine, but increased to control values following clearance and eradication of H. pylori with bismuth and antibiotics.

In order to determine the anatomical and biochemical basis of gastric mucosal hydrophobicity, we studied gastric mucus and mucosa obtained from pigs immediatedly after slaughter. The contact angle of mucus samples spread on glass or polypropylene was independent of the thickness of the layer or the hydrophobicity of the underlying surface and was similar to and correlated with that of the intact mucosa (58° vs 60°, r=0.76, p<0.001). Contact angle of the mucosa correlated with the phosphatidylcholine content (r=.72, p<0.001) and negatively with the lysophosphatidylcholine content (r=.072, p<0.001) of the mucus layer.

We conclude that in man gastric mucosal hydrophobicity can be validly measured on endoscopic biopsy specimens; that it is high in health and reduced in peptic ulcer disease, largely as a result of H. pylori infection. In the pig it is a property of the mucus layer, related to its phospholipid content, and reduced by phospholipolysis, suggesting a possible mechanism whereby the phospholipase activity of H. pylori may impair this property in man.

INTRODUCTION

Although the first axiom of Schwarz's triad [1] - "no acid, no ulcer" -
has stood the test of time, it is clear that acid secretion does not provide the
whole explanation for peptic ulcer disease. Patients with a duodenal ulcer
have an increase in the mean value for peak acid output but there is a
marked overlap with the normal population; and patients with gastric ulcer
have an actual reduction in acid output.

Schwarz's second axiom may provide the explanation for this
paradox, since it lays emphasis on the "self digestion which results from a
loss of the normal balance between the autopeptic power of gastric juice
and the protective forces of the gastric mucus membrane". Our thesis is
that the concept of hydrophobicity may provide a quantifiable assessment
of mucosal resistance to acid/peptic digestion in man.

Hydrophobicity was first demonstrated in animal studies by the
observation that the gastric mucosa forms a high contact angle with saline
drops placed on its surface [2]. This is characteristic of water repellent or
hydrophobic surfaces such as candle wax or polypropylene, which have a
low surface energy and can be wetted by liquid only if these have an even
lower surface free energy [3]. Water has a high surface free energy and is
therefore repelled by low energy polymer surfaces and by gastric mucosa, as
is dilute hydrochloric acid.

Gastric juice, however, is not simply a physiological solution of
electrolytes having the same interfacial properties as water, since it contains
proteins, mucins, lipids and bile acids which are themselves surface active
[4, 5] and could potentially alter the interfacial barrier between gastric juice
and gastric mucosa.

On the basis of their animal studies, Hills and Lichtenberger
postulated that the hydrophobic nature of gastric mucosa is due to a layer
of surface active phospholipids, with their polar ends adsorbed to the apical
cell membrane [2]. Since H pylori has been reported to produce a
phospholipase enzyme [6], and since this would convert phosphatidylcholine
into lysophosphatidylcholine which has detergent properties similar to
those of bile acids [7], the presence of this enzyme might provide a
mechanism by which H pylori could reduce hydrophobicity. But it is a
basic principle of contact angle measurements that it is the free energy of
the surface layer that is being measured, and in the stomach this is the
mucus layer. We therefore postulated that the hydrophobic property of
gastric mucosa is due to phospholipids in the mucus layer.

The aims of our studies have been to develop and validate a method
for measuring the hydrophobicity of human gastric biopsies; to compare this
with similar measurements from other parts of the gastrointestinal tract; to
determine whether a defect in gastric mucosal hydrophobicity can be
detected in peptic ulcer disease and in H pylori infection; to assess the
effect of alterations in the surface tension of gastric juice in patients with
bile reflux; and to study the anatomical and biochemical basis of the
hydrophobic property of gastric mucosa.

SUBJECTS

We studied 228 subjects presenting with abdominal pain or dyspepsia who underwent upper gastrointestinal endoscopy, including 49 with active duodenal ulcer, 17 with active gastric ulcer and 119 with normal upper gastrointestinal endoscopy. We also studied 48 subjects who had undergone gastric surgery for peptic ulcer disease (11 had had a Billroth I gastrectomy, 19 a Billroth II gastrectomy, 17 a vagotomy with drainage procedure and 1 Roux en Y), and 11 patients who underwent diagnostic sigmoidoscopy and biopsy with normal findings.

MATERIALS AND METHODS

Upper GI endoscopy was carried out after overnight fast by an investigator who did not perform the hydrophobicity readings. Following examination of the oesophagus, stomach and duodenum, biopsy specimens were taken from non-ulcerated areas of the stomach, from the antrum (within 2 cm of the pylorus) and from the body (upper greater curve). Two unfixed biopsy specimens from each region were used for hydrophobicity measurements. Two biopsy specimens from each region were fixed in formalin for subsequent histological examination. Gastric juice was collected via the suction channel of the endoscope.   Rectal biopsies were collected at rigid sigmoidoscopy.

MEASUREMENT OF HYDROPHOBICITY

When a liquid drop is applied to a solid, it forms a contact angle that is a resultant of the equilibrium of surface forces at the triple point of contact between the air, solid and liquid phases [3]. The contact angle is inversely related to the surface free energy of the solid by Youngs equation [8]. Thus if water is used as the liquid, on a hydrophobic surface such as candle wax or polypropylene which have a low surface free energy, the drop will bead up to form a high contact angle; whilst on a surface such as glass which has a high surface free energy, the drop will spread out to form a low contact angle. Surface free energy may be calculated from the contact angle [3, 9] and this has been applied to biological tissues [10, 11, 12, 13].

TECHNIQUE

Immediately following collection, biopsy specimens were washed in 0.15M saline, placed on clean glass slides and orientated under a dissecting microscope. They were then placed on the specimen stage of a goniometer (Rame-Hart 100/00), where a saline drop was applied to the surface. The advancing contact angle was measured by aligning the first of two cross-hairs in the eyepiece of the goniometer across the base of the droplet viewed in profile and the second at a tangent to the droplet at the triple point of contact between the liquid solid and air phases. The contact angle could then be read off on a scale encircling the eyepiece.

ANALYSIS OF GASTRIC JUICE

Surface tension of gastric juice was measured using the drop weight method. This method relies on the principle that the weight of a drop of liquid when it falls from a tube of a constant diameter is related directly to the surface tension of the liquid. Thus surface tension was calculated by filling a microsyringe with the gastric juice specimen and collecting and weighing 10 drops formed from a needle tip of known diameter. Using this technique the calculated value for double distilled water was in good agreement with literature values (73.1 vs 72.8 mN/M respectively)

Bile acids were determined by the hydroxysteroid dehydrogenase enzyme assay.

VALIDATION

The effect of drying of the mucosal surface prior to contact angle measurement was determined by measuring the contact angle of freshly applied drops at intervals after preparation. Air drying was also compared with drying under accelerated airflow using a blow dryer and with blotting of the surface with filter paper prior to contact angle measurement. The contact angle of the mucosal surface was compared with that of the serosal surface in paired biopsy specimens.

The surface free energy derived from saline contact angle measurements was compared with that derived from glycerol contact angles on paired biopsy specimens

APPLICATION

COMPARISON OF STOMACH, DUODENUM AND RECTUM.

Contact angles were measured in the stomach body and antrum, duodenal bulb, distal duodenum and rectum in controls without endoscopic or histological evidence of mucosal abnormality.

THERMODYNAMIC EFFECT OF BILE ACIDS IN THE STOMACH.

To determine the effect of bile acids on gastric mucosal hydrophobicity, and interfacial tension we compared gastric mucosal contact angle measurements, and gastric juice surface tension and bile acid concentration in post-gastrectomy patients with a control group of patients with a past history of ulcers that had been healed by medical therapy.

EFFECT OF PEPTIC ULCER DISEASE AND HELICOBACTER PYLORI

We compared gastric contact angle in patients with duodenal ulcer and gastric ulcer with that of patients with normal gastroscopy, and examined the relationship between Helicobacter infection and contact angle.

To determine the effect of clearance and eradication of H. pylori, 28 patients with duodenal ulcer all of whom had H. pylori infection, and 29 patients with H. pylori gastritis, with or without past history of duodenal ulcer were entered into an investigator blind trial of one months treatment with ranitidine vs bismuth (Denol) vs bismuth + amoxycillin for two weeks vs bismuth + metronidazole for 1 week. Contact angle measurements and histology were performed at presentation, at the end of the treatment period, and one month later

ANATOMICAL AND BIOCHEMICAL BASIS OF GASTRIC MUCOSAL
HYDROPHOBICITY IN THE PIG

In order to study the anatomical and biochemical basis for gastric mucosal hydrophobicity, we obtained samples of gastric mucus and mucosa from pigs (n=24) immediately after slaughter. We compared the contact angle of the intact mucosa with that of mucus samples obtained from an adjacent area, and studied the effect on contact angle of the thickness of a layer and of the hydrophobicity of the solid underlying the mucus layer. The contact angle of the mucosa was correlated with the phospholipid content (measured by thin layer chromatography and assay of phosphorus by Bartlett reaction) of mucus samples obtained from an adjacent area.

RESULTS

VALIDATION

EFFECT OF DRYING AND BLOTTING ON CONTACT ANGLE AND REPRODUCIBILITY

Following preparation of the mucosal specimens, contact angle increased with time to reach a plateau value after which it remained constant for up to 60 minutes. When the specimens were viewed under a dissecting microscope during the early drying phase, surface water could be seen first receding into pools leaving dry patches which then increased to cover the whole surface. Attainment of the plateau value coincided with the mucosa assuming a matt dullness associated with evaporation of surface water from the initial shiny surface.

Table 1 compares the plateau value and the percentage of plateau reached by 10 min after washing, washing and blotting, and accelerated drying after washing using biopsy specimens from the antrum. The plateau value was reproducible with a coefficient of variation on paired specimens (n=20) for the same and between two goniometrists of 3.6% and 4.4% respectively when a mean of at least 3 readings per specimen were taken. On the basis of these results, we used the plateau advancing contact angle after washing and drying as our measure of hydrophobicity.

TABLE 1

EFFECT OF THE MODE OF DRYING ON THE PLATEAU VALUE, THE PERCENTAGE
REACHED AFTER 10 MINUTES OF DRYING AND THE COEFFICIENT OF VARIATION
OF PAIRED READINGS AT 10 MINUTES.

	Plateau Value (n = 9)	% of Plateau reached at 10 minutes	Coefficient of variation of paired 10 min values
1. Air drying after washing alone	66.7 ± 2.1	80 ± 11*	37.8
2. Air drying after washing & blotting	65.8 ± 2.4	84 ± 4#	12.0
3. Accelerated drying after washing	66.6 ± 2.3	102 ± 2	9.7

* $p < 0.05$ vs. 3
\# $p < 0.01$ vs. 3

ESTIMATION OF SURFACE FREE ENERGY FROM SALINE & GLYCEROL CONTACT ANGLES.

Table 2 shows that the derived values of surface free energy for the
biopsy specimen surfaces were the same whether saline or glycerol was used
as the dropping liquid.

TABLE 2

VALUES OF SURFACE FREE ENERGY OF GASTRIC MUCOSA DERIVED FROM
MEASUREMENT OF SALINE AND GLYCEROL CONTACT ANGLES ON
SIX DUPLICATE SETS OF ANTRAL BIOPSY SPECIMENS.

	Liquid surface Tension, mN/m	Mucosal contact angle	Surface free energy, mJ/m^2
Saline	72	69.3 ± 2.3	41.1 ± 1.5
Glycerol	63	54.5 ± 3.2	42.4 ± 2.0

APPLICATION

COMPARISON OF STOMACH, DUODENUM AND RECTUM

Figure 1 shows the results of contact angle measurements along the gastrointestinal tract. Mean contact angle of the gastric body (70°) and antrum (70°) was higher than duodenal bulb (62°, $p<0.01$) and distal duodenum (50°, $p<0.001$).

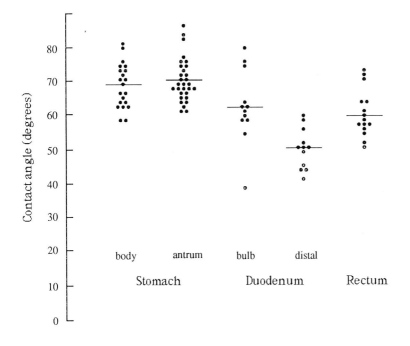

FIGURE 1: *Hydrophobic profile along the human gastrointestinal tract.*

EFFECT OF BILE ACIDS ON GASTRIC MUCOSAL, GASTRIC JUICE AND INTERFACIAL TENSION

The gastric surgery group had higher median fasting gastric bile acid concentrations than the control group with peptic ulcer healed by medical treatment (1.2 vs 0.1 mmol/L; $p<0.0001$))

Mucosal surface tension calculated from saline contact angle measurements correlated with fasting gastric bile acid concentration (r=0.51, p<0.0001), whilst gastric juice surface tension correlated negatively with bile acid concentration (r= 0.6, p<0.0001). Figure 2 shows the relationship between bile acid concentration and the interfacial energy difference between the gastric juice and the mucosa. When the surface tension of gastric juice is less than or equal to that of the mucosa, the interfacial energy difference is negative or zero indicating that the juice will wet the mucosa.

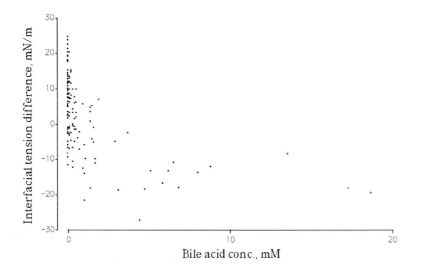

FIGURE 2: *Relationship between bile acid concentration and the interfacial energy difference.*

EFFECT OF PEPTIC ULCER DISEASE AND RELATIONSHIP TO GASTRITIS AND
HELICOBACTER PYLORI INFECTION

The antral contact angles for active duodenal ulcer and gastric ulcer subjects are compared with control subjects in figure 3. Both ulcer groups had significantly lower contact angles than controls (duodenal ulcer 56.8 ± 1.1, gastric ulcer 59.3 ± 2.3 vs. controls 66.2 ± 0.8; p<0.0001). There was no difference within the peptic ulcer groups with respect to site of ulcer.

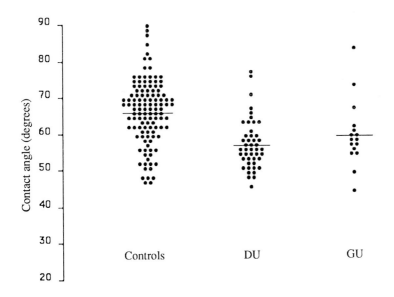

FIGURE 3: *The contact angles of antral mucosa in the active DU and GU subjects and in the non-ulcer controls.*

Figure 4 shows the contact angles of the 15 duodenal ulcer and 5 gastric ulcer subjects who were studied before and after healing with H2 receptor antagonists. There was no change in contact angle compared with pretreatment values (duodenal ulcer 59.1 $\pm$ 2.0 vs. 55.5 $\pm$ 1.5, gastric ulcer 56.9 $\pm$ 3.1 vs. 59.2 $\pm$ 0.9).

The antral contact angles in the subjects with inactive duodenal ulcer (n=29, 57.6 $\pm$ 1.2) and gastric ulcer (n=9, 57.9 $\pm$ 1.2) were not different from the active ulcer groups, but were significantly lower than control subjects (p<0.0001).

In patients without peptic ulcer, those with antral H. pylori positive antral gastritis had lower contact angles than those with H. pylori negative gastritis (58.9 $\pm$ 1.2, n=39 vs 67.5 $\pm$ 1.5, n=14)

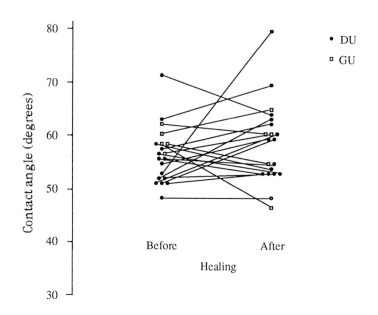

FIGURE 4: *Antral contact angle before and after healing of peptic ulcers
with H_2 receptor antagonists.*

EFFECT OF CLEARANCE AND ERADICATION OF H. PYLORI

In the group of patients entered into this study, contact angle (mean
$\pm$ sem degrees) was reduced in H. pylori positive gastritis ($55.7 \pm .8$, p<0.001)
and H. pylori positive duodenal ulcer ($55.7 \pm .9$, p<0.001) compared with H.
pylori negative controls without gastric pathology ($68.1 \pm .7$). Contact angle
was unchanged following treatment with ranitidine (55.3 ± 1.1 vs 55.0 ± 1.2,
n=16 NS), but increased following treatment with bismuth (55.6 ± 1.3 to
63.2 ± 2.4, p<0.001, n=15), bismuth + amoxycillin (54.6 ± 1.5 to 64 ± 2.4,
p<0.001, n=13) and bismuth + metronidazole ($56.2 \pm .8$ to 67.1 ± 2.7, n=13,
p<0.001) Clearance of H. pylori (31/41 bismuth, 0/16 ranitidine) was
associated with an increase in contact angle ($55.9 \pm .9$ to 67.6 ± 1.4,
p<0.0001). Of 31 patients who had cleared H. pylori at the end of the
treatment period, 20 had become H. pylori positive one month later. In this
group there was a significant fall in contact angle (65.0 ± 1.5 to 54.7 ± 1.3,
p<0.001) to pretreatment levels. In the group that remained H. pylori
negative contact angle remained similar to that of controls (70.1 ± 2.3, n=11).

ANATOMICAL AND BIOCHEMICAL BASIS

The contact angle of mucus samples was similar to and correlated
with that of the intact mucosa (58° vs 60°, r=0.76, p<0.001). The contact
angle of mucus samples spread on glass was the same as on polypropylene

(62° vs 60°) and the individual values correlated (r=.97, p<0.001). Mucus samples 100~m and 1000~m had similar contact angles (60° vs 58°, r=.90, p<0.0001). Contact angle of mucosa correlated with phosphatidylcholine content of mucus both in absolute concentration (r=0.72, p<0.005), and as a percentage of total phospholipids (r=0.66, p<.01), and negatively with lysophosphatidylcholine (LPC) only as a percentage of mucus phospholipids (r=-0.72, p<.005).

DISCUSSION

Our results show that the surface hydrophobicity of human gastrointestinal mucosa can be measured on endoscopic biopsy specimens [14]. We have demonstrated that the contact angle increases with time after exposure of the surface to an air interface to reach a plateau value when the initially glossy surface assumes a matt dullness due to evaporation of surface water. Contact angle studies on blood cells and bacteria [12, 15] have demonstrated that the time taken to reach the plateau can be varied by altering the humidity or the amount of surface water initially present. In agreement with these studies we have shown that the time taken to reach the plateau value can be reduced by use of accelerated air flow or by blotting the surface with filter paper, but the plateau value itself remains unchanged. The plateau contact angle is very reproducible whereas angles read at a fixed time are not [16]. Thus we like others have taken the plateau advancing contact angle as the most relevant angle when assessing the inherent hydrophobicity of a tissue surface [11-13, 15-19].

The hydrophobicity of a surface is inversely related to its surface free energy (or surface tension), and by using an empirical thermodynamic approach [9, 11], the surface tensions of biological surfaces have been derived from the plateau contact angle. We have shown that the calculated surface free energy is the same whether saline or glycerol is used as the dropping liquid, thus validating the method of using contact angles to assess the biophysical properties of a surface.

Our results for the hydrophobic profile of the human gastrointestinal tract do not agree entirely with with the published data on the dog [2]. In particular, the duodenum in humans exhibits appreciable contact angles. Though this may be a species difference, the studies are not comparable since in the canine study, contact angle was measured after a fixed period of time, which was probably before the plateau value was reached.

In our studies on post gastrectomy patients, we have shown that bile reflux is associated with an increase in surface free energy of gastric mucosa (reduced hydrophobicity) and a decrease in that of the gastric juice so that the interfacial energy difference becomes negative and any hydrophobic barrier potential of the gastric mucosa is overcome. This is in keeping with a canine study [2] which demonstrated reduced mucosal hydrophobicity after exposure of the mucosa to bile acids.

Our results also show that the surface hydrophobicity of human gastric mucosa is reduced in subjects with peptic ulcer disease [20] when compared to controls without ulcer, and that this reduction is not dependent upon the site or activity of the ulcer. In order to check on any association between gastritis and hydrophobicity, we divided our control subjects with non ulcer dyspepsia into those with and those without histological evidence of gastritis, and found that those with gastritis had lower contact angles; however the patients with peptic ulcer still had significantly lower contact angles than non-ulcer controls with gastritis, suggesting that gastritis is not the only factor and may be secondary to the changes in hydrophobicity.

We found that the presence of Helicobacter pylori infection was associated with a significant reduction in the contact angle, and that clearance and eradication of the organism was associated with an increase in contact angle to a value similar to that of controls, suggesting that the organism causes the reduction in hydrophobicity rather than reduced hydrophobicity predisposing to infection with H. pylori.

The mechanism by which H. pylori reduces gastric mucosal hydrophobicity is more difficult to ascertain since contact angle measurement does not provide specific information about the molecular configuration at a tissue surface [3, 21]. This could be due to the organism itself within the mucus layer either exerting a direct topical effect that makes the surface appear more hydrophilic, or causing an indirect toxic effect due to release of proteases [22] or phospholipases [6] that could alter hydrophobicity.

Hills attributed gastric mucosal hydrophobicity to an adsorbed monolayer of surface active phospholipids which is thermodynamically stabilized by the mucus layer [23]. However a basic principle of contact angle measurements is that the free energy (surface tension) of the surface of a solid is measured, and gastric mucosa is known to be covered by a complete layer of mucus [24, 25]. This suggests that hydrophobicity of gastric mucosa may be a property of the mucus layer, and mucus itself is known to contain lipids, including phospholipids .

Phospholipids were first recognized in mucus from lung washings where their surface active properties are thought to be important in preventing alveolar collapse. Similar phospholipids (in addition to neutral lipids and free fatty acids) have since been found in mucus from gastric mucosa [26, 27] though in smaller concentrations. In both cases phosphatidylcholine is the predominant species. The importance of surface active phospholipids in gastric mucosal defence is supported by the demonstration that exogenous phospholipids are protective against 0.6N HCl and 100% alcohol [28, 29] in the rat, and against aspirin in the dog [30]. In our studies on porcine gastric mucosa we have demonstrated that the contact angle the mucosa is similar to that of mucus samples scraped from an adjacent area and is related to the phospholipid content of the mucus layer. In particular lysophosphatidylcholine produced by the action of phospholipase on phosphatidylcholine is associated with a reduction in hydrophobicity suggesting a possible mechanism for the action of H. pylori since this organism has been demonstrated to produce a phospholipase A enzyme [6].

ACKNOWLEDGEMENTS

*This work was supported in part by Syntex Pharmaceuticals,
the Cadbury Trust, the Oakdale Trust, Gist Brocades,
the British Digestive Foundation, and Procter and Gamble.*

REFERENCES

1. Schwarz K. Ueber penetrierende Magen- und Jejunalgeschwure. Beitr Klin Chir 1910;67:96-128.

2. Hills BA, Butler BD, Lichtenberger LM. Gastric mucosal barrier: hydrophobic lining to the lumen of the stomach. Am J Physiol 1983;244(5):G561-8.

3. Adamson AW. Physical chemistry of surfaces. (4 ed.). New York: 1982:

4. Van Oss CJ, Absolom DR, Neumann AW, Zingg W. Determination of the Surface tension of proteins. I. Surface tension of native serum proteins in aqueous media. Biochim Biophys Acta 1981;670(1):64-73.

5. Holly FJ, Lemp MA. Wettability and wetting of corneal epithelium. Exp Eye Res 1971;11:239-250.

6. Slomiany BL, Nishikawa H, Piotrowski J, Okazaki K, Slomiany A. Lipolytic activity of Campylobacter pylori: effect of sofalcone. Digestion 1989;43:33-40.

7. Small DM. Surface and bulk interactions of lipids and water with a classification of biologically active lipids based on these interactions. Federal Proceedings 1970;29(4):1320-6.

8. Young T. An Essay on the Cohesion of Fluids. Philisoph Trans Roy Soc London 1805;23:65-87.

9. Neumann AW, Good RJ, Hope CJ, Sepjal M. An equation-of-state approach to determine surface tensions of low energy solids from contact angles. J Colloid Interface Sci 1974;49:291-304.

10. Bell GD, Weil J, Harrison G, et al. 14C-urea breath analysis a non-invasive test for Campylobacter pylori in the stomach [letter]. Lancet 1987;1:1367-8.

11. Neumann FJ, Absolom DR, Francis DW, al e. Measurement of surface tensions of blood cells and proteins. Ann NY Acad Sci 1983;413:276-98.

12. Van Oss CJ, Gillman CF, Neumann AW. Phagocytic engulfment and cell adhesiveness as cellular surface phenomena. New York: Dekker 1975. 1975;

13. Gerson DF, Akin J. Cell surface energy,contact angles and phase partition. 2. Bacterial cells in biphasic aqueous mixtures. Biochim Biophys Acta 1980;602:281-4.

14. Spychal RT, Marrero JM, Saverymuttu SH, Northfield TC. Measurment of surface hydrophobicity of human gastrointestinal mucosa. Gastroenterol 1989;97:104-111.

15. Mege JL, Capo C, Benoliel AM, Foa C, Bongrand P. Nonspecific cell surface properties: contact angle of water on dried cell monolayers. Immunol Commun 1984;13(3):211-27.

16. Absolom DR, Zingg W, Neumann AW. Measurement of contact angles on biological and other highly hydrated surfaces. J Colloid Interface Science 1986;112:599-601.

17. Vissink A, De JH, Busscher HJ, Arends J, 's GE. Wetting properties of human saliva and saliva substitutes. J Dent Res 1986;65(9):1121-4.

18. Chappuis J, Sherman IA, Neumann AW. Surface tension of animal cartilage as it relates to friction in joints. Ann Biomed Eng 1983;11(5):435-49.

19. Hills BA, Cotton DB. Premature rupture of membranes and surface energy: possible role of surfactant. Am J Obstet Gynecol 1984;149:896-902.

20. Spychal RT, Goggin PG, Marrero JM, et al. Surface Hydrophobicity of Gastric Mucosa in Peptic Ulcer Disease: relationship to gastritis and Campylobacter pylori infection. Gastroenterol 1990;98:1-7.

21. Johnson REJ, Dettre RH. Wettability and contact angles. Surface Colloid Sci 1969;2:85-153.

22. Slomiany BL, Bilski J, Sarosiek J, et al. Campylobacter pyloridis degrades mucin and undermines gastric mucosal integrity. Biochem Biophys Res Commun 1987;144(1):307-14.

23. Hills BA. Gastric mucosal barrier: stabilization of hydrophobic lining to the stomach by mucus. Am J Physiol 1985;249:G342-9.

24. Bickel M, Kaufman GLJ. Gastric mucus gel thickness: effect of distension, 16,16-dimethylprostaglandin E2 and carbenoxolone. Gastroenterology 1981;80(4):770-5.

25. Kerss S, Allen A, Garner A. A simple method for measuring the mucus gel layer adherent to rat, frog and human gastric mucosa. Br Med Bull 1978;34:28-33.

26. Wassef MK, Lin YN, Horowitz MI. Molecular species of phospholipids from rat gastric mucosa. Biochimica et Biophysica Acta 1979;573:222-226.

27. Butler BD, Lichtenberger LM, Hills BA. Distribution of surfactants in the canine gastroduodinal tract and their ability to lubricate. Am. J. Physiol. 1983;244(gastrointest. Liver physiol. 7):G645-G651.

28. Dial EJ, Lichtenberger LM. A role for milk phospholipids in protection against gastric acid. Gastroenterol 1984;87:378-85.

29. Szelenvi I, Engler HP-2. Cytoprotective role of gastric surfactant in the ethanol produced gastric mucosal injury of the rat. Pharmacol 1986;33:199-205.

30. Swarm R, 1987;153:48-53 ea. Protective effect of exogenous phospholipid on aspirin-induced gastric mucosal injury. Am J Surg 1987;153:48-53.

NEUROENDOCRINE CONTROL OF MUCOSA PROTECTIVE
FUNCTIONS IN THE DUODENUM

L. Fändriks, A. Hamlet and C. Jönson

Department of Physiology, University of Gothenburg, Sweden

ABSTRACT

In the duodenum, bicarbonate secretion by the surface epithelium is considered to be the most important factor in the protection against luminal acid. This secretion, and other potentially mucosa-protective duodenal functions, are subjected to neuroendocrine control both from the central nervous system and at the local level. The vagal nerves act stimulatory on duodenal bicarbonate secretion using both conventional nicotinic and muscarinic cholinoceptors, as well as non-cholinergic transmission. Local acid-exposure stimulates transepithelial bicarbonate transport by hormones and local synthesis of prostaglandins, as well as by cholinergic and non-cholinergic neural mechanisms. In recent experiments, the acid-induced rise in duodenal bicarbonate secretion remained after acute vagotomy and/or splanchnicotomy, but was blocked by topical application of a local anesthetic. The neural component, therefore, is probably organized as a local nerve reflex within the enteric nervous system (ENS). The data suggest that a low acid-concentration stimulates bicarbonate transport mainly via the neural route and that additional regulatory principles (e.g. prostaglandins) are utilized at higher acidities. The sympathetic splanchnic nerves act inhibitory on duodenal bicarbonate secretion. This effect is not secondary to changes in mucosal blood flow and is exerted by use of peripheral adrenergic neurons and receptors of the alpha-2 subtype. The adrenal glands are probably not involved. Recent experiments on anesthetized cats demonstrate that the acid-induced increased bicarbonate secretion is accompanied with net fluid secretion and an increased duodenal motor activity. All parts of this multiple response was inhibited by sympathetic nerve stimulation.

INTRODUCTION

Acid from the gastric parietal cells is an important factor in the digestive process, but the acid is also a potential threat to the organism itself. Particularly the proximal duodenum, upstreams to the pancreatic inflow, is regularly challenged by acid disposed from the stomach. It is now well established that there exists a bicarbonate secretion by the gastroduodenal surface epithelium which protects against gastric acid [1].

223

Measurements with micro-pH-electrodes have demonstrated a juxta-epithelial pH-gradient (the pH at the cell surface being neutral despite highly acidic luminal contents) which is dependent on a transepithelial transport of bicarbonate. This bicarbonate secretion is probably the most important factor for protection against acid in the duodenum, whereas it plays a more subordinate role in the stomach [1]. The physiological control of the alkaline (bicarbonate) secretion by the duodenal mucosa is complex and involves several regulatory mechanisms including neural and hormonal mechanisms, as well as local synthesis of prostaglandins. Furthermore, mucosal bicarbonate secretion is only one part of an acid-induced functional response pattern. In addition to bicarbonate transport, this multiresponse involves at least also transepithelial net fluid secretion and increased duodenal motor activity, all being potentially mucosa-protective. The present paper summarizes some recent results from this research area.

DUODENAL MUCOSAL BICARBONATE SECRETION

STIMULATORY MECHANISMS.

From a functional point of view, there exist two main neuroendocrine principles for increasing duodenal bicarbonate secretion: 1). a central activation via the vagal nerves to anticipate the cephalic phase of gastric acid secretion, 2). a local response upon direct acid-exposure of the duodenal mucosa.

Central activation. It is evident that stimuli which activate gastric acid secretion in general also stimulate duodenal mucosal alkalinization. For example, central vagal activation by means of sham feeding in dogs [2] and in man [3] have been shown to stimulate duodenal bicarbonate secretion with a partly atropine-sensitive mechanism. Vagotomy lowers duodenal alkaline secretion in anesthetized animals suggesting a central tonic stimulatory influence by these nerves [4]. Furthermore, direct electrical stimulation of the decentralized vagal nerves increases duodenal bicarbonate secretion in several species [4, 5]. In the cat and rat such responses were abolished by hexamethonium, whereas atropine inhibited the response by approximately 50% in the cat and was without effect in the rat [4,5].

The vagal nerves have been centrally activated by means of intracerebro-ventricular (i.c.v.) infusions of various neuropeptides in the rat. TRH (thyrotropin releasing hormone) when given i.c.v. stimulates duodenal bicarbonate secretion [6,7]. This effect was sensitive to hexamethonium and vagotomy, poorly sensitive to atropine but inhibited by a VIP-antagonist [7]. Also other peptides, for example CRF (corticotropin releasing factor), GRP (gastrin releasing peptide) and bombesin, stimulate duodenal bicarbonate secretion when given i.c.v.

Intestinal activation. Exposure of the duodenal mucosa to acid increases the mucosal output of bicarbonate in all species tested, including man (for review see ref 1]. The mechanisms involved in this secretory increase are not fully understood, although synthesis of prostaglandins very likely represent one regulatory factor since pretreatment with either aspirin or indomethacin reduces the acid-induced rise in secretion [8, 9]. Furthermore, a hormonal component is probably involved in the secretory increment in response to acid [1]. For example cholecystokinin, known to be released upon duodenal acidification, stimulates duodenal bicarbonate secretion [10]. Neural factors seem to be important since acid-exposure of the rat duodenal mucosa, after pretreatment with the nicotinic receptor antagonist hexamethonium or the muscarinic receptor antagonist atropine, caused a less pronounced bicarbonate secretion compared to controls [11,12]. In addition, a VIP-antagonist inhibits the response to acid exposure strongly suggesting a role for this neuropeptide in the local regulation of duodenal bicarbonate transport [13]. The neural mediation of acid-induced secretion is primarily due to intrinsic reflexes within the enteric nervous system since the effect is not blocked by bilateral cervical vagotomy and/or splanchnicotomy [12, 14]. Moreover, recent results from our laboratory show that serosal application of the local anesthetic *lidocaine* abolish the acid-induced (10 mM HCl) rise in bicarbonate secretion in anethetized rats (Fig 1).

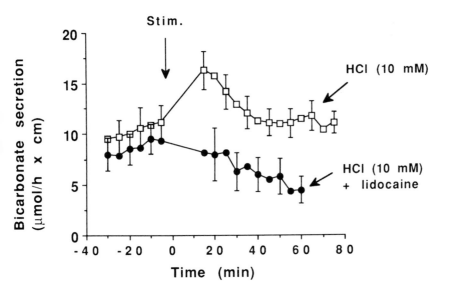

FIGURE 1: *Perfusion of the duodenal lumen with 10 mM hydrochloric acid in chloralose-anesthetized rats increases the bicarbonate secretion (n=6, open squares). Application of the local anesthetic lidocaine (1% w/v) on the serosa of the duodenal segment simultaneously with the luminal exposure to acid, inhibits the increase in bicarbonate transport (n=6, filled circles).*

A local anesthetic administered in such a way has previously been shown to penetrate to the submucosa of the rat small intestine and is considered to block transmission in the enteric nerves without directly influencing the epithelium [15]. The reactivity of the duodenal mucosa in presence of lidocaine was tested by adding prostaglandin E2 (10^{-5} M) to the luminal perfusate. This procedure promptly raised bicarbonate secretion indicating that the epithelium *per se* was not inhibited by the local anesthetic (Fig 2) [14]. Taken together these data suggest that the enteric nervous system plays a key role in the mediation of increases in bicarbonate transport in response to modest concentrations (<50mM) of hydrochloric acid, whereas additional regulatory principles (eg. hormones and synthesis of prostaglandins) are utilized at higher concentrations.

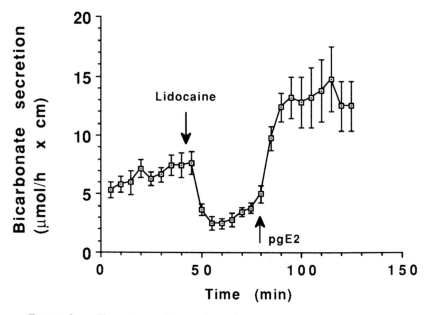

FIGURE 2:   *The effect of serosal application of lidocaine (1% w/v) on basal duodenal bicarbonate secretion in acutely vagotomized anesthetized rats (n=6). Note that luminal administration of prostaglandin E2 (10^{-5} M) stimulates the secretion in presence of lidocaine.*

INHIBITORY MECHANISMS.

Inhibition of duodenal bicarbonate secretion have been observed during e.g. hypovolemia, systemic acidosis or unspecific severe stress conditions [16, 17, 18]. The neuroendocrine mechanisms behind the lowering of duodenal bicarbonate secretion are not fully understood. A central decrease of vagal nerve activity and a peripheral action by the sympathetic nerves and hormonal factors are involved. Systemic acid-base balance as well as local blood supply may be critical during severe conditions.

Sympatho-adrenergic inhibition. Splanchnicotomy raises basal duodenal alkaline secretion and vagally induced increases in duodenal bicarbonate secretion in cats indicating a tonic inhibitory action by these nerves [19]. Direct electrical stimulation of the splanchnic nerves lowers the basal duodenal bicarbonate secretion and inhibits vagally-induced increases in bicarbonate secretion, as well as the response to local exposure to acid [20, 21, 22]. This inhibitory action by the splanchnic nerves on duodenal bicarbonate secretion was sensitive to guanethidine or yohimbine, but resistant to prazosin or propranolol [19, 20, 21, 23]. The data suggest that the sympathetic splanchnic nerves can inhibit duodenal bicarbonate secretion by use of adrenergic neurons and alpha-2-adrenoceptors. Furthermore, this view is supported by the finding that the alpha-2-adrenoceptor agonist clonidine inhibits the secretion by a yohimbine-sensitive mechanism [20, 24, 25].

Sympatho-adrenergic inhibition of duodenal bicarbonate secretion elicited from several "levels" in the CNS has been explored in the anesthetized rat. Electrical stimulation of mesenteric afferents from the jejunum inhibited the bicarbonate secretion in the duodenum. Apparantly, this effect was due to a *spinal reflex* as it was well preserved after cervical cord transection, but it was blocked by bilateral splanchnicotomy [26]. Furthermore, a modest hypovolemia by means of an arterial bleeding of approximately 10% of the total blood volume, lowered duodenal bicarbonate secretion and inhibited the increase in secretion in response to acid exposure [18, 22, 23]. This inhibitory action was probably due to unloading of arterial baroreceptors, and constitutes a reflex via the vasomotor center in the *brain stem* . The opposite situation, a 10% hypervolemia, raised bicarbonate secretion. Interestingly, this effect was not mediated via a neural mechanism, but rather by a humoral factor. Atrial appendectomi of the right heart blocked the hypervolemia-induced increase in bicarbonate secretion suggesting an involvement of atrial natriuretic peptide (ANP) [27]. Higher brain structures could influence duodenal bicarbonate secretion via the sympatho-adrenergic route. Stereotaxic electrical stimulation in the perifornical region of the *hyopthalamus* inhibited the duodenal bicarbonate secretion an effect which could be counteracted by epidural anesthesia or the adrenolytic agent guanethidine [28]. This indicates a mediation via spinal (presumably the splanchnic) nerves and adrenergic transmission. I.c.v. administration of the neuropeptide calciotonin gene related peptide (CGRP) inhibits duodenal bicarbonate secretion in conscious rats [29]. This effect has been shown to be due partly to sympatho-adrenergic inhibition and partly to liberation of vasopressin, in turn inhibiting the duodenal secretory process [29].

Ligation of the adrenal glands increased basal duodenal bicarbonate secretion in the rat [4]. Hypovolemia-induced inhibition of duodenal bicarbonate secretion was, however, not influenced by exclusion of the adrenal glands, suggesting that this response mainly was mediated by direct adrenergic-innervation [18]. The adrenal glands seem to be without importance for the duodenal bicarbonate secretion in the cat [30].

Acid-base balance and blood flow. Experiments with alterations in blood volume and acid-base balance in rabbits suggest that duodenal bicarbonate secretion is directly determined by local blood flow and the arterial bicarbonate concentration [16, 31]. In our laboratory, an arterial bleeding of about 10% of the total blood volume in rats reduced bicarbonate secretion by 44%, duodenal blood flow by 31% and arterial bicarbonate concentration by 11%. The mean arterial pressure fell somewhat (from 135 7 to 123 9 mmHg) [32]. These results thus support the suggestion that the duodenal bicarbonate secretion is correlated to the amount of bicarbonate transported to the mucosa by the blood. However, after bilateral vagotomy or in presence of the alpha-2 adrenoceptor antagonist yohimbine, and despite similar restriction in blood flow and arterial bicarbonate, such a "non-hypotensive" hypovolemia did not reduce duodenal bicarbonate secretion [32]. Consequently, it is possible during certain conditions to separately influence the duodenal blood circulation without influencing the secretory process (presumably by use of discrete sets of fibres within the sympathetic nerves reaching the vessels and the secreting epithelium, respectively).

OTHER MUCOSA-PROTECTIVE FUNCTIONS

The duodenum receives acidified hyper- or hypo-osmolar solutions or even solid material from the stomach and do also handle aggressive digestive factors such as bile and pancreatic secretions. This receptive function, with the digestive process included, demand a "functional alertness" to maintain mucosal integrity. The mucosal net fluid and electrolyte transport can, therefore, change rapidly, together with coordinated motor activity, mixing and moving the luminal contents. Furthermore, highly developed negative feed back systems contribute to regulate the disposal of digestive factors and gastric contents into the duodenum. Although changes in the functional state of the duodenum are primarily related to the digestive process, some of them can be regarded as mucosa-protective. In an attempt to broaden the perspective of functional mucosaprotection we have studied acid-induced changes in, not only mucosal bicarbonate secretion, but also net fluid transport and duodenal wall motility.

METHODS

The experiments were performed on chloralose-anesthetized cats. The splanchnic nerves were bilaterally cut in all experiments in order to block sympatho-adrenergic inhibition of gastroduodenal function due to e.g. the surgical trauma [19, 30]. The common bile duct and the pancreatic duct, respectively, were dissected and cannulated close to the duodenal wall. Biliary and pancreatic secretions were thereby diverted to the outside of the animal. An 2 cm segment of the proximal duodenum was isolated between two luminally situated balloons (the proximal balloon being positioned immediately distal to the pylorus). Each balloon was connected to a barostatic device maintaining a constant pressure within the balloon independently of the degree of contraction. The duodenal segment was perfused with isotonic saline containing C^{14}-PEG (mw: 4000) at a constant rate (1.8 ml/min). The recovered perfusate was sampled in 5 min fractions and analyzed with regard to alkalinity (back titration with HCl during air-bubbling), concentration of C^{14}-PEG (liquid scintillation). Net alkalinization and net fluid transport was calculated with conventional equations. The gastric lumen was perfused with saline containing phenol-red. Occurrence of phenol-red (analyzed with spectrophotometri) in the duodenal perfusate would have indicated leakage from the stomach, but was never observed.

The intra-balloon pressure was set to $+10cmH_2O$ with the barostatic device. This pressure is within a physiological range of intraluminal pressure but still sufficient to prevent leakage from or into the duodenal segment. Volume changes in the proximal balloon was graphically recorded and reflected the contractile activity (during isotonic conditions) in the duodenal wall in immediate association to the luminally perfused segment. The frequency of contractions was used for statistical comparisons.

Basal conditions and the response to 30 mM HCl (n=6).

The recovered duodenal perfusate was sampled in 5 min fractions during a 30 min control period (=basal conditions). To challenge the duodenal mucosa the perfusate was then changed to 30 mM HCl (made isotonic with NaCl) over 15 min after which saline again was utilized during the remaining 40-60 min of perfusion.

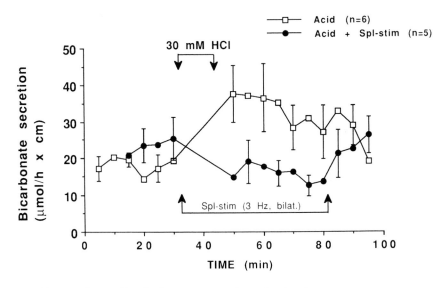

Figure 3:   *Luminal exposure of a duodenal segment to hydrochloric acid stimulates the bicarbonate secretion in a group of chloralose-anesthetized cats (open squares). In another group, simultaneous stimulation of the splanchnic nerves inhibits such an acid-induced increase in secretion (filled circles).*

Basal bicarbonate secretion showed a relatively large variability between the animals in the control group. Independently of the basal level, bicarbonate transport increased by about 100% after exposure of the duodenal mucosa to 30 mM HCl. The titration technique made it impossible to obtain any values of the bicarbonate secretion during the acid exposure (Fig 3). Net fluid transport was close to zero during basal conditions but turned into a marked secretion during the acid exposure. This net fluid secretion decreased immediately after the acid-perfusion but remained elevated during the rest of the experiment (Fig 4).

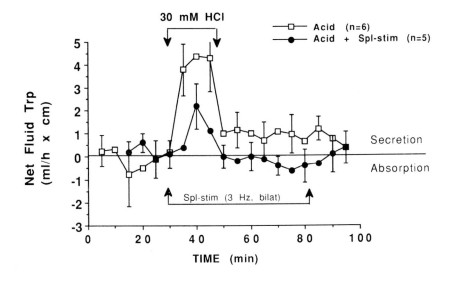

FIGURE 4:   *Chloralose-anesthetized cats. Luminal exposure of a duodenal segment to hydrochloric acid elicits a marked net fluid secretion. The duodenal segment remains in a secretory state after the acid exposure (open squares). In the other group stimulation of the splanchnic nerves inhibits the acid-induced net fluid secretion (filled circles).*

Spontaneous duodenal contractions were present during basal conditions in all animals. Contraction-frequency increased significantly in all animals during the acid-perfusion, but returned immediately to or even below control value when the perfusate again was saline (Fig 5).

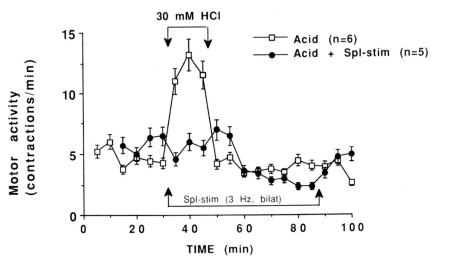

FIGURE 5: *Chloralose-anesthetized cats. Luminal exposure of a duodenal segment to hydrochloric acid increases the frequency of duodenal contractions (open squares). Such acid-induced contractile activity is not obtained during simultaneous stimulation of the splanchnic nerves (filled circles).*

EFFECTS OF VAGOTOMY AND GANGLIONIC RECEPTOR BLOCKADE.

Animals subjected to acute truncal vagotomy (n=4) exhibited a similar response pattern as described above for vagus-intact controls. However, the acid-induced increase in bicarbonate transport was more shortlasting in the vagotomized animals. Blockade of nicotinic cholinoceptor mediated ganglionic transmission with hexamethonium (10 mg/kg x h i.v., n=5) reduced arterial pressure to approximately 85 - 95 mmHg. Basal duodenal bicarbonate secretion was lower in presence of hexamethonium compared to untreated controls and no increase in bicarbonate transport was obtained after exposure to 30 mM HCl. Basal net fluid transport was zero or in an absorptive state but increased promply during acid exposure to a level of about 80% of that seen in the controls. After the acid exposure net fluid transport rapidly returned to its prestimulatory value. Contractile activity was low and irregular in the presence of hexamethonium. Contractions occurred during acid exposure but they were significantly fewer and with smaller amplitude than in the controls.

EFFECTS OF SPLANCHNIC NERVE STIMULATION.

In one group of animals (n=5) splanchnic nerve stimulation was started simultanously with the onset of the acid exposure. Generally, all the recorded acid-induced changes were inhibited by this stimulation: 1). Bicarbonate secretion did not increase after the acid exposure (Fig 3). 2). The net fluid secretion during acid-exposure was small and 3). changed to absorption immediately after the exposure (Fig 4). 4). Acid-induced duodenal contractions did not occur during splanchnic nerve stimulation (Fig 5).

COMMENTS

In the above-mentioned experiments in cats, local acid exposure changed the functional state of the duodenum in several ways: mucosal bicarbonate transport increased, transmucosal fluid movement turned into secretion and duodenal contractions were elicited. These acid-induced responses were resistant to vagotomy (and splanchnicotomy), but sensitive to hexamethonium which suggest that nicotinic cholinergic transmission, within the enteric nervous system, is involved. The marked transepithelial net fluid transport _during_ acid exposure was less sensitive to hexamethonium indicating a different mechanism of mediation. This acid-induced multiple response is interesting from a mucosaprotective point of view. As mentioned in Introduction mucosal bicarbonate secretion protects the duodenal surface epithelium by a chemical neutralization of hydrogen ions close to the mucosa [1]. In addition, mucosal net fluid secretion may be protective by diluting the mucosal microenvironment and thereby reduce the local acidity. It is well known that acid in the duodenum decreases antral motility and increases pyloric tone as parts of the feed back inhibition of gastric emptying. Furthermore, the motility of the proximal duodenum increases in response to luminal acid, probably in order to mix the acid luminal contents or to remove it from an exposed area of the mucosa [33]. The physiological significance of these acid-induced responses remains to be elucidated. It is interesting that activation of the sympathetic splanchnic nerves inhibits all the changes in duodenal function due to acid. A raised activity in the sympatho-adrenal system occurrs during several acute or chronic stress-conditions and such situations are not seldom associated with functional disturbances or even mucosal damage in the upper gastrointestinal tract. It may be speculated that sympathoadrenergic inhibition of duodenal functions contributes to "functional dyspepsia" and/or development of mucosal injury.

ACKNOWLEDGEMENTS

Investigations performed in our laboratory were supported financially by the Swedish Medical Research Council (grants no: 8429 and 8663); the Gothenburg Medical Society.

REFERENCES

1. Flemstrom, G. and Garner A. Secretion of bicarbonate by gastric and duodenal mucosa. In: Handbook of Physiology - The Gastrointestinal System III. Bethesda: American Physiological Society, 1989: p. 309-326.

2. Konturek, SJ., Thor P., Bilski J., Tasler J. & Cieszkowski M. Cephalic phase of gastroduodenal alkaline secretion. Am J Physiol 1987; 252: G742.

3. Ballesteros MA, Hogan DL, Koss MA, Chen HS, Isenberg JI. Vagal stimulation of human duodenal bicarbonate secretion acts by non-cholinergic mechanisms. Gastroenterology 1988; 94: A20 (abstr.)

4. Jönson C, Nylander O, Flemstrom G. & Fändriks L. Vagal stimulation of duodenal HCO_3^--secretion in anaesthetized rats. Acta Physiol Scand. 1986; 128: 65-70.

5. Nylander O, Flemstrom G, Delbro D. & Fändriks L. Vagal influence on gastroduodenal HCO_3^- secretion in the cat in vivo. Am J Physiol 1987; 252: G522-G528.

6. Flemstrom G, & Jedstedt G. Stimulation of duodenal mucosal bicarbonate secretion in the rat by brain peptides. Gastroenterology 1989; 97:412-420.

7. Lenz HJ, Vale WW. & Rivier JE. TRH-induced vagal stimulation of duodenal HCO_3^- mediated by VIP and muscarinic patyhways. Am J Physiol 1989; 256: G677-G682

8. Flemstrom G, Garner A, Nylander O, Hurst BC and Heylings JR. Surface epithelial HCO_3^- transport by mammalian duodenum in vivo. Am J Physiol 1982; 243: G348 - G358.

9. Isenberg JI, Smedfors B. and Johansson C. Effects of graded doses of intraluminal H^+, Prostaglandin E2, and inhibition of endgenous prostaglandin synthesis on proximal duodenal bicarbonate secretion in unanaesthetized rat. Gastroenterology 1985; 88: 303 - 307.

10. Konturek SJ, Bilski J, Tasler J, Laskiewicz J. Gut hormones in stimulation of gastroduodenal alkaline secretion in conscious dogs. Am J Physiol (Gastrointest Liver Physiol 11)1985; 248: G687-G691.

11. Smedfors B. and Johansson C. Cholinergic influence on duodenal bicarbonate response to hydrochloric acid perfusion in the conscious rat. Scand J Gastroenterol 1986; 21: 809-815.

12.   Fändriks L, Jonson C, Nylander O, Flemstrom G. Neural influences
on Gastroduodenal secretion. In: Szabo S, Pfeiffer CJ eds. Ulcer
disease: New aspects of pathogenesis and pharmacology. Boca Raton:
CRC Press, 1989: p. 193-206.

13.   Algazi MC, Chen H-S, Koss MA, Hogan DL, Steinbach J, Pandol
SA.J. and Isenberg JI. Effect of VIP antagonist on VIP-, PGE2-, and
acid-stimulated duodenal bicarbonate secretion. Am J Physiol 1989;
256: G833-G836.

14.   Hamlet A, Jönson C, and Fändriks L. Acid-induced duodenal
alkaline secretion in the anethetized rat; involvement of neural
mechanisms. 1990; subm.

15.   Cassuto J, Siewert A, Jodal M, and Lundgren O. The involvement of
intramural nerves in the cholera toxin induced intestinal secretion.
Acta Physiol Scand 1983; 117: 195-202.

16.   Schiessel R, Starlinger M, Kovats E, Appel W, Feil W, and Simon A.
Alkaline secretion of rabbit duodenum in vivo: its dependence of
acid base balance and mucosal blood flow. In: Allen A, Flemstrm G,
Garner A, Silen W, Turnberg LA, eds. Mechanisms of mucosal
protection in the upper gastrointestinal tract. New York: Raven
Press. 1984, p.267-271.

17.   Takeuchi K, Furuka WAO, Okabe S. Induction of duodenal ulcers
in rats under water-immersion stress conditions. Gastroenterology
1985; 91: 554-563

18.   Jöhnson C. and Fändriks, L. Bleeding inhibits vagally-induced
duodenal HCO_3^- secretion via activation of the splanchnic nerves in
anesthetized rats. Acta Physiol Scand. 1987; 130: 259-264.

19.   Fändriks L. Sympatho-adrenergic inhibition of vagally induced
gastric motility and gastroduodenal HCO_3^--secretions in the cat.
Acta Physiol Scand. 1986; 128: 555-565.

20.   Fändriks L, Jönson C. and Nylander O. Effects of splanchnic nerve
stimulation and of clonidine on gastric and duodenal HCO_3^--
secretion in the anaesthetized cat. Acta Physiol Scand 1987; 130: 251-
258.

21.   Jönson C. and Fändriks L. Splanchnic nerve stimulation inhibits
duodenal HCO_3^- secretion in the rat. Am J Physiol. 1989; 255
(Gastrointest. Liver Physiol.):   G709-G712.

22.   Jöhnson C, Tunback-Hansson P. and Fändriks L. Splanchnic nerve
activation inhibits HCO_3^- secretion from the duodenal mucosa
induced by luminal acid in the rat. Gastroenterology 1989; 96:45-49.

23. Jönson C. and Fändriks L. Bleeding-induced decrease in duodenal HCO$_3^-$ secretion in the rat is mediated via alpha-2 adrenoceptors. Acta Physiol Scand 1987; 130: 387-391.

24. Nylander O and Flemstrom G. Effects of alpha-adrenoceptor agonists and antagonists on duodenal surface epithelial HCO$_3^-$- secretion in vivo, Acta Physiol Scand 1986; 126: 433-441.

25. Knutsson L. and Flemstrom G. Duodenal mucosal bicarbonate secretion in man. Stimulation by acid and inhibition by the alpha-2 adrenoceptor agonist clonidine. Gut 1989; 30, 1708-1715.

26. Jönson C. and Fändriks L. Afferent electrical stimulation of mesenteric nerves inhibits duodenal HCO$_3^-$ secretion via a spinal reflex activation of the splanchnic nerves in the rat. Acta Physiol Scand.1988; 133: 545-550.

27. Jönson C, Fändriks L. and Pettersson A. Increased duodenal HCO3-output after blood volume expansion in the rat: an effect mediated by the atrial natriuretic peptide (ANP)? Acta Physiol. Scand1989; 136: 263-269.

28. Fändriks L, Jönson C, and Lisander B. Hypothalamic inhibition of duodenal alkaline secretion via a sympatho-adrenergic mechanism in the rat. Acta Physiol Scand 1989; 137: 357-363.

29. Lenz HJ, and Brown MR. Cerebroventricular calcitonin gene-related peptide inhibits rat duodenal bicarbonate secretion by release of norepinphrine and vasopressin. J Clin Invest 1990; 85:25-32.

30. Fändriks L. and Jönson C. Influences of the sympatho-adrenal system on gastric motility and acid secretion and on gastroduodenal bicarbonate secretion. Acta Physiol Scand. 1989; 135: 285-292.

31. Starlinger M, and Schiessel R. Bicarbonate (HCO$_3^-$) delivery to the gastroduodenal mucosa by the blood: its importance for mucosal integrity. Gut 1988; 29: 647-654.

32. Jonsson C, Holm L, Jansson T, and Fändriks L. Effects of hypovolemia on duodenal blood flow, arterial HCO$_3^-$ concentration and duodenal alkaline secretion in rats. Am J Physiol 1990; in press.

33. Allescher H-D, Daniel EE, Dent J, Fox JET, and Kostolanska F. Neural reflex of the canine pylorus to intraduodenal acid infusion. Gastroenterology 1989; 96: 18-28.

HUMAN DUODENAL MUCOSAL BICARBONATE SECRETION IN HEALTH AND DISEASE.

Daniel L. Hogan and Jon I. Isenberg

Division of Gastroenterology, UCSD Medical Center, University of California San Diego, San Diego, California.

INTRODUCTION

Transport of bicarbonate by duodenal surface epithelial cells has been studied extensively in bullfrog, rat, rabbit, dog and other species [1-7]. Only recently has bicarbonate secretion by the human duodenal mucosa been studied in any specific detail [8]. Epithelial HCO_3^- transport processes established in amphibian and lower species of mammalian duodenum are of great importance. But these anion transport processes do not always prove directly applicable to the human duodenum, though similarities do exist. Moreover, the rationale for evaluating the transport mechanisms involved is not just to understand how the normal duodenum functions, but to investigate how and why some processes operate abnormally. Thus, our investigations have concentrated on comparing duodenal epithelial bicarbonate production in duodenal ulcer patients as well as in normal healthy subjects. Results so far indicate that the proximal duodenal mucosa of the ulcer patient functions abnormally relative to that of normals. Studies over the past five years evaluating duodenal mucosal bicrbonate secretion in both health and duodenal ulcer disease are summarized.

METHODS

STUDY POPULATION

Approximately 75 healthy volunteers and 40 patients with duodenal ulcer disease have been studied. Some of the ulcer patients have been studied while their ulcer was active and after their ulcer had healed as verified by upper gastrointestinal endoscopy All investigations were approved by the University of California San Diego Human Subjects Committee, and each volunteer gave informed consent.

STUDY PROCEDURES

Isolation of duodenal segments was accomplished with a modified multilumen gastroduodenal tube (Dreiling, Davol, RI, USA). Balloons were positioned under fluoroscopy to occlude a 4 cm segment of either proximal (bulb) or distal (third portion) duodenum. Non-absorbable markers were perfused proximally (phenol red) and distally (vitamin B12) to ensure the segment remained free of gastric and pancreaticobiliary secretions; trypsin was also measured from the isolated loop. The isolated test segment was continuously perfused with 154 mM NaCl (2ml/min, 37°C), and effluents were collected by gravity drainage. Gastroduodenal secretions were aspirated by automatic suction (Stedman pump, ACMI, Stafford, CT, USA).

Measurement of bicarbonate was analyzed by two different methods. In non-acidified samples, $[HCO_3^-]$ was measured by back titration [8]. When the test segment was acidified, samples were collected anaerobically, the pH and PCO_2 measured, and $[HCO_3^-]$ calculated by the Henderson-Hasselbalch equation [9].

Results are summarized and expressed as means ($\pm$ SEM). The standard two-tailed statistical tests were used in the data analysis and differences were considered significant at P <0.05.

RESULTS AND DISCUSSION

BICARBONATE SECRETION IN HEALTH

Resting, basal, proximal duodenal mucosal bicarbonate secretion is approximately 190 μmol/cm-h (N > 100 studies). Bicarbonate secretion in the third portion of the duodenum is about 15% of that in the bulb indicating a gradient from proximal-to-distal duodenum. The duodenal mucosa responds to a variety of agonists and antagonists which are summarized in Table 1.

TABLE 1.

HUMAN DUODENAL MUCOSAL BICARBONATE PRODUCTION

Agonists:

H^+ (25, 50, 100 mM)[a]
PGEs (misoprostol[a], arbacet, trimoprostol,
  natural PGE_2, 10^{-6}-10^{-3} M, i.l.)
VIP (200 and 400 pmol/kg-h, i.v.)
Sham Feeding
Theophylline (10^{-3}-10^{-2} M, i.l.)

Antagonists:

Indomethacin (100 mg p.o.)[a]
Atropine (22 ug/kg, i.v.)
Na_2SO_4

No Effect:

Glucagon (1-8 μg/kg-h, i.v.)
Secretin (0.01-0.18 cu/kg-h, i.v.)[a]
Bethanachol (12.5, 25, 50 μg/kg-h, i.v.)
Na_2HCO_3 (i.l.)

*All agents were tested in the proximal duodenum
(a = distal duodenum also studied);
i.l. = intraluminal administration.*

Luminal acidification with a physiologic dose of 2 mmoles H^+ (20 ml of 100 mM HCl over 5 min) is a potent stimulus increasing bicarbonate secretion 2-3 fold to about 500 μmol/cm-h. Recently, we determined that the pH threshold for duodenal mucosal bicarbonate secretion is pH 3 (Figure 1) [10]. It was also concluded, with the use of citrate buffers, that the mucosa's response was not due to the total acid load (1 to 5 mmol), but to the pH. Indeed, the increase in bicarbonate secretion in response to perfusion with a pH 3 solution was equivalent to that observed with a pH 1 perfusate.

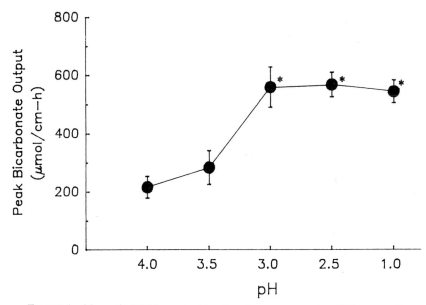

FIGURE 1 *Mean (±SEM) peak bicarbonate responses to different pH solutions. The duodenal mucosa responded significantly at pH 3. The acid loads (1.1 mmol) were equivalent at each pH with the use of citrate buffer; except pH 1 which was 100 mM HCL (1.1 mmol).* * = P < 0.02 *vs basal (saline, pH 6).*

Since acid entering the duodenum stimulates the release of a number of intestinal hormones, it was of interest to examine if the homologous peptides secretin, glucagon and VIP had an effect on bicarbonate secretion. In various animal species each stimulates duodenal bicarbonate secretion, albeit the effect of secretin is conflicting [1,7,11]. Yet, in humans, only VIP significantly increased duodenal mucosal bicarbonate secretion [12].

In addition, prostaglandins of the E class play an important role in regulating duodenal bicarbonate transport. Selling et al [13] demonstrated that luminal acidification increased endogenous PGE_2 output as well as bicarbonate secretion. And, inhibition of endogenous PGE_2 with the cyclooxygenase inhibitor indomethacin (100 mg, orally) significantly decreased both basal and H^+-stimulated bicarbonate output and luminal

PGE_2 release in the proximal and distal duodenum. Furthermore, in another study, inhibition of endogenous prostaglandins enhanced the mucosa's response to luminal PGE_1 administration [14]. This later finding suggests that there is an **increased** sensitivity to PGE after supression of endogenous prostaglandin synthesis. All prostaglandins tested thus far have stimulated duodenal bicarbonate secretion (Table 1). Taken together, these results indicate that E class prostaglandins act locally to regulate bicarbonate secretion.

Duodenal mucosal bicarbonate secretion is also controlled by vagal-cholinergic factors. Muscarinic blockade with the nonspecific anticholinergic atropine (20 ug/kg i.v.) decreased bicarbonate secretion markedly to 20% of basal [15]. On the other hand, cholinergic-stimulation with bethanachol (12.5 - 50 ug/kg-h, i.v.) had no significant stimulatory effect [15]. These data suggest that cholinergic tone is near maximal during basal bicarbonate secretion. Cephalic-vagal stimulation by sham feeding also significantly increased bicarbonate production by 30% [16]. Of interest, cholinergic factors do not seem to regulate the H^+- and vagal-induced bicarbonate responses since atropine had no effect on their respective net stimulated bicarbonate outputs. Also, inhibition of local PGEs with indomethacin did not impair the response to sham feeding. In contrast, studies in rat [17] showed atropine had no effect on basal and decreased the acid-stimulated responses. Results in dog [18], however, were comparable to ours which demonstrated that atropine and indomethacin did not abolish the sham-feeding bicarbonate secretory response. Therefore, in healthy subjects, whereas acid-stimulated bicarbonate transport is most likely regulated by both PGEs and VIP, vagal-stimulated bicarbonate secretion is probably mediated by VIP and/or other non-cholinergic (purinergic) mechanisms.

Studies by Odes at al [19] observed that human duodenal bicarbonate secretion is mediated by an active transport mechanism(s). By eliminating the lumen-to-blood HCO_3^- concentration gradient with a HCO_3^- containing perfusate (24 and 32mM), bicarbonate secretion continued at about 80% of basal. Further, stimulation with either acid or PGE_2 resulted in an increase in bicarbonate secretion equal to the response with the bicarbonate-free saline perfusate.

The intracellular mechanism by which extracellular agonists stimulate human bicarbonate secretion is unknown. In animals, it has been suggested that cAMP is likely the intracellular mediator regulating electrogenic bicarbonate transport [1,2,7]. To examine this question we tested the effect of the phosphodiesterase inhibitor theophylline, which indirectly increases intracellular cAMP, on duodenal bicarbonate secretion. Theophylline ($10^{-2}M$, luminally) significantly increased bicarbonate secretion when given alone, and significantly enhanced the bicarbonate response with PGE_2 co-administration compared to PGE_2 alone (Figure 2)[20]. Moreover, the increases in bicarbonate secretion were accompanied by increases in transmucosal potential difference (basal= -5 mV; peak= -9 mV). Since the interaction of theophylline and PGE_2 produced a synergistic response, the findings agree with the hypothesis that cAMP, in part, mediates human duodenal mucosal bicarbonate secretion.

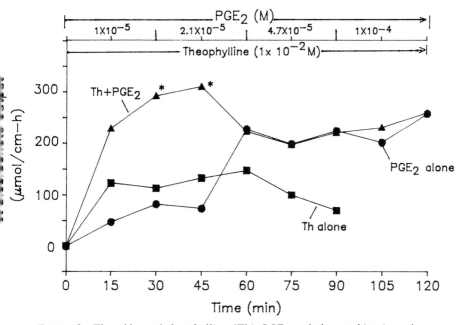

FIGURE 2 *The effect of theophylline (Th), PGE$_2$ and the combination of Th + PGE$_2$ on mean net duodenal bicarbonate secretion. Theophylline was used to increase intracellular cAMP. Since Th significantly enhanced the increase in bicarbonate secretion at the lower doses of PGE$_2$, the results suggest cAMP mediates PGE$_2$-stimulated bicarbonate secretion. * = P < 0.05 versus either Th or PGE$_2$ alone.*

BICARBONATE SECRETION IN DUODENAL ULCER DISEASE.

The first report suggesting that patients with inactive duodenal ulcer (DU) possessed impaired mucosal bicarbonate secretion was in 1987 [21]. Since then, a total of 36 patients have been studied evaluating both basal and acid-stimulated proximal duodenal mucosal bicarbonate secretion (Figure 3). Bicarbonate output in DU is about 50% of that in normal subjects with very little overlap. In addition, patients who were studied while their ulcer was active and after their ulcer healed (the status determined by upper gastrointestinal endoscopy) revealed that basal and acid-stimulated bicarbonate outputs were similar in the presence and absence of an active duodenal ulcer crater. This suggests that the impaired proximal duodenal bicarbonate secretion observed in DU patients is independent of the anatomical defect, and more likely related to a cellular or subcellular phenomenon.

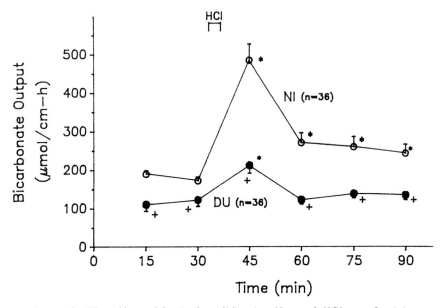

<u>FIGURE 3</u> *The effect of luminal acidification (2 mmol HCl over 5 min)
on mean (± SEM) duodenal bicarbonate output in 36 duodenal ulcer
patients (DU) and 36 normal subjects (NL). In DU, basal and H^+-
stimulated bicarbonate outputs were significantly less compared to NL.
* = P < 0.01 vs basal; + = P < 0.01 vs NL.*

Since prostaglandins are important in bicarbonate regulation, we
hypothesized that there may be deficient duodenal mucosal PGE_2 levels in
DU patients. Further investigations revealed, to our surprise, that DU
patients released significantly greater amounts of endogenous PGE_2 in
response to acidification as compared to normals [22]. Therefore, whereas
DU patients secrete less bicarbonate, they release more PGE_2. This implies
the presence of an altered feedback mechanism or desensitization to PGE_2 in
DU disease.

The next logical question was to examine if exogenous PGE_2
stimulated bicarbonate transport in DU similar to that in normals. PGE_2
was perfused in graded doses (10^{-5}-10^{-4} M) and both bicarbonate secretion
and transmucosal potential difference were measured. The results
demonstrated that, [1] in normals, bicarbonate secretion and potential
difference increased progressively in a dose-response manner; and, [2] in
DU, whereas potential difference increased similar to normals, there was no
significant increase in bicarbonate secretion (Figure 4) [23]. These findings
suggest that while PGE_2 stimulates electrogenic transport of bicarbonate in
normals, there is a defect in bicarbonate transport in DU. The exact
location of this defect has yet to be defined.

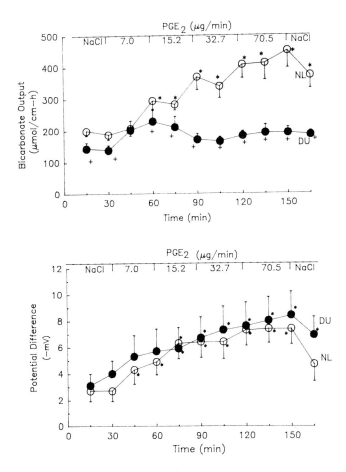

<u>FIGURE 4</u>   *The effect of luminal PGE$_2$ on mean ($\pm$ SEM) duodenal bicarbonate secretion (top) and duodenal transmucosal potential difference (bottom) in 7 duodenal ulcer patients (DU) and 7 normal subjects (NL). See text for details. * = P<0.05 vs basal; + = P<0.05 vs NL.*

The effect of cephalic-vagal stimulation has also been studied in a small number of DU patients (N = 5).   In contrast to normals, there was no response to sham feeding. These results contribute further support that the bicarbonate secretory defect in DU is located at a distal secretory process (i.e., cellular or subcellular).

The impairment in bicarbonate secretion by the proximal duodenal mucosa in duodenal ulcer patients seems to be a global event including diminished basal bicarbonate production as well as being non-responsive to the agonists H^+, PGE_2 and sham feeding.   To explore if the defect could possibly be of morphological origin, biopsies were taken from the duodenal bulb in patients with inactive duodenal ulcer and healthy volunteers.   There were no differences found in quantitative morphometric histology of any parameter between the two groups [24].

The integrity of the duodenal mucosa is maintained by a balance between aggressive and defensive factors.   Increased aggressive factors, such as acid and pepsin, have been associated with duodenal ulcer, but there is a large overlap between ulcer patients and normals in the pathophysiological factors studied thus far [25].   To date, the only substantive observation defining a defect in a major defensive factor is impaired duodenal mucosal bicarbonate secretion.   Other potential defects, such as blood flow, mucus and phospholipids may exist, but need to be investigated.

ACKNOWLEDGEMENTS

The success of this work has been due to major contributions by A. Aly, K. Bukhave, S.P. Feitelberg, M.A. Koss, J.Z. Mu, H.S. Odes, J. Rask-Madsen, J.A. Selling, F.J. Thomas, W.M. Weinstein and J.D. Wolosin.   This work was supported by grant (AM 33491) from the National Institutes of Health.

REFERENCES

1.   Flemstrom G, Heylings JR, Garner A.   Gastric and duodenal HCO_3^- transport *in vitro*: Effects of hormones and local transmitters.   Am J Physiol 1982; 242: G100-110.

2.   Simson JNL, Merhav A, Silen W.   Alkaline secretion by amphibian duodenum: I. General characteristics.   Am J Physiol 1981; 240: G401-408.

3.   Simson JNL, Merhav A, Silen W.   Alkaline secretion by amphibian duodenum: II.   Short-circuit current and Na^+ and Cl^- fluxes.   Am J Physiol 1981; 240: G472-479.

4.   Isenberg JI, Smedfors B, Johansson C.   Effect of graded doses of intraluminal H^+, prostaglandin E_2, and inhibition of endogenous prostaglandin synthesis on proximal duodenal bicarbonate secretion in unanaesthetized rat.   Gastroenterology 1985; 88: 303-307.

5.   Flemstrom G, Garner A, Nylander O, et al.   Surface epithelial HCO_3^- transport by mammalian duodenum *in vivo*.   Am J Physiol 1982; 243: G348-358.

6.   Konturek SJ, Bilski J, Tasier J, et al.   Gut hormones in stimulation of gastroduodenal alkaline secretion in conscious dogs.   Am J Physiol 1985; 248: G687-691.

7. Flemstrom G. Gastric and duodenal mucosal bicarbonate secretion. In: Johnson LR, ed. Physiology of the Gastrointestinal tract. Raven Press, New York. 1987, 1011-1030.

8. Isenberg JI, Hogan DL, Koss MA, Selling JA. Human duodenal mucosal bicarbonate secretion: Evidence for basal secretion and stimulation by hydrochloric acid and a synthetic prostaglandin E_1 analogue. Gastroenterology 1986; 91: 370-378.

9. Isenberg JI, Hogan DL, Thomas FJ. Duodenal mucosal bicarbonate secretion in humans: A brief review. Scand J Gastroenterol 1986; 21(Suppl 125):106-109.

10. Feitelberg SP, Hogan DL, Koss MA, Isenberg JI. pH threshold of human duodenal mucosal bicarbonate secretion is 3. Gastroenterology 1990; 98: A43.

11. Isenberg JI, Wallin B, Johansson C, et al. Secretin, VIP, and PHI stimulate rat proximal duodenal surface epithelial bicarbonate secretion *in vivo*. Regul Pept 1984; 8:315-320.

12. Wolosin JD, Thomas FJ, Hogan DL, Koss MA, O'Dorisio TM, Isenberg JI. The effect of vasoactive intestinal peptide, secretin, and glucagon on human duodenal bicarbonate secretion. Scand J Gastroenterol 1989; 24: 151-157.

13. Selling JA, Hogan DL, Andreas A, Koss MA, Isenberg JI. Indomethacin inhibits duodenal mucosal bicarbonate secretion and endogenous PGE_2 output in human subjects. Ann Intern Med 1987; 106: 368-371.

14. Hogan DL, Ballesteros MA, Koss MA, Isenberg JI. Cyclooxygenase inhibition with indomethacin increases human duodenal mucosal response to prostaglandin E_1. Dig Dis Sci 1989; 34: 1855-1859.

15. Wolosin JD, Hogan DL, Koss MA, Isenberg JI. The effect of cholinergic and anticholinergic agents on human duodenal bicarbonate secretion (DBS) acts by non-cholinergic mechanisms. Gastroenterology 1987; 92: A1698.

16. Ballesteros MA, Hogan DL, Koss MA, Chen HS, Isenberg JI. Vagal stimulation of human duodenal bicarbonate secretion (DBS) acts by non-cholinergic mechanisms. Gastroenterolgoy 1988; 94: A20.

17. Smedfors B, Johansson C. Cholinergic influence on duodenal bicarbonate response to hydrochloric acid perfusion in the conscious rat. Scand J Gastroenterol 1986; 21: 809-815.

18. Konturek SJ, Thor P. Relation between duodenal alkaline secretion and motility in sham fed dogs. Am J. Physiol 1986; 251: G591-96.

19.   Odes HS, Hogan DL, Ballesteros MA, Wolosin JD, Koss MA, Isenberg JI. Human duodenal bicarbonate secretion: Evidence for active transport under basal and stimulated states. Gastroenterology 1988; 94: A329.

20.   Mu JZ, Hogan DL, Koss MA, Isenberg JI. cAMP and prostaglandin E_2 (PGE_2) on human proximal duodenal mucosal bicarbonate secretion. Gastroenterology 1990; 98: A91.

21.   Isenberg JI, Selling JA, Hogan DL, Koss MA. Impaired proximal duodenal mucosal bicarbonate secretion in duodenal ulcer patients. N Engl J Med 1987; 316: 374-379.

22.   Bukhave K, Rask-Madsen J, Hogan DL, Koss MA, Isenberg JI. Proximal duodenal prostaglandin E_2 release and mucosal bicarbonate secretion are altered in duodenal ulcer patients. Gastroenterology 1990: In Press.

23.   Hogan DL, Koss MA, Isenberg JI. Imparied proximal duodenal mucosal bicarbonate secretion in duodenal ulcer patients involves a prostaglandin-mediated cellular defect. Gastroenterology 1990; 98: A60.

24.   Basuk PM, Hogan DL, Marin M, Koss MA, Ballesteros MA, Weinstein WM, Isenberg JI. Diminished duodenal mucosal bicarbonate secretion in duodenal ulcer is independent of mucosal histologic abnormalities. Gastroenterology 1989; 96: A33.

25.   Soll AH. Duodenal ulcer and drug therapy, in Sieisenger MH and Fordtran JS, ed. Gastrointestinal disease. Volume 1. Philadelphia: WB Saunders Co. 1989; 814-878.

REGULATION OF INTRACELLULAR pH (pHi) IN OXYNTICOPEPTIC CELLS: STUDIES IN INTACT AMPHIBIAN GASTRIC MUCOSA

A. Yanaka, K. Carter, P. Goddard, W. Silen

Harvard Medical School, Beth Israel Hospital, Boston, Massachusetts, U.S.A.

ABSTRACT

Gastric mucosal epithelial cells are regularly exposed to enormous concentrations of luminal H^+, with gradients at times as high as 1,000,000:1. The ability of the mucosa to withstand such gradients has properly focused considerable attention on the mechanisms by which the mucosal epithelial cells regulate pHi. While several studies have previously examined the regulation of pHi in surface epithelial cells in intact amphibian antrum [1-6], or in monolayers of chief cells [7], experiments to assess oxynticopeptic cells directly have been limited to isolated cells [8-10] until recently. Since isolated cells invariably lose polarity, and because the interaction of the different types of cells within the complex fundic mucosa may be important [11], we have developed methods to measure pHi in intact amphibian fundic mucosa using the fluorescent dye, BCECF (2',7'-bis-(2-carboxyethyl)-5(6)-carboxyfluorescein) [12-14] Our results have been presented in several previous publications [12-14] and this communication therefore represents an up-to-date synthesis and review of this material.

METHODS AND RESULTS

Initial studies showed that frog *(Rana Catesbeiana)* fundic gastric mucosa exposed to the esterified form of BCECF on the luminal side for 3 hours in an Ussing chamber serendipitously concentrated the fluorescent BCECF in the oxynticopeptic cells and even more selective loading was obtained when both the muscularis propria and the muscularis mucosa were stripped from the mucosa and the tissue was exposed to the BCECF-AM from the basolateral side [13]. The results reported herein are a compilation of the findings in both types of preparation.

Starlinger et al [15] in 1987 demonstrated in isolated rabbit gastric glands that there is autoregulation of pHi in oxyntic cells during exposure to an external pH varying between 6.4 to 7.6. Using the luminally loaded preparation described above, our laboratory found a rapid recovery of pHi over 10 minutes in oxynticopeptic cells exposed to a continuing acidic challenge imposed by changing conditions from HEPES bathing solutions - 100% O_2 to 5% $CO_2^-HCO_3^-$ bathing solutions [12]. Recovery from a more acidic challenge with 10% CO_2 was however prolonged and incomplete [12]. Interestingly, recovery from an alkaline challenge by removal of CO_2 was

247

less rapid and less complete than that from an acidic challenge. This may be relevant to our recent observation that cell death in response to anoxia is greater when intra-cellular pH is high [16].

Subsequent experiments in our laboratory using the doubly stripped mucosa have confirmed the existence of a HCO exchanger on the basolateral membrane of oxynticopeptic cells [13], the presence of which was suggested by others in isolated gastric glands and by us in isolated rabbit parietal cells [10]. This exchanger was readily blocked by the presence of DIDS (an inhibitor of anion exchange) in the nutrient solution or by removal of Cl^- from both the nutrient and luminal solutions [13]. The activity of the HCO_3^-/Cl^- exchanger was greater in stimulated than in inhibited tissues as evidenced by a greater rise in pHi in stimulated tissues exposed to serosal DIDS. Of considerable physiologic interest was the finding that the presence of Cl^- in the luminal solution prevented the rise in pHi observed when Cl^- was removed from both bathing solutions, indicating that luminal Cl^- is available to the basolateral HCO_3^-/Cl^- exchanger [13]. Whether the movement of the luminal Cl^- to the basolateral side is paracellular or through the cells could not be ascertained from these studies.

Forskolin-stimulated mucosae bathed in nutrient HCO_3^- solutions maintain a pHi of about 7.03 when the luminal pH is 7.2. This pHi was unchanged by luminal acidifiction to pH 1.5, but further luminal acidification to 1.0 caused a decrease in pHi to ~ 6.85. The decrease in pHi was somewhat greater in stimulated tissues bathed in HEPES nutrient solutions, but pHi returned to control levels when luminal pH was restored to 7.2. Similar results were obtained in resting tissues, i.e. those pre-treated with the H^+/K^+ ATPase inhibitor, omeprazole. In resting tissues bathed in HEPES, the decrease in pHi induced by increasing luminal $[H^+]$ was exaggerated by serosal amiloride, an inhibitor of Na^+/H^+ exchange but not by serosal H_2-DIDS. In resting tissues bathed in HCO_3^-, the decrease in pHi induced by lowering luminal pH was not altered by either amiloride or H_2-DIDS alone but was accentuated by a combination of these two agents. Amiloride did not alter the changes in pHi induced by increasing luminal $[H^+]$ in resting tissues bathed in Cl^- free HCO_3^- but H_2-DIDS enhanced the decrease in pHi and partially inhibited the recovery at luminal pH 7.2. The amiloride-insensitive, Cl^- independent recovery of pHi in the presence of serosal HCO_3^- was completely inhibited either by removal of ambient Na^+ or by the addition of serosal H_2-DIDS. We concluded from these recent studies that pHi in oxynticopeptic cells in intact sheets of frog mucosa exposed to high luminal $[H^+]$ is maintained more readily in the stimulated state than in the resting state, and that serosal HCO_3^- protects oxynticopeptic cells from a major decrease in pHi during exposure to high luminal $[H^+]$. In addition, our data clearly demonstrate that both a basolateral Na^+/H^+ exchanger and basolateral Na^+-HCO_3^- co-transport are involved in the recovery of pHi from exposure to low luminal pH [17].

Since others have shown in antral mucosa that basolateral acidification is much more deleterious to the mucosal cells than is luminal acidification, we studied the effects of acidification of the nutrient solution in intact sheets of fundic mucosa [14]. Interestingly, lowering the pH of an unbuffered nutrient solution from 7.2 to 3.5 acidified pHi in oxynticopeptic cells from 7.05 only to 6.44 without a change in potential difference or resistance, and with a striking increase in acid secretion from 0.86 to 1.88 μEq/cm^2/hr. By light and electron microscopy, oxynticopeptic cells appeared normal despite the nutrient pH of 3.5. pHi returned to normal values upon return of the nutrient pH to 7.2 in untreated and forskolin stimulated tissues, whereas pHi was irreversibly lowered to 6.26 and 6.44 by the nutrient pH 3.5 in omeprazole and cimetidine treated tissues respectively. In the latter tissues, oxynticopeptic and smooth muscle cells of the muscularis mucosa showed extensive morphologic damage. These data indicate that per se a pHi as low as 6.4 is not deleterious in the secreting mucosa, whereas the inhibited fundic mucosa is much more susceptible to a similar degree of basolateral acidification.

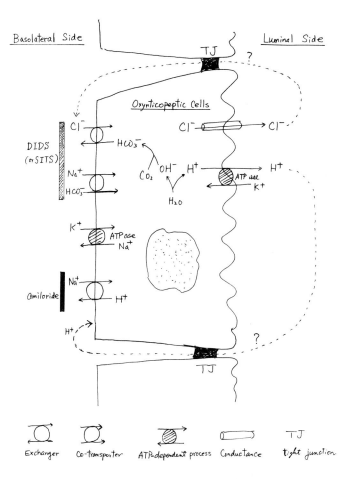

FIGURE 1   (See Discussion and Summary)

While we have not specifically examined the relative tolerance to acidification of oxynticopeptic and surface cells, our studies have suggested that oxynticopeptic cells may be more susceptible to an acid challenge than surface cells. For example, the decrease in pHi in response to a challenge with change of gassing from 100% O_2 to 95% O_2- 5% CO_2 was much greater in fundic oxynticopeptic cells than in antral surface cells [12]. In addition, we have observed a much more profound morphologic injury of oxynticopeptic than to surface cells during basolateral acidification. Most investigators have naturally focused attention on surface cells as the initial site of ulceration since these cells are most superficially located and are therefore presumably more exposed to luminal acid. Since systemic acidification, however, has been shown to be so injurious, and because luminal acidification is well tolerated by both surface and oxyntic cells, we must begin to focus on the oxyntic cell as perhaps the initial site of damage under conditions of sytemic acidication.

DISCUSSION AND SUMMARY

Figure 1 is a schematic diagram of our current concepts of regulation of pHi in the amphibian oxynticopeptic cell. On the basolateral membrane, we have shown the presence of a HCO_3^-/Cl^- exchanger, a Na^+/H^+ exchanger, and a co-transport of Na^+-HCO_3^-. The HCO_3^-/Cl^- exchanger is poised to extrude HCO_3^- and to alkalinize the basolateral surface when it is exposed to an acidic challenge or to back-diffusion of luminal H^+, especially in the stimulated fundic gastric mucosa. The presence of HCO_3^- in the nutrient solution serves a similar purpose, probably because of Na^+-HCO_3^- co-transport. Luminal Cl^- can participate in the operation of the basolateral HCO_3^-/Cl^- exchanger after diffusion of the Cl^- through the mucosa. Strong acidification of the luminal surface of the mucosa is better tolerated than acidification of the nutrient solution, with minimal lowering of pHi, probably because of the relatively impermeant nature of the apical membrane to H^+. It appears that the damaging effect of luminal H^+ occurs mainly after back-diffusion of H^+ to the basolateral side. The response to an alkaline challenge which is mediated solely by the HCO_3^-/Cl^- exchanger is less brisk and less complete than that to an acidic challenge.

REFERENCES

1.   Kivilaakso E, Kiviluoto T. Intracellular pH in isolated Necturus antral mucosa in simulated ulcerogenic conditions. Gastroenterology. 95: 1198-1205.

2.   Kiviluoto T, Coipio J, Kivilaakso E. Subepithelial tissue pH of rat gastric mucosa exposed to luminal acid, barrier breaking agents, and hemorrhagic shock. Gastroenterology 1988; 94: 695-702.

3.   Ashley S.W., Soybel D.I., Cheung L.Y. Measurements of intra-cellular pH in Necturus antral mucosa by microelectrode technique. Am J Physiol. 1986; 250 (Gastrointest. Liver Physiol. 13): G625-G632.

4.   Ashley SW, Soybel DI, Moore D, Cheung LY. Intracellular pH (pHi) in gastric surface epithelium is more susceptible to serosal than mucosal acidification. Surgery 1987; 371-379.

5. Kiviluoto T, Paimela H, Mustonen H, Kivilaakso E. Intracellular pH in isolated necturus antral mucosa exposed to luminal acid. Gastroenterology 1990; 98: 901-908.

6. Kivilaakso E. Contribution of ambient HCO_3^- to mucosal protection and intracellular pH in isolated amphibian gastric mucosa. Gastroenterology 1983; 85: 1284-1289.

7. Sanders MJ, Ayalon A, Roll M, Soll AH. The apical surface of canine chief cell monolayer resist H^+ back-diffusion. Nature 1985; 313: 52-54.

8. Paradiso AM, Townsley MC, Wentzl E, Machen TE. Regulation of intracellular pH in resting and in stimulated parietal cells. Am. J. Physiol. 1989; 257 (Cell Physiol. 26): C554-C561.

9. Townsley MC, Machen TE. Na^+-HCO_3^- co-transport in rabbit parietal cells. Am J Physiol. 1989; 257 (Gastrointest. Liver Physiol. 19): G350-G356.

10. Seidler U, Carter K, Ito S, Silen W. Effect of CO_2 on pHi in rabbit parietal, chief, and surface cells. Am J Physiol. 1989; 256 (Gastrointest. Liver Physiol. 19): G466-G475.

11. Curci S, Debellis L, Fromter E. Evidence for rheogenic sodium bicarbonate co-transport in the basolateral membrane of oxyntic cells of frog gastric fundus. Pflugers Arch. 1987; 408: 497-594.

12. Carter KJ, Saario I, Seidler U, Silen W. Effect of PCO_2 on intracellular pH in in vitro frog gastric mucosa. Am J Physiol. 1989; 256 (Gastrointest. Liver Physiol. 19): G206-213.

13. Yanaka A, Carter KJ, Lee HH, Silen W. Influence of Cl^- on pHi in oxynticopeptic cells in in vitro frog gastric mucosa. Am J Physiol (Gastrointest. Liver Physiol.) (In press)

14. Arvidsson S, Carter KJ, Yanaka A, Ito S, Silen W. The effect of basolateral acidification on the frog oxyntico-peptic cell. Am. J Physiol. (Gastrointest. Liver Physiol.) Submitted.

15. Rowe PH, Starlinger MJ, Kasdon E, Hollands MJ, Silen W. Parenteral aspirin and sodium salicylate are equally injurious to the rat gastric mucosa. Gastroenterology 1987; 93: 863-871.

16. Lee HH, Carter K, Yanaka A, Goddard P, Ito S, Silen W. Intracellular acidosis enhances the viability of rabbit gastric glands during "chemical hypoxia". Gastroenterology 1990; 98:A77.

17. Yanaka A, Carter KJ, Goddard P, Heissenberg M, Ito S, Silen W. Role of Na^+-HCO_3^- co-transport in the regulation of intracellular pH (pHi) in oxynticopeptic cells in frog gastric mucosa exposed to luminal acid. Gastroenterology, 1990; 98: A151.

pH$_i$-REGULATING ION TRANSPORT SYSTEMS IN ISOLATED RABBIT PARIETAL, CHIEF AND SURFACE CELLS

U. Seidler, S. Roithmaier, V. Schusdziarra,
M. Classen, and W. Silen

*II Med. Klinik der Techn. Universitat Munchen and Department of Surgery,
Beth Israel Hospital, Harvard Medical School, Boston, USA*

ABSTRACT

We have studied the ion transport mechanisms in isolated rabbit parietal, chief and surface cells that are capable of regulating the pH$_i$ with special emphasis on the role of the HCO$_3^-$ ion in pH$_i$-regulation. Our data suggest that proton entry into isolated gastric cells in the presence of a low extracellular pH occurs predominantly via the Na$^+$/H$^+$ exchanger. pH$_i$-Recovery from an intracellular acid load is also mediated predominantly by Na$^+$/H$^+$ exchange in the presence as well as the absence of CO$_2$/HCO$_3^-$ in all three cell types. Due to the higher intracellular buffering capacity, a given acid load will result in a much smaller decrease in pH$_i$ in the presence of CO$_2$/HCO$_3^-$ compared to its absence. pH$_i$-Recovery from an alkaline load is very fast in parietal cells and mediated predominatly by the Cl$^-$/HCO$_3^-$ (OH$^-$) exchanger, whose main physiological role is the exchange of intracellularly produced base of extracellular Cl$^-$ destined for apical secretion during HCl secretion. This exchanger is absent in chief and surface cells.

The Na$^+$/H$^+$ exchanger, which is located on the basolateral side of the gastric epithelial cells, was further characterized. In all three cell types, the dependency of H$^+$-efflux rate on pH$_i$ showed a strong inverse correlation (demonstrating the strong dependency of the Na$^+$/H$^+$ exchange rate on the pH$_i$) and the results of Hill plot analyses were compatible with the presence of two internal binding sites for H$^+$, one transport site and one serving as an activation site. No change in the kinetic parameters by a stimulation of intracellular cAMP generation was observed.

Determination of the steady-state pH$_i$ at different pH$_0$ revealed that gastric cells are able to maintain a considerable transmembrane pH-gradient. This transmembrane pH-gradient is maintained by the operation of several ion transport systems, the kinetic energy for all of which is ultimately derived from the action of the Na$^+$/K$^+$-ATPase.

INTRODUCTION

The gastric mucosa provides the secretory juice which initiates food digestion. The acid, protease-containing juice then digests not only the food in the stomach, but may injure the gastric mucosa itself. Our present appreciation of the physiological mechanisms involved in mucosal resistance to acid comes from studies utilizing a variety of methodological approaches. All of them are artificial systems, and all of them have their problems. While is is theoretically always desirable to use models that are as close to the physiological situation as possible, results obtained in complex systems are often too difficult to explain without previously studying simpler systems. This is exactly the reason why we have studied ion transport systems involved in cellular pH_i-regulation in isolated, purified rabbit mucosal cell populations. To use isolated cell populations has some very obvious disadvantages, because by disrupting the epithelial structure, the cells loose their polarity, and we cannot distinguish between processes localized to the apical and those localized to the basolateral membrane. On the other hand, using isolated purified cell population, one can conveniently localize an ion transport system to a specific cell type. manipulate intra- and extracellular ion concentrations and simultaneously assess the effect of such manipulations on cell function and viability, and perform experiments on multiple aliquots of one homogenous cell population.

In this overview we will present an excerpt from studies we have done recently in an attempt to identify and characterize ion transport mechanisms in rabbit gastric mucosal cells that are involved in the maintenance of pH-homeostasis in the gastric mucosa. This overview shall not attempt to give a complete account of our findings, but shall focus on the different types of experiments one can perform in isolated cell systems in order to address different questions aimed at a more complete understanding of proton and base handling of the different epithelial cells in the gastric mucosa.

METHODS

CELL ISOLATION

Parietal cells were isolated and purified as previously described in detail [26,28]. In brief, male New Zealand white rabbits were anesthetized and the stomach perfused under high pressure via the aorta for 15 min with oxygenated Hepes-saline, excised, and the mucosa scraped from the submucosa and minced into small pieces. The cells were enzymatically dispersed by successive incubations in 100 ml buffer A containing 0.5g/l Pronase E (Sigma) for 30 min followed by incubation in 50 ml buffer A containing 0.8 g/l Collagenase 1A (Sigma) for 20-30 min. Buffer A consisted of (in mM) 98 NaCl, 20 $NaHCO_3$, 20 HEPES-Tris, 3 KH_2PO_4, 2 K_2HPO_4, 1.2 $MgSO_4$, $1CaCl_2$, 11 glucose, 1 g/l bovine serum albumin, pH 7.4). When the cells were 100% dispersed, they were washed 3 times with buffer B (118 NaCl, no $NaHCO_3$), dispersed in 20% Percoll (Pharmacia)/buffer B, and layered on top of a preformed 40% Percoll gradient, and spun for 20 min at 2000 rpm. After removing the bottom and the cell layer at the interface of the 20/40% percoll with a syringe, the interface cell layer was subjected to the same procedure again. The interface cell layer of that second spin was enriched in mucous and parietal cells and virtually free of chief cells. The cells of the interface layer and the cells of the pooled bottom layer of the first and second spin were then purified to approx. 95% homogeneity in a Beckman elutriator rotor as previously described. Cell characterization was performed as previously described [26,28].

Parietal cells obtained this way showed very low basal AP-uptake ratios even in the absence of H_2 blockers or omeprazole, and displayed a 20-25 fold stimulation of ^{14}C-AP uptake with 10^{-5}-10^{-4}M histamine alone (without addition of IBMX). The viability of the isolated cells was routinely tested by Trypan blue exclusion and by inspecting aliquots of the cell suspension that had been loaded with fura-2 or BCECF under the microscope. Bright intracellular fluorescence with BCECF indicated viable cells, which were always trypan-blue negative, and cells which had lost the bright fluorescence from BCECF were always trypan-blue positive. These findings were similar to results described by Lemasters et al, whose group has extensively studied the relationship between cellular integrity and a number of parameters including BCECF fluorescence [13,18].

^{14}C-AMINOPYRINE UPTAKE

^{14}C-Aminopyrine uptake was measured as follows: the cells were gently dispersed to a concentration of 0.8-1 x 10^{-6} cells/ml in oxygenated BSA-containing buffer B containing 0.1 uCi/ml ^{14}C-aminopyrine (New England Nuclear), and preincubated for 20 min at 37°C. 5 ml Aliquots were pipetted into liquid scintillation vials to which the appropriate test drugs had been added, and incubated with 80 cycles/min either in a New Brunswick incubator shaker or a Braun-Melsungen Certomat U equipped with an incubation hood. Every 10 min for up to 40 min 1 ml of cell suspension was removed from the vial, centrifuged in an Eppendorf tube, the pellet was resuspended and the cells washed once with puffer, repelleted, and dissolved in 100 ul of 1 N KOH and counted in liquid scintillation fluid in a conventional betacounter. Nonspecific trapping and uptake ratios were determined exactly as previously described [26].

MEASUREMENT OF pH_i

The cells were incubated with 2.5 uM BCECF/AM (Molecular probes, Eugene, Or) in Buffer B under oxygen and gentle shaking at 25°C for 30-45 min. The cells were then washed twice, resuspended in buffer B and kept in suspension until use within the next two hours. Immediately before use the cells were spun down at 400 rpm and the medium removed. The cells were resuspended in the respective test medium, immediately placed into the fluorometer, and the first reading taken within 5 s of the medium change. Fluorescence was measured in a processor-controlled LS-3 or LS-5 Perkin-Elmer spectrofluorometer equipped with a magnetic stirrer. Excitation wavelengths were rapidly changed between 490 and 439 nm, emission wavelength was 540 nm. A ratio of the fluorescence intensity at the 490 nm excitation wavelength and that at the 439 nm excitation wavelength was obtained every 12 sec for 15 min. If longer reading times were necessary, the cells were pelleted and resuspended in fresh test solution of identical composition. To assess dye leakage, the cells were pelleted after 15 min and resuspended in fresh test solution. If significant dye leak had occurred (difference in apparent pH_i more than 0.5%), the ratios were corrected for the dye leak. This was necessary when ion substitutions were performed that inflicted marked volume changes on the parietal cells. To measure the equilibrium or steady-state pH_i, cell aliquots were suspended in the appropriate buffer, placed in plastic scintillation vials, the fluid was overlayed with the appropriate gas mixture (oxygen or carbon dioxide/oxygen mixtures, capped and sealed with teflon tape, incubated at $37^{\circ}C$ for 30 min, 1 and 3 hours with constant shaking in a New Brunswick incubator shaker or a Braun-Melsungen Certomat U/HK. At the indicated times the cells were pelleted, resuspended in the identical medium, an placed into the fluorometer. Calibration was performed by suspending cell aliquots in solutions containing (in mM) 125 KCl, 20 HEPES-Tris, 2 K_2HPO_4, 3 KH_2PO_4, 1 $CaSO_4$, 1.2 $MgSO_4$, 11 glucose, and 10 uM of the K^+/H^+ ionophore nigericin, and at 5 different pH-values between 6.4 and 7.8. The addition of Nigericin causes pH_i to become equal to the extracellular pH (pH_o), if K^+_o is approximally equal to K^+_i. The calculated fluorescence ratio at each pH_o is then plotted against pH_o (=pH_i under the calibration conditions). The fluorescence ratio was linearly correlated to pH_i between 6.4 and 7.8, and linear regression analysis of the obtained values resulted in a function that allowed transformation of the obtained fluorescence ratios to pH_i values.

DETERMINATION OF INTRACELLULAR BUFFERING CAPACITY

We have used CO_2 addition (cell permeable acid) and NH_4Cl addition (the cell-permeable base is NH_3) to measure intracellular buffer capacity. Because of the known pH_i-dependency of the intrinsic as well as the CO_2/HCO_3^-buffer system [25], it is necessary to obtain small increases or decreases in $[H^+_i]$. This was performed by the addition of small amounts of 1 M NH_4Cl (pH_i-increase) or sequentially transferring the cells in buffer gassed with 1, 2.5, 5, 10, 20, 25%CO_2/rest O_2. The extracellular pH was kept at 7.4 for all experiments. In order to prevent pH_i-recovery to occur from cellular ion transport, cells whose pH_i was lowered below 7.4 were suspended in a Na^+-free buffer and cell whose pH_i was elevated above 7.4 were suspended in a Cl^--free buffer. This approach was most suitable to obtain a steady plateau of pH_i after each addition of acid or base. NH_4Cl is known to enter the cell in a variety of cell types via different transporters, and we have found that, if at all, this occurs at pH_i-values above 7.4. This would lead to an overestimation of the buffer capacity at high pH_i values, and this is exactly what was observed to happen at high pH_i-values, where we calculated an apparent rise of β_i above 7.5, a clearly erroneous finding, when compared with results obtained in a variety of other cell types [5,34]. We have therefore measured β_i at high pH_i with CO_2-pulses. The calculations that are necessary to obtain the intracellular buffer capacity have been described several times in detail [4,5,25,34].

STATISTICAL ANALYSIS

Values are given as means   SE, n is always the number of experiments with different rabbits. The Student's t-test for paired samples was used for statistical evaluation if not otherwise indicated. Unless otherwise indicated, our results are statistically significant with p values below 0.05.

All test solutions for pH_i measurements contained the following (in mM): 20 HEPES-Tris, 2 K_2HPO_4, 3 KH_2PO_4, 1 $CaSO_4$, 1.2 $MgSO_4$, and 11 glucose. In addition, medium gassed with 100% oxygen contained one of the following: 120 NaCl, 120 Nagluconate (Cl^--substitution), 120 trimethylammonium (TMA)Cl (Na^+-substitution), 120 mM Kgluconate or 120 mM TMAgluconate. Medium gassed with CO_2/O_2 contained, depending on the CO_2-content of the gas and pH, varying concentration of $NaHCO_3$ (Na^+-containing) or choline HCO_3 (Na^+-free), together with the appropriate concentration of NaCl or TMACl to obtain isoosmolarity. Amiloride (Merck, Sharp & Dohme or Sigma) was dissolved in dimethyl sulfoxide (DMSO) at a final DMSO concentration of 0.5%, the same concentration was added to the control. DIDS (Sigma) was dissolved in water. A stock solution of Nigericin was made in ethanol (100 mM) and for each experiment 5 ul of this stock was diluted with 245 ul of buffer, 20 ul of this solution was added to each 4 ml cuvette.

RESULTS AND DISCUSSION

PROTON PERMEABILITY

Protons may enter the gastric epithelial cells both through the apical or the basolateral membrane. The apical membranes of gastric epithelial cells appear to be extraordinarily impermeable to protons, and it is still unclear whether a physiological situation exists where protons enter the cells through the apical membrane. Alternatively, the tight junctions may become proton-permeable and protons may enter the epithelial cells from the basolateral side. It is known that the basolateral membrane is far more proton-permeable than the apical membrane, but the mechanism of proton entry has not been elucidated [2]. It is obviously impossible to obtain any information about apical proton permeability in isolated cells in suspension, but as most of the exposed cell membrane is of basolateral origin in isolated cells, on can study basolateral proton-entry mechanisms.

We have performed a number of studies to see if protons enter the cell primarily through a proton conductance, or through one or several proton/base transporters that are located in the basolateral membrane.

Table 1 shows the rate of proton influx during the first 10 min occuring in rabbit parietal cell that had been incubated at pH_o 7.4, under five different conditions: control cells (incubated in NaCl-buffer), Na^+-loaded cells (incubated in 100 uM ouabain), Na^+-depleted cells (incubated in TMA-Cl) and Na^+ and Cl^- depleted cells where the membrane potential was or was not clamped to zero with valinomycin (incubated in Kgluconate and TMAgluconate, respectively). The total transmembrane Na^+ and H^+-gradient $[Na^+_o]/[Na^+_i] + [H^+_o]/[H^+_i]$ was set to approximately 10 for all experiments. $[Cl^-_o]$ was 120 mM except in the Kgluconate buffer. Although the driving force for proton entry was therefore roughly equal in all four conditions, the proton efflux rate was clearly highest in the ouabain-treated cells, and very low in the Na^+-depleted cells. The absence or presence of Cl^- did not influence the results, indicating that a Cl^-/base exchanger had little role in transporting protons into the cells. 1 mM Amiloride did not significantly affect the rate of acidification in parietal cells and inhibited acidification in chief cells slightly. We interpret these finding as an indication that proton entry into the cells in a low pH surrounding (absence of open CO_2/HCO_3^- buffer system) occurs predominantly in exchange with intracellular Na^+ ions. In the presence of identical driving forces (sum of the transmembrane gradients for Na^+ and H^+) and low pH_o, the availibility of Na^+_i appears to be rate limiting for proton entry. 1 mM Amiloride, which inhibits Na^+-influx through the Na^+/H^+ exchanger, does not significantly inhibit proton influx, because in contrast to the affinity for Na^+, the affinity for H^+ to the external transport site is be very much higher than for amiloride. Thus, in a low basolateral pH surrounding, the maintenance of a low Na^+_i protects the cells from rapid basolateral proton entry.

TABLE 1

	Proton influx (mM/5 min)	
Cells Preincubated in:	1st 5 min	2nd 5 min
NaCl	1.92	1.75
NaCl + ouabain	4.56	2.80
TMA-Cl	0.68	0.69
TMA-gluconate	0.72	0.71
K-gluconate + valinomycin	0.96	0.81

Proton influx into parietal cells incubated in buffer with a low pH (as the driving force for Na^+/H^+ exchange $[Na^+_o]/[Na^+_i]$ + $[H^+_o]/[H^+_i]$ was kept constant in all 5 conditions, pH_o varied between 6.4 and 6.0). The intracellular Na^+ concentration $[Na^+_i]$ was measured by atomic absorption spectroscopy and estimated at 24 mM in control conditions, 89 mM in ouabain-treated cells and 4 mM in Na^+-depleted cells. n=4. It is obvious that the proton influx rate is highest in the presence of a high $[Na^+_i]$ and low at low $[Na^+_i]$, suggesting that H^+_o is exchanged for Na^+_i. The absence or presence of Cl^- or high K/valinomycin does not influence the results much, suggesting that a Cl^-/base or a proton conductance play little role in proton entry.

PROTON BUFFERING

The degree of intracellular acidification that a transmembrane proton flux will cause depends very much on the intracellular buffering power. The intracellular buffering capacity can be measured by adding a certain amount of cell-permeable acid or base and measuring the resulting pH_i-change, and calculating $\Delta[H^+_i]/\Delta$ pH. Fig. 1 shows the intracellular buffer capacity in rabbit parietal cells in mM/pH-unit at different pH_i. β_i in the absence of CO_2/HCO_3^- decreased with increasing pH_i. In CO_2/HCO_3^-, β_i increased dramatically with increasing pH_i (at constant pCO_2) and further with increasing pCO_2 and HCO_3^- concentrations (at constant pH_i). the results in the other cell types are qualitatively similar.

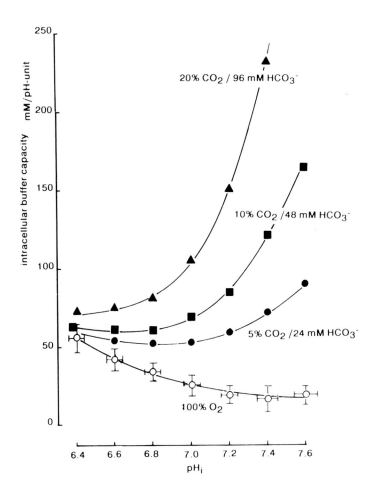

FIGURE 1: *Intracellular buffer capacity in mM/pH-unit in parietal cells in the absence and presence of different pCO_2/HCO_3^- and different pH_i. The buffer capacity was determined as described in the method section. Data were averaged for 0.5 pH_i-unit groups. n=9*

Due to this difference in β_i, a much higher intracellular acid load is required to acidify the cytoplasm to the same pH_i in the presence than the absence of CO_2/HCO_3^-. This extremely high buffering capacity of the

CO_2/HCO_3^- buffer system at neutral pH and above may be the main if not the whole explanation for the fact that the in vitro or in vivo gastric mucosa is more resistant to acid injury in the presence of high basolateral HCO_3^- concentrations [9,15]. If the apical membrane and tight junctions were absolutely impermeable to protons, the intracellular or interstitial buffering capacity would be irrelevant. As soon as there is any permeability of the epithelial layer under physiological or pathological conditions, it will depend mainly on the buffering power of the cytoplasm and the interstitial fluid if and where those protons will be neutralized.

PROTON EXTRUSION IN THE ABSENCE AND PRESENCE OF CO_2/HCO_3^-

If a significant amount of protons has managed to enter the cell and the buffering capacity was not strong enough to prevent a fall in pH_i, pH_i-regulation becomes important.

Imposing an intracellular acid load in the presence and absence of CO_2/HCO_3^-

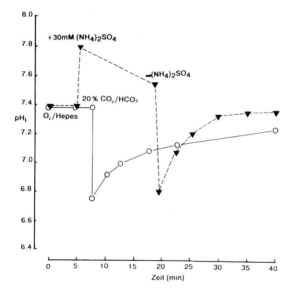

FIGURE 2:   *Typical trace of a pH_i-recovery curve in parietal cells that have been acidified, either by the so-called "ammonium prepulse" technique or by introducing them in a CO_2/HCO_3^- containing buffer. In the first instance, a cell-permeable base (NH_3) causes a selective increase in pH_i, pH_i-recovery sets in and a pH_i-undershoot results when all the base is removed again. In the second instance, a cell-permeable "acid" (CO_2) causes a selective decrease in pH_i. Proton efflux rates can be calculated by multiplying the pH_i-recovery rate dpH/min with the buffering capacity β_i at the given pH_i.*

We have extensively studied pH_i-recovery mechanisms from an acid load in the past three years with special emphasis on the question whether in the presence of HCO_3^- additional acid extrusion mechanisms may be operative. Fig. 2 shows a typical trace of pH_i-recovery curve in parietal cells that have been acidified, either by the so-called "ammonium prepulse" technique or by introducing them in a CO_2/HCO_3^- containing buffer. In the first instance, the principle is that a cell-permeable base causes a selective increase in pH_i, pH_i recovery sets in, by whatever mechanisms, then all the base is removed again and a pH_i-undershoot results. In the second instance, a cell-permeable "acid" causes a selective decrease in pH_i. Both methods have the advantage that the external pH is kept constant. Other methods of acidification are also used, such as preincubation in buffer with a low pH, with or without the use of ionophores [19,33]. The application of the latter methods result in higher subsequent proton efflux rates, for unclear reasons. By multiplying the initial pH_i-recovery rate dpH/min with the intracellular buffer capacity β_i at the given pH_i, the proton efflux rate $J_{[H^+]}$ is obtained. With this type of experiment one identifies different acid extrusion mechanisms that may be involved in pH_i-recovery from an acid load. An example is given in Table 2 and Fig. 3. In order to find out if acid extrusion mechanisms other than the Na^+/H^+ exchanger may be involved in pH_i-recovery from intracellular acidification in the presence of CO_2/HCO_3^-, we acidified parietal cells as shown in Fig. 2, measured pH_i-recovery rates and calculated proton efflux rates in the absence and presence of CO_2/HCO_3^- under a variety of different conditions (see Table 2, for a 20% $CO_2/80\%$ O_2, 90 mM $MaHCO_3^-$ or choline HCO_3^-). In the presence of Cl^- in cells and buffer, there was a markedly higher initial proton efflux rates in the presence of CO_2/HCO_3^- compared to its absence (see table 2, first row).

TABLE 2

Parietal cells	Proton efflux (mM/min)	
Initial pH_i6.7, pH_o7.4	$-CO^2/HCO^{3-}$	CO^2/HCO^{3-}
NaCl	9.7	14.2
Na-gluconate (Cl-depleted)	9.0	8.4
TMA-Cl	0.7	4.3
TMA-gluconate (Cl-depleted)	0.3	0.4

Proton efflux rates in mM/min in parietal cells that had been acidified in the absence and presence of 20% CO_2/90 mM HCO_3^- as described in Fig. 2 and the text. pH_i-Recovery rates were measured in the absence and presence of Na^+_o in Cl^--containing and Cl^--depleted cells. Note that the markedly larger proton extrusions rates in the presence of CO_2/HCO_3^- as compared to its absence were only observed in the presence of Cl^-_i, but this difference was independent of the presence of Na^+ (third row) and abolished by 2 mM DIDS. The most likely explanation is that, because of the high $[HCO_3^-]_o$ and relatively low $[Cl^-]_o$, the Cl^-/HCO_3^- mediates base uptake. n=6

Three different types of ion transporters have been identified in different cell types that could explain this finding: an electrogenic Na^+-HCO_3^- co-transporter [14,17], a Na^+-coupled [6] or, although not previously described as a transporter mediating proton efflux, a Na^+-independent Cl^- /HCO_3^- exchanger [8,16,23]. In order to differentiate between the three possibilities, we compared the proton efflux rates in the presence and absence of CO_2/HCO_3^- in a) buffer that contained both Na^+ and Cl^-, b) buffer that contained no Cl^-(cells previously Cl^--depleted), c) buffer that contained Cl^- but no Na^+, and d) buffer that contained neither, in cells had been Cl^--depleted. In b) all Cl^--dependent transport processes are blocked, but a Na^+-HCO_3^- cotransporter could be operative in addition to the Na^+/H^+ exchanger. In c), a Cl^-/HCO_3^- exchanger could operate, and in d) all transporters are blocked. The results were unexpected: as seen in Table 2, there was no difference in the proton efflux rate with or without CO_2/HCO_3^- in the absence of Cl^-. This suggests that the observed effect is not due to a Na^+-HCO_3^- co-transporter. The Na^+-coupled Cl^-/HCO_3^- exchanger also cannot explain the higher proton efflux rate in CO_2/HCO_3^- and NaCl containing buffer, because the effect can still be seen in the absence of Na^+. We therefore tentatively concluded that the Na^+-independent Cl^-/HCO_3^- exchanger may reverse its normal transport direction and import base in exchange for Cl^-_i. This was curious, because it was then thought that the Cl^-/HCO_3^- exchanger was inactive at pH_i values below 7.0 [16,21,23]. In order to further clarify this question we performed the experiments shown in Fig. 3. By increasing the driving force for the reversal of the Cl^-/HCO_3^- exchanger by reducing Cl^-_0 to zero at the time of CO_2/HCO_3^-introduction, a much larger initial pH_i-increase was observed (Fig. 3a). This showed that Cl^-/HCO_3^-exchange could indeed occur at this low pH_i, and the similar time course with pH_i-recovery in NaCl/HCO_3^- buffer suggested that the initial pH_i-recovery phase in the presence of CO_2/HCO_3^- was indeed dominated by Cl^-/HCO_3^- exchange. Whether this exchanger has a role in pH_i-recovery from an acid load *in vivo* remains to be determined.

Subsequent pH_i-recovery could be inhibited by 1 mM amiloride and was therefore most likely due to Na^+/H^+ exchange. In Fig. 3b, pH_i-recovery in the presence of Na^+_0 and 1 mM amiloride was similar to that in the absence of K^+. This suggests that a Na^+-HCO_3^- co-transporter contributes little, if any, to pH_i-recovery in this experimental conditions. In chief and surface cells, pH_i-recovery was mediated by the Na^+/H^+ exchanger in the absence and presence of CO_2/HCO_3^-, in accordance with our results demonstrating the absence of any detectable Cl^-/HCO_3^- exchange in these cell types [27,28].

ANION EXCHANGE IN GASTRIC EPITHELIAL CELLS

During acid secretion, the parietal cell generates large amounts of intracellular base. A Cl^-/base exchanger in the parietal cell basolateral membrane exports base in exchange for Cl^- ions needed for apical HCl secretion [11]. The characteristics of this exchanger, which is also capable of mediating a rapid pH_i-recovery from an intracellular alkaline load, have been studied by us and others [7,19,23,27,28,32,34] and will not be reviewed in this manuscript. Of note is that neither chief and surface cells demonstrate any Cl$^-$/base exchange activity under any of the experimental conditions that we applied.

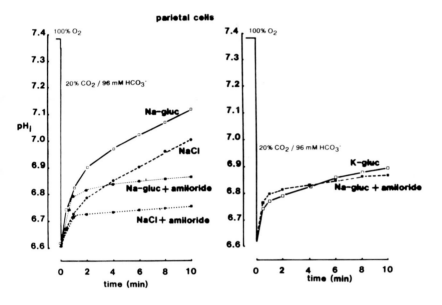

FIGURE 3A: The pH_i-recovery curves in parietal cells acidified by introduction into a buffer gassed with 20% CO_2/80%O_2, containing 90 mM HCO_3^-, 50 mM of either Cl$^-$ or gluconate, and 1 mM amiloride where indicated. The initial rapid pH_i-rise was enhanced by removing all Cl$^-$ from the buffer (a maneuver that would enhance Cl$^-$ efflux though the Cl$^-$/HCO_3^- exchanger), and the second phase of recovery was inhibited by the Na$^+$/H$^+$ exchange inhibitor amiloride.

FIGURE 3B: The pH_i-recovery curve in the presence of Na$^+$ and HCO_3^- plus 1 mM amiloride (Na$^+$/H$^+$ exchanger inhibited but Na$^+$-HCO_3^-, if operative, unaffected) is compared with that in the absence of Na$^+$. There is no major difference between the two curves, arguing against the participation of a Na$^+$-HCO_3^- cotransporter in pH_i-recovery.

REGULATION OF ION TRANSPORTERS

Extensive evidence exists in the literature that the activity of many ion transporters is subjected to hormonal control. It has been suggested that Na^+/H^+ and Cl^-/base exchange is activated during stimulation of acid formation with agonists that stimulate the adenylate cyclase [20,22].

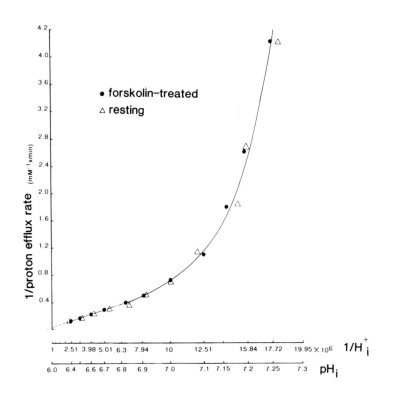

FIGURE 4: *Lineweaver-burke transformation of the initial proton efflux rates in forskolin ($5x10^{-6}M$)-treated ($\triangle$) and resting ($\bullet$) cells after acidification to pH_i-values from 6.5 to 7.2. The intersection of the curves with the y-axis gives the V_{max}, and the intersection with the x-axis should give the apparent K_m for the internal H^+ transport site. The curves for forskolin-stimulated and resting cells are identical. Hill analysis of the data revealed a straight line with a slope of 1.85 (almost 2), indicating that two binding sites for H^+ exist. The results are compatible with the existence of an internal modifier site, to which H^+-ions bind, thus activating the exchanger, but are not transported. cAMP does not appear to regulate the parietal cell Na^+/H^+ exchanger. The curves were constructed from experiments with cells from eleven different rabbits.*

The measured "activity" of an exchanger can be altered by a conformational change in the transport molecule with a change in the affinity (K_m) or maximal transport capacity (V_{max}) or both, or by an change in the transmembrane ion gradients. Fig. 4 shows the results of a series of experiments in which we determined if a rise in intracellular cAMP affects a conformational change in the parietal cell Na^+/H^+ exchanger. The pH_i-recovery rates after intracellular acidification to pH_i-values from 6.5 to 7.2 were measured in forskolin-stimulated and resting parietal cells and the proton efflux rates were calculated. A Lineweaver-Burke transformation of the data resulted in the curves shown in Fig. 4.

The intersection of the curves with the y-axis gives the V_{max}, and the intersection with the x-axis the apparent K_m for the internal H^+ transport site. It is apparent that the curve is not a straight line. With decreasing pH_i the proton efflux rates in crease in a more than linear fashion. Hill analysis of the data revealed a straight line with a slope of 1.85 (almost 2), indicating that two binding sites for H^+ exist, (we know from the electroneutrality of the exchange process that only one functions as a transport site). The results are compatible with the existence of an internal modifier site, to which H^+-ions bind, thus activating the exchanger. [1,12].

The curves for forskolin-stimulated and resting cells were identical (forskolin caused an up to 30fold stimulation of ^{14}C-uptake compared to resting cells and a strong stimulation of adenylate cyclase activity). Therefore, cAMP does not appear to regulate the parietal cell Na^+/H^+ exchanger. We are now in the process of determining if other second messengers do.

STEADY-STATE pH_i REGULATION

A different approach to studying pH_i-regulation is to determine the equilibrium pH_i. Fig. 5, a-d shows experiments where we have measured the steady-state pH_i after 1-3 hours of incubation in the buffers indicated in the figure legends. The cells are able to maintain a considerable transmembrane pH-gradient for many hours. If amiloride was added (Fig. 5a), the whole curve was shifted to a lower pH_i-level, but the transmembrane gradient was maintained. Also, when DIDS or SITS was added (data not shown), Cl^- taken out (Fig. 5b), CO_2/HCO_3^- added (Fig. 5c), the curve was shifted, but the transmembrane pH_i-gradient was not abolished. However, when sodium pump was blocked, either by ouabain or by high extracellular K^+, or cellular energy metabolism poisoned, the transmembrane pH-gradient was eventually abolished (Fig. 5d).

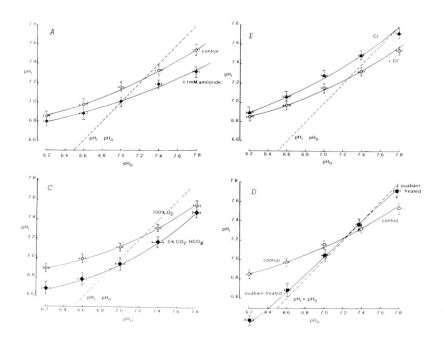

FIGURE 5: *Steady-state pH_i at different pH_o in parietal cells had had
been incubated for 1 and 3 hours in buffer with different pH-values,
under control conditions and 1 mM amiloride (Fig. 5a), in Cl^--free (Fig.
5b), $5\% CO_2/22$ mM HCO_3^- or 100 uM ouabain. In Fig. 5a-c, the cells are
able to maintain a substantial transmembrane pH-gradient under all
experimental conditions, although the overall pH_i-level is shifted
downward or upward by the inhibition (Fig. 5a, b) or stimulation (Fig.
5c) of certain ion transport processes. After the inhibition of the Na^+/K^+
and therefore the dissipation of the transmembrane Na^+-gradient and the
membrane potential, the pH-gradient also dissipates. n=8*

The maintenance of a transmembrane gradient is active, energy-dependent
cellular pH_i-regulation. While all the energy required for active pH_i
regulation appears to be stored in the transmembrane Na^+ and K^+ gradients,
this energy is used to operate a number of ion transport systems involved in
the mainentance in this transmembrane gradient, and depending on the
internal and external pH, different pH_i -regulation systems are operative,
and we are still in the process of finding and characterizing them.

SUMMARY

Let us apply the knowledge that has accumulated in the last few years on the regulation of intracellular pH in gastric epithelial cells to construct a hypothesis on gastric mucosal proton handling:

1. Proton Permeability:

The apical membranes of gastric epithelial cells appear to be extraordinarily impermeable to acid. This may be due to the lack of ion transport mechanisms capable of transporting protons into the cell, a specialized membrane composition, or other factors. When the pH on the basolateral side falls, a Na^+/H^+ exchanger in the basolateral membrane is able to import protons into the cells. A number of agents, the so-called "barrier breakers", are able to increase apical membrane permeability. It is not yet clear if, an under what conditions, the tight junctions between the epithelial cells become proton permeable.

2. Proton Buffering

The gastric epithelial cells have "intrinsic" buffer systems as well as, under physiological conditions, the CO_2/HCO_3^- buffer system. Whereas the intrinsic buffering capacity β_i increases strongly with decreasing pH_i, the CO_2/HCO_3^- buffer system buffers well at neutral pH and above. This extremely high buffer capacity of the CO_2/HCO_3^- buffer system is likely to explain the observed protection of high mucosal HCO_3^- concentrations against gastric injury by acid.

3. Proton Extrusion

When the gastric barrier is broken, protons may enter the mucosa. If the cellular and interstitial buffering capacity is overwhelmed, the pH_i falls. All three major epithelial cell types possess a Na^+/H^+ exchanger that is activated by a drop in pH_i and can exchange large amounts of protons for Na^+_o as long as the basolateral pH remains high. If the basolateral pH falls by acid back diffusion through tight junctions or the lack of extracellular neutralization of basolaterally extruded protons, H^+_o, with a much higher affinity than Na^+, competes with Na^+_o for binding at the external transport site and the proton extrusion rate rapidly falls. Therefore, HCO_3^- in the interstitial fluid may serve to keep the basolateral pH high, an essential factor for gastric pH_i homeostasis.

4. Anion Exchange

Parietal cells generate intracellular base during acid secretion and exchange this base for Cl^- on the basolateral side. This locally generated base may serve as a protective buffer and is used for bicarbonate secretion by the surface cells. The ion transporters that mediate both basolateral HCO_3^- uptake into surface cells and apical secretion remain to be elucidated.

REFERENCES:

1.   Aronson, P.A., J. Nee, und M.A. Suhm. 1982. Modifier role of internal H^+ in activating the Na^+/H^+ exchanger in renal microvillus membrane vesicles. J. Biol. Chem. 258:6767-6771

2.   Ashley, S.W., D.I. Soybel, D. Moore, and L.Y. Cheung. 1987. Intracellular pH (pH_i) in gastric surface epithelium is more susceptible to serosal than mucosal acidification. Surgery 102:371-379

3.   Boron, W.F. 1983. Transport of H^+ and of ionic weak acids and bases. J. Membr. Biol 72:1-16

4.   Boron, W.F. 1986. Intracellular pH-regulation. In. Physiology of membrane disorders. Andreoli, T.E., Hoffman, J.F., Fanestil, D.D., Schultz, S.G. eds. 2nd ed. New York: Plenum Publishing Corporation. pp 423-435

5.   Boyarsky, G., M.B. Ganz, R.B. Sterzel, und W.F. Boron. 1988 Intracellular pH-regulation in single glomerular mesangial cells. I. Acid extrusion in the absence and presence of HCO_3^-. Am. J. Physiol. 255:C857-C869

6.   Boyarsky, G., M.B. Ganz, R.B. Sterzel, und W.F. Boron. 1988. Intracellular pH-regulation in single glomerular mesangial cells. II. Na^+-dependent and -independent $Cl-HCO_3$ exchangers. Am J. Physiol. 255:C844-C856

7.   Carter, K.J., I. Saario, U. Seidler, und W. Silen. 1989. Effect of pCO_2 on intracellular pH in in vitro frog gastric mucosa. Am. J. Physiol. 256:G206-G213

8.   Chaillet, J.R., K. Amsler, und W.F. Boron. 1986. Optical measurements of intracellular pH in single $LLC-PK_1$ cells: Demonstration of Cl^--HCO_3^-exchange. Proc. Natl. Acad. Sci. USA, 83:522-526

9.   Cheung, L.Y., und G. Porterfield. 1979. Protection of gastric mucosa against acute ulceration by intravenous infusion of sodium bicarbonate. Am. J. Surg. 137:106-110,

10. Curci, S., L. Debellis, und E. Frmter. 1987. Evidence for rheogenic sodium bicarbonate cotransport in the basolateral membrane of oxyntic cells of frog gastric mucosa. Pflgers Arch. 408:497-504

11. Forte, J.G., and T.E. Machen. 1986. Ion transport by gastric mucosa. In: Physiology of membrane disorders. Andreoli, T.E., Hoffman, J.F., Fanestil, D.D., Schultz, S.G. eds. 2nd ed. New York: Plenum Publishing Corporation, pp535-558

12. Grinstein, S, und A. Rothstein. 1986. Mechanisms of regulation of the Na^+/H^+ exchanger. J. Membrane Biol. 90:1-12

13.   Herman, B., A.-L. Niemen, G.J. Gores, and J.J. Lemasters. 1988. Irreversible injury in anoxic hepatocytes precipitated by an abrupt increase in plasma membrane permeability. FASEB J. 2:146-151

14.   Jentsch, T.J., P. Schwartz, B.S. Schill, B. Langner, A.P. Lepple, S.K. Keller, und M. Wiederholt. 1986. Kinetic properties of the sodium bicarbonate (carbonate) symport in monkey kidney epithelial cells (BSC-1). J. Biol. Chem. 261:10673-10679

15.   Kivilaakso, E. 1983. Contribution of ambient HCO_3^- to mucosal protection and intracellular pH in isolated amphibian gastric mucosa. Gastroenterology 85: 1284-1289

16.   Kurtz, I., und K. Golchini. 1987. Na^+-independent Cl^-/HCO_3^- exchange in Madin-Darby canine kidney cells. Role in intracellular pH-regulation. J. Biol. Chem. 262:4516-4520

17.   L'Allemain, G., S. Paris, und J. Pouyssgar. 1985. Role of a Na^+-dependent Cl^-/HCO_3^- exchange in regulation of intracellular pH in fibroblasts. J. Biol. Chem. 260:4877-4883

18.   Lemasters, J.J., J.D. DiGuiseppi, A.-L. Niemen, B. Herman. 1987. Blebbing, free Ca^{2+}, and mitochondrial membrane potential preceding cell death in hepatocytes. Nature 325:78-81

19.   Muallem, S, C. Burnham, D. Blissard, T. Berglindh, and G. Sachs. 1985. Electrolyte transport across the basolateral membrane of parietal cells. J. Biol. Chem. 260:6641-6653

20.   Muallem, S., D. Blissard, E.J. Cragoe, und G. Sachs. 1988. Activation of the Na^+/H^+ and Cl^-/HCO_3^- exchange by stimulation of acid secretion in the parietal cell. J. Biol. Chem. 263:14703-14711

21.   Olsnes, S, T.I. Tonnessen, and K. Sandvig. 1986. pH-regulated anion antiport in nucleated mammalian cells. J. Cell Biol. 102:967-971

22.   Paradiso, A.M., M.C. Townsley, E. Wenzl, and T.E. Machen. Regulation of intracellular pH in resting and stimulated parietal cells. Am. J. Physiol. 257:C554-561, 1989

23.   Paradiso, A.M., R.Y.Tsien, J.R. Demarest, and T.E. Machen. 1987. Na-H and Cl-HCO_3 exchange in rabbit oxyntic cells using fluorescence microscopy. Am. J. Physiol. 253:C30-C36

24.   Reuss, L., and J.S. Stoddard. 1987. Role of H^+ and HCO_3^- in salt transport in gallbladder epithelium. Annu. Rev. Physiol. 49:35-49

25.   Roos, A, und W. Boron. 1981. Intracellular pH. Physiol. Rev. 61:296-434

26. Seidler, U., Beinborn, M. and K.-Fr.Sewing. 1989. Inhibition of acid formation in rabbit parietal cells by prostaglandins is mediated by the PGE_2 receptor. Gastroenterology 96:314-320

27. Seidler, U., and W. Silen. 1989. Control of steady-state intracellular pH in rabbit parietal, chief and surface cells in the presence of HCO_3^-: Role of Cl^-/HCO_3^- exchange and a Cl^--independent mechanism. Gastroenterology 96 (abstract)

28. Seidler, U. K. Carter, and W. Silen. 1989. Effect of CO_2 on pH_i rabbit parietal, chief and surface cells. Am J. Physiol 256:G466-G475

29. Seidler, U., und W. Silen. 1989. Evidence for Na^+-HCO_3^- cotransport during pH-recovery from acidification in isolated frog oxyntopeptic cells. Gastroenterology 96 (abstract)

30. Seidler, U., S. Roithmeier, V. Schusdziarra, M. Classen, and W. Silen. Influence of the acid secretory state on Cl^-/base, Na^+/H^+ exchange and intracellular pH_i in isolated rabbit parietal cells. (submitted)

31. Starlinger, M.J. A.M. Paradiso, and T.E. Machen. Steady-state regulation of intracellular pH in isolated rabbit gastric glands. Gastroenterology 92:957-965, 1987

32. Tanaka, A., K.J. Carter, H.-H. Lee, and W. Silen. Influence of Cl^- on pH_i in oxyntopeptic cells of in vitro frog gastric mucosa. Am. J. Physiol. in press

33. Wall, S.M., J.A. Kraut, und S. Muallem. 1989. Modulation of Na^+/H^+ exchange activity by intracellular Na^+, H^+, and Li^+ in IMCD cells. Am. J. Physiol. 255:F331-F339

34. Wenzl, E., T.E. Machen. 1989. Intracellular pH dependence of buffer capacity and anion exchange in the parietal cell. Am. J. Physiol. 257:G741-G747

INTRACELLULAR pH IN ACID-EXPOSED GASTRIC MUCOSA

E. Kivilaakso, T. Kiviluoto, H. Mustonen and H. Paimela

II Department of Surgery,
Helsinki University Central Hospital, Finland

ABSTRACT

Regulation and maintenance of intracellular pH in acid-exposed gastric mucosa was investigated in isolated Necturus antral mucosa using microelectrode technique. Acidification of the luminal perfusate from pH 7 to pH 3 had no influence on intracellular pH, but exposure to luminal pH 2 (10 mM HCl) provoked a rapid initial acidifiction of pH_i, which was followed by a steady state pH_i recording. This suggests that compensatory pH_i regulatory mechanisms were activated and that they were efficient enough to maintain a stable pH_i despite continuous acid exposure. The first-line of defence against luminal acid seems to be a HCO_3^--dependent, partially SITS-sensitive extracellular mechanism, serosal HCO_3^- being transported to the epithelial surface, where it forms an "alkaline" buffer layer to prevent or impede the entry of luminal H^+ inside the surface cells. When this mechanism fails or is eliminated e.g. by removal of serosal HCO_3^-, a second-line Na^+-dependent, amiloride-sensitive mechanism, presumably Na^+/H^+ antiport, is activated and becomes the critical regulator of pH_i. Ulcerogenic barrier breaking agents, such as taurocholate, acetylsalicylic acid or ethanol, promote intracellular acidification in acid-exposed mucosa by enhancing the conductance of the apical cell membrane of surface cells to H^+ (and other ions). On the other hand, pretreatment with exogenous surface active phospholipid protects the mucosa against luminal acid and acidified barrier breaking agents, presumably by decreasing the conductance of the apical cell membrane of surface cells to H^+ (and other ions).

INTRODUCTION

The gastric mucosa is continuously exposed to strong luminal acid, which implies efficient regulatory and protective mechanisms in surface epithelial cells to maintain intracellular pH within physiologic ranges. This paper reviews some of these homeostatic mechanisms and describes how some ulcerogenic and protective agents modulate the response of intracellular pH to luminal acid.

MATERIALS AND METHODS

Necturus (*Necturus maculosus*) antral mucosa was stripped of its seromuscular coat and mounted mucosal side up in a perfusion chamber. Both sides of the mucosa were perfused individually with Ringer's solutions, having serosal side buffered to 7.3 with HCO_3^-/CO_2 or $HEPES/0_2$. Mucosal side was always gassed as was the serosal side. Intracellular pH in surface epithelial cells was measured with two single or one double-barrelled liquid sensor pH- and conventional PD-microelectrodes [1]. Intraepithelial resistances were measured by passing current pulses across the mucosa and using the amiloride exposure technique [2].

RESULTS AND DISCUSSION

EFFECT OF LUMINAL ACID

In the absence of luminal acid, intracellular pH in surface epithelial cells was 7.22 $\pm$ 0.02 (n = 27). Acidification of the mucosal perfusate from pH 7.0 to pH 3.0 had no influence on pH_i (pH_i from 7.24 $\pm$ 0.04 to 7.21 $\pm$ 0.04, n = 8), but luminal pH 2 (10 mM HCl) provoked a rapid intracellular acidification of 0.2 - 0.3 pH-units. This was usually followed by a partial recovery, whereafter a steady state pH_i at a somewhat lower level than the baseline was obtained (pH_i 6.93 $\pm$ 0.07, n = 8). After removal of luminal acid, pH_i returned to the baseline level within 2-4 min [1].

MAINTENANCE OF pH_i DURING ACID EXPOSURE

The initial reversal and partial recovery of pH_i with subsequent steady state pH_i suggests that some kind of compensatory pH_i regulatory mechanism(s) is/are activated in the mucosa following exposure to luminal acid, and that these mechanisms are efficient enough to maintain a steady state pH_i despite continuous exposure to acid. In the following experiments [3] this model, with pH_i regulators activated and (sub)maximally strained by luminal acid, was used in order to elucidate the nature of these compensatory pH_i regulatory mechanisms. The working hypothesis was that blocking of the function of the critical pH_i regulator(s) would manifest as further intracellular acidification.

In all vertebrate cells so far studied the main regulator of intracellular pH (against intracellular acidosis) seems to be Na^+/H^+ exchanger, which extrudes protons from the cell by the force of the inward-directed electrochemical gradient of Na^+. However, obstructing the function of this exchanger by removal of Na^+ from the perfusates had no influence on pH_i (pH_i from 6.97 $\pm$ 0.07 to 6.96 $\pm$ 0.07 in 15 min, n = 7). Similarly, addition of a specific inhibitor of this exchanger, amiloride (1 mM), to the serosal perfusate had no influence on pH_i (pH_i from 6.84 $\pm$ 0.17 to 6.81 $\pm$ 0.17 in 15 min, n = 4). These findings suggest that the Na^+/H^+ exchanger is not the critical pH_i regulator that maintains steady state pH_i during acid exposure in the present model. In contrast, when HCO_3^-/CO_2 was removed from the serosal perfusate a rapid and profound intracellular acidification occurred (pH_i from 7.02 $\pm$ 0.03 to 6.45 $\pm$ 0.15 in 15 min, n = 10; Figure 1a). Similarly, when HCO_3^- transport across the basolateral cell membrane was blocked by adding SITS (0.5 mM) to the serosal perfusate, a similar but somewhat weaker acidification of cell interior occurred (pH_i from 6.97 $\pm$ 0.06 to 6.58 $\pm$ 0.26 in 15 min, n = 6).

The outcome was different when the two ions were removed successively, HCO_3^- first and Na^+ thereafter. In these experiments a slightly weaker luminal acid, pH 2.7, had to be used in order to get a stable pH_i in the absence of serosal HCO_3^-/CO_2. Figure 1b shows that removal of serosal HCO_3^-/CO_2 in this situation induced an initial acidification of pH_i, which was, however, rapidly reversed and partially recovered, whereafter a stable pH_i was obtained. This suggests that, again, a compensatory but now HCO_3^--independent pH_i regulatory mechanism was activated. Yet, when also Na^+ was removed from the serosal perfusate, a progressive acidification of pH_i occurred, pH_i decreasing from 7.00 $\pm$ 0.07 to 6.48 $\pm$ 0.10 in 15 min (n = 6, Figure 1b). An essentially similar result was obtained when an inhibitor of Na^+/H^+ exchanger, amiloride (1 mM), was added to the serosal perfusate (pH_i from 6.85 $\pm$ 0.06 to 6.32 $\pm$ 0.10 in 15 min, n = 5). Our interpretation of these findings is that there are two separate mechanisms contributing to the maintenance of physiologic pH_i in acid exposed gastric mucosa, a first-line HCO_3^--dependent, partially SITS-sensitive mechanism and a second-line, Na^+-dependent and amiloride-sensitive mechanism.

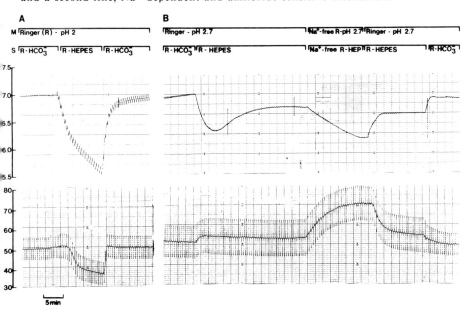

FIGURE 1 Effect of HCO_3^-/CO_2 and Na^+ removal on intracellular pH (pH_i) in isolated Necturus antral mucosa exposed to luminal acid. M, mucosal perfusate; S, serosal perfusate. The mucosal perfusate was always gassed as was the serosal perfusate.
A. The mucosa was continuously exposed to luminal pH2. Removal of serosal HCO_3^-/CO_2 (R-HEPES) provoked a profound but reversible acidification of pH_i.
B. The mucosa was continuously exposed to luminal pH 2.7. Removal of, first, HCO_3^-/CO_2 from the serosal perfusate provoked an initial acidification of pH_i followed by steady state pH_i recording at somewhat lower level than the baseline. Subsequent removal of also Na^+ from the serosal perfusate (Na^+-free R-HEPES) provoked a progressive but still reversible acidification of pH_i.

Gastric mucosa is known to actively secrete (or transport) HCO_3^- and it is assumed that the secreted HCO_3^- forms together with the surface mucus gel a protective "alkaline" buffer layer against luminal acid at the epithelial surface [4]. In order to explore whether serosal HCO_3^- contributes to the maintenance of intracellular pH_i in acid-exposed mucosa by the same mechanism, intracellular pH and extracellular epithelial surface pH were measured simultaneously using two double-barrelled pH-PD microelectrodes. It turned out that in mucosae exposed to luminal pH 2.5, a distinct pH-gradient existed between the luminal bulk solution (pH 2.5) and the epithelial surface (pH_s 5.8 ± 0.1, n = 5) (Figure 2). However, when HCO_3^- /CO_2 was removed from the serosal perfusate, this pH-gradient dissipated, pH_s decreasing <3 (where the measurements become inaccurate), and this was followed by acidification of intracellular pH (Figure 2). This finding suggests that serosal HCO_3^- does, at least in part, contribute to the maintenance of intracellular pH in acid-exposed mucosa extracellularly by forming an "alkaline" buffer layer at the epithelial surface, which prevents or impedes the access of luminal H^+ inside the surface epithelial cells. To what extent serosal HCO_3^- contributes to the maintenance of pH_i also intracellularly, e.g. by enhancing the cytosolic buffer capacity of the cell, cannot be deduced on the basis of the present data.

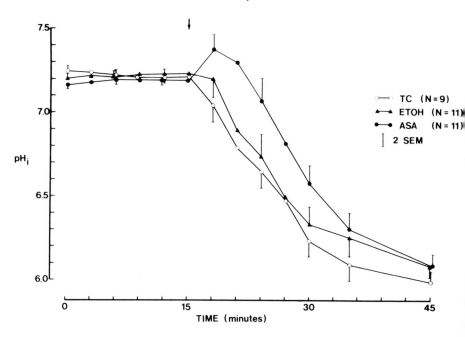

FIGURE 2.   Effect of barrier breaking agents on intracellular pH in acid-exposed gastric mucosa. The mucosa was first exposed to weak luminal acid (pH3), which alone has no effect on pH_i. Addition of one of the three barrier breaking agents studied (10mM taurocholate, 20% ethanol and 10mM acetylsalicylic acid) to the luminal perfusate provoked a profound acidification of pH_i.

Simultaneous measurement of intracellular pH and [Na$^+$] indicates that the intracellular acidification following exposure to luminal acid is associated with a rapid transient increase in intracellular Na$^+$ and in the absence of serosal Na$^+$ no reversal of the initial intracellular acidification occurs but pH$_i$ rapidly falls below 6 after acid exposure (unpublished data). These findings suggest that the initial reversal and partial recovery of pH$_i$ in acid-exposed surface cells is accomplished by the proton extruding action of Na$^+$/H$^+$ exchanger. However, it seems that the initial intracellular acidification also activates the epithelial HCO$_3^-$ transport mechanism (luminal acid is known to be a potent stimulator of epithelial HCO$_3^-$ transport, [4]), and that this mechanism is efficient enough to prevent the access of luminal H$^+$ inside the surface cell, since when the steady state pH$_i$ was attained, blocking of the proton extruding action of the Na$^+$/H$^+$ exchanger had no more influence on pH$_i$.

EFFECT OF BARRIER BREAKING AGENTS

Barrier breaking agents are ulcerogenic compounds, which by disrupting the "gastric mucosal barrier" are assumed to facilitate the entry of luminal acid inside the mucosa and thereby to provoke mucosal damage. However, the exact mechanism of their action at the cellular level still remains largely obscure. The following experiments [2] were undertaken to explore how these agents possibly affect intracellular pH and intraepithelial resistances in acid-exposed gastric mucosa. It turned out that in mucosae exposed to relatively weak luminal acid (pH3), which alone has no effect on intracellular pH, addition of one of the three barrier breaking agents studied, 10 mM taurocholate, 20% (v/v) ethanol or 10 mM acetylsalicylic acid (ASA), provoked a rapid and profound intracellular acidification in surface epithelial cells (Figure 3). Yet, the behaviour of pH$_i$ was different in each instance and characteristic to the agent used: taurocholate induced an immediate acidification of pH$_i$, ethanol acidified pH$_i$ after a delay of 4-6 min, while in ASA treated tissue a paradoxical intracellular alkalinization preceded acidification of pH$_i$. Measurement of intraepithelial resistances suggests that the main target in the damaging and acidifying action of all three agents is the apical cell membrane of surface cells, since reduction of the ratio of apical and basolateral cell membrane resistances always preceded intracellular acidification. Yet, the effects on intraepithelial resistances were, again, different in each instance and characteristic to the agent used: taurocholate primarily decreased cellular (in particular apical cell membrane) resistance and had no primary influence on paracellular resistance, ethanol mainly decreased paracellular resistance but also decreased cellular resistance, while ASA primarily increased cellular (in particular apical cell membrane) resistance, which was followed by a decrease in both cellular and paracellular resistances. These findings strongly suggest that at least one mechanism by which the ulcerogenic barrier breaking agents provoke mucosal damage is to increase the conductance of the apical cell membrane of surface epithelial cells to H$^+$ (and other ions) with resultant excessive accummulation of luminal H$^+$ inside the cell during acid exposure.

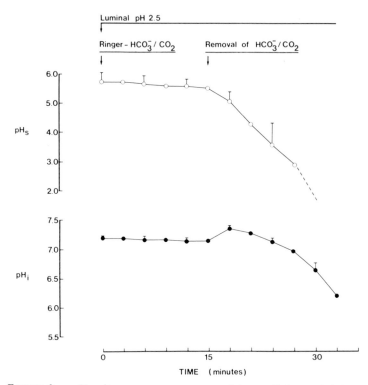

FIGURE 3.   *Simultaneous measurement of intracellular pH (pH_i) and extracellular, epithelial surface pH (pH_s) in acid-exposed gastric mucosa. The mucosa was continuously exposed to luminal pH 2.5. In the presence of serosal HCO_3^-, a distinct pH gradient existed between the luminal bulk solution (pH 2.5) and the epithelial surface (pH_s 5.8). Removal of HCO_3^-/CO_2 from the serosal perfusate dissipated this gradient, and this was followed by acidification of intracellular pH.*

EFFECT OF SURFACE ACTIVE PHOSPHOLIPID

The gastric mucosa has a hydrophobic lining, which is assumed to have a protective function against luminal acid as well as intrinsic and extrinsic ulcerogenic agents [5]. It is also assumed that the hydrophobicity of the mucosal lining is attributable to a surfactant-like phospholipid monolayer adsorbed to the gastric mucosal surface and that the hydrophobic lining might, in fact, functionally correspond to the "gastric mucosal barrier", which prevents "back diffusion" of luminal acid inside the mucosal tissue [6]. Indirect evidence to support the view that this lining might, indeed, have a protective function is provided by the findings that exogenously administered surface active phospholipids do protect the gastric mucosa against damage induced by strong acid [7], or acidified barrier breaking agents [8,9] and that the loss of excessive gastric sensitivity to luminal acid coincides with the appearance of a hydrophobic lining in the stomach of a developing rat [10]. The following experiments [11] were undertaken to investigate how exogenous surface active phospholipid possibly modulates the response of intracellular pH to exposure to luminal acid and barrier breaking agents.

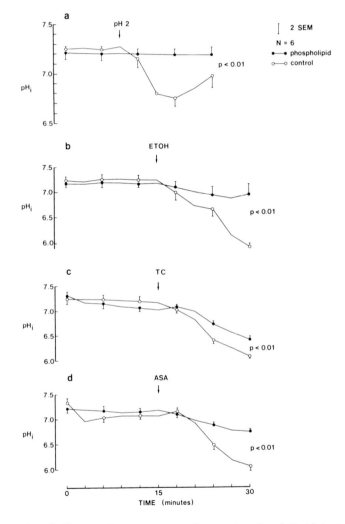

FIGURE 4. Influence of exogenous surface active phospholipid in intracellular pH in isolated gastric mucosa exposed to luminal acid and barrier breaking agents. Pretreatment with pulmonary surfactant-like phospholipid mixture completely abolished the intracellular acidification normally provoked by exposure to luminal acid (pH2) and significantly protected against the intracellular acidosis provoked by the acidified barrier breaking agents.

A 20 min pretreatment of the mucosa with pulmonary surfactant-like phospholipid mixture [7] completely abolished the acidotic response of intracellular pH normally seen in surface cells during exposure to luminal acid (pH2)(Figure 4a). Likewise, phospholipid pretreatment completely abolished the acidotic response of intracellular pH elicited by acidified ethanol (20% v/v, pH 2.5), and significantly alleviated the responses elicited by acidified taurocholate (10 mM, pH 2.5) and ASA (10 mM, pH 2.0)(Figure 4b,c,d,). The findings that phospholipid pretreatment completely abolishes the acidifying influence of luminal H^+ alone or that of acidified ethanol, and that it also abolishes the increase in the ratio of apical and basolateral cell membrane resistances normally seen in acid-exposed mucosa [3,11], suggest that exogenous phospholipid (almost?) completely prevents the entry of H^+ inside the cell. On the other hand, the finding that it opposes only partially (but significantly) the acidotic effects of acidified taurocholate and ASA, suggests that exogenous phospholipid may allow a relatively free entry of the lipid-soluble barrier breaking agents inside the cell, since, being weak acids, taurocholate and ASA can act as protonophores carrying H^+ inside the cell in their protonated form (a property that ethanol, being a neutral molecule, does not possess). Further support to the view that exogenous phospholipid protects the surface epithelial cells mainly by decreasing the conductance of apical cell membrane to H^+ (and other ions) is provided by the finding that phospholipid pretreatment markedly enhances cellular, especially apical cell membrane resistance (by +108%), but has no effect on paracellular resistance.

REFERENCES

1. Kivilaakso E, Kiviluoto T. Intracellular pH in isolated Necturus antral mucosa in simulated ulcerogenic conditions. Gastroenterology 1988; 95: 1198-1205.

2. Kiviluoto T, Mustonen H, Kivilaakso E. Effect of barrier-breaking agents on intracelular pH and epithelial membrane resistances: Studies in isolated Necturus antral mucosa exposed to luminal acid. Gastroenterology 1989; 96: 1410-1418.

3. Kiviluoto T, Paimela H, Mustonen H, Kivilaakso E. Intracellular pH in isolated Necturus antral mucosa exposed to luminal acid. Gastroenterology 1990; 98: 901-908.

4. Flemstrom G. Gastric and duodenal mucosal bicarbonate secretion. In: Johnson KR, ed. Physiology of the gastrointestinal tract. 2nd ed. New York: Raven, 1987; 1011-1029.

5. Hills BA, Butler BD, Lichtenberger LM. Gastric mucosal barrier: hydrophobic lining to the lumen of the stomach. Am J Physiol 1983; 244(5): G561-568.

6. Davenport HW. Gastric mucosal injury by fatty and acetylsalicylic acids. Gastroenterology. 1964; 46: 245-253.

7.   Lichtenberger LM, Graziani LA, Dial EJ, Butler BD, Hills BA. Role
     of surface-active phospholipids in gastric cytoprotection. Science
     1983; 219: 1327-1329.

8.   Swarm RA, Ashley SW, Soybel DI, Ordway FS, Cheung LY.
     Protective effect of exogenous phospholipid on aspirin-induced
     gastric mucosal injury. Am J Surg 1987; 153: 48-53.

9.   Szelenyi I, Engler H. Cytoprotective role of gastric surfactant in the
     ethanol-produced gastric mucosal injury of the rat. Pharmacology
     1986; 33: 199-205.

10. Dial EJ, Lichtenberger LM. Surface hydrophobicity of the gastric
     mucosa in the developing rat. Effects of corticosteroids, thyroxine,
     and prostaglandin E2. Gastroenterology 1988; 94: 57-61.

11. Kiviluoto T, Paimela H, Mustonen H, Kivilaakso E. Exogenous
     surface active phospholipid protects Necturus gastric mucosa against
     luminal acid and barrier breaking agents. Gastroenterology (in
     press).

INTRACELLULAR pH REGULATION IN THE DUODENAL MUCOSA

M. Starlinger, M. Weinlich, R. Kinne

Chirurgische Universitatsklinik Tubingen and Max-Planck-Institut fur Systemphysiologie, Dortmund, FRG

ABSTRACT

Similar to the situation in the stomach, the duodenum is periodically exposed to a high transmural proton gradient. In contrast to the stomach the duodenum secretes large amounts of bicarbonate, that buffer most of the acid intraluminally. However this buffering process creates a high luminal pCO_2. This CO_2 may rapidly diffuse into the duodenal mucosa and be converted to carbonic acid inside the cell. Two basic mechanisms have been described in intestinal epithelial cells to participate in intracellular pH regulation; 1) the Na/H exchanger (acid extruder) and 2), the Cl/HCO_3 exchanger (acid loader). Work on isolated duodenal cells could not identify the polarized nature of pH regulating mechanisms. We have thought to circumvent these potential deficiences by using confocal laserscan fluoroscopy and *in vitro* intracellular labelling of intact sheets of rat duodenal mucosa with pH sensitive fluorescent dyes. However, the utilisation of this new technology creates new technical problems, which so far we have been unable to solve. Preliminary data from isolated duodenal cells have verified the existance of a Na/H exchanger in the cell membrane. In intact epithelial layers the pH regulation after NH_4Cl pulses was slowed down, probably due to barrier functions.

INTRODUCTION

Regulation of intracellular pH is a necessary function of all living cells. Cells usually have a large inside negative membrane potential and passive distribution of H-ions across the cell membrane, which according to electrochemical equilibrium, would create an acid intracellular pH incompatible with normal metabolic functions [1]. Epithelial cells of the gastrointestinal tract are exposed to transepithelial gradients of H-ions and CO_2, a freely diffusible volatile form of acid. This is particularly true of cells in the gastric and duodenal epithelium. In the duodenum luminal pH periodically drops below pH 3 as HCl is emptied from the stomach. Most of this acid is neutralized in the lumen by HCO_3 derived from biliary, pancreatic and duodenal epithelial secretions [2]. This neutralization process creates large amounts of CO_2 and partial pressures of up to 500 mmHg have been described postprandially [3]. This CO_2 may diffuse into the cells and combine with water to create carbonic acid. The reaction is catalysed by carbonic anhydrase, an enzyme that is known to be abundantly present in the gastroduodenal mucosa [4]. The expected lumen to cytosol gradient of pCO_2 in the proximal duodenum is considerably greater than that resulting from bathing cells in 5% CO_2 gassed solutions (pCO_2 = 33 mmHg). Upon institution of this relatively small CO_2 gradient, a transient acidification has been observed in gastric mucosal cells [5] and IEC-6 cells, an intestinal cell line [6]. Apart from the obvious necessity for duodenal epithelial cells to possess efficient acid extruding mechanisms, these cells are also exposed to osmotic gradients after a meal [7] and they secrete HCO_3. Transport processes, that mediate acid extrusion are known to be also involved in volume regulation and electrolyte secretion [8,9]. Two distinct electroneutral ion exchangers have been described in a variety of enterocytes and are supposed to participate in intracellular pH regulation, namely the Na/H and Cl/HCO_3 exchanger. Recently a third mechanism, $Na-HCO_3$ cotransport, has been described in isolated IEC-6 cells, a cultured intestinal cell line [6]. This cotransporter functions to alkalinize the cells and if positioned on the basolateral membrane may contribute to alkaline secretion by facilitating HCO_3 entry into the cell. A basolaterally located Na/H exchanger recently described to be present in rat duodenal bruch border membrane vesicles [10]. Such a model has been evoked to explain changes in intracellular pH in response to extracellular ion substitution and specific inhibitors of the ion exchangers in IEC-6 cells. This scheme is very similar to that drawn to explain HCO_3 secretion by ileal crypt cells [11]. Whether these regulatory mechanisms contribute to the regulation of intracellular pH, volume and transepithelial HCO_3 secretion in the duodenal mucosa is unknown.

One reason for this is methodological problems. Studies on isolated membrane vesicles such as mentioned above, can identify and locate ion transport mechanisms on the basolateral membrane, but they are unable to evaluate their relative contribution to intracellular pH regulation in the intact cell or the transepithelial ion transport in the intact epithelium. Moreover ion transport mechanisms may be differentially expressed in various types of enterocytes. Crypt cells have a distribution of ion exchangers that is likely to be different from that of villus cells, according to their different properties of secretion and absorption [11]. Thus specific isolation of villus and crypt cell membranes may be necessary.

Work with isolated intestinal cell is hampered by difficulties to isolate them in a viable form and these preparations lack cellular polarity, that is normally present in the intact epithelium. Furthermore, the above mentioned argument regarding differences between the various cell types of the intestinal mucosa (crypt versus villus cells) also applies to isolated cells. Methods applicable to the intact epithelium are either technically difficult, especially in the small mammalian enterocytes (pH sensitive microelectrodes) or cannot differentiate between different cell types (nuclear magnetic resonance).

We have therefore set out to develop a model that would enable us to study intracellular pH regulation in single cells in an intact sheet of duodenal mucosa. The combination of the recently developed confocal laser scan microscopy [12] with the application of a fluorescent pH sensitive dye seemed to fulfill the necessary prerequisites. 1) Confocal laser scan microscopy can collect images from single cells irrespective of the surrounding signals; 2) intracellular fluorescent dyes have repeatedly been shown to reliably record intracellular pH [13].

METHODS

Isolated Rat Duodenal Enterocytes

Duodenal enterocytes were isolated from a 5 cm segment of proximal duodenum from male Wistar rats anaesthetized with pentobarbital. The segment was rinsed with NaCl-Ringers buffered to pH 7,40 with 20 mM HEPES at $37^{o}C$. The segment was then filled with 27 mM citrate solution pregassed with 100% 0_2, clamped at both ends and incubated in citrate (100% 0_2) for 15 min [14]. Luminal solution, containing isolated cells was collected and centrifuged twice at 20g. Cells from 100 ul samples were then centrifuged on glass cover slips and placed in a micro perfusion chamber. Loading of cells on cover slips was performed by incubation with 4 uM BCECF-AM, the fluorescent pH-sensitive dye, in HEPES-Ringer.

Intact Stripped Duodenal Mucosa

Duodenal segments, as described above, were mounted on icecold glass rods. With fine forceps the serosa and muscle layer was stripped from the underlying mucosa, which was then mounted horizontally in a microchamber with a hydrostatic perfusion system (bicarbonate Ringers gassed with 95% 0_2/5% CO_2). Intact duodenal mucosa was loaded with BCECF-AM in two ways:

1. An *in vivo* duodenal segment was filled luminally with 40 uM BCECF containing Ringers and closed at both ends. After 20 minutes the segment was excised, rinsed with Ringers and prepared for mounting as described above.

2. BCECF-AM at a concentration of 40 uM in Ringers was micro-injected in the submucosa of a villus in already prepared and mounted duodenal mucosa using glass micropipettes (tip diameter 8 um) and a micromanipulator under microscopic control [15].

Confocal Laser Scan Microscopy

An MRC-500 Confocal Laserscan Imaging System [16] (Bio-Rad, Boston, Mass.) and a Nikon Labophot epifluorescent microscope was used (Figure 1). The excitation light at 488 nm (pH-dependent fluorescence) was provided by an argon ion laser (Ion Laser Technology, Utah). For double excitation experiments a second 442 nm (pH independent fluorescence) He-Cd ion laser (Liconix) was adapted to the system [17,17]. The laser beam was scanned by two galvanometer mirrors in a raster pattern across the surface of the tissue. The fluorescent signal emitted by the excited dye was collected by the objective and descanned by the same galvanometric mirrors. Passing an emission filter (OG 515 LP) and the variable confocal pinhole, the fluorescent signal was measured by a photomultiplier. Confocal laserscan microscopy allowed the measurement of fluorescent signals in a defined horizontal plane of focus. Signals above or below this plane were not detected by the photomultiplier due to the effect of the confocal pinhole. The digitalized photomultiplier output was collected on a Nimbus AX personal computer. A special program was designed to collect fluorescence data in set time intervals and store picture frames on hard disc. Further data processing was performed using the Bio-Rad software. Arbitrary fluorescent units were calculated as the mean pixel intensity in a rectangular area in one image.

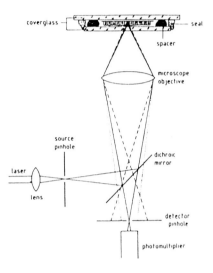

<u>FIGURE 1</u>:   *The technique of confocal laserscan microscopy allows to collect fluorescence signals from a defined horizontal plane of focus. This is done with a laser beam and a pinhole in front of the photomultiplier. Fluorescence signals above or below the focal plane cannot pass the pinhole.*

RATIOMETRIC MEASUREMENTS

The dual wavelength excitation of BCECF allowed ratiometric calculations. Separate fluorescence images, exposing the loaded cells to each laser light (442 and 488 nm) were collected. Dividing the mean pixel intensity at 488 nm (pH-dependent) by the intensity at 442 nm (pH-independent) gives a new pH-dependent image, the so-called ratio image. The relationship between the ratio image and intracellular pH is linear over a range of at least pH 6.5 to 7.5 [17,18].

RESULTS

ISOLATED RAT DUODENAL CELLS (SINGLE EXCITATION AT 488 NM)

In single duodenal cells an uneven BCECF fluorescence signal distribution was visible within the cells. The brightest signals were seen in the nucleus. In the cytoplasm a slight compartmentalisation could be noticed. Experiments on kidney and colon cells revealed that this uneven distribution of the dye is due to different dye concentrations that appeared to be actively accumulated in these compartments (i.e. nucleus), rather than differs pH in these compartments. In kidney cells (TALH) accumulation of dye in the endoplasmatic reticulum surrounding the nucleus, was observed (unpublished observation). Dead cells (trypan blue positive) were indicated by a complete lack of nuclear dye accumulation.

BCECF loaded duodenal cells showed almost no change in fluorescence signal over a 15 min time period in oxygenated HEPES Ringers at 37°C. Therefore the assumption was made that in the resting state intracellular pH is constant and dye leakage minimal. To preliminary test the feasibility of using BCECF and confocal laser scan microscopy, the following experiment was made. Resting duodenal cells were exposed to 25 mM HC4Cl buffer, which caused a 20% increase in fluorescence signal. A slow decline of the signal was then discernible in NH4Cl medium, but did not reach baseline. Changing NH4Cl buffer to Na-free Ringers caused an abrupt 50% decrease in fluorescence signal. Over a period of 2 minutes in Na-free Ringers no increase of the signal was noticed. Changing back to the original Na containing buffer caused an immediate increase of the fluorescence signal almost back to baseline values, indicating an Na-dependent pH recovery (Figure 2). Volume changes of the cells were not visible during the experiments.

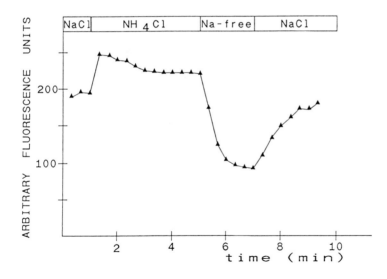

FIGURE 2: *Evidence of a Na-dependent pH regulatory mechanism in isolated rat duodenal cells. Cells were exposed to 25 mM NH_4Cl Ringers buffer, causing an increase in intracellular pH. Changing to Na-free Ringers buffer (Na replaced by N-methyl-glutamine) led to a srong acidification of the cells. In Na-containing Ringers buffer a back-regulation of intracellular pH was evident.*

The following conclusions were made: 1) Confocal laser scan microscopy in combination with BCECF is a potent tool to measure intracellular pH changes.   This method is comparable to microspectrofluorimetry;   2) for absolute pH measurements a second excitation at the isosbestic wavelength (440 nm) is necessary; 3) the above experiments indicated the presence of an Na-dependent pH regulatory mechanism in duodenal enterocytes; and 4) in isolated cell experiments the location of the exchanger for pH regulation (apical or basolateral membrane) cannot be identified.

<u>INTACT DUODENAL RAT MUCOSA (DOUBLE EXCITATION)</u>

In vivo loading with luminal BCECF application showed almost equal distribution of the dye in the mucosal layer. However the dye concentration was very low and not sufficient for pH measurements in individual cells.

The method using micropipette injection into the subepithelial layer and therefore loading the cells via the basolateral membrane gave a much brighter signal in a set of 10 to 20 cells around the injection site.   The fluorescence signal was much stronger than autofluorescence, which was automatically substracted.   This method was then used for further experiments using ratio imaging.

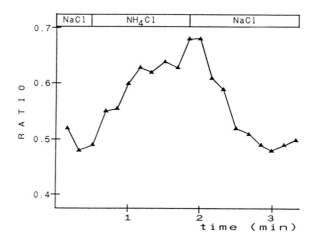

FIGURE 3: *Effect of NH_4Cl pulse on intracellular pH in intact duodenal epithelium with removed mucus layer. Luminal NH_4Cl exposure caused a slow increase in intracellular pH.   The expected acidification after NH_4Cl removal did not occur, as seen in isolated cell experiments.*

Every 10 seconds a couplet of confocal images - excited at 488nm and 442 nm - was collected. To induce pH changes within the cells, the mucosa was luminally exposed to 25 mM NH_4Cl Ringers. In contrast to experiments on isolated duodenal enterocytes, pH did not change immediately after the perfusion change. A slow increase of pH could be seen starting after 1 minute. After removal of NH_4Cl intracellular pH did not acidify immediately, but a slow decrease over several minutes to baseline was observed. An immediate increase in intracellular pH was seen after NH_4Cl exposure, when the mucus layer was removed at the beginning of the experiment (Figure 3).

Even though these observations could be explained by the diffusion barrier of the mucus overlying the epithelial cells or an apical membrane relatively impermeable to NH_4/NH_3, several methodological problems may also play a role. The major problem in using confocal laser scan microscopy and intact intestinal mucosa is motion. Even with fixation of the epithelium on a nylon mesh by hydrostatic pressure, peristaltic movements of villi could be observed which were in the range of up to 30 um. Fluorescent cells escaped the confocal plane and the fluorescent signal decreased strongly. This shift led to changes in the ratio (R-I_{488}/I_{442}) which were not due to changes in intracellular pH. In NH_4Cl experiments the ratio changes due to pH changes were more intense than the ratio changes due to motion. Another uncertainty of this new method is the loading procedure. The only method giving useful dye concentrations within the cells was microinjection of the dye directly into the subepithelial layer of the villus. This manouvre led to destruction of parts of the villus and the mucus layer at least temporarily. Even though the trauma was distant to the measured cells, its influence on the barrier properties of the epithelial layer is yet unknown.

CONCLUSIONS

Confocal laser scan microscopy is a promising new method to evaluate intracellular pH regulation in intact epithelia. In isolated cells, the main advantage over microspectrofluorimetry lies in better anatomical resolution, allowing evaluation of different cell compartments. In intact epithelium, confocal laserscan microscopy so far seems to be the only method to study intracellular pH in single duodenal cells. Experiments indicated that fast intracellular pH response to NH_4Cl in isolated cells were slowed down in intact tissue, probably due to barrier functions, which need to be elucidated. However major methodological problems still need to be solved before application of this method to the study of barrier function of duodenal epithelium to H-ions.

REFERENCES

1. Boron WF. Intracellular pH regulation in epithelial cells. Ann Rev Physiol 1986; 48: 377-388.

2. Flemstrom G. Gastric and duodenal mucosal bicarbonate secretion. In: Johnson LR, ed. Physiology of the Gastrointestinal Tract. Volume 2. 2nd edition. New York: Raven Press. 1987; 1011-1029.

3.   Lonnerholm G, Knutson L, Wistrand PJ, Flemstrom G.   Carbonic anhydrase in the normal rat stomach and duodenum and after treatment with omeprazole and ranitidine.   Acta Physiol Scand 1989; 136: 253-262.

4.   Rune SJ, Henriksen FW.   Carbon dioxide tensions in the proximal part of the canine gastrointestinal tract.   Gastroenterology 1969; 56: 758-762.

5.   Seidler U, Carter K, Ito S, Silen W.   Effect of CO_2 on pH_i in rabbit parietal, chief, and surface cells.   Am J Physiol 1989; 256: G466-G475.

6.   Wenzl E, Sjaastad MD, Weintraub WH, Machen TE.   Intracellular pH regulation in IEC-6 cells, a cryptlike intestinal cell line.   Am J Physiol 1989; 257: G732-740.

7.   Miller L, Malagelada J, Go V.   Postprandial duodenal function in man.   Gut 1978; 19: 699-706.

8.   Hoffmann EK, Simonsen LO.   Membrane mechanisms in volume and pH regulation in vertebrate cells.   Physiol Rev. 1989; 69: 315-382.

9.   Seifter JL, Aronson PS.   Properties and physiologic roles of the plasma membrane sodium-hydrogen exchanger.   J Clin Invest 1986; 78: 859-864.

10.   Brown CDS, Dunk CR, Turnberg LA.   Cl-HCO3 exchange and anion conductance in rat duodenal apical membrane vesicles.   Am J Physiol 1989; 257: G61-G67.

11.   Knickelbein RG, Aronson PS, Dobbins JW.   Membrane distribution of sodium-hydrogen and chloride bicarbonate exchangers in crypt and villus cell membranes from rabbit ileum.   J Clin Invest 1988; 82: 2158-2163.

12.   Shotton D, White N.   Confocal scanning microscopy: three-dimensional biologic imaging.   TIBS 1989; 14: 435-439.

13.   Paradiso AM, Tsien RY, Demarest JR, Machen TE.   Na-H and Cl-HCO_3 exchange in rabbit oxyntic cells using fluorescence microscopy.   Am J Physiol 1987; 253: C30-C36.

14.   Hegazy E, Del Pino VL, Schwenk M.   Isolated intestinal mucosa cells of high viability from guinea pig.   Eur J Cell Biol 1983; 30: 132-136.

15.   Capasso G, Kinne-Saffran E, De Santo NG, Kinne R.   Regulation of volume reabsorption by thyroid hormones in the proximal tubule of rat: Minor role of luminal sodium permeability.   Pfluegers Arch 1985; 403: 97-104.

16.   Shotton DM,   Confocal scanning optical microscopy and its applications for biological specimens.   J Cell Sci 1989; 94: 175-206.

17. Wang X, Kurtz I. Intracellular pH (pHi) regulation in the rabbit cortical collecting duct using inverted confocal fluorescence microscopy. Clin Res 1989; 37(2): 504A.

18. Wang X, Kurtz I. Basolateral membrane H+/base transport in single principal cells (PC) studied with dual excitation confocal fluorescence imaging. Kidney Int 1990; 37 (NI): 548.

MICROVASCULATURE OF THE GASTRIC
AND DUODENAL MUCOSA

Bren Gannon

Department of Anatomy & Histology, Flinders University of South Australia
School of Medicine, Flinders Medical Centre, Bedford Park, South Australia

ABSTRACT

The stratified oesophageal epithelium is underlain by a sparse planar plexus of continuous, non-fenestrated capillaries; the presence of a substantial subepithelial vascular plexus at the lower (as well as the upper) oesophageal sphincter is clearly of significance if this is exposed to gastric reflux.

In the gastric body, arteriolar supply to the fenestrated mucosal capillaries is at the mucosal base; capillaries cross connect, but run principally towards the luminal surface in close proximity to the gastric glands, especially the oxyntic cells. Drainage is to infrequent intramural venules originating subjacent to the gastric lumen. In the antrum, the arterioles penetrate well into the mucosa, giving rise to two capillary plexuses - a tortuous basal plexus of fine capillaries, and a superficial plexus of slightly larger capillaries. There are fewer cross anastomoses in the plexuses of the antrum than in that of the body.

In the duodenum, blood supply to the villi is largely direct, and is not via a local portal system from Brunner's glands, as might be expected by analogy with the lower small intestine.

The explanation of the differing microvascular architectures, and their abrupt transition in the upper GI tract, may lie in the requirements for efficient supply of HCO_3^- to luminal surface enterocytes required to resist the differing luminal acid loads; the differing relative susceptibilities in this region to ischaemia and other insults may also lie in their differing microvascular organizations.

INTRODUCTION

Over the last ten years, the possible importance of the gastric microvasculature in mucosal protection against luminal acid erosion has been frequently suggested. In this time there have been several accounts of the microvascular architecture of gastric mucosa in several species, including humans [1-5]. An account of the duodenal microvascular architecture presents a strikingly different arrangement from that of the gastric corpus, while in two species with a squamous epithelially lined forestomach, there is again a markedly different mucosal microvascular

291

arrangement [3,7].   Given the apparent interspecies differences in eg. gastric corpus mucosal microvascular architecture, [eg. 1 of 4], reported regional differences between corpus and antrum [4], and even disagreement about gastric corpus mucosal microvascular architecture in humans, it appears that any attempt to distil a synthetic understanding from these varying accounts is unlikely to succeed.

This article reviews the microvascular architectures reported for the various regions of the upper GI tract in different species, attempting to focus on the site of the acid load, HCO_3^- secretion, and mucosal ulceration as pointers towards a synthetic view of the differing mucosal microvascular architectures.

MATERIALS AND METHODS

Recent microangioarchitectural studies of the upper GI tract have commonly used scanning electron microscopy of acrylic injection replicas of the mucosal microvascular networks [1-7].   These studies have been supplemented by light microscopy [5], tissue scanning electron microscopy [1], transmission electron microscopy [1] and intravital microscopy [1]. Whole stomachs have usually been prepared in experimental animals; whole or partial samples of human stomachs of cancer and ulcer patients [5] or small gastric body samples from healthy but obese patients undergoing gastric reduction surgery [2] have been utilized.

RESULTS AND DISCUSSION

In the gastric corpus of rat, human and hamster [1,2,3] the microvascular architecture is as illustrated in Figure 1. Short mucosal arterioles, derived from the submucous arterial plexus, penetrate the muscularis mucosa and ramify into capillaries in the lamina propria at the bases of the gastric glands. The capillaries proceed luminally through the mucosa, but have frequent cross-anastomoses to connect with a polygonal array of microvessels surrounding the necks of the gastric glands just subjacent to the gastric luminal epithelium.   This subsurface polygonal capillary network, which contains vessels which could be considered post capillary venules, is drained by infrequent mucosal venules which pass through the mucosa to the submucous venous plexus without receiving any direct capillary tributaries en route. In human corpus, occasional smaller, obliquely oriented mucosal venular tributaries may join the main mucosal venules in the mucosa, but these small mucosal venules themselves only receive capillary tributaries at their most luminal ends - i.e. at the polygonal subsurface plexus.

The frequent cross anastomoses between capillaries of the gastric corpus [1,2] may be important in providing alternative flow pathways to permit the continuation of perfusion of the mucosa subjacent to a surface erosion; without such cross connections, such a surface erosion would inevitably lead to stasis of the basal capillaries also, and presumably to full thickness erosion. The relative lack of such cross anastomoses in the antral mucosa has been suggested as a partial explanation of the relative susceptibility of this mucosa to ulceration [9].

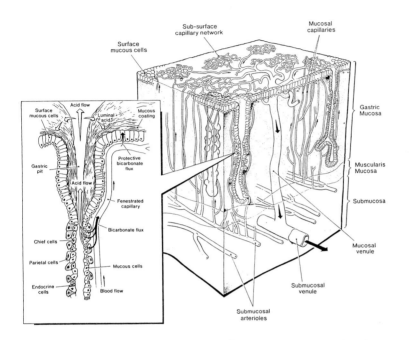

FIGURE 1: *Schematic diagram of the vascular organization in oxyntic mucosa (right) and the proposed mechanism for vascular transport of HCO_3^-, toward the surface mucus cells, from deeper within the mucosa (inset left). Reprinted from [2] by permission of Gastroenterology.*

Rasche et al [5] have, however, reported a dual system of mucosal arterioles in human gastric corpus: short mucosal arterioles with a branching pattern similar to that described above for the basal two-thirds of the mucosa, and long mucosal arterioles which directly supply capillaries of the luminal third of the mucosa. Mucosal drainage is reported similar to that described above, with the capillaries of the basal mucosa draining to the superficial capillaries (Figure 2.)

This study questioned the accuracy of previous reports of human [2] and rat [1] gastric corpus. Prokopiw et al [8] recently reported equivalent mucosal microvascular architecture in dog gastric body to that earlier reported for human [2] and rat [1] gastric corpus (see Figure 1), but reported a dual system of short and long mucosal arterioles in the gastric antrum, similar to that reported by Raschke (Figure 2) for human corpus.

It is tempting to speculate that the differences between the reports for human gastric corpus microvascular architecture between Raschke et al [5] and Gannon et al [2] may lie in the different patient groups sampled; Raschke's patients had carcinoma or ulceration, whereas Gannon's samples came from obese but otherwise gastrically normal patients. Perhaps the presence of substantial gastric pathology sufficient to warrant gastrectomy induces changes in gastric corpus mucosal microvasculature to that of the gastric antrum. Alternatively, the tissue samples available to Raschke may have been predominantly antral mucosa, or perhaps there are two different forms of gastric corpus mucosal microvascular architecture in humans? Prokopiw et al [9] points out that the India ink studies of TsuChiHashi et al [10] in normal human mucosa have shown the same differences between gastric corpus and antral mucosa in humans which they found in dogs and conclude that the microvasculature of human gastric body is as described in Figure 1 [2].

The finding by Piasecki et al [8] that ligation of individual mucosal arterioles en route to the mucosa in guinea-pigs causes full thickness gastric erosion strongly suggests that these are end-arteries supplying the whole mucosal thickness in this species, and probably that there is unlikely to be two levels of arterial supply to the gastric mucosa in this species. Unfortunately, however, Piasecki did not indicate precisely in which region of the stomach the ligations were performed, other than in the anterior gastric wall; it seems unlikely that this was in the gastric corpus, but this cannot be definitely determined from the paper.

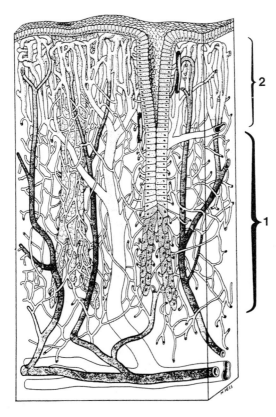

FIGURE 2:

Scheme of the microangioarchitecture of human corpus mucosa (arterioles = dark-coloured; venules = light-coloured). Short arterioles branch into a basal capillary network (1) reaching from the base to the isthmus of the gastric glands. Long arterioles ascend into the mucosa and branch into a layer of wide, apical capillaries (2). Reprinted from [5] by permission of Acta Anatomica.

The mucosal microvascular architecture of rabbit gastric corpus contains both short and long arterioles [4] as reported by Raschke for humans (Figure 2) while in the hamster antral mucosa the apparently single network of microvessels are grouped into tufts, each supplying a mucosal fold. Thus, the microvascular arrangement in the gastric corpus of rabbit and the antral mucosa of the hamster appear to differ significantly from the arrangements predominantly described above, perhaps for reasons of a herbivorous as compared to an omnivorous diet.

In species with a forestomach lined with stratified squamous epithelium (rat-1 and hamster-3) this layer is underlain by a single planar array of continuous, unfenestrated capillaries. This arrangement has been proposed as a model for the subepithelial microvascular plexus of the oesophagus [11].

In the rat duodenum, there are separate arteriolar supplies to the bicarbonate secreting Brunner's glands, to the bases of groups of intestinal glands, and to the apices of each duodenal villus lamina proprial core [6] (see Figure 3).

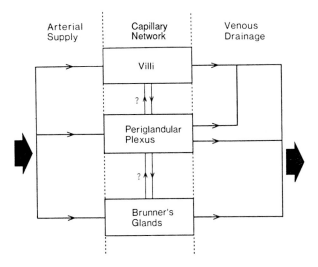

FIGURE 3: *Block diagram of the rat gastro-duodenal junction, illustrating the pattern of intramural blood supply and drainage of intestinal mucosa and Brunner's glands in the proximal duodenum. Reprinted from [6] by permission of Biomedical Research*

In gastric corpus mucosa, the fenestrated mucosal capillaries lie in close proximity (<0.2 um) to the abluminal membranes of the parietal cells, which are often arrayed in vertical rows along an individual capillary [1]. As previously pointed out [2] and illustrated in Figure 1, this arrangement together with the infrequency of mucosal venules must result in the interstitial secretion of bicarbonate by the parietal cells (stoichiochemically equal to their luminal secretion of acid [12]) being picked up by the capillaries and carried to the basal surfaces of the surface mucous cells which secrete HCO_3^- into the surface mucous gel. This arrangement of a local mucosal portal system for bicarbonate presumably explains why the gastric corpus, the surface of which is exposed to the highest H^+ concentration, is rarely the site of ulceration [13]. The explanation of the absence of such a microvascular based intramucosal HCO_3^- translocation system for the forestomach may be that this part of the rodent stomach is normally exposed to substantially lower H^+ levels, due to the buffering action of the routinely maintained forestomach gastric bolus [14]. In rats denied access to solid food but given a liquid diet, the forestomach surface pH falls [14] and the region ulcerates [15].

For the gastric antrum, again there is no availability of mucosally generated HCO_3^- (as there is in the corpus) and so it makes sense that a more luxuriant blood supply may be needed for the antral than the corpus mucosa, perhaps provided by direct arterial supply close to the surface mucous cells. In this situation, the reason for a separate short arteriolar supply to the basal mucosa is not clear and must await further investigation.

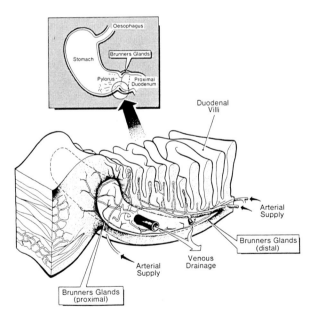

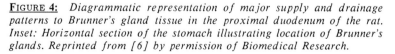

FIGURE 4: *Diagrammatic representation of major supply and drainage patterns to Brunner's gland tissue in the proximal duodenum of the rat. Inset: Horizontal section of the stomach illustrating location of Brunner's glands. Reprinted from [6] by permission of Biomedical Research.*

The separate arteriole supplies to the HCO_3^- secreting Brunner's gland region and to the villi of the duodenum may at first sight appear to be necessary due to the spatial separation of these structures. However, just as acid secretion by the parietal cells must result in a bicarbonate rich plasma of raised pH in the gastric corpus, so the abstraction of HCO_3^- from the blood by the Brunner's gland cells must result in a lowering of the pH of the venous effluent of the Brunner's gland microvessel network. Supply of such blood to the duodenal mucosa, (as does happen for blood effluent from the perglandular plexus of the intestine distal to the bile duct entry) would presumably be suboptimal, as this layer is subject to a high H^+ load on gastric emptying. Thus, the anatomical arrangement of separate blood supplies of Brunner's glands and duodenal villi may be explicable in terms of HCO_3^- secretion by the glands, and a simultaneous requirement to withstand a H^+ load by the duodenal villi.

The apparent differences in microvascular architecture of the rabbit gastric corpus [4] (dual short and long arterioles) and hamster antrum [3] may be due to dietary differences in herbivores which may result in the gastric mucosa of these regions being exposed to lower H^+ loads. Comparative measurements of mucosal surface pH in the different regions of the stomach [13] in fed and fasting herbivores compared to omnivores may provide further insight into the design requirements of the gastric mucosal microvasculature in the different regions of the upper GI tract.

REFERENCES

1. Gannon B, Browning J, O'Brien P. The microvascular architecture of the glandular mucosa of rat stomach. J Anat 1982; 135: 6667-683.

2. Gannon B, Browning J, O'Brien P, Rogers P. Mucosal microvascular architecture of the fundus and body of human stomach. Gastroenterology 1984; 84: 866-875.

3. Imada M, Tatsumi H, Fujita H. Scanning electron microscopy of vascular architecture in the gastric mucosa of the golden hamster. Cell Tissue Res. 1987; 250: 287-293.

4. Ohtsuka A, Ohtani O. The microvascular architecture of the rabbit stomach corpus in vascular corrosion casts. Scan Electron Microsc 1984; IV: 1951-1956.

5. Raschke M. Lierse W, Van Ackeren H. Microvascular architecture of the mucosa of the gastric corpus in man. Acta Anat 1987; 130: 185-190.

6. Browning J, Gannon B. The microvascular architecture of rat proximal duodenum, with particular reference to Brunner's glands. Biomed Res 1984; 5: 245-258.

7.   Browning J, Gannon BJ, O'Brien P. The microvasculature and gastric
      luminal pH of the forestomach of the rat: a comparison with the
      glandular stomach. Int J Microcirc Chin Exp 1983; 2: 109-118.

8.   Piasecki C, Thrasivoulou C, Rahim A. Ulcers produced by ligation of
      individual   gastric   mucosal   arteries   in   the   guinea-pig.
      Gastroenterology 1989; 97: 1121-1129.

9.   Prokopiw I. Hynna-Liepert TT, Dinda PK, Prentice RSA, Beck IT.
      The microvascular anatomy of the canine stomach. A comparison
      between the body and the antrum. Gastroenterology 1990 (In press).

10.   Tsuchihashi Y, Tani T, Maruyama K, et al. Structural alterations of
      mucosal microvascular system in human chronic gastritis. In: Manabe
      H, Szeifach BW, Messmer K. (eds). Microcirculation in circulatory
      disorders. Tokyo: Springer-Verlag, 1988: 171-178.

11.   Gannon BJ, Perry MA. Histoanatomy and ultrastructure of the
      microvasculature of the alimentary tract. In: Handbook of
      Physiology Section 6 (ed Schultz SG), Vol 1 (ed Wood JD) pt. 2: 1301-
      1334. American Physiological Society, Bethesda, MD 1989.

12.   Teorell T. The acid-base balance of the secreting isolated gastric
      mucosa. J Physiol 1951; 114: 267-276.

13.   Oi M, Oshida K, Sugimura S. The location of gastric ulcer.
      Gastroenterology 1959; 36: 45-56.

14.   Browning J, O'Brien P, Gannon BJ. Low forestomach acidity in the
      rat and the role of the gastric bolus. Comp Biochem Physiol 1984;
      78A; 63-5.

15.   Kokue E, Kurebayachi Y. Rat forestomach ulcer induced by
      drinking glucose solution as an experimental model of
      gastroesophageal ulcer in swine. Jap J Vet Sci 1980; 42: 395-399.

PHYSIOLOGICAL AND PATHOLOGICAL RESPONSES IN THE GASTRIC MUCOSAL BLOOD FLOW

Nobuhiro Sato, Sunao Kawano, Shingo Tsuji,
Tatsuo Ogihara, Hisato Kitagawa

*The First Department of Medicine, Osaka University
Medical School, Osaka, Japan*

INTRODUCTION

A functional vasodilator mechanism might exist so that sufficient nutrient and oxygen would be available to meet increased metabolic demands and would allow for the removal of by-products associated with the rise in metabolic rate. For example, stimulation of acid secretion by histamine or gastrin might result in a concomitant increase in mucosal blood flow [1,2]. Thus defending roles of mucosal circulation against various aggressive factors have been emphasized [3].

In the last decade, basic concept of organ blood flow has been revised in view of tissue microcirculation. According to this view, various stimuli in arterioles and venules may enhance or disturb capillary circulation. It has been found that certain mediators, prostaglandins, for example, may increase gastric blood flow without apparent increase in gastric metabolic demands [2]. It is believed that such a regulator protects the mucosa from various aggressive factors. Mediators disturbing mucosal circulation may damage tissue without enhancing aggressive factors. In the present paper, the authors re-evaluate the regulatory mechanism of mucosal microcirculation and mucosal oxygenation in various pathophysiological conditions.

EXPERIMENTAL METHODS

IN VIVO MICROSCOPIC OBSERVATION OF MUCOSAL CAPILLARIES AND COLLECTING VENULES

A microscope (BH2, Olympus Co., Tokyo, Japan) with x4-x25 objective lenses for observing the gastric mucosal microcirculation were connected to a high-speed video camera (NAC, Osaka, Japan), a video camera (Yokosha, Tokyo, Japan) or a movie camera (Aliflex, France). The videocameras were connected to a videotape recorder (Sony VO5800, Panasonic AG2850, or NAC MHS-200) and to an image analyzer (ED1181, EDEC, Tokyo, Japan) controlled by a microcomputer (PC9801, NEC, Toyko, Japan). The information stored on a videotape recorder were also analysed to obtain the blood velocity by a cross-correlator using photodiodes and a workstation (PS-9000, Yokokawa-Hewlett-Packard, Tokyo, Japan).

Male Sprague-Dawley rats weighing 200-250g were purchased from Nihon Dobutsu Inc., Osaka, Japan. They were fasted for 24 hours but allowed free access to water. They were anaesthetized with pentobarbital sodium (35-40 mg/kg i.p.)   The abdomen of the animal was opened with a midline incision, and the gastric anterior wall was opened by a cautery knife (Thermoknife, Natsume Instrument Co., Tokyo, Japan).   The animal was placed on a special stage left side down, so that the posterior wall of the stomach was gently extended over the window of the stage. The gastric wall was kept moistened with saline, and the animal was kept at a temperature of $37^{\circ}C$ by a heating pad

IN VIVO MICROSCOPY OF GASTRIC SUBMUCOSAL LAYER.

The gastric serosa and gastric muscle layer were carefully removed and the gastric submucosal layer was illuminated by a tungsten lamp (1000W) via a condenser (Olympus, long distance working type).   Gastric arterioles and venules were observed and recorded in the video tape recorder.

LASER DOPPLER FLOWMETRY

Laser Doppler flowmeter (BPM-403, TSI Inc., St. Paul, MN, USA) was used to estimate mucosal blood flow velocity.   The optical probe of the laser Doppler flowmeter combined with the probe of organ reflectance spectrophotometer was held vertically and gently of the mucosal surface using an x,y,z-manipulator (Narishige, Tokyo, Japan) with the balancer to minimize the pressure on the mucosa.

HYDROGEN GAS CLEARANCE METHOD

A platinum electrode (Unique Medical Co., Osaka, Japan) was inserted into the mucosa. Hydrogen gas was inspired by the animal for 2 min.

ESTIMATION OF SURFACE MUCOSAL BLOOD VOLUME AND SURFACE MUCOSAL BLOOD HEMOGLOBIN OXYGENATION USING REFLECTANCE SPECTROPHOTOMETRY.

The changes of the blood volume and the blood hemoglobin oxygenation at surface mucosa of the stomach were estimated by organ reflectance spectrophotometry developed in collaboration with Sumitomo Electronic Industry Ltd., Osaka, Japan (Type TS-200) [4]. The hemoglobin concentration in the mucosal tissue, i.e. the index of mucosal blood volume and mucosal blood hemoglobin oxygenation were automatically calculated from the spectra. The instrument detected the hemoglobin signals within 0.4-1.0 mm from the surface of the tissue.

EXPERIMENTAL PROTOCOL

ISCHEMIA AND REPERFUSION OF THE GASTRIC MUCOSAL CIRCULATION DURING STRESS: ROLES OF EDRF AND PAF.

Right carotid artery of the rat was cannulated with PE-50 polyethylene tube which was connected to a blood reservoir. A pressure transducer (TP-101T, Nihon Kohden Corp., Tokyo, Japan) was also connected to the tube and the mean arterial pressure was measured. Blood was removed from the carotid artery and the mean arterial pressure was controlled by changing position of the blood reservoir. The mucosal blood flow, the mucosal blood volume, and the mucosal blood hemoglobin oxygenation were measured at various mean arterial pressures. Small volume (<0.1ml) of the blood was routinely taken from the catheter, so that the blood hematocrit was maintained between 38-40%. Effect of intra-gastric arterial infusion of acetylcholine (Ach), $NaNO_2$ and papaverine was studied before and after ischemia-reperfusion procedure.

Platelet activating factor (PAF) is reported to exist in rat gastric mucosa [5], although PAF per se is hardly found in circulating plasma. The physiological roles of PAF were examined using PAF receptor antagonists such as CV-3988 [6]. Rats were treated with PAF intravenously or intragastric-arterially. In another experiment, rats were pretreated with intravenous infusion of CV-3988 (a genuine gift from Takeda Chemical Industry Co., Osaka, Japan, 10 mg/kg) or saline.

ROLE OF PROSTAGLANDINS AND LEUKOTRIENES IN ETHANOL-INDUCED MICRO-CIRCULATORY INSUFFICIENCY IN THE STOMACH.

In the experiment for studying the role of arachidonate and its derivatives in ethanol-induced acute gastric mucosal lesion, *in vivo* microscopy was employed to observe the circulation of gastric mucosa and submucosa. Organ reflectance spectrophotometry, hydrogen gas clearance method and laser Doppler flowmetry were also applied. After the measurement of basal state, the ethanol solution at concentrations of 20, 30, 40, 50, 70 or 99.5% was administered into the stomach. Various doses (0-1000 ug/kg) of PGD_2, 20 mg/kg of indomethacin, 40 mg/kg of AA-861 (a 5-lipoxygenase-specific inhibitor) or its vehicle was administered topically to the gastric mucosa in order to elucidate the role of arachidonate and its derivatives. Thirty minutes after the administration of the above agent, 1 ml of ethanol solution at various concentrations was administered to the gastric mucosa.

RESULTS AND DISCUSSION

REGULATION OF MUCOSAL MICROCIRCULATION UNDER VARIOUS STRESSES: A ROLE OF EDRF IN ISCHEMIA-REPERFUSION.

Gastric hypersecretion was not generally observed in the experiments of stress ulceration induced by hemorrhagic shock, burn and water immersion restraint condition in animals [4]. Thus the development of gastric damage under these conditions may be related with mucosal ischemia and changes in mucosal metabolism under stresses. Previous experiments using various stress models have suggested a decreased energy charge in the mucosal tissue during stresses [7], which also induces mucosal ischaemia [4],

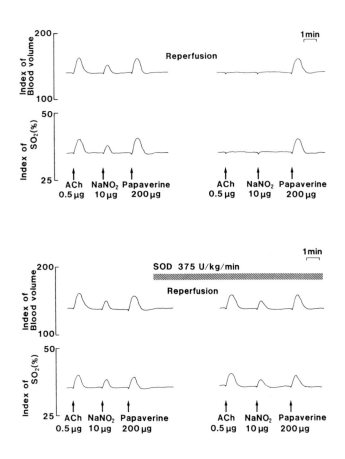

FIGURE 1: *Changes in mucosal blood volume and mucosal oxygenation caused by acetylcholine (ACh), NaNO$_2$ and papaverine in rat stomach. The changes caused by Ach and NaNO$_2$ were prohibited by ischaemia-reperfusion of rat gastric mucosa. They were also prohibited by removal of vascular endothelia using collagenase (data were not shown) suggesting they were endothelium-dependent vascular responses. In rats pretreated with SOD, the endothelium-dependent responses were preserved after the ischaemia-reperfusion stress.*

production of oxygen-derived free radicals [8] and of lipid peroxides in gastric mucosa at reperfusion process [9], and resecretion of gastric acid during mucosal reperfusion [4]. Thus, the disturbed gastric circulation may be of importance in gastric damage caused by shock, and various somatic stresses.

The factors regulating the mucosal microcirculation during stresses appear to affect 1) arterioles, 2) venules, 3) mucosal capillaries, or 4) interaction between blood cells and vascular endothelial cells as well as 5) systemic circulation.   Direct damage in vascular endothelial cells also modifies endothelium-dependent vasoactive substances.   If endothelium-derived factors increase after the mucosal damage, they may aggravate or attenuate the development of the damage without aggravating factors such as hydrochloric acid, and taurocholate.

Normally, infusion of acetylcholine (Ach) (0.5μg), NaNO$_2$ (10μg) and papaverine (200μg) into the gastric artery via the catheterization into the left gastric artery via the splenic artery in rats induces a prompt increase in the index of surface mucosal blood volume and blood oxygenation (Figure 1).   After the ischaemia (30 min) followed by reperfusion, this reaction except for effect of papaverine disappears completely, suggesting that the endothelium is damaged during these processes.   Pretreatment with SOD (375U/kg/min), but not the vehicle (DSMO), before and during ischaemia-reperfusion procedure reverses the response of mucosal circulation to Ach and NaNO$_2$: Ach and NaNO$_2$ increase the surface mucosal blood volume index and oxygenation index as normally.   Thus it seems that during ischaemia (hypotension) or reperfusion process, the endothelium-derived relaxing factor (EDRF) may be inactivated by radical formation [10], and SOD protected the endothelium from the radical-induced inactivation of EDRF.

A ROLE OF PLATELET ACTIVATING FACTOR (PAF) IN THE GASTRIC MUCOSAL CIRCULATION IN HYPOTENSION

Gastric mucosal blood flow *in vivo* may also be modified by various factors including neural stimulation and various hormones. In this study, the role of PAF on mucosal microcirculation was examined in rats under normotension and hemorrhage-induced hypotension. Intravenous and intra-arterial infusion of PAF decreases gastric mucosal blood flow as evidenced by *in vivo* microscopy [11].   Intravenous administration of PAF (01. ug/kg/min) causes an abrupt decrease of arterial blood pressure as well as the decreases of indices of gastric mucosal blood volume and blood oxygenation and blood flow velocity (Figure 2-a). In contrast, intra-gastric arterial infusion of PAF (0.1 ug/kg/min) causes a decrease in surface mucosal blood flow velocity and blood oxygenation (Figure 2-b). The data suggest that exogenous PAF may disturb mucosal microcirculation as arachidonate in resting stomach is negligible.

LOCAL REGULATION AT GASTRIC ARTERIOLES, CAPILLARIES AND VENULES DURING ETHANOL INGESTION.

After administration of ethanol at a concentration of 40 or 50%, the capillaries and venules showed partial congestion. Surface gastric mucosal flow heterogeneously decreased in 10-30 seconds. Grossly, no lesion was

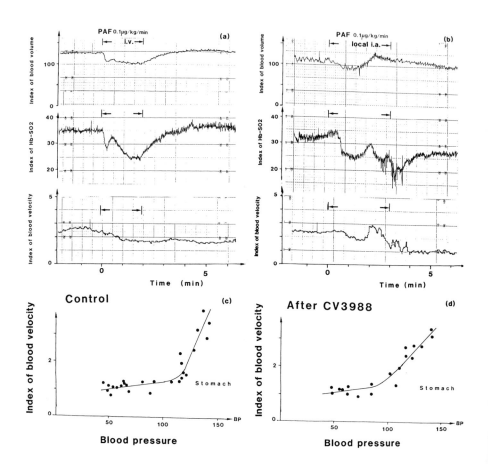

FIGURE 2: *Changes in mucosal blood volume, mucosal oxygenation and mucosal blood flow velocity in rats treated with PAF (Fig. 2-a and 2-b). Relationship between mean arterial pressure and mucosal blood flow velocity in rats pretreated with saline or CV-3988 (Fig 2-c and 2-d).*

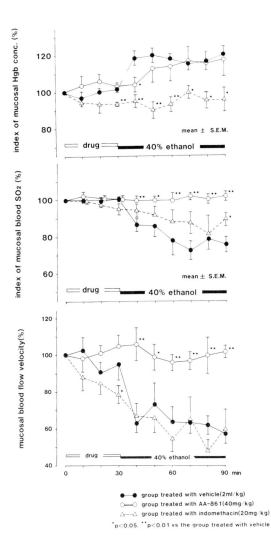

FIGURE 3: *Changes in mucosal blood volume, mucosal oxygenation and mucosal blood flow velocity in rats teated with 40% solution of ethanol. The rats were pretreated with indomethacin, AA-861 or vehicle.*

observed except for hyperemic and congestive streaks. Arterioles in gastric submucosa appeared dilated and some portions of venules in the submucosa and muscle layer appeared constricted in *in vivo* microscopy.

Changes in gastric mucosal blood volume, mucosal blood hemoglobin oxygenation and mucosal blood flow after intraluminal administration of 40-60% ethanol were also assessed by organ reflectance spectrophotometry, hydrogen gas clearance method and laser Doppler flowmetry. While the index of mucosal blood volume increased, mucosal blood hemoglobin oxygenation estimated spectrophotometrically and mucosal blood flow measured by hydrogen clearance method decreased. In contrast, gastric submucosal blood flow clearly increased, as evidenced by *in vivo* microscopy. The indices of mucosal blood volume and blood oxygenation at submucosal layer also increased after intraluminal ethanol load, suggesting an opening of shunting at submucosal layer.

The above change in gastric mucosal and submucosal hemodynamics is similar to the change caused by topical administration of LTC_4 [11,13]. It is well known that ethanol ingestion increases mucosal content of prostaglandins and leukotrienes [14]. In this study, the effects of PGD_2, indomethacin, and AA-861 were examined. Organ reflectance spectrophotometry and laser Doppler flowmetry revealed that AA-861 prohibited the decrease in mucosal blood flow and mucosal oxygenation (Figure 3). PGD_2 which is reported to antagonize several arachidonate receptors also prohibited the ethanol-induced decrease of gastric mucosal blood flow and mucosal oxygenation. While indomethacin did not attenuate nor aggravate the development of ethanol-induced mucosal damage, both PGD_2 and AA-861 prohibited the development of mucosal damage. Thus it appears that receptors of leukotriene C_4 and prostaglandin D_2 relate to gastric mucosal congestion caused by ethanol.

CONCLUDING REMARKS.

Gastric mucosal microcirculation is regulated by various factors such as arterial pressures, and vasoconstriction and vasodilation of gastric arterioles, venules and possibly capillaries. In hemorrhage-induced hypotension and reperfusion of gastric circulation, the mucosal blood flow is influenced by EDRF and PAF. Ingestion of ethanol at high concentrations increases endogenous production of leukotrienes which causes mucosal blood congestion. PGD_2 may also mediate the ethanol-induced mucosal microcirculatory disturbance.

The other aspects of mucosal circulation on mucosal protection may be on mucosal regeneration. Recently the authors have examined sequential expression of proto-oncogenes, c-myc and c-Ha-ras in gastric mucosa after indomethacin-induced gastric mucosal damage. C-myc gene is expressed 3 h after, and c-Ha-ras is expressed 6-12 h after the initiation of gastric injury by indomethacin (50 mg/kg). Disturbance followed by recovery of gastric mucosal microcirculation may alter the proliferation process of mucosal cells.

REFERENCES

1. Thompson J, Vane J. Gastric secretion induced by histamine and its relationship to the rate of blood flow. J Physiol (Lond) 1953; 121: 433.

2. Main IHM, Whittle NHJ. A study of the vascular and acid-secretory response of the rat gastric mucosa to histamine. J Physiol (Lond) 1976; 257: 407-18.

3. Guth PH, Leung FW. Physiology of the gastric circulation. In: Johnson LR. Ed. Physiology of the Gastrointestinal Tract. Vol. 1. 2nd Ed. New York: Raven Press. 1987; 1031-53.

4. Sato N, Kamada T, Shichiri M, Kawano S, Abe H, Hagihara B. Measurement of hemoperfusion and oxygen sufficiency in gastric mucosa in vivo: evidence of mucosal hypoxia as the cause of hemorrhagic shock-induced gastric mucosal lesion in rats. Gastroenterology 1979; 776: 814-9.

5. Sugatani J, Fujimura K, Miwa M, Mizuno T, Sameshima Y, Saito K. Occurrence of platelet-activating factor (PAF) in normal rat stomach and alteration of PAF level by water immersion stress. FASEB J 1989; 3: 65-70.

6. Terashita Z, Tsushima S, Yoshioka Y, Nomura H, Inada Y, Nishikawa K. CV-3988-a specific antagonist of platelet activation factor (PAF). Life Sci 1983; 32: 1975-82.

7. Menguy R, Desbaillets L, Masters YF. Mechanism of stress ulcer: influence of hypovolemic shock on energy metabolism in the gastric mucosa. Gstroenterology 1974; 66: 46-55.

8. Ito M, Guth PH. Role of oxygen-derived free radicals in hemorrhagic shock-induced gastric lesions in the rat. Gastroenterology 1985; 88: 1162-7.

9. Tsuji S, Kawano S, Sato N, Kamada T. Role of calcium ion influx, lipid peroxidation and intraluminal acid in stress ulceration in rats. In: Tsuchiya M, et al., Eds. Free radicals in digestive disease. Amsterdam: Elsevier Science Publishers 1987; 105-10.

10. Gryglewski RJ, Palmer TMJ, Moncada S. Superoxide anion is involved in the breakdown of endothelium-derived vascular relaxing factor. Nature, London 1986; 320: 454-6.

11. Kawano S, Sato N, Tsuji S, Kamada T, Satoh H, Inatomi N. Gastric microcirculatory changes associated with physicochemical and ionic mediators. In: Manabe H, Zweifach BW, Messmer K, Eds. Microcirculation in Circulatory Disorders. 1st Ed. Tokyo: Springer-Verlag, 1988; 189-94.

12.   Tsuji S, Kawano S, Sato N, Kamada T. Roles of endogenous prostaglandins and endogenous leukotrienes in ethanol-induced gastric mucosal lesion in rats. Clin J Gastroenterol 1990 (in press).

13.   Oates PJ and Hakkinen JP. Studies on the mechanism of ethanol-induced gastric damage in rats. Gastroenterology 1988; 94: 10-21.

14.   Peskar BM, Lange K, Hoppe V, Peskar BA. Ethanol stimulates formation of leukotriene C4 in rat gastric mucosa. Prostaglandins 1986; 31: 283-93.

EFFECTS OF AGING ON GASTRIC SECRETION
AND BLOOD FLOW IN RATS

Yutaka Masuda, Tomochika Ohno, Hiroshi Uramoto and Takafumi Ishihara

Laboratory of Experimental Pharmacology,
Suntory Institute for Biomedical Research, Osaka, Japan

ABSTRACT

The purpose of this study was to characterize the effects of aging on gastric acid and pepsin secretion and on gastric mucosal blood flow in rats. Young (2-3 month old) and aged (24-25 month old) Fischer 344 rats were anaesthetized with urethane and underwent surgery for the preparation of a gastric chamber. The fluid in the chamber was removed at 30 min intervals for measurements of gastric acid and pepsin and replaced with 2 ml saline. Gastric mucosal blood flow was measured in the same preparation using the H2 gas clearance technique and laser-doppler flowmetry. Papaverine, histamine and pentagastrin were given intravenously, and the left vagal nerve was efferently stimulated at the cervical level. In aged rats, the basal acid secretion decreased, but the secretory responses to histamine and pentagastrin and vagal nerve stimulation were preserved or rather increased compared with those in young rats. Basal pepsin secretion in aged rats was almost the same as observed in young rats, but pentagastrin- and vagal stimulation-induced secretions increased in aged rats. Basal mucosal blood flow decreased in aged rats and % increases of blood flow in response to papaverine, pentagastrin and vagal nerve stimulation were almost the same or rather lower than those in young rats. In conclusion, responses of gastric acid and pepsin secretion, but not gastric mucosal blood flow, to various stimuli were preserved or rather increased, which may be involved in the mechanism of higher incidence of gastric ulceration in aged rats.

INTRODUCTION

Aging has been shown to represent one of the most important factors in affecting the progress of gastric ulcer. Several studies have been published showing that the incidence of gastric ulcer is higher [1,2], healing is slower [3-5] and risk of relapse is greater in the elderly [6]. However, there have been few reports on the effect of aging on peptic ulceration in animals and the mechanisms responsible for such alterations are unclear. We have previously reported that gastric mucosal injury produced by restraint and water-immersion stress is more severe in aged rats, which is considered to be concerned with an inadequate microvascular network in stomachs and preservation of gastric acid and pepsin secretion [7]. To extend this study, we have further studied the influence of aging on gastric secretion and mucosal blood flow in rats.

MATERIALS AND METHODS

Young (2-3 month old) and aged (24-25 month old) male Fischer 344 rats were fasted overnight in individual cages with mesh bottoms but allowed free access to water. Animals were anaesthetized with urethane (1.25 g/kg i.p.). The trachea was intubated and the esophagus was ligated at the neck without disturbing the vagal nerves. The left femoral artery was cannulated with a polyethylene tube to monitor blood pressure with the aid of a pressure transducer (Nihon Koden, MPU-0.5-290-0-III). Heart rate was measured using a cardiotachometer (Nihon Koden, AT-600) triggered by the R wave of the limb lead II electrocardiogram. An *ex vivo* gastric chamber preparation was constructed according to the method of Wallace et al [8]. Briefly, a laparotomy was performed, and the stomach was exteriorized. The pylorus was ligated with care taken to avoid damage to the vascular and neural supplies to the stomach. The stomach was pulled through the aperture of a plexiglass plate, opened by an incision along the greater curvature, and pinned out, mucosal side up, onto the plexiglass plate. A plexiglass cylinder (height, 1.0 cm; diameter, 2.0 cm) was clamped onto the stomach forming a chamber with the gastric mucosa comprising the bottom. The surface was lavaged and filled with warmed saline (37°C).

DETERMINATION OF GASTRIC ACID AND PEPSIN SECRETION.

The fluid in the chamber was removed at 30 min intervals and replaced by 2 ml saline. The secretory volume was calculated as the change in weight between the instilled and removed solutions. H^+ secretion was determined with the aid of an automatic titrator (Hiranuma, Comtite-101) by titrating instillated and recovered samples to pH 7.0 with 0.1 N NaOH. Pepsin secretion was determined by the method of Anson and Mirsky [9].

DETERMINATION OF GASTRIC MUCOSAL BLOOD FLOW

H2 gas clearance and laser-doppler flowmetry were used for measurements of blood flow of the gastric corpus mucosa at the same focal point. Two experiments were performed, the first one to measure the basal blood flow by H2 gas clearance method [10], where a platinum black electrode (Unique Medical Co) was placed in contact with the corpus mucosa and the reference Ag/AgCl electrode (Unique Medical Co) in the abdominal cavity, both of which were connected to an amplifier (MT Giuken, PHG-300) coupled to the chart recorder. Pure H2 gas was then administered at a rate of 0.5 l/min for about 60 sec through a funnel-shaped mouthpiece allowing some mixing of the gas with room air. Under these conditions, femoral arterial blood pressure and heart rate did not show any changes. Hydrogen saturation-desaturation curves were obtained and mucosal blood flow was expressed as ml/min/100g tissue. In the second experiment, laser-doppler flowmetry was used for continuous measurement of gastric mucosal blood flow. A 3 mW helium-neon laser probe (1 mm diameter) was placed in contact with the mucosal surface using a balancer, which enables avoidance of excess contact pressure, and was connected to a detector (Advance, ALF-2100) and a pen recorder. Since calibration in absolute units has not been clearly achieved, the gastric mucosal blood flow was expressed as percent change from control levels before treatments with drugs or nerve stimulation.

DRUGS AND NERVE STIMULATION

Papaverine HCl (0.3-3.0 mg/kg, Nacalai Tesqu), histamine 2HCl (0.1-1.0 mg/kg, Nacalai Tesque) and pentagastrin (1-10µg/kg, Sumitomo Pharmac) were dissolved in saline and intravenously administered through a polyethylene cannula inserted into the tail vein at a volume of 0.1 ml/100g. Vagal nerve stimulation was carried out at 0.2 mA, 2 msec duration and 5 Hz for 10 min through a bipolar platinum electrode placed on the peripheral cut of the left cervical vagus [11]. The nerve stimulation induced reproducible responses of gastric acid and pepsin secretion and mucosal blood flow without considerable changes in blood pressure and heart rate.

STATISTICS

Data are presented as the mean ± S.E. of values obtained from 6 or 7 rats per group. Statistical analysis was performed using a two-tailed Dunnett's multiple comparison test [12] and p values less than 0.05 were regarded as significant.

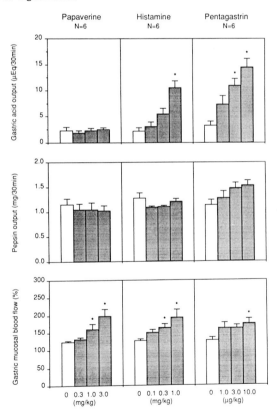

FIGURE 1   Dose-response studies of papaverine, histamine and penta-gastrin on gastric acid and pepsin secretion amd mucosal blood flow in chambered stomachs of anaesthetized young rats. * P<0.05 vs saline control.

RESULTS

In young rats, intravenous injections of papaverine, histamine or pentagastrin dose-dependently increased gastric mucosal blood flow (Figure 1). Histamine and pentagastrin, but not papaverine, increased gastric acid secretion in a dose-dependent manner. Pentagastrin tended to increase pepsin secretion, but papaverine and histamine did not exert any effect. Since cardiovascular responses were marked and considered to affect gastric secretion and mucosal blood flow at the highest dose of each drug, the median doses were used in the following comparative experiments in young and aged rats. Typical responses of gastric mucosal blood flow, blood pressure and heart rate in young rats to intravenous bolus injections of saline, papaverine (1 mg/kg), pentagastrin (3ug/kg) and histamine (0.3 mg/kg), and vagal nerve stimulation are shown in Figure 2.

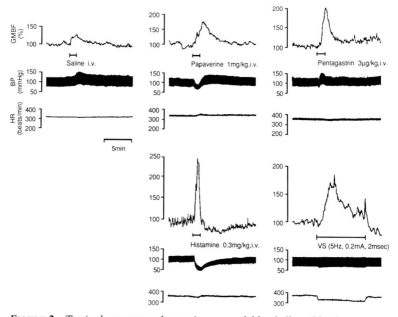

FIGURE 2 *Typical patterns of gastric mucosal blood flow, blood pressure and heart rate in response to papaverine, pentagastrin, histamine and vagal nerve stimulation in chambered stomachs of anaesthetized young rats.*

Papaverine- and pentagastrin-injection and vagal nerve stimulation remarkably increased gastric mucosal blood flow. Histamine caused a transient increase followed by decrease in blood flow. The late decrease was accompanied by hypotension. Basal acid output (BAO) was measured in saline-treated rats. As shown in Figure 3, BAO was significantly lower in aged rats (1.14 ± 0.17 uEq/30 min) compared to that of young rats (2.97 ± 0.46uEq/30 min).

However, there was no signficant difference in the histamine-induced increase of gastric acid output between aged (6.58 ± 1.14uEq/30 min) and young (7.33 ± 0.98uEq/30 min) rats.

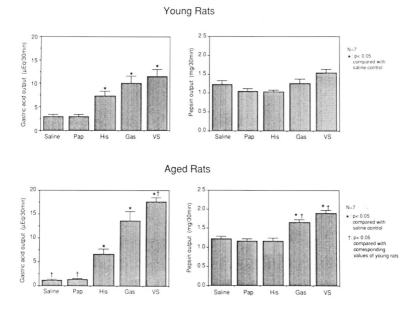

FIGURE 3 *Gastric acid and pepsin secretory responses to papaverine (Pap; 1 mg/kg i.v.), histamine (His; 0.3 mg/kg i.v.), pentagastrin (Gas; 3ug/kg i.v.) and vagal nerve stimulation (VS; 5 Hs, 0.2 mA, 2 msec, 10 min) in anaesthetized young and aged rats. Each column represents mean ± S.E. from 7 rats. * P<0.05 vs saline control, + P<0.05 vs young rats.*

Gastric acid output in response to pentagastrin and vagal nerve stimulation in aged rats was 13.61 ± 1.92 and 17.55 ± 0.93uEq/30 min, respectively, the response to pentagastrin was slightly larger than in young rats (10.01 ± 1.55uEq/30 min), and the value in the case of vagal nerve stimulation was significantly larger than in young rats (11.47 ± 1.49uEq/30 min). Basal pepsin output in aged rats (1.22 ± 0.07 mg/30 min) was almost the same as observed in young rats (1.23 ± 0.10 mg/30min). Administration of papaverine and histamine did not increase pepsin output both in young and aged rats. However, pepsin output in response to pentagastrin and vagal nerve stimulation was significantly increased in aged rats, at 1.66 ± 0.07 and 1.89 ± 0.08 mg/30 min, respectively. In contrast, pepsin secretory responses in young rats to pentagastrin and vagal nerve stimulation were not statistically significant.

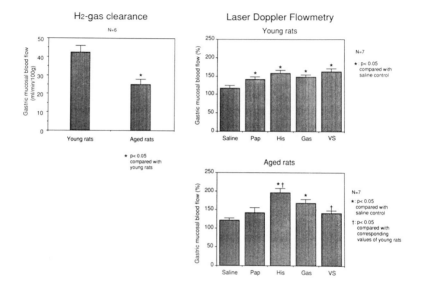

FIGURE 4 *Basal and stimulated mucosal blood flow in young and aged rat stomachs. Basal blood flow was measured by H2 gas clearance technique, and the maximal responses to papaverine (Pap; 1 mg/kg i.v.), histamine (His; 0.3 mg/kg i.v.), pentagastrin (Gas; 3ug/kg i.v.) and vagal nerve stimulation (VS; 5 Hz, 0.2 mA, 2 msec, 10 min) were measured by laser-doppler flowmetry. Each column represents mean + S.E. from 6 or 7 rats. * P<0.05 vs saline control, + P<0.05 vs young rats.*

As shown in Figure 4, basal mucosal blood flow in aged rat stomachs (23.9 $\pm$ 3.9 ml/min/100 g) was lower by 44% compared with that in young rats (42.7 $\pm$ 3.4 ml/min/100 g). Intravenous administration of papaverine (1 mg/kg), histamine (0.3 mg/kg) or pentagastrin (3 ug/kg) and vagal nerve stimulation significantly increased mucosal blood flow in young rats by 41.9 $\pm$ 6.1, 58.1 $\pm$ 8.7, 48.1 $\pm$ 5.6, 63.0 $\pm$ 7.4%, respectively. In aged rats, percentage increases of blood flow in response to papaverine and pentagastrin were almost the same as those in young rats. However, vagal nerve stimulation did not significantly increase the blood flow in aged rats. Histamine increased the blood flow more markedly in aged rats than young rats and the difference was statistically significant. However, the increase was transient and was followed by a decrease in association with more serious hypotension in aged rats.

DISCUSSION

Deterioration of gastrointestinal function is a common symptom associated with the aging process. Studies on gastric acid secretion demonstrated a progressive decrease in both basal and stimulated secretion with aging in humans [13-15]. The decrease of gastric secretion in the elderly is attributed to a loss of parietal cells that occurs with atrophic gastritis, the incidence of which increases steadily with aging [16-18]. However, it is difficult to determine if the changes, if any, in gastric function or mucosal structure in aged humans are due to aging and not due to secondary effects of dietary irritants, alcohol, and/or injurious medications [19,20]. Indeed, gastric acid secretion remains normal in elderly humans with normal gastric mucosa [18]. Furthermore, it is now generally believed that approximately 20% of the population over the age of 70 has hypochlorhydria, whereas the remainder has acid production no different from young adults [21]. In the present study in rats, basal acid secretion decreased, but the secretory responses to histamine, pentagastrin and vagal nerve stimulation were well preserved or rather increased in aged rats compared to young rats. In contrast, Khalil et al [22] reported that gastric acid secretion in aged rats (32 months old) was significantly decreased compared to young rats not only under basal conditions, but also in response to exogenous gastrin in fistula rats. The reasons for this discrepancy may be due to differences in the preparation used to measure acid secretion and/or the age of rats used.

Basal pepsin secretion in aged rats was much the same as observed in young rats, but pentagastrin-and vagal nerve stimulation-induced increases in pepsin secretion were more marked in aged rats than in the young. In a histochemical examination, parietal cell density in aged rat stomachs has been shown to be almost equivalent to that of young rats, but the chief cell density was higher in aged rats than in the young [7]. These findings might account for the disparity between the basal acid output and the basal pepsin output in aged rats as observed in the present study.

In microvascular cast examinations, deficiencies of the gastric capillary network have been demonstrated in aged rats [7]. This finding strongly suggests a decrease in gastric mucosal blood circulation. Indeed, the basal gastric mucosal blood flow in aged rats decreased as compared with that in young rats. The increases of the blood flow in response to papaverine, pentagastrin and vagal nerve stimulation were almost the same in aged and young rats or rather decreased in aged rats compared with young rats. Histamine increased the blood flow much more markedly in aged rats. However, since the basal gastric mucosal blood flow in aged rats was remarkably lower than that in young rats, the absolute value of the blood flow in response to histamine was considered to be not enough to perfuse the whole gastric mucosa on a weight basis. Bernick et al [23] reported that a focal area of PAS (periodic acid-Schiff)-positive material developed in the media of arterioles and small arteries and increased in extent and severity with age, and that the adventitial layer of nonmuscular venules, which is PAS-positive due to the mucopolysaccharide coating of collagen fibers, became more intensely PAS-positive with age in rats. In 26 month-old rats, the media of arterioles and small arteries were extensively hyalinized and became intensely PAS -positive [23]. The effect of hyalinization of the arteriolar wall on its compliance is not known [23] but may be concerned with the resultant stiffening of the arterial wall and subsequent decrease of gastric mucosal blood flow.

In conclusion, in aged rats the responses of gastric acid and pepsin secretion, but not gastric mucosal blood flow, to various stimuli were preserved or rather increased, which may be involved in the mechanism of higher incidence of gastric ulcer during aging.

REFERENCES

1.   Bonnevie O. The incidence of gastric ulcer in Copenhagen county. Scand J Gastroenterol 1975; 10: 231-239.

2.   Bonnevie O. Changing demographics of peptic ulcer disease.   Dig Dis Sci 1985; Suppl 30: 8-14.

3.   Nakajima T. Studies on factors affecting healing of gastric ulcer. Am J Gastroenterol 1976; 66: 150-155.

4.   Piper DW, Hunt J, Heap TR.   The healing rate of chronic gastric ulcer in patients admitted to hospital. Scand J Gastroenterol 1980; 15: 113-117.

5.   Okada M, Yao T, Fuchigami T, Imamura K, Omae T.   Factors influencing the healing rate of gastric ulcer in hospitalized subjects. Gut 1984; 25: 881-885.

6.   Battaglia G, DiMario F, Piccoli A, Vianello F, Farinati F, Naccarato R. Clinical markers of slow healing and relapsing gastric ulcer.   Gut 1987; 28: 210-215.

7.   Ohno T, Uramoto H, Masuda Y, Kubota H, Ishihara T. Influence of aging on stress ulcer formation in rats. Gastroenterology 1989; 96: A374 (abstract).

8.   Wallace JL,   Morris GP, Krausse EJ, Greaves SE.   Reduction by cytoprotective agents of ethanol-induced damage to the rat gastric mucosa: a correlated morphological and physiological study.   Can J Physiol Pharmacol 1982; 60: 1686-1699.

9.   Anson ML, Mirsky AE. The estimation of pepsin with hemoglobin. J Gen Physiol 1932; 16: 59-63.

10.   Murakami M, Moriga M, Miyake T, Uchino H.   Contact electrode method in hydrogen gas clearance technique: a new method for determination of regional gastric mucosal blood flow in animals and humans. Gastroenterology 1982; 82: 457-467.

11.   Ohno T, Uramoto H, Ishihara T, Okabe S. Effects of 16, 16-dimethyl prostaglandin E2 on surface epithelial cell damage in the rat stomach induced by vagal nerve stimulation. Japan J Pharmacol 1987; 43: 429-439.

12.   Dunnett CW. A multiple comparison procedure for comparing several treatments with a control. J Am Stat Assoc 1955; 50: 1096-1121.

13.   Baron JH. The clinical use of gastric function test. Scand J Gastroenterol 1970; Suppl 6: 9-46.

14.   Grossman MI, Kirsner JB, Gillespie IE. Basal and histalog-stimulated gastric secretion in control subjects and in patients with peptic ulcer or gastric cancer. Gastroenterology 1963; 45: 14-26.

15.   Miyoshi A, Ohe K, Inagawa T, Inoue M, Uraki S, Tatsugami M, Noguchi A, Onda M, Yokoya H, Shirakawa H. A statistical study on the age distribution of gastric secretion in patients with peptic ulcer. Hiroshima J Med Sci 1980; 29: 21-28.

16.   Kimura K. Chronological transition of the fundic-pyloric border determined by stepwise biopsy of the lesser and greater curvatures of the stomachs. Gastroenterology 1972; 63: 584-592.

17.   Strickland RG, Mackay IR. A reappraisal of the nature and significance of chronic atrophic gastritis. Am J Dig Dis 1973; 18: 426-440.

18.   Kekki M, Samloff IM, Ihamaki T, Varis K, Siurala M. Age- and sex-related behaviour of gastric acid secretion at the population level. Scand J Gastroenterol 1982; 17: 737-743.

19.   Caruso I, Porro GB. Gastroscopic evaluation of anti-inflammatory agents. Brit Med J 1980; 280: 75-78.

20.   Meyers BM, Smith JL, Graham DY. Effect of red pepper and black pepper on the stomach. Am J Gastroenterol 1987; 82: 211-214.

21.   Holt PR, Rosenberg IH, Russell RM. Causes and consequences of hypochlorhydria in the elderly. Dig Dis Sci 1989; 34: 933-937.

22.   Khalil T, Singh P, Fijimura M, Townsend CM, Greeley GH, Thompson JC. Effect of aging on gastric acid secretion, serum gastrin, and antral gastrin content in rats. Dig Dis Sci 1988; 33: 1544-1548.

23.   Bernick S, Sobin SS, Lindal RG. Changes in the microvasculature with age. Microvascular Res 1978; 16: 215-223.

ROLE OF INCREASED BLOOD FLOW AFTER MUCOSAL INJURY

K. Svanes and J.E. Grønbech

*Surgical Research Laboratory, Department of Surgery,
University of Bergen, Bergen, Norway*

INTRODUCTION

The surface mucous cells probably play an important role in protection of normal gastric mucosa, owing to secretion of mucus and HCO_3^- and the ability of the cells to rapid regeneration. It is also well known, however, that after destruction of the epithelial lining the mucosa usually has the capacity to withstand further damage and to heal. Not much is known about the mechanisms of protection of damaged mucosa. However, some evidence has been provided that increased mucosal blood flow after damage may contribute to protect the mucosa during the early phase of repair [1].

It has been shown in many studies that the gastric mucosa may respond to injury by increasing the local blood flow [2-6]. Probably the blood flow increases when the injury is superficial so that most of the mucosal blood vessels are left intact, while the blood flow decreases after severe deep injury accompanied by vascular damage [7-9].

Recently a histologically well defined lesion was obtained in our laboratory by exposing the *in vivo* cat gastric mucosa to 2M NaCl for 10 min [10]. This caused damage or detachment of approximately 80% of the surface mucous cells and the upper part of the pits, but minimal damage to the glands. The damage was followed by a two- or threefold increase in mucosal blood flow.

The significance of the hyperemic response in protection and repair of damaged mucosa can be tested by exposing 2M NaCl-injured mucosa to a second injurious agent, in animals with intact hyperemic response to 2M NaCl, and in animals where the hyperemic response has been abolished by partial clamping of the celiac artery. In the present study two injurious substances will be tested; strong hydrochloric acid (pH 1.0) which is the most common and important aggressor of the gastric mucosa, and absolute ethanol which is known to cause deep lesions in the mucosa.

METHODS

Cats weighing 2.2-4.2 kg were anaesthetized with 40 mg/kg pentobarbital, tracheotomized and kept at spontaneous respiration. A cannula (ID 1.02 mm) was inserted into the left femoral vein for infusion of Ringers acetat (10 ml:kg^{-1} min^{-1}). Another cannula was passed into the left femoral artery and was used for measurement of arterial pressure and heart rate and for withdrawal of blood samples. A third cannula inserted into the left ventricle of the heart, was used for injection of microspheres.

The experimental setup is shown in Figure 1. The stomach was perfused with isotonic saline kept at pH 1.0 by pH-stat titration. Mucosal blood flow was determined by radioactive microspheres 15 ± 1 u in diameter [11,12]. Celiac artery blood flow was measured continuously by Doppler ultrasound [13]. Gastric blood flow could be reduced by tightening a vessel loop placed around the celic artery.

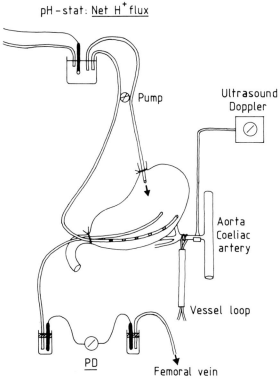

FIGURE 1: *Saline maintained at pH 1 by pH-stat titration was circulated from a reservoir via an esophageal tube into the stomach and returned to the reservoir via a duodenal tube at rate of 5 ml/min. Transmucosal potential difference (PD) was measured by means of agar bridges inserted into the stomach and the right femoral vein and connected via calomel electrodes to a voltmeter. A vessel loop and an ultrasound Doppler probe were placed around the celiac artery allowing reduction of celiac artery blood flow in a controlled manner.*

MUCOSAL DAMAGE:

Superficial mucosal damage was induced by instillation of 30 ml of 2M NaCl into the stomach for 10 min. Deep mucosal lesions were produced by application of 30 ml of absolute ethanol into the stomach for two min. Before and after exposure to 2M NaCl or ethanol the stomach was perfused with saline at pH 1.0.

MORPHOLOGIC EXAMINATION

After completion of an experiment initial fixation of the mucosa was performed by instillation of 30 ml of Bouin's solution for 10 min. The stomach was then opened, inspected and photographed. After this the stomach was fixed in Bouin's solution for at least two days, and samples from the anterior and posterior walls of the corpus were prepared for microscopic examination. Microscopically the mucosal lesions were graded according to the classification recommended by Lacy and Ito [14]: I = damage to surface mucous cells; II = damage to gastric pits in addition to extensive luminal surface cell damage; III = damage to gastric glands in addition to grad I- and II-damage.

RESULTS

EFFECT OF STRONG ACID (PH 1.0) ON 2M NaCl-DAMAGED MUCOSA WITH INTACT OR INHIBITED HYPEREMIC RESPONSE.

Exposure of the cat gastric mucosa to hypertonic saline (2M NaCl) results in damage to the surface epithelium and the upper part of the pits accompanied by increased mucosal blood flow, and restitution of the mucosa occurs within 90 min, even in the presence of strongly acidic luminal solution [10]. The present experiment was undertaken to test the hypothesis that the increased blood flow after mucosal damage is important for the rapid mucosal repair.

Two experimental groups were used. In a group of 8 animals the stomach was perfused with saline at pH 1.00 for 30 min, after which the perfusion was stopped and the mucosa exposed to 2M NaCl for 10 min, followed by washout and re-establishment of gastric luminal perfusion at pH 1.0 for 90 min. Mucosal blood flow was determined before mucosal damage and 15 and 90 min after the damage. In a second group of 8 cats the celiac artery flow was reduced by about 60% by partial clamping of the artery, immediately after mucosal exposure to 2M NaCl. Apart from this, the experiment was conducted in the same way as in the first group.

The blood flow values of the corpus mucosa are recorded in Table 1. The corpus blood flow increased markedly (p<0.001) after treatment with 2M NaCl in Group 1. Partial clamping of the celiac artery in Group 2 inhibited the hyperemic response after mucosal exposure to 2M NaCl.

TABLE 1

pH 1.0 EXPERIMENT

Corpus mucosal blood flow (ml: $min^{-1} g^{-1}$)

	Before 2M NaCl	After 2M NaCl 15 min	After 2M NaCl 90 min
Group 1 (n=8)	0.33 ± 0.05	0.94 ± 0.12	0.76 ± 0.09
Group 2 (n=8)	0.44 ± 0.06	0.54 ± 0.10	0.42 ± 0.06

Mean values ± SEM.

Group 1:   *Mucosal exposure to 2M NaCl for 10 min and gastric luminal perfusion with saline at pH 1.0 before and after 2M NaCl.*

Group 2:   *Exposure to 2M NaCl followed by gastric perfusion at pH 1.0 and 60% reduction of celiac artery blood flow.*

Microscopic examination of the corpus mucosa 90 min after treatment with 2M NaCl (Group 1) revealed epithelial restitution in most of the mucosa (Table 2). Only one percent of grade III lesions was found. However, when the celiac artery blood flow was reduced after treatment with 2M NaCl (Group 2), about 13% of the mucosa showed grade III lesions.

TABLE 2

pH 1.0 EXPERIMENT

Microscopic lesions in cat corpus mucosa exposed to 2M NaCl for 10 min followed by luminal perfusion at pH 1.0 for 90 min and intact (Group 1) or reduced (Group 2) celiac artery blood flow (percent of surface lengths).

	Grade of mucosal damage 0	I + II	III	Epithelial Restitution
Group 1	16.2 ± 6.0	7.5 ± 0.4	1.0 ± 0.4	77.1 ± 5.5
Group 2	16.4 ± 5.4	7.5 ± 2.7	13.6 ± 3.5	62.6 ± 6.6

Mean values ± SEM

Effect of Ethanol on 2M NaCl-Damaged Mucosa With Intact or Inhibited Hyperemic Response

It is well known that exposure of normal gastric mucosa to absolute ethanol may result in deep mucosal lesions [14]. In the present study we want to find out how gastric mucosa, which is already injured by hypertonic saline, responds to ethanol, and in particular we want to test the importance the hyperemic response occurring after application of 2M NaCl.

Three groups of anaesthetized cats were used for the experiment. In 5 animals (Group 1) the gastric mucosa was exposed to 2M NaCl for 10 min, and 20 min later the animals were sacrificed to obtain information about the condition of the mucosa at a time interval corresponding to that of ethanol application in Groups 2 and 3. In a second group of 8 animals (Group 2) the gastric mucosa was exposed to 2M NaCl for 10 min, followed after 20 min by mucosal exposure to absolute ethanol for two min. The animals were killed 15 min after ethanol application. A third group of 8 animals (Group 3) was treated as Group 2 except that celiac artery blood flow was reduced by about 60% about 8 min before and during ethanol treatment. The second injection of microspheres was given during celiac artery flow reduction.

As shown in Table 3 the corpus mucosal blood flow increased markedly ($p < 0.001$) after mucosal exposure to 2M NaCl. The subsequent application of absolute ethanol did not cause further increase in blood flow (Group 2). A 60% reduction of celiac artery blood flow (Group 3) inhibited the hyperemic response after appliction of 2M NaCl.

TABLE 3

Ethanol Experiment

Corpus mucosal blood flow (ml:min^{-1} g^{-1})

	Before 2M NaCl	15 min After 2M NaCl	10 min After Ethanol
Group 1 (n=5)	0.58 ± 0.20	1.21 ± 0.28	
Group 2 (n=5)	0.39 ± 0.07	0.97 ± 0.13	1.03 ± 0.10
Group 3 (n=5)	0.42 ± 0.04	0.39 ± 0.05	$.62 \pm 0.08$

Mean values ± SEM

Group 1:   *Mucosal exposure to 2M NaCl for 10 min.*

Group 2:   *Treatment with 2M NaCl followed after 20 min by exposure to absolute ethanol for two min.*

Group 3:   *Treatment with 2M NaCl followed by exposure to ethanol during celiac artery flow reduction.*

A summary of the microscopic findings is given in Table 4. Twenty min after treatment with 2M NaCl (Group 1) the mucosa showed extensive damage of the surface epithelium while most of the glands were intact. In animals with intact hyperemic response to 2M NaCl (Group 2) the application of absolute ethanol did not cause further mucosal damage. About 9% of grade III lesions were obtained both in Group 1 and Group 2. When the hyperemic response to 2M NaCl was inhibited (Group 3) grade III lesions were found in 39% of the mucosal surface, which differed significantly from the value obtained in Group 2 (p<0.005).

TABLE 4

ETHANOL EXPERIMENT

Microscopic lesions in cat corpus mucosa
(per cent of surface lengths).

	0	Grade of mucosal damage I	II	III	Epithelial Restitution
Group 1	6 ± 4	65 ± 5	10 ± 4	9 ± 5	9 ± 3
Group 2	10 ± 4	44 ± 6	14 ± 4	9 ± 5	24 ± 5
Group 3	2 ± 1	36 ± 8	12 ± 4	39 ± 8	11 ± 4

Mean values ± SEM

Same groups as in Table 3.

Group 1:   *20 min after mucosal exposure 2M NaCl.*

Group 2:   *15 min after ethanol which was applied 20 min after*
mucosal exposure to 2M NaCl.

Group 3:   *Same as Group 2 except that ethanol was applied during*
celic artery flow reduction.

Figures 2 and 3 show representative examples of microscopic lesions in corpus mucosa of Groups 2 and 3.

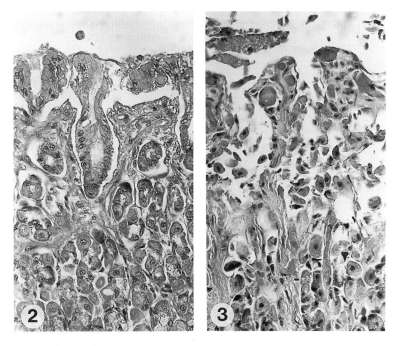

FIGURE 2 AND 3: *Cat corpus mucosa exposed to 2M NaCl for 10 min followed after 20 min by exposure to absolute ethanol for 2 min, with intact (Fig. 2) or 60% reduction of celiac artery blood flow (Fig. 3). Figure 2 shows mucosa with damaged surface epithelium and upper part of a pit, but with intact glands. Figure 3 shows necrosis of the luminal part of corpus mucosa including the upper part of the glands.*

DISCUSSION

In the present experiment cat gastric mucosa injured by exposure to hypertonic saline was used as a model to study resistance of damaged mucosa against aggressive agents.

Since 2M NaCl causes extensive damage to the surface epithelium, the present experimental model can not be used to study effects of strong acid or ethanol on surface mucous cells. On the other hand the model is well suited to study changes in the glandular layer of damaged mucosa.

Cat gastric mucosa, which had already been damaged by 2M NaCl, showed surprisingly high resistance against strong acid (pH 1.0) and even absolute ethanol neither of which caused damage to the glandular layer as long as the hyperemic response to hypertonic saline was intact. On the other hand both strong acid and ethanol caused extensive damage to the glandular layer (III-damage) when the hyperemic response was inhibited.

It should be noticed that by 60% reduction of the celiac artery blood flow the hyperemic response after application of 2M NaCl was eliminated. The gastric mucosal blood flow was reduced to about the same level as that obtained before the administration of 2M NaCl. However, the stomach was not ischaemic.

The mucosal damage caused by 2M NaCl is associated with increased flux of H^+ from the lumen into the mucosa when the luminal pH is low [10]. The protection provided by increased blood flow is probably due to increased elimination of H^+ ions and improved supply of HCO_3^- by the high mucosal blood flow.

The rapid development of deep mucosal lesion after instillation of absolute ethanol into the stomach indicates that ethanol is transported rapidly into the mucosa. The protection offered by the high blood flow after application of 2M NaCl may be explained as a result of rapid elimination of ethanol by the blood stream.

In conclusion the results of the present studies show that the hyperemic response occurring after gastric mucosal injury is of vital importance for protection of the mucosa during the early phase of restitution.

REFERENCES

1.   Grønbech JE, Matre K, Stangeland L, Svanes K, Varhaug JE. Gastroenterology 1988; 95: 311-20.

2.   Cheung LY, Moody FG, Reese RS. Surgery 1975; 77: 786-92.

3.   McGreevy JM, Moody FG. Surgery 1981; 89: 337-41.

4.   Cheung LY, Chang N. J Surg Res 1977; 22: 357-61.

5.   Whittle BJR. Br J Pharmacol 1977; 60: 455-60.

6.   Puurunen J. Eur J Pharmacol 1980; 63: 275-80.

7.   Svanes K, Grønbech JE, Varhaug JE. Mucosal blood flow. In: Cheli R, Berri F, Molinari F, Parodi MC, Eds. Gastric Protection, New York: Raven, 1988: 1-11.

8.   Pihan G, Majzoubi D, Haudenschild C, Trier JS, Szabo S. Gastroenterology 1986; 91: 1415-26.

9.   Leung FW, Robert A, Guth PH. Gastroenterology 1985; 88: 1948-53.

10.   Grønbech JE, Grong K, Varhaug JE, Lekven J, Svanes K. Gastroenterology 1987; 93: 753-64.

11.   Heyman MA, Payne BD, Hoffman JIE, Rudolph AM. Progr Cardiovasc Dis 1977; 20: 55-79.

12.   Varhaug JE, Svanes K, Svanes C, Lekven J. Am J Physiol 1984; 247:G468-G479.

13.   Matre K, Segadal L, Engedal H. J Biomed Eng 1985; 7: 84-8.

14.   Lacy ER, Ito S. Gastroenterology 1982; 83: 619-25.

QUANTITATIVE HISTOLOGY IN THE ASSESSMENT OF GASTRIC MUCOSAL INJURY AND PROTECTION

Gary M. Frydman, Cathy Malcontenti, Angela G. Penney, Paul E. O'Brien

Monash University Department of Surgery,
Alfred Hospital, Melbourne, Australia

Since the original description of gastric cytoprotection by prostaglandins there have been many studies which have sought to further characterize this phenomenon. The initial report was based on the macroscopic assessment of the rat stomach after injury by ethanol as well as other injurious agents [1]. Subsequently many reports have appeared which have extended the observations of Robert *et al* using similar methods of assessment of damage. Lacy and Ito [2], in a careful histological evaluation of the process of cytoprotection demonstrated that macroscopic assessment of the gastric mucosa was misleading. Macroscopic assessment of the gastric mucosa relies upon visual expressions of injury which consist mainly of haemorrhage into the mucosa, bleeding onto the surface, or the presence of slough and desquamated tissue. This does not allow for assessment of deep mucosal injury. It is therefore believed that some form of histological assessment of the gastric mucosa is required to make a valid estimate of the extent of tissue injury.

We have developed a reproducible technique for quantitative histological evaluation of the amount of gastric mucosa injured following application of an injurious agent to the stomach. This technique provides a measure of the surface area of the stomach damaged expressed as a percentage of total surface area, and a measure of the volume of mucosa damaged as a percentage of the total volume of the gastric mucosa.

We have utilized this technique to re-assess the proposed protective properties of a variety of agents used in the treatment of peptic ulcer disease against ethanol injury. These agents include the histamine H_2 receptor antagonists cimetidine and ranitidine, the substituted benzimidazole compound omeprazole, colloidal bismuth subcitrate, the sulphated aluminium sucrose compound, sucralfate, and the antimuscarinic drug pirenzepine. We have also used this technique of quantitative histology to assess the influence of time after injury on the histological expression of gastric mucosal injury. It is possible that full expression of the extent of injury has not occurred following a short period of time such as 15 to 30 minutes after ethanol injury. during this period.

Underestimation of mucosal injury after a short time period may be due to inadequate time for tissues to develop histological evidence of cell death or for killed cells to be excluded from the gastric mucosa gastric mucosa. The possibility of tissue fixation by the irritant must also be

327

considered. Saario et al [3] proposed that application of 100% ethanol to the isolated amphibian gastric mucosa resulted in fixation of the tissue with the persistence of a normal histological appearance at a time when physiological parameters indicated tissue death. Schmidt and Miller have previously eluded to the possibility of fixation of the gastric mucosa following 100% ethanol exposure in the intact animal [4]. However this has not previously been rigourously tested. We have therefore tested the effect of time on the expression of gastric mucosal injury following various concentrations of ethanol in rats pretreated with either saline or prostaglandin utilizing quantitative histology.

MATERIALS AND METHODS

Adult Long-Evans rats (200-300 gram) were purchased from the Monash Central Animal Breeding Unit and maintained on standard rat chow prior to experiments. Each animal was fasted for 24 hours and deprived of water for two hours prior to the experiment.

PREPARATION OF TEST AGENTS

Prostaglandin E_2 (PGE) was purchased from Sigma (St. Louis) as a crystalline powder, which was dissolved in 100% ethanol to give a concentration of 1 mg/ml, which was stored as a stock solution at $-4^{\circ}C$. Immediately prior to use, a test solution was prepared by the addition of an aliquot of the stock solution to normal saline to provide a final concentration of 25 ug/ml. Enprostil, a synthetic analogue of PGE_2, was a gift from Syntex Research and was stored as a solid at $-10^{\circ}C$. The test solution was prepared by dissolving Enprostil in ether (0.4 ml/mg) and then mixing with Tween 80 (0.02 ml/mg). The ether was completely evaporated with nitrogen gas and the residue mixed with Sorensen's phosphate buffer at pH 6.8 to make a final concentration of 0.25 ug Enprostil per ml. of Sorensen's buffer. Cimetidine (Smith, Kline & French) was obtained as a solution of 200 mg/2 ml. An aliquot of this solution was taken and made up with normal saline to give a strength of 20 mg/ml. Ranitidine (Glaxo) was obtained as a solution containing 50 mg/ml. An aliquot of this solution was taken and made up with normal saline to provide a test solution containing 10 mg/ml. Colloidal bismuth subcitrate (De-Nol, Parke Davis) was obtained as tablets containing 107.7 mg of bismuth. Each tablet was crushed and dissolved in normal saline to prepare a stock solution of 4 mg/ml. Sucralfate (DuPont) was obtained as tablets containing 1 g Sucralfate. Each tablet was crushed and dissolved in saline to prepare a test solution of 10 mg/ml. Pirenzepine was a gift from Boehringer Ingelheim Pty. Ltd. as pure substance. It was dissolved in normal saline to make up two test solutions containing 0.4 mg/ml or 4 mg/ml. Omeprazole, a gift from Astra Pharmaceuticals as a pure substance, was added to a solution of normal saline containing 0.5% hypermellose and raised to pH 9.0 with the addition of sodium bicarbonate. The final concentration in the test solution was 4 mg/ml. All test solutions were prepared on the day of experiment.

HISTOLOGICAL PREPARATION

After one hour in buffered formalin the stomach was opened along the greater curvature, pinned flat adjacent to a calibration ruler and photographed. After overnight fixation in buffered formalin the specimens were prepared for histology by dividing the flattened stomach in the following standard manner. Two transverse strips, each approxiametly 6mm wide were cut from the stomach with the upper line of section based on the fundo-rumenal junction as shown in Figure 1. The lower margin of strip A contained only gastric fundic mucosa. The lower margin of strip B contained a segment of antral mucosa. These A and B strips were then divided into two segements to allow for easy embedding and subsequent sectioning. These cut edges were then embedded in paraffin by standard techniques, and mounted in such a way that sections showing the full length of the gastric glands, from the surface epithelium to the muscularis mucosa, could be obtained. Three micron sections were cut and the sections stained with haematoxylin and eosin.

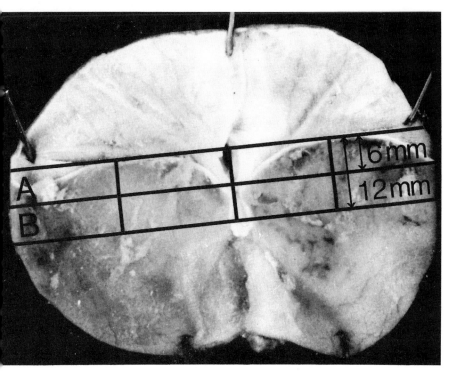

FIGURE 1: *photograph of the opened rats stomach showing the whitish forestomach superiorly, separated by the forestomach ridge from the darker gastric corpus. An overlying ridge shows the sites of samplying. Sections were cut from the full width of the lower margin of the A strip and B strip.*

QUANTITATIVE ASSESSMENT

The extent of microscopic damage was assessed by techniques previously described in detail [5]. On histological examination, the criteria for damage were the absence or gross disruption of gastric mucosal cells. The length of the damaged surface epithelium was used as a measure of the area of the gastric mucosa damaged, and the area of each section showing damage was used as a measure of the volume of the mucosa damaged. These were assessed by the use of a drawing attachment to the microscope (Olympus BH with a S-Plan Apochromat objective and an Olympus BH-D drawing attachment). Using the drawing attachment, tracings were made of the muscularis mucosa and the surface epithelium. If the surface epithelium was intact a solid line was drawn and where the mucosa was damaged a broken line was drawn. A line was then drawn through the mucosa indicating the interface of damaged and intact mucosa (Figure 2).

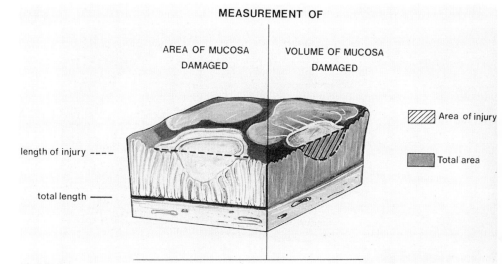

FIGURE 2: *Schematic diagragm of the gastric mucosa showing the method of histological quantification. On the left hand side of the diagram the dotted line corresponds to the length of damaged mucosa. The solid line represents the total mucosal length. The ratio of these lengths gives the percentage of damaged mucosal surface area. On the right hand side of the diagram the hatched area corresponds to the volume of mucosa injured. This figure is divided by the total mucosal area and expressed as the percentage volume of mucosa injured.*

Using an IBM computer digitising system attached to a HIPAD digitiser and the software package "MEASURE", version 2.15 (Capricorn Scientific, Melbourne) the extent of mucosal damage was quantified. The length of the damaged surface epithelium was measured and divided by the total mucosal length. This figure was then used as a measure of the surface area of the damaged gastric mucosa and expressed as a percentage of total mucosal area. The volume of mucosal damaged was quantified and divided by the total mucosal volume. This was the measure of total mucosal volume damaged and expressed as a percentage of total mucosal volume. The amount of mucosal damage seen in the A1 and A2 sections were then averaged and expressed as the amount of injury seen in that experimental animal. A previous study showed that there was no difference in the amount of injury seen whether 2 or 8 sections were taken therefore only A1 and A2 sections were cut [5].

EXPERIMENTAL PROCEDURES

Animals were briefly anaesthetised with 100% CO_2 to allow for instillation of the test drug via an oro-gastric tube (Table 1). Eight minutes later rats were anaesthetised with methohexitone sodium (Lily) in a dose of 75mg/kg via intraperitoneal injection. The abdomen was then opened via a left subcostal incision and a small bulldog vascular clamp placed across the oesophagus and duodenum.

Part 1: Assessment of anti-ulcer agents

In the study to assess the protective properties of the anti-ulcer agents rats were subjected to instillation of 100% ethanol intragastrically in a dosage of 10 ml/kg body weight, 30 minutes after instillation of the test agent. Fifteen minutes later, the ethanol was removed from the stomach and the stomach inflated with fixative, removed and placed in further fixative.

Part 2: Effect of time on expression of injury

In the experiments to assess the effect of time on the expression of histological injury either 50% or 100% ethanol was instilled into the stomach in a dose of 5ml/kg body weight 15 minutes after instillation of the either PGE_2 or saline. Control groups of rats were given normal saline in similar volumes. After the mucosa was exposed to the ethanol for 15 minutes, the ethanol was aspirated from the stomach via a needle placed in the gastric rumen. Fixation of the stomach was performed either at 30 minutes or at 24 hours after instillation of ethanol. For the early fixation group the animal was kept anaesthetised and after 30 minutes, fixation was achieved by inflating the stomach with 5 mls of phosphate buffered formalin (pH 7.2) followed by removal of the stomach and its immersion in further formalin. For the animals in the late fixation groups, the stomach was initially reinfused with 0.5 mls of normal saline to replace gastric fluid volume and the abdomen was then closed with 3/0 silk sutures. Each rat was sacrificed at 24 hours and the stomach was inflated with 5 mls of phosphate buffered formalin and removed.

ANALYSIS OF DATA

Group data are expressed as mean $\pm$ SEM. The significance of differences between groups was estimated using Mann-Whitney U-test for unpaired nonparametric data.

RESULTS

Part 1: Assessment of anti-ulcer agents

The effects of ethanol alone and after pretreatment by prostaglandins are shown in Figure 3. Ethanol alone causes extensive loss of the surface epithelium and a loss of 14% of the volume of the mucosa. Pretreatment with prostaglandin, either as natural PGE_2 or the synthetic analogue Enprostil, significantly reduced the amount of gastric superficial injury following 100% ethanol exposure compared to saline control animals. This involved a reduction in the amount of surface injury from 76.5% of the mucosa in saline treated animals to 40.0% and 46.9% of the mucosal surface in PGE_2 and Enprostil treated rats respectively. Both prostaglandins were associated with a marked reduction of the volume of the mucosa damaged. Colloidal bismuth subcitrate showed a clear protective effect against the development of the deep necrotic lesions with a total volume of mucosa damaged being only 2.7% (Figure 3).

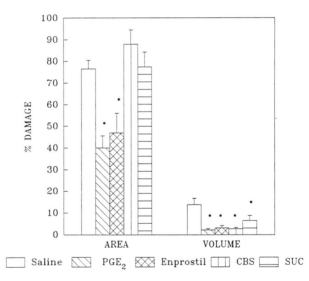

FIGURE 3 *This shows the extent of surface and mucosal epithelial damage by ethanol after pretreatement with saline, natural PGE_2, Enprostil, CBS, or SUC. * $p <0.05$ compared with saline controls. Values expressed as mean $\pm$ sem.*

This effect is comparable to that of natural PGE_2 and Enprostil. In contrast to these prostaglandins, however, no protection against surface epithelial damage was present. The use of a higher dose of colloidal bismuth subcitrate (350 mg/kg) was not associated with any further improvement in the protective effect. At this dosage, $78 \pm 28\%$ of the area of the mucosa was damaged and $6.0 \pm 6.2\%$ of the volume of the mucosa was damaged. These values are not significantly different from those achieved with the lower dosage. Sucralfate also showed a protective effect against the formation of deep necrotic lesions with a significant reduction in the volume of mucosa damaged (Figure 3). finding that increased dosage of sucralfate does not appear to show a more protective effect. At a dosage of 500 mg/kg the extent of surface epithelial damage was 61.1 $\pm$ 30% and 2.5 $\pm$ 3.0% of the volume of the mucosa was damaged. If sucralfate was acting as a simple physical barrier it might be expected that an increase of dosage by 20-fold would lead to a more marked protective effect but this was not seen. The histamine H_2 receptor antagonists, cimetidine and ranitidine, the anti-muscurinic drug, pirenzepine, and the substituted benzimidazole compound Omeprazole, showed no protective effects (Figure 4).

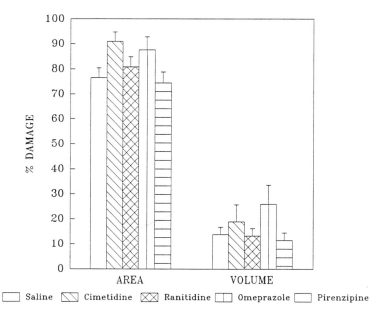

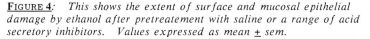

FIGURE 4: *This shows the extent of surface and mucosal epithelial damage by ethanol after pretreatement with saline or a range of acid secretory inhibitors. Values expressed as mean $\pm$ sem.*

Part 2 Effect of time on expression of injury

Injury with 100% Ethanol

In studies in which rats were pretreated with normal saline prior to 100% ethanol exposure histological assessment of injury 30 minutes after ethanol exposure grossly underestimated the amount of mucosal damage seen when the mucosa was assessed after 24 hours (Table 1, Figure 5).

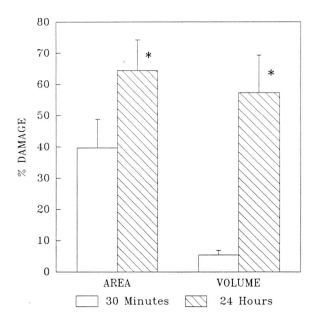

FIGURE 5: *The surface area and volume of gastric mucosa damaged following application of 100% ethanol following saline pretreatment. Values expressed as mean ± sem.* * *indicates significant difference from the thirty minute group*

The histological appearance of the gastric mucosa 24 hours after ethanol exposure was that of either full thickness cell loss to the level of the muscularis mucosa or that of an intact mucosa. In some mucosal areas that appeared intact, the surface cells appeared flattened and attenuated indicating prior mucosal restitution. When the gastric mucosa was pretreated with PGE_2 the amount of deep mucosal damage was again underestimated when assessment was performed at 30-minutes compared to 24 hours after ethanol exposure. However at 24 hours the amount of deep mucosal damage seen is significantly less than the volume of mucosa destroyed when no pretreatment with PGE_2 was given (Figure 6).

No difference was seen in the amount of mucosal surface area damaged after PGE_2 pretreatment when assessed either at 30 minutes or 24 hours (Table 1). Once again the extent of surface area damaged in the groups sacrificed at 24 hours after injury shows that in animals pretreated with PGE_2 a small but significant reduction in injury is noted compared to the equivalent group of rats not treated with PGE_2 (Table 1).

TABLE 1

TREATMENT GROUPS AND EXTENT OF DAMAGE, EXPRESSED
AS A PERCENTAGE OF TOTAL AREA AND VOLUME.
VALUES ARE MEAN ± SEM.

		TREATMENT PROTOCOL			EXTENT OF DAMAGE	
Group	N	Pretreat	%ETOH	Sacrifice	Area	Volume
1	12	Saline	100%	30min	39.7± 9.1	5.4± 1.5
2	12	Saline	100%	24hrs	64.4± 9.9	57.3±12.0
3	10	PGE_2	100%	30min	48.1± 8.1	6.4± 1.7
4	12	PGE_2	100%	24hrs	44.4± 7.7	33.4± 7.7
5	10	Saline	50%	30min	67.6± 6.1	16.8± 3.2
6	14	Saline	50%	24hrs	42.9± 8.3	23.8± 8.1
7	8	PGE_2	50%	30min	35.9±10.3	6.8± 3.6
8	13	PGE_2	50%	24hrs	14.3± 4.3	3.8± 1.4
9	5	Saline	25%	30min	9.4± 1.7	0.3± 0.2
10	8	Saline	25%	24hrs	17.3± 6.2	0.6± 0.3

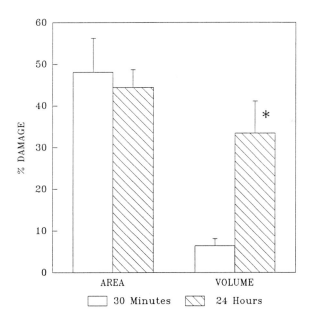

FIGURE 6: *The effect of PGE_2 assessed at 24 hours following 100%
ethanol exposure on the amount of surface area and volume of mucosa
damaged. Values expressed as mean ± sem. * indicates significant
difference from the thirty minute group*

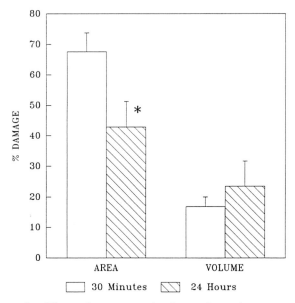

FIGURE 7: *The surface area and volume of gastric mucosa damaged following application of 50% ethanol following saline pretreatment. Values expressed as mean ± sem. * indicates significant difference from the thirty minute group*

Injury with 50% ethanol

There was no disparity in the extent of deep mucosal injury seen after 50% ethanol exposure when the mucosa is assessed histologically at either 30 minutes or 24 hours. However, the extent of surface area damage is significantly less at 24 hours, a change which could be attributable to restitution occurring during that time (Figure 7). Pretreatment with PGE_2 significantly reduced the amount of both suferficial and deep mucosal injury seen when assessed at either 30 minutes or 24 hours after 50% ethanol exposure although this is more apparant when assesses at 24 hours.

DISCUSSION

We have utilized a quantitative histological technique to re-evaluate the cytoprotective properties of a range of drugs used in the treatment of peptic ulcer disease. We have shown that PGE_2, enprostil, CBS and SUC protect the gastric mucosa from ethanol injury. In contrast we have been unable demonstrate any protective action for cimetidine, ranitidine, omeprazole or pirenzepine to reduce the extent of ethanol injury.

PGE_2 and the stable prostaglandin E_2 analogue, Enprostil, demonstrated a profound ability to reduce ethanol induced injury. At a dose of 1 ug/kg enprostil reduced both the area of the mucosa damaged and the volume of mucosal damage to an extent equivalent to that achieved by 100ug/kg of natural PGE_2. As the dosage of both agents is insufficient to cause inhibition of acid secretion, the protective effect is presumed to be achieved through augmentation of gastric mucosal defence mechanisms [6]. In previous studies we have demonstrated a direct protective effect of Enprostil on the structure and permeability of the mucosal microvasculature [7], thereby promoting the maintenance of an intact microcirculation. The relative importance of this and other defence mechanisms in the process of cytoprotection remains to be established.

Our findings that both these prostaglandins reduce the amount of gastric mucosal surface damage following ethanol instillation has not been previously reported. Most histological studies are unable to measure any detectable surface protection following ethanol injury however we have repeatedly been able to detect surface protection following pretreatment with prostaglandins. These studies also clearly and repeatedly indicate that both PGE_2 and Enprostil significantly reduce the extent of surface epithelial damage to the gastric mucosa following ethanol instillation. In the original histological studies of Lacy and Ito [2] such protective effect was not noted. Subsequently, it has been frequently stated that whilst the protective effect of prostaglandins against deep necrotic lesions is accepted, no protection against the extent of surface epithelial damage can be expected. Our studies provide, by using quantitative histological methods, a clear definition of protection of the surface epithelium. The extent of this protection is less than the extent of protection against the volume of mucosa damaged, but is a consistent and clear finding. In a recent report Henegan *et al* [8] was able to demonstrate that prostaglandins administered prior to aspirin exposure reduced the amount gastric mucosal surface injury.

CBS and SUC were able to reduce the amount of deep mucosal injury seen after 100% ethanol exposure. The extent of reduction is equivalent to that achieved by natural or synthetic prostaglandin E_2. However CBS and SUC whilst being able to protect the gastric mucosa from deep ethanol damage are unable to reduce the amount of ethanol induced surface mucosal damage. As CBS and sucralfate are potent protective agents against acute irritants and potent stimuli for the healing of peptic ulcer, study of the possible mechanisms of action of theses agents are appropriate. Despite using oral doses of cimetidine, ranitidine and omeprazole which are sufficient to cause some inhibition of acid secretion, thereby excluding the possibility of missing a "cytoprotective" effect due to inadequate doses we were unable to protect any protective effects of these agents. Tarnawski reported similar results for cimetidine and ranitidine [9]. Reports which describe the protective properties of omeprazole have utilized only macroscopic assessment of the stomach [10-12]. No histological study to confirm the extent of injury has previously been performed.

Similarly we ahve been unable to demonstrate any protective effect of pirenzipine on ethanol induced gastric mucosal injury. This agent has previously been reported to protect the gastric mucosa against ethanol in the rat [13-14]. Anti-secretory effects for pirenzepine can be noted in the rat at concentrations of 6 mg/kg [20]. None of these studies indicated a protective effect against ethanol damage at doses of less than this antisecretory dose. Furthermore macroscopic criteria for damage were utilized in each study. It

should therefore be concluded that on current data a cytoprotective effect
for pirenzepine against ethanol damage has not been proven.   In the second
part of the study, however we have shown that there is insufficient
expression of cell death when the mucosa is examined histologically 30
minutes after 100% ethanol exposure. This involves the underestimation of
the amount of injury of both surface area as well as the mucosal volume. Of
greater importance however is the extent of the volume of mucosa damaged
as this indicates penetrating injury to the gastric mucosa which will require
repair by cell division.

Saario et al [3] showed that application of 100% ethanol to isolated
sheets of amphibian gastric mucosa rapidly and instantaneouly killed the
gastric mucosal cells when measured by physiological parameters.
Histological examination however of the gastric mucosa revealed the
appaerance of an intact gastric mucosa. They proposed that 100% ethanol
acted as a fixative and that the killed mucosal cells had been fixed to the
basement membrane.

Application of 100% ethanol to the gastric mucosa causes cessation of
gastric mucosal blood flow [16-20]. This reduction in mucosal perfusion
would render the stomach at least in part ischaemic. This cessation of blood
flow following 100% ethanol is focal in nature, precedes epithelial cell
necrosis [20], and can be seen to occur in areas which show subsequent
mucosal erosion [17,20].

We propose that the reduction of mucosal perfusion that occurs in the
intact animal following 100% ethanol exposure allows for the fixation of
gastric mucosal cells, as can be demonstrated following 100% ethanol
exposure to isolated gastric mucosal tissue.

Previous studies of the influence of time on histological expression of
injury have not shown the discrepancy noted in this study. Schmidt et al [21-
22] was unable to detect any difference in the amount of histological
damage seen 5, 20, 60 minutes and at 2, 8 and 24 hours after 100% ethanol
exposure. They used a lower dose of ethanol than used in our studies which
would become more prone to dilution by gastric juices.

Tarnawski et al [23] used a dosage of 100% ethanol similar to that
used in this study reported that 46% of the gastric mucosa was injured 15
minutes after 100% ethanol exposure. By 16 hours later 68% of the gastric
mucosa was reported to be injured. This suggests that 22% of the gastric
mucosa which was assessed as being un-injured was later thought to be
injured. These findings although not showing the extent of underestimation
shown in this study do support the proposal that early histological
assessment of injury following 100% ethanol injury is incomplete.

When 50% ethanol was used as the injurious agent, no difference
could be seen in the amount of deep mucosal damage seen after the two time
periods. In contrast however, there was a substantially significant reduction
in the extent of superficial damage seen 24 hours after injury. This
difference is probabaly due to restitution of areas of minor damage of the
gastric mucosal surface.

The process of cytoprotection generated a vast amount of work and interest into the process of this phenomenon. The original description as well as early studies into this process relied exclusively on macroscopic assessement. Since the landmark finding of Lacy and Ito some form of histological assessement is often used to assess the protective properties of various agents. With the use of a quantitative histological technique, we have confirmed the cytoprotective effect of natural and synthetic prostaglandin E_2, colloidal bismuth subcitrate and sucralfate. The prostaglandin agents appear to be able to reduce the amount of surface mucosal damage seen after ethanol damage. No cytoprotective effect for ethanol damage to the rat stomach has been shown in this study for cimetidine, ranitidine, omeprazole or pirenzepine.

Injury by 100% ethanol, although being criticised as being inappropriately severe [24], remains a standard form of injury. We have shown that histological assessment of the gastric mucosa 30 minutes after 100% ethanol exposure was grossly underestimated, probabaly due to fixation by 100% ethanol. This finding does not suggest that all results obtained using 100% ethanol as an injurious agent are not valid, but does provide a reason for the re-evaluation of certain crucial pieces of data and of anomalous results.

ACKNOWLEDGEMENT

This study was supported by a Grant from the
National Health and Medical Research Council of Australia.

REFERENCES

1.   Robert A, Nezamis JE, Lancaster C, Hanchar AJ. Cytoprotection by prostaglandins in rats. Gastroenterology 77:433-43, 1979

2.   Lacy ER, Ito S. Microscopic analysis of ethanol damage to rat gastric mucosa after treatment with a prostaglandin. Gastroenterology 83:619-25, 1982

3.   Saario I, Rosen S, Carter K, Silen W. Effect of ethanol on frog gastric mucosa: Electrophysiologic and morphologic correlations. Gastroenterology 94:638-46, 1988

4.   Schmidt KL, Miller TA. Ultrastructural aspects of prostaglandin cytoprotection in an alcohol injury model. J Clin Gastroenterol 10:S84-S92, 1988

5.   O'Brien P, Schultz C, Gannon B. An evaluation of the phenomenon of cytoprotection using quantitative histological criteria. J Gastroenterol Hepatol 2:113-121, 1987

6.   Miller TA. Protective effects of prostaglandins against gastric mucosal damage: current knowledge and proposed mechanisms. Am J Physiol 245:G601-G623, 1983

7.   O'Brien P, Schultz C, Gannon B, Browning J. Protective effects of the synthetic prostaglandin Enprostil on the gastric microvasculature after ethanol injury to the rat. Am J Med 81:12-17, 1986

8.   Henegen JM, Scmidt KT, Miller TA. Prostaglandin prevents aspirin injury in the canine stomach under in vivo but not in vitro conditions. Gastroenterology 97:649-659, 1989

9.   Tarnawski A, Hollander D, Gergely H, Stachura J. Comparison of antacid, sucralfate, cimetidine, and ranitidine in protection of the gastric mucosa against ethanol injury. Am J Med 79:19-23, 1985.

10.   Kollberg B, Isenberg JI, Johansson C. Cytoprotective effect of omeprazole on the rat gastric mucosa. In: Mechanisms of Mucosal Protection in the Upper Gastrointestinal Tract. Ed: A. Allen et al. Raven Press, New York. 1984; pp 351-356.

11.   Okabe S, Miyake H, Awane Y. Cytoprotective effects of NC-1300 and omeprazole on HCl-ethanol-induced gastric lesions in rats. Japan J Pharmacol 42:123-133, 1986

12.   Konturek SJ, Brzozowski T, Radecki T. Protective action of omeprazole, a benzimidazole derivative, on gastric mucosal damage by aspirin and ethanol in rats. Digestion 27:159-164, 1983

13.   Konturek SJ, Brzozowski T, Radecki T, Piastucki I. Gastric cytoprotection by pirenzepine: Role of endogenous prostaglandins. Scand J Gasteroent 17:255-259, 1982

14.   Takeda F, Kitagawa H, Kohei H. Gastric cytoprotection by pirenzepine in rats: Evaluating method for cytoprotective activity by antisecretory agents. Japan J Pharmacol 38:337-346, 1985

15.   Martinotti E, Bernardini C, Del Tacca M, Pellegrini M, Soldani G, Bertelli A. Gastric cytoprotection by pirenzepine is not mediated by catecholamines. Acta Physiologica Hungarica 64:219-224, 1984

16.   Oates PJ, Hakkinen JP. Studies on the mechanism of ethanol-induced gastric damage in rats. Gastroenterology 94:10-21, 1988

17.   Guth PH, Paulsen G, Nagata H. Histologic and microcirculatory changes in alcohol-induced gastric lesions in the rat: effect of prostaglandin cytoprotection. Gastroenterology 87:1083-1091, 1984

18.   Ohya Y, Guth P. Ethanol induced gastric mucosal blood flow and vascular permeability changes in the rat. Dig Dis Sci 33:883-888, 1988

19. Pihan G, Majzoubi D, Haudenschild C, Trier J, Szabo S. Early microcirculatory stasis in acute gastric mucosal injury in the rat and prevention by 16,16-dimethyl prostaglandin E_2 or sodium thiosulfate. Gastroenterology 91:1415-1426, 1986

20. Bou-abboud C, Wayland H, Paulsen G, Guth P. Microcirculatory stasis precedes tissue necrosis in ethanol induced gastric mucosal injury in the rat. Dig Dis Sci 33:872-877, 1988

21. Schmidt KL, Bellard RL, Smith GS, Henagan JM, Miller TA. Influence of prostaglandin on rat stomach damaged by absolute ethanol. J Surg Res 41:367-377, 1986

22. Schmidt KL, Henagan JM, Smith GS, Hilburn PJ, Miller TA. Prostaglandin cytoprotection against ethanol-induced gastric injury in the rat: a histologic and cytologic study. Gastroenterology 88:649-659, 1985

23. Tarnawski A, Hollander D, Strachura J, Krause WJ, Gergeley H. Prostaglandin protection of the gastric mucosa against alcohol injury - a dynamic time-related process. Gastroenterology 88:334-352, 1985

24. Silen W. Experimental models of gastric ulceration and injury. Am J Physiol 255:G395 - G402, 1988

INTERCELLULAR MATRIX IN THE GUT:
PUTATIVE ROLES IN GASTRIC PROTECTION

O.W. Wiebkin, D. Hillen, S.C. Wiebkin, D.J.C. Shearman

Department of Medicine, University of Adelaide,
Royal Adelaide Hospital, Adelaide, South Australia

ABSTRACT

Characterization of intercellular matrices of different tissues reveals that the populations of macromolecular protein-polysaccharides (proteoglycans) as well as glycoproteins fulfill many structural and functional roles. An understanding of these molecules in the gut has been largely ignored. The present study shows that distinct pools of proteoglycans can be identified such that tissue-specific distribution would imply tissue-specific function. While connective-tissue (lamina propria)-derived proteoglycan pools from stomach, jejunum and duodenum are similar, pools for epithelium of two gastric sites (body and antrum) and jejunum are different. The study focuses on a proteoglycan peak rich in heparan sulphate and dermatan sulphate. The hypothesis is that this is a glycosaminoglycan hybrid and is represented by a slow turnover pool described in metabolic studies in vitro. A role in gastro-protection is presented.

INTRODUCTION

Degradation, modification and alteration of the intercellular matrix have been recognized as important in several degenerative or inflammatory diseases e.g. osteo- and rheumatoid arthritis, periodontal disease and nephritis [1]. Such conditions commonly demonstrate a loss of tissue integrity. Even though microvasculature, prostaglandin E levels and mucus production, luminal pH and epithelial restitution are but few of the major factors that are quoted as responsible for aspects of gut protection, it is surprising that little or no attention has been paid to the role of the intercellular matrix in the intrinsic protection of the gut. Nor do we know to what extent disease-modified matrix in the gastric mucosa compromises repair or protection.

We have previously implied that the intercellular matrix is yet another pivotal component of the "mucosal barrier" [2]. Following that preliminary report, the present study attempts to further address the dearth of information about a class of intercellular macromolecules, the proteoglycans, in the gastric mucosa. Quantitatively these proteoglycans represent the major components of the intercellular matrix within which the constituent cells and fibrous proteins are embedded. Furthermore, it is within this highly charged aqueous-polymer matrix that all extracellular

343

biochemical events actually occur e.g. antibody-antigen reactions, hormone to receptor interactions, enzymatic digestion and matrix turnover in development and wound healing.

By analogy with known functions of the matrix components of other tissues, we offer putative roles for these molecules which we are now identifying in the gastric mucosa. Moreover, since we can compare and contrast tissue-specific differencs in the intercellular proteoglycans from other gastrointestinal sites we will especially focus on their role in maintenance of tissue integrity.

MATERIALS AND METHODS

MATERIALS

DEAE Sephacel and Sepharose CL4B were purchased from Pharmacia LKB, Uppsala, Sweden, tissue culture materials from Flow Laboratories, Va, US, and [^{35}S]-sulphate from Amersham Radiochemicals, UK. Cellulose acetate electrophoresis strips were supplied by Chemitron Milan, Italy. While all supplies of Alcian blue were satisfactory for electrophoresic staining, only Gurr Batch No. 870827 (BDH, Poole, UK) did not precipitate out at the higher molarities of $MgCl_2$ necessary for histochemistry. Testicular hyaluronidase, trypsin and chondroitinase ABC were purchased from Sigma Chemical Co., Mo, US or Seikagaku Kogyo, Tokyo, Japan. International standards of glycosaminoglycan were kindly supplied by Dr. M. Matthews, Chicago, U.S.A.

Human gastrointestinal tissues were clinically and histopathologically healthy and processed for histochemistry or biochemistry within 2 h of resection. Tissues used for metabolic studies were used immediately, either washed in Dulbecco's Modified Eagles Medium (DMEM) or undisturbed. Control tissues were snap frozen in 80% ethanol (-57°C). To separate epithelium from connective tissue, fresh gastrointestinal tissues freed of fat, were incubated in 10mM EDTA [3]. The jejunum and duodenum yielded clean separation of epithelial cells and lamina propria uncontaminated with fibroblasts or epithelial cells respectively. Stomach separations resulted in a discrete separation of the epithelium from about two thirds down the crypt. Connective tissue preparations must, therefore, be regarded as "predominantly lamina propria". Three independent separations were generally made for gastric specimens and wet weights obtained for each of them.

EXTRACTION AND DIGESTION OF INTERCELLULAR MATRIX POLYSACCHARIDES

Sequential exhaustive overnight extractions in 0.5 M Na acetate (pH5.6) and 4M guanidinium chloride (4M GuHCl) (pH 5.6) or direct 4M GuHCl extraction for chemical analysis were undertaken.

Intercellular-matrix digestion was achieved with testicular hyaluronidase, (1mg/ml) or trypsin, (650u/ml), pH6.5 60°C and 37°C for 90 min or 3 hours respectively.

CHROMATOGRAPHY AND ELECTROPHORESIS AND ASSAYS

All chromatographic fractionation was performed on ethanol precipitated extracts (4 vols). Pellets were resuspended in either 0.5-5ml of 4M GuHCl or in 16 mls 7M Urea/Tris. In spite of the viscous nature of the denatured insoluble residue, glycosaminoglycan was identified in only one gastric-epithelial sample. Material dissolved in 9 mls 7M urea was applied to DEAE Sephacel. After equilibration, elution with a continuous linear gradient was undertaken to achieve 2M NaCl.

Both material dissolved in 2.5 ml 4M GuHCl or hydrolysed samples (0.3N NaOH) were fractionated on Sepharose CL-4B with 4M GuHCl. Electrophoresis on cellulose acetate of hydrolysed fraction was performed in 0.2M Ca Acetate buffer containing 17% ethanol (pH7.2) [4]. Standards, enzyme elimination and nitrous acid reduction were used to identify specific glycosaminoglycans.

Glycosaminoglycans were assayed with dimethyl methylene blue [5] and uronic acid [6] and protein with micro Biuret or at A280. Chondroitin sulphate and bovine serum albumin were standards. [^{35}S]-sulphate incorporation was measured in ethanol-precipitated hydrolysed tissue samples with carrier glycosaminoglycan.

IN VITRO METABOLIC STUDIES

Tissue pieces were incubated for 24 h and 48 h in [^{35}S]-sulphate (carrier-free) supplemented DMEM with 5% FCS. [^{35}S]-sulphate released into radioactive-free media was monitored over the subsequent 7 days. Viability was determined periodically by post incorporation of [^{3}H]-leucine into trichloracetic acid precipitates.

HISTOCHEMISTRY

Histology was performed at all stages of tissue preparation. Fixation was achieved by immersing tissue into 80% ethanol at -56°C. Limited mobility of water-soluble materials occurs during thawing. Alcian blue staining at the critical electrolyte concentrations, 0.06M to 0.8M $MgCl_2$, was undertaken as was enzyme elimination with hyaluronidase (<5TRU) or chondroitinase ABC (0.25u). Positive and negative controls included rat tongue and cartilage and heat-inactivated enzyme or buffer alone.

RESULTS AND DISCUSSION

STRUCTURAL ROLES OF MATRIX

Of those extrinsic factors which determine the maintenance of gastric-mucosal integrity, the purely physicochemical molecular arrangements at the epithelial/luminal surface appear to be important. These arrangements include rheologically relevant glycoprotein entanglements of the mucus, the presence of surfactants and the buffering protection against acid damage by "entrapped" bicarbonate. In other mucosal tissues such as the gingivae or bladder, which are mainly devoid of mucus, the role of intercellular proteoglycans has long been described as fulfilling such physicochemical protection [7,8]. In the mucosa of the gut where the presence of mucus is predominant, proteoglycans have been largely ignored.

The extraction of intercellular matrix materials from the gastric mucosa under aqueous conditions, especially in the presence of a cocktail of exogenous protease inhibitors [9], yields proteoglycans which are substantially intact. Other soluble glycoproteins and some fibrous proteins are also liberated. Unlike the residual tissue-bound components such as cell surface trans-inserted macromolecules, and structural scaffold molecules, the "soluble" molecules represent the intercellular polymer matrix amongst which intercellular events occur. The ease with which these matrix macromolecules can be extracted reveals something about both their size and about the simplicity of their binding to other tissue compartments.

TABLE 1

EXTRACTION AND DIGESTION OF INTERCELLULAR MATRIX
PROTEOGLYCAN FROM THE INTERCELLULAR MATRIX OF GASTRIC MUCOSA

a. Extractant conditions	% of total uronic acid	
	Epithelium	Lamina Propria
EDTA 10mM (30 min)[1]	not detectable	
Sequential		
- 0.5 MNaAc (associative)[2]	74	43
- 4MGuHCl (dissociative)[2]	26	55

[1]conditions for separating epithelium from connective tissue [3].
[2]exhaustive sequential

> **N.B.** *Epithelium released material more easily than the connective tissue. The dissociative conditions necessary indicates ionic organisation in the intercellular matrix.*

b. Enzyme	% [^{35}S] of total[3] intact gastric pieces
Hyaluronidase[4]	54.5
Trypsin[5]	69.8

[3] gastric mucosa pre-incubated in [^{35}S]
[4] testicular hyaluronidase degrades hyaluronate, chondroitin sulphate A and C.
[5] limited hydrolysis (lysine/argine residues)

> **N.B.** *Both hyaluronidase and trypsin have limited capacity to remove all intercellular proteoglycan suggesting a non chondroitin sulphate, tightly bound cryptic and orderly proteoglycan component in the intercellular matrix.*

Preliminary data on aqueous extractability of uronic acid-rich components (glycosaminoglycans) show that the short (30 min) chelating process necessary for separating epithelium from underlying connective tissue in 10mM EDTA is mild enough to avoid detectable extraction of matrix. However, exhaustive overnight extraction of the separated tissue, achieved under mild associative conditions (0.5 M Na acetate), shows that the gastric epithelium retains only a quarter of its uronic acid, while the connective tissue retains about one half (Table 1). The subsequent exposure of the tissue to more severe dissociative conditions (4M GuHCl) shows that ionically-mediated entanglement plays a major role in maintaining the orderly arrangement of these components in their intercellular compartments. About half of the total sulphated glycosaminoglycan-rich complement in intact [35S]-sulphate labelled tissue, is susceptible to testicular hyaluronidase. This suggests that hyaluronate and chondroitin sulphate 4 and 6 are major carbohydrate moieties. The former is not represented by [35S]-sulphate but its presence may play a role in the integrity of the intercellular polymer network of the stomach. Indeed, the clear observation that the bulk of proteoglycans in both epithelium and connective tissue is of large hydrodynamic size (Figure 1) which will elute at Kavs of 0.85 and variously beyond 0.5 respectively, and that they are rich in chondroitin sulphate, implies a structural function. In conclusion, these findings, which are broadly similar to those in other tissues, point to equivalent space-filling and structural roles for large proteoglycans in the gastric mucosa.

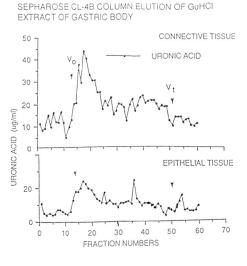

FIGURE 1: *Chromatography on Sepharose CL-4B of proteoglycans extracted in 4M GuHCl from gastric mucosal (a) connective tissue (b) epithelium.*

BIOLOGICAL FUNCTIONS OF THE PROTEOGLYCAN

Apart from the protective role that the physicochemical presence of proteoglycans around cells might play, many biological functions have also been attributed to these macromolecules. Some of the more important biological functions demanded by the gut mucosa might include the regulation of cell adhesion, ligand binding on cell surface receptors for hormones and growth factors [10], substrata for epithelial migration [11] and regulators of enzyme action [12]. Proteoglycans can be directly implicated in all these functions [13]. Relevant to the microvasculature is the role of thrombin-binding octasaccharide on heparin or the specific binding affinity for fibronectin or thrombospondin of cell surface heparan sulphate proteoglycans [14,15]. The lymphocyte homing receptor CDw44, is also a proteoglycan [16].

Thus the biological functions of the proteoglycans can be exploited by specific tissues or their tissue compartments. To accommodate this range of functions the family of proteoglycans contains a structurally diverse membership. Although proteoglycans are represented by such a very wide spectrum of macromolecular structures, all consist of a substantially basic parent form; a linear protein core generally containing the serines which might be variously 0- or N-glycanated with a glycosaminoglycan. Glycosaminoglycans are unbranched sulphated polysaccharides, generally consisting of repeating disaccharides of uronic acid or galactose and hexosamine. Chondroitin-, dermatan- and heparan sulphates and heparin contain uronic acid or iduronic acid whilst keratan sulphate is unique by having galactose substituted for the uronic acid.

Heparan sulphate proteoglycans (HSPG) have been shown to occupy all cell surfaces and, increasingly, their structures and functions are being recognized. Other groups of intercellular polymers are described for intercellular compartments and sites more remote from cells. These range from hyaluronate (3×10^6 D) (a proteo-free glycosaminoglycan) in the synovial fluid and in the vitreous of the eye, to the large aggregating chondroitin sulphate-rich proteoglycans of cartilage which interact with hyaluronate to produce massive (30×10^6 D) aggregates (aggrecans). Other smaller proteoglycans containing only one or two glycosaminoglycans are specifically associated with collagen (decorin) and other fibrous proteins (biglycan). While HSPG can be found inserted in the plasma membrane and function to bind transferrrin or growth factors, they can also be isolated from basement membranes. Since the epithelium of the gastric mucosa is a component of the mucosal barrier, the relevant intercellular components such as basement membrane HSPG or other members of the heparan sulphate family are likely to play a role in gastric protection. We now describe preliminary characterization of these components.

ION EXCHANGE CHROMATOGRAPHY

The proteoglycan-rich material extracted under dissociative aqueous conditions (4M GuHCl) from gastric-body epithelium is easily separated from any neutral glycoproteins and less highly charged hyaluronate into two populations on DEAE Sephacel. The epithelia of gastric antrum revealed a more polydispersed profile while jejunum, which has a different structure and function, showed yet a different and more discrete profile (Figure 2).

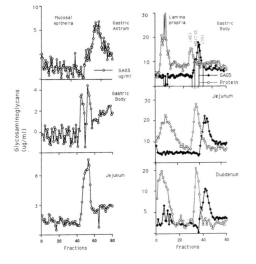

FIGURE 2: *DEAE Sephacel: ion exchange chromatography of 4M GuHCl extracts from (a) mucosal epithelium: gastric - body and antrum and jejunum; and (b) lamina propria: gastric, duodenal and jejunum.*

Conversely the proteoglycan population distribution in the lamina propria of all the gastrointestinal tissues sampled, suggested a similar "blue print" throughout these underlying connective tissues. The underlying connective tissue from stomach, jejunum and duodenum contained one polydispersed population of proteoglycans.

Electrophoretic separation of 0.3N NaOH hydrolysates shows that both the epithelium and the connective tissue contained both dermatan- and chondroitin sulphate proteoglycans. In another proteoglycan fraction isolated from both gastric epithelium and connective tissue, both heparan sulphate and chondroitin sulphate appear to be so closely associated in a single ion-exchange peak that the presence of a proteoglycan hybrid, similar to syndecan [17], is proposed. The special roles for syndecan in providing a specific substratum for epithelial mobility [11] and its effect on epithelial differentiation [18] make this an important candidate component for mucosal integrity.

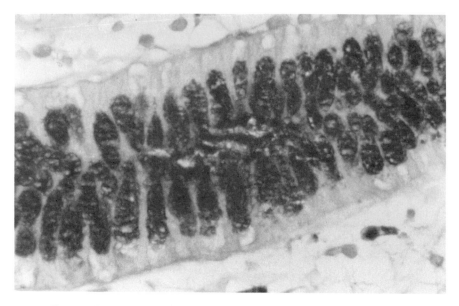

FIGURE 3:   *Mucosal epithelium stained with Alcian blue for (a)
glycoprotein (PAS), proteoglycan at 0.1M MgCl$_2$ (Alcian blue)(b) goblet
Alcian blue staining is abolished at 0.3M MgCl$_2$ but note basement
membrane and luminal retention.*

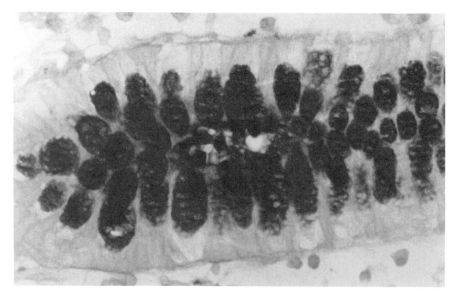

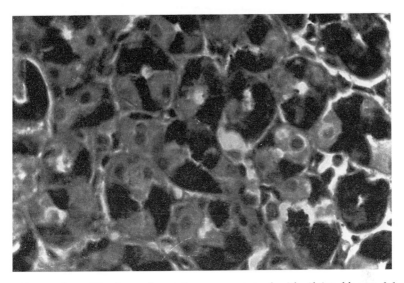

FIGURE 4a: *Histology of gastric mucosa stained with Alcian blue at 0.1 M MgCl$_2$ to feature chondroitin sulphate, dermatan sulphate, heparan sulphate and/or heparin.*

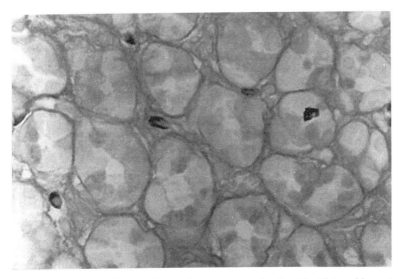

FIGURE 4b: *Histology of gastric mucosa stained with Alcian blue at 0.3M MgCl$_2$ elimates staining of hyaluronate, chondroitin- and dermatan sulphates (residual stain is susceptible to nitrous acid reduction).*

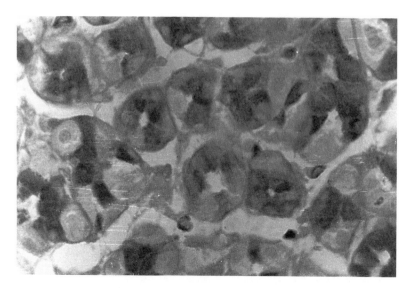

FIGURE 4c: *Histology of gastric mucosa stained with Alcian blue at 0.2M $MgCl_2$ to leave detmatan and heparan sulphates alone.*

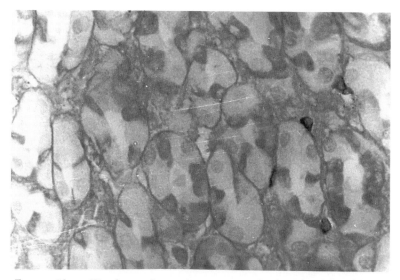

FIGURE 4d: *Histology of gastric mucosa stained with Alcian blue at 0.2M $MgCl_2$ after chondroitinase ABC to remove dermatan sulphate and to leave heparan sulphate. N.B. residual heparin/disulphated chondroitin containing mast cells in b and d.*

LOCALIZATION OF SPECIFIC PROTEOGLYCANS

We are yet to analyse the small proteoglycans or to bind anti-syndecan, -biglycan or -decorin monoclonal antibodies to them, either on PAGE or in tissue sections, but other histological evidence is available. Periodic acid Schiff-positive glycoproteins are vacariously localized in gastric and intestinal lining cells as are the proteoglycans which can be stongly stained with conventional Alcian blue techniques (Figure 3).

Although the histology shows that most gastric epithelial cells contain both proteoglycan and mucus, presumably destined for secretion, some are relatively devoid of proteoglycan. Either these cells are able to differentially eject or deplete their total stores of proteoglycan, or they differentially synthesize it. In other studies in progress, we have separated distinct hyaluronate and chondroitin sulphate bands on cellulose acetate electrophoresis from the glycoprotein of the mucus secreted by these cells. Again we must pose questions about the gastro-protective function and special regulation of these macromolecules in a milieu of mucus. However, it is the postulated roles for proteoglycan in the gastric mucosa itself that are fundamentally involved with maintenance of the tissue's integrity. Indeed in other experiments in which small pieces of pre-labelled [^{35}S]-sulphate human and rat gastric mucosae have been incubated for periods up to 36 hours, the turnover of the pre-labelled [^{35}S]-proteoglycan is very slow despite wholesale secretion of mucus. Maximal release does not appear until after 72 hours incubation [19]. The retention in the basement membrane of a discrete Alcian blue-binding substrate at CEC beyond 0.3 M $MgCl_2$, which shows milder susceptibility to chondroitinase ABC and little or no elimination with testicular hyaluronidase, suggest heparan- and dermatan sulphate components (Figure 4). The localization of a heparan sulphate/dermatan sulphate variant of the syndecan; the unique hybrid proteoglycan which has been identified and localised by others on the baso-lateral surfaces of simple epithelium [11] is suggested. Since the metabolic experiments do not show a ready loss of this molecule into the media of gastric-mucosal incubations, we believe that this hybrid proteoglycan may provide the mechanism whereby epithelial cells, liberated during restitution or following injury, will migrate (and differentiate) through a basket of this plasma-membrane associated material. It would remain essentially intact, ready to facilitate the migration and differentiation of subsequent daughter epithelial cells.

In summary, the hydrodynamically-large macromolecules which are likely to be integral in a water-logged supportive structure, will affect the diffusion of cell products and nutrients. Furthermore, this network of polymers can also interfere with the rates of reactions of say, degradative enzymes within it [12,20]. In pathology, breakdown of such fine structures are likely to have adverse consequences. In addition, we can emphasize the important biological roles being ascribed to the "minor" proteoglycans. Because we can only identify a presence of heparan sulphate and other hitherto poorly identified glycosaminoglycans and proteoglycans in intercellular gastric compartments, we can but wait for verification of their putative protective role.

ACKNOWLEDGEMENTS

The N.H. & M.R.C. funding to support S.C.Wiebkin and the project as well as consolidated funds from the Department of Medicine to support D.Hillen is gratefully acknowledged. We thank Mrs. Mary Marucci for typing of the manuscript and Mr. Peter Devitt for regular supply of human tissue. Ms. Susan Clare has been most helpful in histological matters.

REFERENCES

1. Harris ED. Rheumatoid Arthritis: Pathophysiology and Implication for Therapy. New Eng J Med 1989; 322: 1277-1289.

2. Wiebkin OW, Shearman DJC. Maintenance of gastric mucosal integrity. Active role for tissue specific intercellular matrix. Gastroenterol and Hepatol 1989; Supl:20-26.

3. Bartold PM, Wiebkin OW, Thonard JC. Glycosaminoglycans of human gingival epithelium and connective tissue. Connect Tiss Res 1989; 9: 99-106.

4. Bartold PM, Wiebkin OW, Thonard JC. Molecular weight estimation of sulphate glycosaminoglycan in human gingivae. Connect Tiss Res 1982; 9: 165-172.

5. Farndale RW, Buttle DJ, Barrett AJ. Improved quantitation and discrimination of sulphated glycosaminoglycans by use of dimethylmethylene blue. Biochim Biophys Acta 1986; 883: 173-177.

6. Blumenkrantz N, Asboe-Hansen G. A new method for quantitative determination of uronic acid. Anal Biochem 1973; 54: 484-489.

7. Bartold PM, Wiebkin OW, Thonard JC. The active role of gingival proteoglycans in periodontal disease. Med Hypoth 1983; 12: 377-387.

8. Morris B, Lambrano D. Transitional epithelium of urinary tract in normal and dehydrated rats. Z Zelforsch 1968; 85: 165-182.

9. Oegema TR, Hascall VC, Eisenstein R. Characterisation of bovine aorta proteoglycan extracted with guanidine hydrochloride in the presence of protease inhibitors. J Biol Chem 1979; 254: 1312-1318.

10. Termanini B, Nardi RV, Finan TM, Parikh I, Korman LY. Insulin-like growth factor I receptors in rabbit gastrointestinal tract: Characterisation and autoradiogrphic localisation. Gastroenterology 1990; 90: 51-60.

11. Bernfield M, Trelstad R. An epithelial cell-surface proteoglycan. In: Functions of the Proteoglycans. Ciba Foundation Symposium 1986; 124: 184.

12. Wiebkin OW. Regulation of the rates of reaction of enzymes within concentrated polymeric solutions (e.g. Hyaluronate). Proc Fed Europ Conn Tiss Soc 1986; 77.

13. Gallagher JT. The extended family of proteoglycans: social residents of the pericellular zone. Curr Opin Cell Biol 1989; 1: 1201-1218.

14. Kaesberg PR, Ershler WB, Esko JD, Masher DF. Chinese hampster ovary cell adhesion to human platelet thrombospondin is dependent on cell surface heparan sulphate proteoglycans. J Clin Invest 1989; 994-1001.

15. Sanders S, Bernfield M. Cell surface proteoglycan binds mouse mammary epithelial cell to fibronectin and behaves as a receptor for interstitial matrix. J Cell Biol 1988; 106: 423-430.

16. Coombe DR, Tider CC. Lymphocyte homing receptor cloned - a role for anionic polysaccharides in lymphocyte adhesion. Immunol Today 1989; 10: 289-291.

17. Rapraeger A, Jakanen M, Endo E, Koda J, Bernfield M. The cell surface proteoglycan from mouse mammary epithelial cells bears chondroitin sulphate and heparan sulphate glycosaminoglycans. J Biol Chem 1985; 260: 11046-11052.

18. Kato M, Kokenyensi R, Sanders S, Nguyen H, Bernfield M. Syndecan is required for epithelial morphology 1990 (unpublished report).

19. Wiebkin OW, Wiebkin SC, Shearman DJC. Mechanisms of peptic ulcer healing. Falk Symposium No. 59. Oct. 1990. (in press).

20. Laurent TC. Enzyme reactions in polymer media. Europ J Biochem 1971; 21: 498-506.

GASTRIC ADAPTATION TO REPEATED ADMINISTRATION OF A NECROTIZING AGENT

A. Robert, C. Lancaster, A.S. Olafsson, W. Zhang

*Safety Pharmacology, The Upjohn Company
Kalamazoo, Missouri, U.S.A.*

ABSTRACT

Oral administration of 0.2 M NaOH to fasted rats produced gastric mucosal necrosis, haemorrhages and edema. However, when 0.2 M NaOH was given repeatedly, every other day, gastric adaptation developed: the lesions became less severe as the number of treatments increased. Adaptation was first noticed after the second administration of NaOH, and was maximal after four treatments. This tolerance to NaOH disappeared after a six day rest during which the animals were not receiving NaOH. Histologically, the necrosis, hemorrhages and edema, seen after a single oral treatment, were no longer present during adaptation; instead, the gastric mucosa regenerated in spite of continued exposure to NaOH. The necrotic areas were replaced by granulation tissue, and new glands formed. During adaptation, the mucosal synthesis of prostaglandin E_2, 6-Keto PGF_1 and thromboxane B_2, was markedly increased. Pretreatment with indomethacin prevented the adaptation. Gastric acid secretion was not changed during adaptation. We conclude that the stomach has the ability to withstand damage by a necrotizing agent when the latter is administered repeatedly. The mechanism of this gastric adaptation is unknown, but is partially due to increased formation of prostaglandins by the mucosa.

INTRODUCTION

Short term administration of nonsteroidal anti-inflammatory drugs can produce gastroduodenal erosions and bleeding in animals [1,2,3] and humans [4,5]. However, long-term treatment with aspirin or indomethacin was shown to induce tolerance to the development of gastric lesions, both in animals [6,7,8] and humans [9,10]. Similarly, a single intragastric administration of mild irritants, e.g., 20% ethanol, 0.3 M HCl, 0.075 M NaOH, 4% NaCl, 10 mM taurocholate, prevents the formation of gastric mucosal necrosis produced by oral administration, 15 minutes later, of strong irritants such as 100% ethanol, 0.6 M HCl, 0.2 M NaOH, 25% NaCl [11], or acidified 80 mM taurocholate [12]. The damage to the rat gastric fundic mucosa following acute oral administration of 50% ethanol was reported to be significantly less in animals given ethanol chronically than in rats receiving ethanol acutely [13].

The mechanism by which gastric adaptation occurs is not known. In the case of certain mild irritants, the release of prostaglandins by the stomach has been implicated, and prostaglandin mediation was proposed as a

mechanism of protection [11,14,15]. In other studies, such mediation was not
demonstrated [16,17,18]. Certain drugs, such as sucralfate [19], bismuth
subsalicylate [20] acetazolamide [21] and diethyl maleate [22] exert gastric
cytoprotection against necrotizing agents while stimulating endogenous
prostaglandin release, whereas others, such as certain antibiotics [23],
meciadanol [24] and sulfhydryls [25], seem to protect the stomach by a
mechanism independent of prostaglandin release.

In the present studies, we investigated whether a necrotizing agent,
0.2 M NaOH, would induce gastric adaptation in rats upon continued
administration, and whether the mechanism of such adaptation involved
endogenous prostaglandins or changes in gastric acid secretion.

METHODS

SINGLE ADMINISTRATION OF 0.2 M NaOH

Female Sprague-Dawley rats of an average body weight of 230g were
fasted overnight. On the next morning, they received 1 ml of 0.2 M NaOH,
or water, orally and were killed one hour later. Their stomachs were
excised, opened along the greater curvature and examined with a 5 x
magnifier, without knowledge of the treatment. The necrotic lesions were
counted, and for each group was expressed as average number of lesions per
stomach. The method for assessing gross damage using the number of
lesions had been validated earlier by comparing the number of lesions
produced by aspirin [26] with the planimetric measurement of the damaged
areas. The correlation was very good: $r = 0.77$, $P = 0.03$. The stomachs were
fixed in 10% buffered formaldehyde, and 5 μm sections were stained with
hematoxylin-eosin, PAS and toluidine blue. The slides were coded before
examination.

REPEATED ADMINISTRATION OF 0.2 M NaOH

One ml of 0.2 M NaOH, or water, was given orally, and the treatment
was repeated every other day according to the following schedule. One hour
after the first treatment, the animals were given food and water *ad libitum*
until the next day at 3.00 p.m. at which time they were again fasted
overnight. On the next morning, 0.2 M NaOH was administered for the
second time, followed by refeeding one hour later. This schedule of 0.2 M
NaOH, refeeding and fasting every other day was repeated for a total of 4
times. Approximately 32 hours after the fourth administration of 0.2 M
NaOH, the animals were fasted overnight (at 3.00 p.m.) for the last time, and
on the following morning they received 1 ml of 0.2 M NaOH orally for the
fifth time (termed the "challenging dose"). Control animals received one ml
of water every other day instead of 0.2 M NaOH.

EFFECT OF INDOMETHACIN

One ml of 0.2 M NaOH was given orally every other day as described
above. On the day of the challenging dose of NaOH, indomethacin, 5 mg/kg
in one ml 1% $NaHCO_3$, was injected intraperitoneally. Ninety minutes later,
the animals received the challenging dose of 0.2 M NaOH orally, and they
were killed one hour later. This was done to determine whether gastric

adaptation would persist in the virtual absence of endogenous prostaglandins.

EFFECT OF REPEATED 0.2 M NaOH ON GASTRIC PROSTAGLANDINS

In a parallel study, the generation of PGE_2, by the gastric mucosa (corpus) was determined by radioimmunoassay, using an *ex vivo* method [27,11]. The PGE_2 content was expressed as ng/g of wet tissue.

ONSET AND DURATION OF GASTRIC ADAPTATION TO 0.2 M NaOH

For the onset of adaptation, groups of animals were killed after 1, 2, 4 and 6 treatments of 0.2 M NaOH, given every other day following an overnight fast. For the duration of adaptation, the animals were first treated with 0.2 M NaOH every other day for a total of 4 times, as described above, to achieve a state of gastric adaptation. A challenging dose of 0.2 M NaOH (1 ml) was then administered to separate groups of animals at various time intervals, from 1 to 6 days, after gastric adaptation had developed.

GASTRIC SECRETION DURING ADAPTATION TO 0.2 M NaOH

One ml of 0.2 M NaOH (or water) was given orally every other day for a total of 4 times, as described above. A challenging dose of 1 ml of 0.2 M NaOH was then given orally after an overnight fast. One hour later, the pylorus was ligated under ether anesthesia, and the animals were killed 4 hours later. A control group received 0.2 M NaOH (or water) only once, 1 hour before pylorus ligation. Gastric juice was collected through a cut in the forestomach. The volume was measured, and acidity was titrated with 0.01 M NaOH to pH7 with an automatic titrator (Zymark Robotics, Hopkinton, MA). The volume was expressed in ml/4 hours, the acid concentration in mEq/L, and the acid output in uEq/4 hours.

STATISTICAL ANALYSIS

The data were evaluated by analysis of variance, the Student t-test, and the Fisher exact test. Differences between groups with a P value of less than 0.05 were considered significant. The number of animals per group is indicated in the legends for Figures.

RESULTS

SINGLE ADMINISTRATION OF 0.2 M NaOH

Gastric lesions produced by a single oral administration of 0.2 M NaOH appeared as elongated black streaks located in the corpus mucosa (Figure 1-B). Histologically, the lesions consisted of mucosal necrotic tissue occupying up to four fifths of the mucosal thickness but not penetrating the muscularis mucosae (Figure 2-B). Hemorrhages within the necrotic tissue and intense vasocongestion at its periphery were prominent (Figure 2-C). The necrotic mass contained no recognizable cellular structures. Outside of the necrotic areas, the surface epithelium showed extensive exfoliation. The submucosa of the entire stomach was markedly edematous (Figure 2-B).

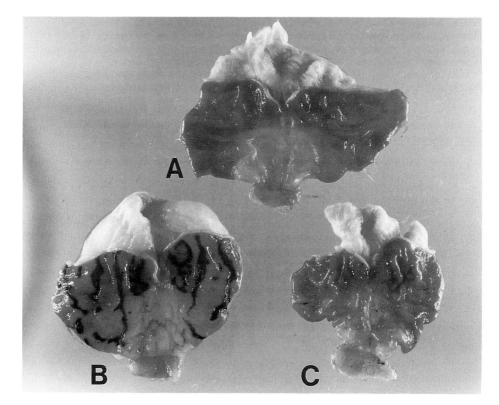

FIGURE 1   *Gastric adaptation to 0.2 M NaOH: gross lesions. Stomachs opened along the greater curvature. A. Normal stomach, opened along the greater curvature. B. Single oral administration of 0.2 M NaOH (1ml). Multiple lesions in the corpus mucosa. C. 0.2 M NaOH given orally 4 times, every other day, followed by a challenging dose of 0.2 M NaOH. Normal appearance of the gastric mucosa, demonstrating gastric adaptation.*

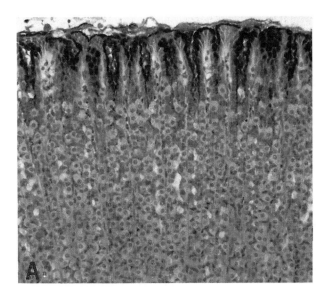

FIGURE 2A.   *Gastric histology during gastric adaptation to 0.2 M NaOH. A. Normal gastric mucosa. PAS, 40 x.*

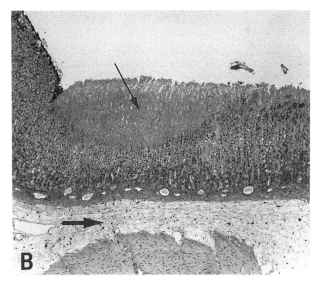

FIGURE 2B.   *0.2 M NaOH (1 ml) orally, animal killed 1 hour later. Large necrotic area of the mucosa (thin arrow). Submucosal edema (thick arrow). PAS, 16 x.*

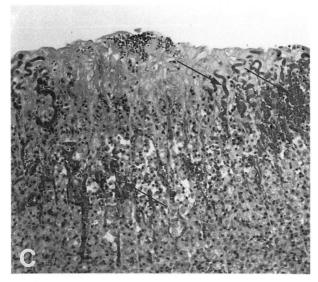

FIGURE 2C.   Same treatment as B. Intense vasocongestion at the margin
of the necrotic mass and in the tissue surrounding it (arrows). H & E,
40 x.

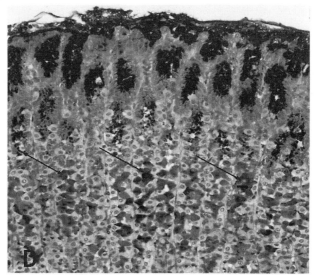

FIGURE 2D.   0.2 M NaOH (1ml) given orally 4 times (every other day),
followed by a challenging dose of 0.2 M NaOH. Normal looking mucosa.
Large number of mucus neck cells (arrows). PAS, 40 X.

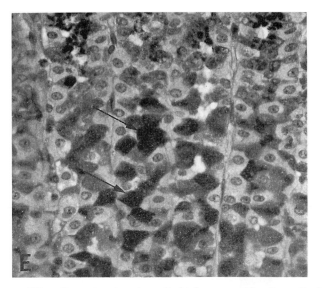

FIGURE 2E. *Same treatment as D, higher magnification. Proliferation of mucus neck cells containing PAS-positive cytoplasmic granules (arrows). PAS, 100 X.*

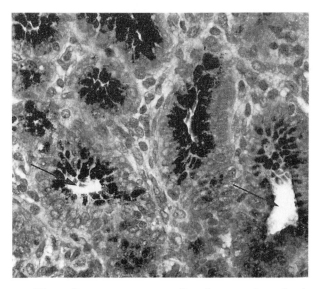

FIGURE 2F. *Same treatment as D. Regenerating glands with cyst formation (arrows). PAS, 100 X.*

REPEATED ADMINISTRATION OF 0.2 M NaOH

0.2 M NaOH given orally every other day for a total of 4 times reduced by 91% (P<0.001) the number of gross necrotic lesions by comparison with animals receiving 0.2 M NaOH only once (Figure 3). Fifty percent of the animals treated wih 0.2 M NaOH every other day had no gross lesion by comparison with an incidence of 100% in the controls (P<0.05). Figure 1-C illustrates the gastric adaptation to repeated 0.2 M NaOH. Administration of water every other day combined with fasting did not reduce gastric damage caused by a challenging dose of 0.2 M NaOH.

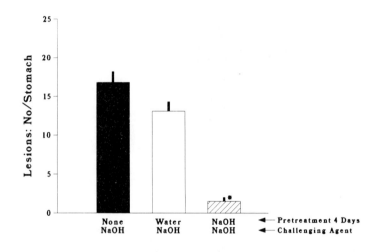

FIGURE 3.   Gastric adaptation to 0.2 M NaOH.   Animals given 0.2 M NaOH 4 times have 90% less gross lesions than animals given 0.2 M NaOH only once, or water 4 times. *P<0.001, n = 10.

Histologically, there was no necrosis, no hemorrhages, and no evidence of vasocongestion or submucosal edema (Figure 2-D). In PAS-stained sections, the amount of mucus in the surface epithelial cells appeared normal, but some portions of the surface epithelium were exfoliated; however, this change was less pronounced than in amimals given 0.2 M NaOH only once. The mucosa was 12% thinner (P<0.05) than that of control animals.   Three histological alterations were noticeable: a) Granulation tissue had developed in areas that had become necrotic earlier, that is when the mucosa was exposed to 0.2 M NaOH for the first time, and new glands had formed over the granulation tissue.   b) There was a proliferation of mucus neck cells. These were located above and within the parietal cell region, and their cytoplasm was PAS positive (Figure 2-E, 2-F). c) Several new glands had a cystic appearance (Figure 2-F), and were lined with cells whose cytoplasm stained positive with PAS. They probably are mucus cells.

<u>EFFECT OF INDOMETHACIN</u>

Pretreatment with indomethacin, 90 minutes before the challenging dose of 0.2 M NaOH, markedly reduced the degree of gastric adaptation (Figure 4).

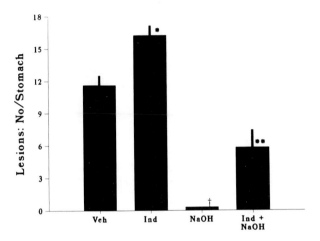

<u>FIGURE 4.</u>   *Prevention of gastric adaptation by indomethacin. 0.2 M NaOH given 4 times produced total adaptation of the gasric mucosa to a challenging dose of 0.2 M NaOH. Indomethacin, 5 mg/kg given 90 minutes before the challenging dose, markedly reduced the degree of adaptation. *P<0.05 and **P<0.01, vs. vehicle group. P<0.01 vs. all groups. n = 10.*

<u>PROSTAGLANDIN GENERATION DURING GASTRIC ADAPTATION TO 0.2 M NaOH.</u>

The generation of eicosanoids by the gastric mucosa was increased by repeated administration of 0.2 M NaOH by comparison to the values of control animals (either untreated or receiving a single administration of 0.2 M NaOH). The increases over values of untreated controls were: 25% for 6-keto $PGF_{1\alpha}$ (P<0.05), 32% for thromboxane B_2 (P<0.05), and 144% for PGE_2 (P<0.01, n = 8). (Figure 5).

<u>ONSET AND DURATION OF GASTRIC ADAPTATION</u>

Adaptation was first noted when the challenging dose of NaOH was given 24 hours after one pretreatment with 0.2 M NaOH (35% reduction of the number of lesions) (Figure 6). When two and four pretreatments were administered on alternate days, the inhibition rose to 70% and 79%, respectively.

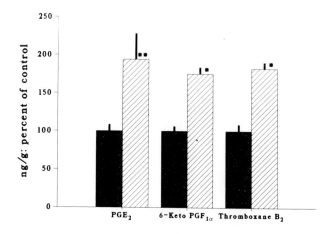

FIGURE 5. *Effect of repeated 0.2 M NaOH on eicosanoid generation by the gastric mucosa. Solid bars: water given orally. Hatched bars: 0.2 M NaOH (1 ml) given orally 4 times (every other day). Marked stimulation of eicosanoid synthesis. *P<0.05. **P<0.01. n = 8.*

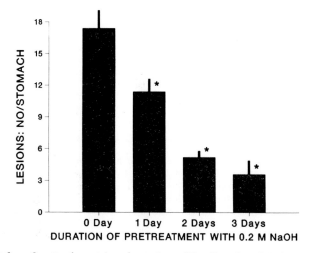

FIGURE 6. *Onset of gastric adaptation. The first bar ("0 day") shows the number of gastric lesions after a single administration of 0.2 M NaOH. The other bars refer to lesions obtained after repeated administration of NaOH, every other day. 1 day: 2 treatments. 2 days: 3 treatments. 4 days: 5 treatments. Gastric adaptation was related to the number of treatments with 0.2 M NaOH. *P<0.001. n = 8.*

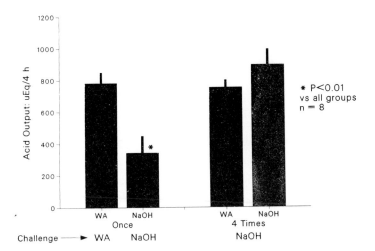

FIGURE 7. Duration of gastric adaptation. The first bar ("NaOH Once")
shows the number of gastric lesions after a single administration of 0.2
M NaOH. The other bars refer to animals that received NaOH 4 times,
every other day, and were rechallenged at various time intervals (1 to 6
days) thereafter. * and **P<0.05 and P<0.01, respectively, vs. first
group.

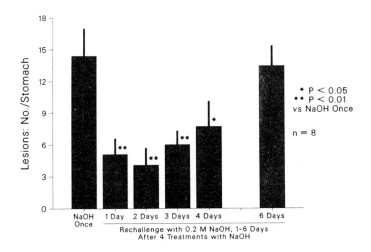

FIGURE 8. Gastric secretion during adaptation to 0.2 M NaOH. A single
administration of NaOH decreased acid secretion by 56%, whereas, NaOH
given 4 times prior to challenge with a fifth dose prevented such
inhibition.

Once gastric adaptation had been achieved by giving 0.2 M NaOH 4 times every other day, it lasted at least four days. (Figure 7). The response to a challenge dose of 0.2 M NaOH given after 1 to 4 days of rest still showed the same reduction in the number of gastric lesions (60-70% inhibition, $P<0.01$, n = 8); however, gastric adaptation was lost when the challenge with NaOH was given after 6 days.

GASTRIC SECRETION DURING GASTRIC ADAPTATION TO 0.2 M NaOH

A single oral administration of 0.2 M NaOH reduced gastric acid secretion by 56% ($P<0.01$) (Figure 8). However, repeated treatment (4 times) with NaOH prevented this inhibition of acid secretion.

DISCUSSION

The present results show that upon repeated exposure to 0.2 M NaOH, the rat gastric mucosa undergoes progressive adaptation to that necrotizing agent. Gastric adaptation is nearly complete after four treatments given every other day, and vanishes when the challenging dose of NaOH is administered 6 days after a 4 day treatment.

Gastric adaptation to 0.2 M NaOH seems to be largely dependent on endogenous prostaglandins. This was shown in two studies. First, the adaptation was prevented by pretreatment with indomethacin, an inhibitor of prostaglandin synthesis. Second, the generation of prostaglandins by the gastric mucosa was increased by repeated (4 times) administration of 0.2 M NaOH, that is, at a time when adaptation to the necrotizing agent was maximal. Since, however, gastric adaptation occurs also for aspirin [6,7,9,10] and indomethacin [8], two inhibitors of prostaglandin synthesis, it is likely that factors other than prostanoids also play a role.

The histological appearance of the gastric mucosa when adaptation had developed showed minimal damage. The changes characteristic of acute contact with 0.2 M NaOH (massive mucosal necrosis, hemorrhages, vasocongestion, edema) were absent. The only damage still present was limited to the surface epithlial monolayer, which showed spotty exfoliation. Deeper in the mucosa, granulation tissue in previously necrotic areas, and cystic formations in regenerating glands were noticeable; these changes indicate active repair of the areas that had been necrotic. The abundance of mucus neck cells is another sign of active regeneration of gastric glands.

The present results are consistent with findings reported by Ivey et al [13] that gastric adaptation develops in rats upon chronic administration of 50% ethanol. The major differences between their and our studies, in addition to the fact that they used ethanol whereas we used NaOH, are that in their study the animals were fed throughout, and the stomachs were examined eight hours after the last treatment with ethanol. In our studies, the animals were fasted overnight prior to each administration of the necrotizing agent, and they were killed one hour after the challenging dose.

The mechanism of gastric adaptation remains unexplained. Whether it involves changes in gastric mucosal blood flow, the elaboration of protective factors by the stomach in response to repeated administration of the necrotizing agent, changes in mucus secretion, increased secretion of epidermal growth factor by the salivary glands, or changes in gastric motility are possibilities that have not been explored. The reduced acid secretion by a single oral administration of 0.2 M NaOH is probably due to the extensive destruction of parietal cells. The fact that repeated treatment with NaOH prevented the inhibition of acid secretion elicited by a single treatment indicates that not only were parietal cells intact by histological examination but they were also functionally normal. We concluded, therefore, that gastric adaptation is not due to reduced acid secretion.

REFERENCES

1. Whittle BJR. Mechanisms underlying gastric mucosal damage induced by indomethacin and bile salts, and the actions of prostaglandins. Br J Pharmacol 1977; 60: 455-460.

2. Rainsford KD. Asynergistic interaction between aspirin, or other nonsteroidal anti-inflammatory drugs, and stress which produces gastric mucosal damage in rats and pigs. Agents Actions 1975; 5: 553-558.

3. Robert A. Antisecretory, antiulcer, cytoprotective and diarrheogenic properties of prostaglandin. Adv. Prostaglandin Thromboxane Res. 1976; 2: 507-520.

4. Lanza F, Royer G, Nelson R. An endoscopic evaluation of the effects of nonsteroidal anti-inflammatory drugs on the gastric mucosa. Gastrointest Endosc. 1975; 21: 103-105.

5. Hoftiezer JW, O'Loughlin JC, Ivey KJ. Effects of 24 hours of aspirin, Bufferin, paracetamol and placebo on normal human gastroduodenal mucosa. Gut 1982; 23: 692-697.

6. St. John DJB, Yeomans ND, McDermott FT, Boer WGRM. Adaptation of the gastric mucosa to repeated administration of aspirin in the rat. Am J Dig Dis. 1973; 18: 881-886.

7. Robert A, Lancaster C, Gilbertson-Beadling S, Olafsson AS, Guth PH. Gastric adaptation to aspirin-induced gastric erosions in rats. Gastroenterology 1989; 96: A418.

8. Shorrock CJ, Prescott RJ, Rees WDW. The effects of indomethacin on gastroduodenal morphology and mucosal pH gradient in the healthy human stomach. Gastroenterology 1990; 99: 334-339.

9. Graham DY, Smith JL, Dobbs SM. Gastric adaptation occurs with aspirin administration in man. Dig Dis Sci 1983; 28: 1-6.

10. Graham DY, Smith JL, Spjut HJ, Torres E. Gastric adaptation. Studies in humans during continuous aspirin administration. Gastroenterology 1988; 95: 327-333.

11. Robert A, Nezamis JE, Lancaster C, Davis JP, Field SO, Hanchar AJ. Mild irritants prevent gastric necrosis through "adaptive cytoprotection" mediated by prostaglandins. Am J Physiol. 1983; 245: G113-G121.

12. Chaudhury TK, Robert A. Prevention by mild irritants of gastric necrosis produced in rats by sodium taurocholate. Dig Dis Sci. 1980; 25: 830-836.

13. Ivey KJ, Tarnawski A, Stachura J, Werner H, Mach WT, Burks M. The induction of gastric mucosal tolerance to alcohol by chronic administration. J Lab Clin Med 1980; 96: 922-932.

14. Konturek SJ, Brzozowski T, Piastucki I, Radecki T, Dembinski A, Dembinska-Kiec A. Role of locally generated prostaglandins in adaptive gastric cytoprotection. Dig Dis Sci 1982; 27: 967-971.

15. Kobayashi K, Arakawa, Nakamura H. Adaptive cytoprotection by prostaglandins. Adv. Prostaglandin Thromboxane Leukotriene Res 1985; 15: 651-653.

16. Hawkey CJ, Kemp RT, Walt RP, Bhaskar NK, Davies J, Filipowicz B. Evidence that adaptive cytoprotection in rats is not mediated by prostaglandins. Gastroenterology 1988; 94: 948-954.

17. Smith GS, Parks LL, Myers SI, Miller TA. Increased prostaglandin synthesis is not responsible for ethanol-induced adaptive cytoprotection in the rat. Gastroenterology 1989; 96: A478.

18. Wallace JL. Increased resistance of the rat gastric mucosa to hemorrhagic damage after exposure to an irritant. Role of the "mucoid cap" and prostaglandin synthesis. Gastroenterology 1988; 94: 22-32.

19. Tarnawski A, Hollander D. Krause WJ, Zipser RD, Stachura J, Gergely H. Does sucralfate affect the normal gastric mucosa? Histologic, ultrastructural, and functional assessment in the rat. Gastroenterology 1986; 90: 893-905.

20. Konturek SJ, Radecki T, Piastucki I, Drozdowicz D. Advances in the understanding of the mechanism of cytoprotective action by colloidal bismuth subcitrate. Scand J Gastroenterol 1986; 21 (Suppl. 122): 6-10.

21. Robert A, Lancaster C, Davis JP, Kolbasa KP, Nezamis JE. Ulcer formation and cytoprotection by acetazolamide. Eur J Pharmacol 1985; 118: 193-201.

22. Robert A, Eberle D, Kaplowitz N. Role of glutathione in gastric mucosal cytoprotection. Am J Physiol 1984; 247: G296-G304.

23. Satoh H, Guth PH, Grossman MI. Role of bacteria in gastric ulceration produced by indomethacin in the rat: cytoprotective action of antibiotics. Gastroenterology 1983; 84: 483-489.

24. Konturek SJ. Kitler ME, Brzozowski T, Radecki T. Gastric protection by meciadanol. A new synthetic flavonoid-inhibiting histidine decarboxylase. Dig Dis Sci 1986; 31: 847-852.

25. Szabo S, Trier JS, Frankel PW. Sulfhydryl compounds may mediate gastric cytoprotection. Science 1981; 214; 200-202.

26. Robert A. Leung FW, Kaiser DG, Guth PH. Potentiation of aspirin-induced gastric lesions by exposure to cold. Gastroenterology 1989; 97: 1147-1158.

27. Whittle BJR. Higgs GA, Eakins KE, Moncada S, Vane Jr. Selective inhibition of prostaglandin production in inflammatory exudates and gastric mucosa. Nature 1090; 284: 271-273.

LOCAL AND REFERRED PROTECTION IN THE GASTRIC MUCOSA: PROSTAGLANDIN-INDEPENDENT AND PROSTAGLANDIN-DEPENDENT MECHANISMS

G.P. Morris, C.L. Donaldson, C.A. Holitzner,
K.H. Tufts, T.E. Williamson

*Gastrointestinal Disease Research Unit & Department of Biology,
Queen's University, Kingston, Ontario, Canada*

INTRODUCTION

The concept of cytoprotection has undergone a series of revisions since its articulation by Robert [1]. It was initially assumed that cytoprotective agents, particularly the prostaglandins (PG), strengthened or protected the "gastric mucosal barrier" and, by association, the luminal epithelium. Subsequent studies demonstrated that protection by PG against the development of hemorrhagic erosions did not necessarily involve preservation of the integrity of surface epithelial cells [2,3]. Further studies by Robert and his colleagues [4,5] introduced the concept of "adaptive cytoprotection" in which prior exposure of the gastric mucosa to an "irritant" provided protection of the same type as direct administration of PG. Since this protection was abolished by prior inhibition of cyclooxygenase by treatment with indomethacin, it was hypothesized that adaptive cytoprotection resulted from irritant-induced elevations in rates of mucosal PG synthesis [5]. This concept has also been modified subsequent to a series of studies which demonstrated that adaptive cytoprotection can occur under conditions in which cyclooxygenase activity is suppressed [6-8].

The mechanism that causes increased resistance of the gastric mucosa to necrotizing agents remains unclear. Stimulation of PG synthesis is, as noted above, not necessary. The formation of a protective coat of mucus and cell debris by exposure to irritants has been suggested [6], but another study has shown that removal of the mucus cap did not abolish the protective effect of exposure to hypertonic saline [7]. We have previously suggested tht irritant-induced mucosal edema could be protective by preventing gastric contractions and subsequent constriction of mucosal veins [9]. Alternatively, mucosal edema may be an incidental effect of topical exposure to irritants or PG and not necessary for protection.

The present study was designed to further investigate some of the physiological and morphological changes which are produced in the gastric mucosa following contact with protective concentrations of irritants. In particular, we have developed a model of adaptive cytoprotection in which certain agents protect the regions of the mucosa with which they are in contact (local protection) and also confer protection on regions of the mucosa which were not exposed to the irritant (referred protection). This model thus affords an opportunity to distinguish between those effects of protective agents which are central to prevention of gastric erosions and those changes in mucosal structure or function which are irrelevant consequences of topical exposure to the agents. Furthermore, the comparison of different necrotizing agents and the variable extent to which agents produce local or referred protection enables us to resolve some of the conflicting findings of earlier studies.

METHODS

Female Sprague-Dawley rats weighing between 175 and 225 g were denied food but not water for 18-24 h prior to the start of experiments. All experiment groups contained 5 or more animals. Anaesthesia was achieved by intraperitoneal injection of sodium pentobarbital (Somnotol, 60 mg/kg body weight) and an *ex-vivo* gastric chamber was prepared as described previously [2].

DEMONSTRATION OF LOCAL AND REFERRED PROTECTION

Each experiment consisted of 3 sequential 10-minute periods during which the gastric chamber contained 10 ml of either 0.2 M mannitol (Man) or 0.05 M HCl in 0.2 M mannitol (HCl). Man was used during the first 3 periods when the effects of concentrated ethanol were examined, and HCl was used when sodium taurocholate was used as a necrotizing agent. During the fourth period, which was 5 minutes long, the entire chamber apparatus (including the rat) was tilted to either the left or the right at a 30° angle. During this period, 1 ml of either irritant (4% NaCl, 12% NaCl, 0.25 M HCl, 20% (v/v) ethanol), or control solution (0.9% NaCl) was placed on the lower half of the chambered mucosa. This volume covered only half of the mucosa, leaving the other half uncovered. Experience showed that 5 min was sufficient for the development of protection while ensuring that the uncovered half of the mucosa remained wet. The irritant was then removed with a syringe, the mucosa was rinsed, and the apparatus returned to the horizontal position. Subsequently, when referring to the side which was or was not exposed to 1.0 ml of irritant or control solution during period 4, the terms "covered half" and "uncovered half" will be used. During all other periods, both sides of the mucosa were covered.

During the fifth period either 5 or 10 ml of necrotizing agent (80 mM sodium taurocholate in 50 mM HCl or 40% ethanol) were placed in the chamber for 10 min, followed by 3 successive 10-minute exposures to 0.05 M HCl. The effect of inhibition of PG synthesis was examined by pretreating animals with indomethacin (s.c. at a dose of 5 mg/kg 1 h prior to the start of experiments).

At the end of each experiment, the chambered mucosa was photographed with color transparency film. The fraction of grossly damaged glandular mucosa (lesion area) was determined from coded tracings of the photographs, using a digital image analyzer.

Histological observations

At the end of each experiment or, in some experiments, at the end of period 4 (after exposure of half of the mucosa to irritant or control solution for 5 min), the gastric pedicle was severed and the chamber removed. The stomach was pinned out on a wax surface and fixed for 2 h in buffered 2.5% glutaraldehyde, post-fixed in 1% osmium tetroxide, processed by routine methods and embedded in Epon for subsequent light and electron microscopy. Semi-thin sections were cut at 1.0 μm, mounted on coded glass slides, and stained with toluidine blue for light microscopy.   Selected samples were sectioned and stained by routine methods for electron microscopy. The fraction of the interfoveolar (luminal) surface epithelium that was destroyed and the extent and depth of subepithelial edema were determined in some groups as described previously [9].

Effects of irritants on thickness of layer of extracellular mucus

The tilted gastric chamber protocol, as described above, was employed. Three groups of 5 animals each were exposed on one side of the mucosa for 5 min to one of 4% NaCl, 0.25 M HCl, or 0.2 M mannitol.   At the end of period 4, the animals were killed, the stomachs removed and 2 sections of unfixed mucosa, each 1 cm long x 1 mm wide, were cut with paired scalpel blades separated by a spacer, from each of the covered and uncovered sides of the fundic mucosa. The thickness of the apparent extracellular mucus coat was measured, at 100x magnification, using phase contrast optics, at 500 μm intervals according to the technique of McQueen et al. [10]. Sections of fundic mucosa from the same stomachs were also removed, fixed in 2.5% glutaraldehyde, processed as described above, and embedded in Epon.   Semi-thin sections were cut, stained with toluidine blue, placed on coded slides, and the thickness and extent of the extracellular mucus layer determined by light microscopy as described previously [11].

Measurement of the thickness and magnitude of the juxtamucosal pH gradient

The thickness (in μm) and magnitude (in pH units) were measured using antimony microelectrodes with tip diameters of 25 to 40 μm, as described previously [12].   The microelectrodes were mounted in a micromanipulator capable of x-axis movement in 10 μm increments. Microelectrodes were calibrated daily using standard solutions of known pH. The antimony microelectrode was advanced from the luminal solution towards the mucosal surface while under continuous observation with a modified dissecting microscope at a magnification of 63x. Measurements were carried out on mucosae which had been exposed for three consecutive 10-min periods to 0.05 M HCl. Four measurements were obtained from each half of the mucosa. The chamber was then tilted and 1 ml of 0.25 M HCl was placed in the chamber for 5 min, after which the chamber was returned to the horizontal position and 0.05 M HCl was placed in the chamber. Four measurements were then obtained within a 5 min period from each of the previously covered and uncovered sides. We have established in unpublished studies that the effectiveness of referred protection against ethanol by 0.25 M HCl was not affected by either prior exposure to 0.05 M HCl during periods 1 to 3 or by a subsequent 10 min exposure to 0.05 M HCl. The beginning of the pH gradient was recorded as the distance above the mucosa at which there was an increase in pH of 0.05 pH units above that of the luminal solution. The depth of the gradient is defined as the distance from the beginning of the gradient to a point 10 um or less above the mucosal surface. The change in pH across the entire gradient is referred to as the magnitude of the gradient.

STATISTICAL ANALYSIS

All data are expressed as mean $\pm$ SEM. Statistical comparisons between 2 groups were performed using Student's two-tailed t-test for unpaired data. Comparisons between more than 2 groups were made using analysis of variance (ANOVA) for unbalanced groups. The least significant difference of means was used to determine significant differences between groups. With all statistical analyses, an associated probability (p value) of $\leq 5\%$ was considered significant.

RESULTS AND DISCUSSION

IS ADAPTIVE CYTOPROTECTION AGAINST 40% ETHANOL LIMITED TO SITES OF CONTACT BETWEEN THE MILD IRRITANT AND THE GASTRIC MUCOSA?

The irritants which were tested differed in their abilities to produce protection which extended beyond the point of contact with the mucosa (defined as referred adaptive cytoprotection or, more simply, referred protection). 20% ethanol and 4% NaCl protected only those regions of the mucosa which were contacted by the irritants, while 0.25 M HCl and 12% NaCl produced referred protection (Figure 1). It is not clear why some agents produce only local protection while others produce referred protection. There is unlikely to be a qualitative difference in the effects of the various agents tested since, at progressively increasing concentrations, an agent such as NaCl can be ineffective (0.9%), locally protective (4%) or produce both local and referred protection (12%). We did not examine the effects of concentrations of ethanol higher than 20% since this agent produces significant ulceration at concentrations between 25% and 40%, but we have shown that the extent of protection afforded by topical exposure to a prostaglandin E_1 analog (Rio-prostil) increases in a similar concentration-dependent fashion [13].

Some of the conflicting results of previous studies in which agents did or did not protect against ethanol after inhibition of cyclooxygenase activity could reflect differences in technique which would affect the extent to which irritants were in contact with all of the mucosa which was subsequently exposed to concentrated ethanol. Studies in which the volume of irritant used or the method of application (such as a gastric chamber) allowed complete coverage of the mucosa would produce protection which was not abolished by indomethacin pretreatment.

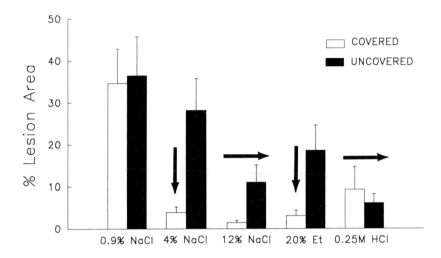

FIGURE 1. *Mean (± SEM) lesion areas for "covered" and "uncovered" sides of mucosae exposed to 40% ethanol. Covered sides were exposed to 1 ml of the indicated solutions for 5 minutes prior to exposure of the entire mucosa to 40% ethanol. The lesion area of all covered sides was significantly less than that of the 0.9% NaCl control. Local protection is indicated by vertical arrows, while significant protection of both sides (local and referred protection) is indicated by horizontal arrows. n = 10 for all groups.*

Is Either Local or Referred Protection Depdendent on Elevated Levels of Prostaglandin Synthesis?

It is likely that local protection is accomplished by mechanisms which do not depend on elevated prostaglandin synthesis. In the tilted chamber preparation, exposure for 5 min to 0.25 M HCl reduced the lesion area on the covered side whether or not the animals had been pretreated with indomethacin. However, indomethacin pretreatment abolished referred protection (Figure 2). These results are consistent with other studies carried out by us and by others. We have found, using the gastric chamber preparation, that indomethacin pretreatment does not abolish local protection conferred by 0.25 M HCl against acidified 80 mM sodium taurocholate or by sucralfate against 40% ethanol [14]. Similarly, Wallace [7] and Hawkey et al [6] have demonstrated that hypertonic NaCl and 20% ethanol, respectively, are protective against concentrated ethanol in indomethacin-pretreated animals.

Robert [15] also recognized, more than 10 years ago, that certain "irritants" such as sodium salicylate produce adapative cytoprotection by mechanisms which do not involve stimulation of prostaglandin synthesis. We found that 0.1 M sodium salicylate in neutral solution was equal in effectiveness to 0.25 M HCl in production of both referred and local protection against 40% ethanol [13].

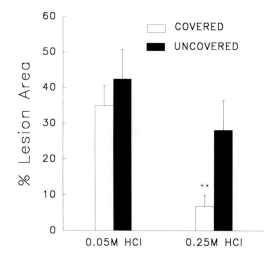

FIGURE 2.   Mean lesion areas of indomethacin-pretreated (5 mg/kg) groups exposed for 5 minutes to 1 ml of 0.05 M HCl or to 1 ml of 0.25 M HCl before exposure to 40% ethanol. Significant (p<0.01) protection was only present on the covered side, after exposure to the irritant.

IS REFERRED PROTECTION BY 0.25 M HCl EFFECTIVE
AGAINST AGENTS OTHER THAN CONCENTRATED ETHANOL?

We have used the tilted chamber model to test the effects of various irritants against 40% ethanol, 80 mM sodium taurocholate in 50 mM HCl (see Figure 3), and 80 mM ASA in 160 mM HCl. Both 4% NaCl and 0.25 M HCl provided local protection against all three necrotizing agents but referred protection has only been produced against 40% ethanol.

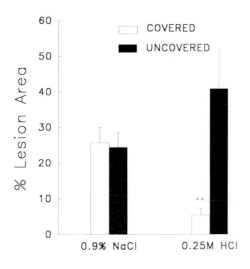

FIGURE 3.   *Mean lesion areas for groups exposed on covered sides to 1 ml of 0.9% NaCl or to 1 ml of 0.25 M HCl before exposure to 80 mM sodium taurocholate in 0.5 M HCl.   The irritant produced significant (p<0.01) protection only on the covered side.*

Is Local or Referred Protection Associated with Increases in Thickness of Either the Layer of Extracellular Mucus or the Juxtamucosal pH Gradient/Unstirred Layer?

We examined the effects on the extracellular mucus coat of an agent which produced only local protection (4% NaCl) and of an agent which was consistently capable of producing referred protection against 40% ethanol (0.25 M HCl).   The mean measured thickness of the mucus layer varied between groups from ~90 μm to 130 μm.   There were no significant differences in the measured thickness of the mucus coat when the sides exposed to 0.25 M HCl or to 4% NaCl were compared to either their respective uncovered sides or to mucosae exposed only to 0.2 M mannitol (Table 1). The effects of 12% NaCl on the thickness of the mucus coat were not examined although it was apparent from grossly visible changes that this irritant was stimulating mucus release at sites of contact with the mucosa.

The results obtained from measurements of the mucus coat on semi-thin plastic sections were similar to those taken from the thick, unfixed slices in that there was no significant difference between the mean thickness over regions exposed to 0.25 M HCl (24.4 $\pm$ 1.4 μm) and the mean thickness of the mucus layer on the uncovered sides (25.2 $\pm$ 1.7 μm).   The mean thicknesses of the extracellular mucus coat over these specimens matched closely those obtained using similar techniques (either thick, unfixed slices or semi-thin plastic sections) in previous studies of control mucosae [10,11,16]. The increased thickness of the mucus coat obtained by measurement of thick, unfixed slices is due to exudation of mucus from the cut edges of the slices and of superimposition effects [17].

TABLE 1

THICKNESS OF EXTRACELLULAR MUCUS LAYER OVER THICK, UNFIXED MUCOSAL
SLICES FROM COVERED AND UNCOVERED REGIONS OF THE MUCOSA.

Group	Solution[a]	Mean ($\pm$ SEM) Thickness of Mucus Layer (um)	
		Covered Half	Uncovered Half
1	0.2 M MAN	115.9 $\pm$ 6.7	126.6 $\pm$ 8.0
2	0.25 M HCl	128.6 $\pm$ 8.3	110.7 $\pm$ 8.2
3	4% NaCl	89.6 $\pm$ 6.9	102.9 $\pm$ 7.2

[a]*Solution present on the covered half of the mucosae immediately prior to assessment of thickness of mucus layer. MAN, Mannitol.*

The effects of exposure of half of the mucosa to 0.25 M HCl on the magnitude and thickness of the juxtamucosal pH gradient were similar to those seen in the mucus coat. That is, there was no significant effect of exposure to the irritant on either the covered or the uncovered side. The mean depth of the pH gradient over these mucosae varied (non-significantly) between about 900 and 1000 um, while the magnitude of the gradient was between 1.25 and 1.50 pH units in the presence of 0.05 M HCl (Table 2).

TABLE 2

MEAN ($\pm$ SEM) THICKNESS (IN um) AND MAGNITUDE (IN pH UNITS) OF THE
JUXTAMUCOSAL pH GRADIENT ON COVERED AND UNCOVERED SIDES OF
GASTRIC MUCOSA, BEFORE AND AFTER EXPOSURE OF THE COVERED SIDE OF
THE MUCOSA TO 0.25 M HCl. N = 20 FOR ALL GROUPS

Covered Side	Before 0.25 M HCl	After 0.25 M HCl
Thickness	990 $\pm$ 132	918 $\pm$ 164
Magnitude	1.35 $\pm$ 0.25	1.30 $\pm$ 0.25
Uncovered Side	Before 0.25 M HCl	After 0.25 M HC l
Thickness	1036 $\pm$ 170	963 $\pm$ 155
Magnitude	1.50 $\pm$ 0.30	1.25 $\pm$ 0.20

CONCLUSIONS

Referred protection against 40% ethanol and local protection against both ethanol and sodium taurocholate occurred in regions of gastric mucosae which did not show detectable changes in the constituents of the "mucus-bicarbonate barrier". Furthermore, the most effective protective agents such as 0.1 M sodium salicylate and 0.25 M HCl did not produce significant damage to the luminal epithelium on either covered or uncovered sides, whereas 4% NaCl, which was incapable of referred protection, produced obvious morphological effects at the sites of contact. The only consistent change in mucosal morphology was the production of some degree of subepithelial edema on the covered sides of mucosae. There was no effusion of mucus on the uncovered sides and the thickness and magnitude of the juxtamucosal pH gradient/unstirred water layer were unaffected on both covered and uncovered sides in the case of 0.25 M HCl. Neither local nor referred protection can be attributed simply to the production of a protective mat of mucus and cells, or to elevated bicarbonate secretion or release.

In studies subsequent to those described herein we found that referred protection gainst ethanol was abolished by (in addition to indomethacin pretreatment) parenteral administration of the dopamine (DA2) receptor-antagonist haloperidol and by topical exposure to the substance P receptor-antagonist spantide. Our current hypothesis is that referred protection involves a sequence of: (1) irritant-induced mediator release on the covered side; (2) impulse transmission by the enteric nervous system; (3) mast cell/nerve interactions which result in a reduction of the release of vasoactive mediators during subsequent exposure to concentrated ethanol.

Mucosal resistance ("cytoprotection") can, of course, be produced by parenteral as well as topical administration of protective agents. High concentrations of parenterally administered prostaglandins have been shown to be protective against indomethacin [18] and against ethanol [19], and parenteral sodium salicylate has been shown to be protective against both aspirin and concentrated ethanol [15]. It remains to be determined whether the effects of these parenterally administered agents resemble those observed at the "covered" or the "uncovered" sites in the present model.

The protective effects of laparotomy, in which the abdominal incision confers resistance to orogastric administration of 75% ethanol, may be considered as a form of referred protection [20]. Yonei et al, propose that protection by laparotomy results from somatovisceral or viscerovisceral axon reflex of afferent neurons with collateral nerve endings in both the abdominal wall and the gastric mucosa. It is of interest that laparotomy protection is abolished by pretreatment with indomethacin but unaffected by atropine. We have found in our (unpublished) studies that referred protection is not affected by atropine.

Another example of referred protection is provided by the study of Raugstad et al [21] on the ability of prior chronic injury to modify the severity of acute injury in the rat stomach. They found that the presence of a pre-existing, chronic-type acetic-acid ulcer protected the immediately adjacent fundus (and, in some cases, the entire mucosa) from erosions produced by i.p. injection of the vasoconstrictor, epinephrine.

Referred protection was, in our studies, limited to ethanol. This presumably reflected the ability of concentrated ethanol to produce vascular congestion at the mucosal base; possibly by venous constriction subsequent to mast cell degranulation [22]. Acidified sodium taurocholate causes damage by destroying surface epithelial cells and exposing the subepithelial blood vessels to direct damage by acid and by bile salt [23] and thus the vascular damage and stasis which precede hemorrhage are produced by different mechanisms; mechanisms which are not affected by changes which occur at the sites responsible for referred protection.

Local protection could result from one or more of several mucosal responses to protective agents or "irritants". The mucosa responds to local application of most irritants and to prostaglandins with a localized color change which could indicate transient hyperemia, and there is variable loss of mucosal folding, and significant but transient decreases in the transmucosal potential difference. Histological inspection reveals subepithelial edema and this could constitute part of the "dilutional barrier" [24] which may attenuate the severity of the initial assault by necrotizing agents. Effects of protective irritants on local mediator synthesis and on stored mediators in mast cells could also affect the resistance of the microvasculature to necrotizing agents, the extent of post-injury hyperemia, and the thickness of the unstirred water layer. The net result is attenuation of initial damage, preservation of microvascular integrity, and provision of a microenvironment (at the mucoal surface) in which rapid repair by restitution can occur.

ACKNOWLEDGEMENT

*This research was supported by the
Medical Research Council of Canada.*

REFERENCES

1. Robert A. Antisecretory, antiulcer, cytoprotective and diarrheogenic properties of prostaglandins. In: Samuelsson B, Paoletti R, eds. Advances in Prostaglandins and Thromboxane Research. Vol. 2. New York: Raven Press. 1976; 507-520.

2. Wallace JL, Morris GP, Krausse EJ, Greaves SE. Reduction by cytoprotective agents of ethanol-induced damage to the rat gastric mucosa: a correlated morphological and physiological study. Can J Physiol Pharmacol. 1982; 60: 1686-1699.

3.   Lacy ER, Ito S. Microscopic analysis of ethanol damage to rat gastric mucosa after treatment with a prostaglandin. Gastroenterology 1982; 83: 619-625.

4.   Robert A, Nezamis JE, Lancaster C, Davis JP, Field SO, Hanchar AJ. Mild irritants prevent gastric necrosis through "adaptive cytoprotection" mediated by prostaglandins. Am J Physiol 1983; 245: G113-G121.

5.   Chaudhury TK, Robert A. Prevention by mild irritants of gastric necrosis produced in rats by sodium taurocholate. Dig Dis Sci. 1980; 25: 830-836.

6.   Hawkey CJ, Kemp RT, Walt RP, Bhaskar NK, Davies J, Filipowicz B. Evidence that adaptive cytoprotection in rats is not mediated by prostaglandins. Gastroenterology 1988; 94: 948-954.

7.   Wallace JL. Increased resistance of the rat gastric mucosa to hemorrhagic damage after exposure to an irritant. Role of the "mucoid cap" and prostaglandin synthesis. Gastroenterology. 1988; 94: 22-32.

8.   MacNaughton WK, Williamson TE, Morris GP. Adaptive cytoprotection by 0.25 M HCl is truly "cytoprotective" and may not depend upon elevated levels of prostaglandin synthesis. Can J Physiol Pharmacol 1988; 66: 1075-1081.

9.   Morris GP, Keenan CM, Shriver DA. Morphological and physiological effects of a cytoprotective prostaglandin analog (rioprostil) on the rat gastric mucosa. Clin Invest med 1987; 10: 121-131.

10. McQueen S, Allen A, Garner A. Measurement of gastric and duodenal mucus gel thickness. In: Allen A, Flemstrom G, Garner A, Silen W, Turnberg LA. eds. Mechanisms of Mucosal Protection in the Upper Gastrointestinal Tract. New York: Raven Press. 1984; 215-221.

11. Morris GP, Harding PL. Mechanisms of mucosal recovery from acute gastric damage: roles of extracellular mucus and cell migration. In: Allen A, Flemstrom G, Garner A, Silen W, Turnberg LA. eds. Mechanisms of Mucosal Protection in the Upper Gastrointestinal Tract. New York: Raven Press. 1984; 215-221.

12. Morris GP, Williamson TE, Hynna TT. Prostaglandins and mucosal defensive mechanisms. Can J Gastroenterol 1990; 4: 95-107.

13. Donaldson CL, Morris GP. Local and "referred" cytoprotection by mild irritants and a PGE$_1$ analog (abs). Gastroenterology 1988; 94: A614.

14. Morris GP, Keenan CM, MacNaughton WK, Wallace JL, Williamson TE. Protection of rat gastric mucosa by sucralfate: Effects of luminal stasis and of inhibition of prostaglandin synthesis. Am J Med. 1989; 86(suppl 6A): 10-16.

15.   Robert A.   Gastric cytoprotection by sodium salicylate.
Prostaglandins 1981; 21(suppl): 139-146.

16.   Morris GP, Harding RK, Wallace JL.   A functional model for
extracellular gastric mucus in the rat.   Virchows Arch (Cell Pathol)
1984; 46: 239-251.

17.   Morris GP. The myth of the mucus barrier. Gastroenterol Clin Biol.
1985; 9: 106-107.

18.   Van Kolfschoten AA, Hagelen F, Hillen FC, Jager LP, Zandberg P,
Van Noordwijk J.   Protective effects of prostaglandins against
ulcerogenic activity of indomethacin during different stages of
erosion development in rat stomach: role of acid and bicarbonate
secretion. Dig Dis Sci 1983; 28: 1127-1132.

19.   Puurunen J. Effect of prostaglandin E2, cimetidine, and atropine on
ethanol-induced gastric mucosal damage in the rat.   Scand J
Gastroent. 1980; 15: 485-488.

20.   Yonei Y, Holzer P, Guth PH. Laparotomy-induced gastric protection
against ethanol injury is mediated by capsaicin-sensitive sensory
neurons. Gastroenterology 1990; 99: 3-9.

21.   Raugstad TS, Svanes K, Molster A. Interaction between acute gastric
ulcer and epinephrine-induced mucosal erosions in the rat. Eur Surg
Res. 1977; 9: 67-73.

22.   Oates PJ, Hakkinen JP. Studis on the mechanism of ethanol-induced
gastric damage in rats. Gastroenterology 1988; 94: 10-21.

23.   Morris GP, Lacy ER, Cohen MM.   Effects of bile on the gastric
mucosa. In: Wallace JL, ed. Endogenous Mediators of Damage in the
Gastrointestinal Tract. Boca Raton, Florida. CRC Press, 1989: 1-27.

24.   Szabo S, Hollander D. Pathways of gastrointestinal protection and
repair: Mechanisms of action of sucralfate. Am J Med. 1989; 86(suppl
6A): 23-31.

INTRACISTERNAL INJECTION OF CALCITONIN-GENE RELATED PEPTIDE INHIBITS EXPERIMENTAL GASTRIC ULCERS

Yvette Tache

Center for Ulcer Research and Education, VA Wadsworth Medical Center, Department of Medicine & Brain Research Institute, UCLA, Los Angeles, USA

ABSTRACT

Rat α-calcitonin gene-related peptide (CGRP) acts in the brain to inhibit gastric acid secretion, emptying and contractility and to stimulate gastric mucosal blood flow [1]. In the present study, intracisternal injection of CGRP (1.4 nmol) was demonstrated to reduce gastric erosions induced by cold restraint stress or central injection of the stable thyrotropin-releasing factor (TRH) analog, RX 77368, in conscious fasted rats. CGRP injected intravenously was inactive. The preventive effect of intracisternal CGRP may be mediated through the inhibition of vagal outflow to the stomach and associated changes in gastric secretory and motor function previously described. Moreover intracisternal injection of CGRP (0.08-80 pmol) dose dependently prevented gastric lesions produced by 40% ethanol in conscious rats. The cytoprotective effect of central CGRP was peptide specific since intracisternal injection of corticotropin- releasing factor (CRF), calcitonin or bombesin, at doses known to inhibit gastric acid secretion, motility and hemorrhagic lesions induced by cold restraint stress or central TRH did not prevent lesions produced by ethanol. The underlying mechanisms of the cytoprotective effect of intracisternal CGRP are not dependent on prostaglandin pathways and may involve an increase in gastric mucosal blood flow. These studies further support the concept that gastric ulcer formation is influenced by central injection of neuropeptides and show that intracisternal CGRP can induce cytoprotection independently from prostaglandin pathways.

INTRODUCTION

CGRP was one of the first examples of a biologically active peptide to be identified by recombinant DNA and molecular biological approach [2,3]. It was also the first example of tissue-specific alternative processing of a gene. In central or peripheral neural tissues, the RNA transcript from the calcitonin gene resulted in a mRNA which encodes the 37-residue peptide called CGRP or α-CGRP [2]. In thyroidal cells, the calcitonin gene generates a mRNA which encodes a calcitonin precursor protein expressing the calcium-regulating hormone, calcitonin [2]. The same mechanism of specific alternate RNA processing was described in human tissues [4,5]. Although rat α-CGRP was originally identified in the absence of biological information, the first report on its characterization showed the ubiquitous distribution of CGRP-like immunoreactivity with dense representation in forebrain and medullary nuclei, and in pathways modulating ingestive behaviour and autonomic outflow [2]. In the periphery, CGRP-LI is present in neurons associated with blood vessels and visceral organs including the gastrointestinal tract [2]. The neuroanatomical distribution of the peptide prompted us to investigate CGRP actions on gastric function. We initially reported that rat α-CGRP exerts potent central and peripheral inhibitory effects on gastric acid secretion and emptying in rats [6,7] and dogs [8]. In the present study, we report the protective effect of intracisternal injection of CGRP on experimental ulcers in rats.

METHODS

Male Sprague Dawley albino rats (Simenson Laboratories, Gilroy, CA), weighing 200-220g, were maintained *ad libitum* on Purina Laboratory Chow and tap water. They were housed under conditions of controlled temperature ($20 \pm 1^{\circ}C$) and lighting (06:00 h to 18:00 h). All experiments were performed in rats deprived of food for 24 h but given free access to water up to the beginning of experiments.

TREATMENTS

The following drugs were used, rat α-CGRP (generously provided by Dr. J. Rivier, Salk Institute, La Jolla, CA), RX 77368 pGlu-His-(3,3'-dimethyl)-ProNH$_2$, Reckitt Colman, Kingston-Upon-Hull, England, and indomethacin (Sigma Chemical Co.). Just before the experiments, CGRP in powder form was dissolved in saline for intracisternal injection and saline with 0.1% BSA for intravenous injection. Indomethacin was dissolved in 1% sodium bicarbonate and given intraperitoneally. The stable TRH-analog, RX 77368, was aliquoted at a concentration of 0.01 mg/100ul, stored at -20°C and diluted in saline to the required concentration at the time of the experiment. Intracisternal injections were performed on rats placed on a stereotaxic instrument and under light ether anesthesia. Peptides and saline were delivered in 10ul with a 50ul Hamilton syringe. Intravenous injections were delivered through the jugular vein in 1 ml/kg. Oro-pharyngeal administrations of ethanol were given through a stainless steel tube in conscious rats.

EXPERIMENTAL PROTOCOLS

Groups of rats were injected intracisternally or intravenously with saline or CGRP, 5-7 min before exposure to one of the following ulcerogenic treatments: cold by placing rats at 5°C for 3 h in individual cylindrical restraining metallic cages ; intracisternal injection of the TRH stable analogue, RX 77368, at 1ug dose; oro-pharyngeal administration of 1 ml of ethanol 40%. Rats were sacrificed by CO_2 inhalation at the end of cold restraint exposure, 4 h after intracisternal injection of TRH analog, and 1 h after ethanol administration. Then stomachs were removed, rinsed with ice-cold saline, opened along the greater curvature, and scored for lesions by an observer not knowing the treatment group to which the stomach belonged. The length and width of each lesion were measured to the nearest 0.2 mm and calculated as an ellipse (length x width x /4). The total area was summated and expressed in square mm as in a previous study [9].

STATISTICAL ANALYSIS

The data are presented as means ± SE. The statistical analysis of the results was performed using t-tests and ANOVA. Values of P<0.05 were regarded as significant.

RESULTS AND DISCUSSION

CENTRAL CGRP PREVENTS STRESS- AND CENTRAL TRH-INDUCED GASTRIC EROSIONS

Intracisternal injection of the stable TRH analog, RX 77367 and exposure for 3 h to cold restraint stress in rats injected intracisternally with saline induced gastric lesions as previously reported [9,10]. Intracisternal injection of α-CGRP (1.4 nmol) inhibited gastric lesions produced by central injection of RX 77368 and cold restraint by 59% and 70% respectively in conscious rats (Fig. 1). When the same dose of CGRP was given intravenously, the protective effect against cold restraint stress or central RX 77368 was no longer observed (data not shown). These results suggest that CGRP acts centrally to decrease gastric erosions induced by central TRH or cold restraint stress. CGRP can be added to the list of several other peptides including calcitonin, bombesin, CRF, opioid peptides and neurotensin which prevent cold restraint stress- or central TRH-induced gastric lesions through centrally-mediated action [11,12].

Convincing evidence indicates that endogenous release of TRH plays a role in cold restraint-stress induced gastric lesions in fasted rats [13,14]. The present findings show that central CGRP prevents the ulcerogenic actions of exogenous and endogenous TRH. One mechanism whereby central injection of TRH and cold restraint stress induce gastric lesions, involves the stimulation of vagal activity and associated increase in gastric secretory and motor function [11,15,16]. Central CGRP may act by preventing TRH action on vagal outflow to the stomach [17,18]. This is supported by electrophysiological, surgical and pharmacological studies demonstrating that central CGRP inhibits gastric function through vagal pathways. We recently reported that intracisternal injection of α-CGRP inhibits multiple- and single-unit efferent discharges recorded from the gastric branch of the vagus in fasted rats [19]. The inhibitory effect is dose-related in terms of both the magnitude and duration [19]. Furthermore, intracisternal injection of rat α-CGRP inhibits gastric acid secretion stimulated by central vagal activation induced by TRH [20,21]. Central injection of CGRP-induced inhibition of stimulated gastric acid secretion was also shown to be mediated by the vagus and not to involve the sympathetic nervous system [6,20]. Lastly, microinjection of CGRP into medullary nuclei regulating vagal outflow to the stomach, such as the dorsal vagal complex, [22], inhibits gastric acid secretion stimulated by pentagastrin and vagal activation, but does not inhibit the peripherally acting muscarinic agonist bethanechol [23,24]. Likewise central CGRP inhibits gastric motor function partly through vagal pathways [7,25,26]. Further studies will be needed to evaluate the interactions between TRH and CGRP on neuronal activity in the dorsal vagal complex. TRH excites unit activity of preganglionic vagal neurons projecting to the stomach [17] whereas the influence of α-CGRP on extracellular activity of single neurons in rats is predominantly inhibitory, at least in the forebrain [27].

EFFECT OF INTRACISTERNAL INJECTION OF CGRP
ON VARIOUS MODELS OF GASTRIC LESIONS

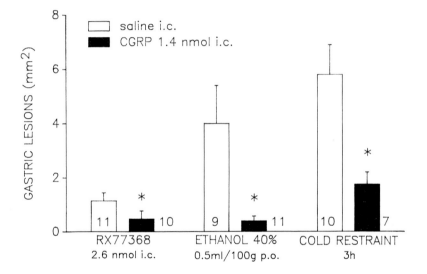

FIGURE 1. *Effect of intracisternal injection of CGRP on experimental ulcers in fasted rats. Rats were lightly anesthetized with ether and injected intracisternally with saline or CGRP (1.4 nmol) alone or combined with RX 77368 (2.6 nmol). When rats recovered from anesthesia they were either left at room temperature, exposed at $4^{0}C$ in restraining individual cages for 3 h or given by oro-pharyngeal intubation ethanol (40%, 1 ml). Gastric lesions were monitored 1 and 4 h after ethanol and RX77368 injection, and at the end of cold restraint exposure. Each column represents the mean ± SE of number of rats indicated at the bottom of column.*

INTRACISTERNAL CGRP PREVENTS GASTRIC LESIONS INDUCED BY ETHANOL

Oro-pharyngeal administration of 40% ethanol (1 ml) induced average gastric lesions of 4.9 $\pm$ 0.8 mm^2 in fasted rats injected intracisternally with saline. Macroscopic gastric lesions induced by ethanol were completely prevented by intracisternal injection of α-CGRP (1.4 nmol) (Fig. 1). CGRP injected at intracisternal doses of 0.08, 8 and 80 pmol inhibited ethanol lesions by 14%, 76% and 97% respectively (Fig. 2). The ability of intracisternal CGRP to prevent ethanol-induced gastric damage is quite unique to CGRP since intracisternal injection of bombesin (0.31-3.1 nmol), CRF (63 pmol), or salmon calcitonin (0.03-1.5 nmol) at doses which inhibited stress ulcer [28-30] do not prevent (bombesin, CRF) or even aggravate (calcitonin) ethanol-induced gastric lesions [9,31] (Table 1). Interestingly, intracisternal injections of calcitonin and CGRP exert opposite effects on ethanol-induced gastric lesions at doses established for both peptides to inhibit gastric acid secretion and emptying [6,7,9,25].

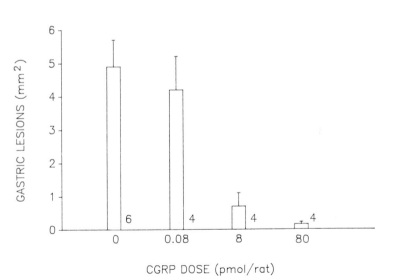

FIGURE 2. Dose related inhibition of ethanol-induced gastric lesions by intracisternal injection of CGRP in fasted rats. For other details, see legend of Fig. 1.

The mechanisms by which central CGRP induces cytoprotection are not prostaglandin mediated since indomethacin pretreatment (5 mg/kg, ip, -1 h) did not alter the protective effect of intracisternal injection of CGRP (8 pmol) (Fig. 3). Since other centrally acting peptides such as calcitonin, bombesin or CRF injected intracisternally at a dose inhibiting gastric acid secretion and motor function, did not protect against experimental ulcers induced by ethanol [28-30] (Table 1), CGRP action is not primarily related to its effects on gastric acid secretion and motor function.

TABLE 1

Treatment[a] Lesions[b]	Dose pmol	N	Gastric mm^2
Saline		13	5.3 ± 1.0
CRF	63	5	4.7 ± 2.0
Calcitonin	29	5	10.1 ± 0.8*
CGRP	8	4	0.7 ± 0.4*

[a]*Fasted rats under light ether anesthesia were injected intracisternally with saline or peptides. When recovered from anesthesia, ethanol 40% was given through oro-pharyngeal administration and gastric lesions were monitored 1 h later.*

[b]*Mean ± SE; P<0.05 compared with saline-treated group.*

These findings further confirm previous studies showing that cytoprotection is not related to the antisecretory properties of drugs [32]. The pathogenesis of ethanol lesions appear to involve changes in microcirculation [33]. Recent findings support the view that activation of capsaicin sensitive neurons in the gastric mucosa lead to CGRP release and increase gastric mucosal blood flow [34,35]. Mobilization of such mechanisms play an important protective role against ethanol-induced lesions [34-36]. Intracisternal injection of CGRP-induced cytoprotection may involve similar pathways since it has recently been reported that central injection of CGRP stimulates gastric mucosal blood flow through the local release of CGRP [37,38]. In further agreement with such a possibility is the demonstration that the capsaicin-sensitive pathways mediating protection against ethanol lesions does not depend on prostaglandin formation [34]. Likewise, we observed that central CGRP-induced protection against ethanol is not modified by indomethacin pretreatment.

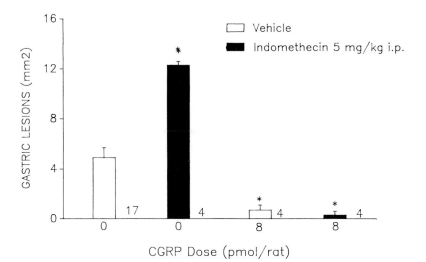

FIGURE 3. *Effect of indomethacin on intracisternal CGRP-induced inhibition of gastric lesions induced by ethanol in fasted rats. Indomethacin was given intraperitonially one hour prior to intracisternal injection of saline or CGRP. For oter details, see legend of Fig. 1.*

CONCLUSIONS

The present findings demonstrate that intracisternal injection of CGRP decreases gastric lesions induced by cold restraint stress and central injection of stable TRH analog. The mechanism underlying such protective effects may be related to the inhibitory effect of CGRP on vagal outflow to the stomach and associated decrease in gastric secretory and motor function. The protection against cold restraint stress and exogenous TRH is communly induced by other peptides (bombesin, CRF, calcitonin, neurotensin, opioid peptides) acting centrally to inhibit gastric acid secretion and motor function. However, CGRP is the only peptide so far established to prevent ethanol-induced gastric lesions when injected intracisternally. Intracisternal injection of bombesin and CRF had no effect and calcitonin even aggravated ethanol-induced lesions. The mechanisms whereby the cytoprotective effect of central CGRP is exerted is not related to prostaglandins and may involve stimulation of mucosal blood flow.

The physiological role of CGRP in the central regulation of gastric function is still to be defined. However, existing information on CGRP-immunoreactivity and receptor distribution in specific subsets of medullary (dorsal vagal complex, parabranchial nucleus) and forebrain nuclei (hypothalamus, central amygdala) receiving visceral information and influencing autonomic outflow provide anatomical substrate for such a role [39-42]. The recently developed CGRP antagonist, human CGRP8-37 [43], will provide a useful tool to assess physiological relevance of this peptide in relation to central regulation of gastric function.

ACKNOWLEDGEMENT

The work was supported by the National Institute of Arthritis, Metabolism and Digestive Disease, Grants AM 30110 and 33061 and the National Institute of Mental Health, Grant MH-0063.

The author thanks Mrs Elizabeth Kolve for expert technical assistance and Dr. Jean Rivier (Clayton Foundation Lab., Salk Institute, la Jolla, CA) for the generous donation of rat a-CGRP. The author also wishes to thank Paul Kirshbaum for his editorial assistance.

REFERENCES

1.   Tache Y, Raybould H Wei JY. Central and peripheral actions of calcitonin-gene related peptide on secretory and motor function. In: Brugioni D Maggi CA. eds. Sensory nerves and neuropeptides in gastroenterology: from basic sciences to clinical perspective. : Plenum Press, 1990:in press.

2.   Rosenfeld MG, Mermod J-J, Amara SG, et al. Production of a novel neuropeptide encoded by the calcitonin gene via tissue-specific RNA processing. Nature 1983;304:129-135.

3.   Amara SG, Arriza JL, Leff SE, Swanson LW, Evans RM, Rosenfeld MG. Expression in brain of a messenger RNA encoding a novel neuropeptide homologous to calcitonin gene-related peptide. Science 1985;229:1094-1097.

4.   Steenbergh PH, Hoppener JWM, Zandberg J, Visser A, Lips CJM, Jansz HS. Structure and expression of the human calcitonin/CGRP genes. FEBS Lett 1986;209:97-103.

5.   Steenbergh PH, H ppener JWM, Zandberg J, Lips CJM, Jansz HS. A second human calcitonin/CGRP gene. FEBS 1985;183:403-407.

6.   Tache Y, Gunion M, Lauffenberger M, Goto Y. Inhibition of gastric acid secretion by intracerebral injection of calcitonin gene related peptide in rats. Life Sci 1984;35:871-878.

7.   Raybould HE, Kolve E, Tache Y. Central nervous sytem action of calcitonin-gene related peptide to inhibit gastric emptying in the conscious rat. Peptides 1988;9:735-737.

8.   Tache Y, Pappas T, Lauffenburger M, Goto Y, Walsh JH, Debas H. Calcitonin gene-related peptide: potent peripheral inhibitor of gastric acid secretion in rats and dogs. Gastroenterology 1984;87:344-349.

9.   Tache Y, Kolve E, Maeda-Hagiwara M, Kauffman G. CNS action of calctionin to alter experimental gastric ulcers in rats. Gastroenterology 1987;41:651-655.

10. Goto Y, Tache Y. Gastric erosions induced by intracisternal thyrotropin-releasing hormone (TRH) in rats. Peptides 1985;6:153-156.

11. Tache Y Ishikawa T. Role of brain peptides in the ulcerogenic response to stress. In: Tach Y, Morley JE Brown MR. eds. Hans Selye Symposia on neuroendocrinology and stress: Neuropeptides and stress. New York: Springer-Verlag, 1989:146-157.

12. Tache Y. Central nervous system action of neuropeptides to influence or prevent experimental gastroduodenal ulceration. In: Szabo S Pfeiffer CJ. eds. Ulcer disease: new aspects of pathogenesis and pharmacology. Boca Raton: CRC Press, Inc., 1989:179-191.

13. Tache Y, Stephens RL Ishikawa T. Stress-induced alterations of gastrointestinal function: involvment of brain CRF and TRH. In: Weiner H, Florin I, Hellhammer D Murison M. eds. IV. New Frontiers of Stress Research. : Hans Huber, 1989:1-11.

14. Basso N, Bagarani M, Pekary E, Genco A, Materia A. Role of thyrotropin-releasing hormone in stress ulcer formation in the rat. Dig Dis Sci 1988;33:819-823.

15. Tache Y, Stephens RL, Ishikawa T. Central nervous system action of TRH to influence gastrointestinal function and ulceration. Ann N Y Acad Sci 1989;553:269-285.

16. Tache Y. Stress and gastric ulcer formation. In: Brown MR, Rivier C Koob G. eds. Neurobiology and neuroendocrinology of stress. New York: Marcel Dekker Inc., 1990:549-564.

17. McCann MJ, Hermann GE, Rogers RC. Thyrotropin-releasing hormone:effects on identified neurons of the dorsal vagal complex. J Autonom Nerv Syst 1989;26:107-112.

18. Rogers RC, McCann MJ. Effects of TRH on the activity of gastric inflation-related neurons in the solitary nucleus in the rat. Neurosci Lett 1989;104:71-76.

19.   Wei JY, Tache Y. Alterations of efferent discharges of the gastric branch of the vagus nerve by intracisternal injection of peptides influencing gastric function in rats. Gastroenterology 1990;98:A531. (Abstract)

20.   Lenz HJ, Mortrud MT, Rivier JE, Brown MR. Central nervous system actions of calcitonin gene-related peptide on gastric acid secretion in the rat. Gastroenterology 1985;88:539-544.

21.   Hughes JJ, Levine AS, Morley JE, Gosnell BA, Silvis SE. Intraventricular calcitonin gene-related peptide inhibits gastric acid secretion. Peptides 1984;5:665-667.

22.   Shapiro RE, Miselis RR. The central organization of the vagus nerve innervating the stomach of the rat. J Comp Neurol 1985;238:473-488.

23.   Goto Y, Tache Y, Debas H, Novin D. Gastric and vagus nerve response to GABA agonist baclofen. Life Sci 1985;36:2471-2475.

24.   Ishikawa T, Tache Y. Inhibitory effect of α-CGRP microinjected into the dorsal vagal complex on gastric acid secretion in the rats. Dig Dis Sci 1989;34:979-(Abstract).

25.   Lenz HJ. Calcitonin and CGRP inhibit gastrointestinal transit via distinct neuronal pathways. Am J Physiol 1988;254:G920-G924.

26.   Raybould HE, Kolve E, Tache Y. Central nervous system action of calcitonin gene-related peptide (CGRP) to inhibit gastric motor function by adrenergic mechanisms in the rat. Gastroenterology 1989;96:A410.

27.   Twery MJ, Moss RL. Calcitonin and calcitonin gene-related peptide alter the excitability of neurons in rat forebrain. Peptides 1985;6:373-378.

28.   Gunion MW, Kauffman GL, Tache Y. Intrahypothalamic microinfusion of corticotropin-releasing factor elevates gastric bicarbonate secretion and protects against cold-stress ulceration in rats. Am J Physiol 1990;258:G152-G157.

29.   Ishikawa T, Tache Y. Intrahypothalamic microinjection of calcitonin prevents stress-induced gastric lesions in rats. Brain Res Bull 1988;20:415-419.

30.   Tache Y, Simard P, Collu R. Prevention by bombesin of cold-restraint stress induced hemorrhagic lesions in rats. Life Sci 1979;24:1719-1725.

31.   Lesiege D, Tache Y. Inhibition of gastric acid secretion by intracisternal bombesin in rats: independence from interaction with prostaglandins. Gastroenterology 1983;84:1228-Abstract.

32. Robert A, Nezamis JE, Lancaster C, Hanchar AJ. Cytoprotection by prostaglandinss in rats. Prevention of gastric necrosis produced by alcohol, HCL, NaOH, hypertonic saline, and thermal injury. Gastroenterology 1979;77:433-443.

33. Oates PJ, Haakkinen JP. Studies on the mechanism of ethanol-induced gastric damage in rats. Gastroenterology 1988;94:10-21.

34. Holzer P, Pabst MA, Lippe ITh, et al. Afferent nerve-mediated protection against deep mucosal damage in the rat stomach. Gastroenterology 1990;98:838-848.

35. Holzer P, Lippe ITh, Pabst MA, et al. Role of sensory neurons in the control of gastric mucosal blood flow and protection. In: Szabo S. ed.Hans Selye Symposia on Neuroendocrinology of gastrointestinal ulceration. : Springer Verlag, 1991:in press.

36. Lippe IT, Lorbach M, Holzer P. Close arterial infusion of calcitonin gene-related peptide into the rat stomach inhibits aspirin- and ethanol-induced hemorrhagic damage. Regul Pept 1989;26:35-46.

37. Bauerfeind P, Cucala M, Hof RP, et al. Calcitonin gene-related peptide mediates CNS regulation of gastric secretion and blood flow. Gastroenterology 1987;92:1311.

38. Bauerfeind P, Koerfer J, Armstrong D, Hof R, Fischer JA, Blum AL. Intravenous anti-CGRP inhibits the increase of gastric blood flow caused by centrally administered CGRP. Gastroenterology 1989;96:A34.

39. Kruger L, Mantyh PW, Sternini C, Brecha NC, Mantyh CR. Calcitonin gene-related peptide (CGRP) in the rat central nervous system: patterns of immunoreactivity and receptor binding sites. Brain Res 1988;463:223-244.

40. Skofitsch G, Jacobowitz DM. Autoradiographic distribution of 125I calcitonin gene-related peptide binding sites in the rat central nervous system. Peptides 1985;4:975-986.

41. Schwaber JS, Sternini C, Brecha NC, Rogers WT, Card JP. Neurons containing calcitonin gene-related peptide in the parabrachial nucleus project to the central nucleus of the amygdala. J Comp Neurol 1988;270:416-426.

42. Morishima K, Takagi H, Akai F, et al. Light and electron microcopic studies of calcitonin gene-related peptide immunoreacte neurons and axon terminals of the nucleus of the tractus solitarius of the rat. Brain Res 1985;344:191-195.

43. Dennis T, Fournier A, Cadieux A, et al. hCGRP8-37, a calcitonin gene-related peptide antagonist revealing CGRP receptor hetero-geneity in brain and periphery. J Pharmacol Exp Ther 1990;in press:

CHRONIC CHALLENGE WITH HYPEROSMOLAR SALT PROTECTS THE RAT GASTRIC MUCOSA AGAINST ACUTE HEMORRHAGIC LESIONS: RESPONSE OF ANTRAL MUCOUS CELLS

Eric R. Lacy, Kathryn S. Cowart and Jan S. King

Department of Anatomy & Cell Biology, Medical University of South Carolina, Charleston, SC. U.S.A.

INTRODUCTION

Clinical and laboratory investigations have shown that chronic luminal insult "strengthens" the gastric mucosa against damage. The mechanisms for this progressive mucosal protection are unknown. Although the relative importance of mucus in protecting the gastric mucosa is controversial [1], it appears to facilitate restitution and may play a role in preventing deep hemorrhagic damage. The purposes of this study were to determine whether chronic superficial damage to the gastric mucosa 1) produced long-term protection against a strong necrotizing agent, 2) induced changes in cellular mucin or the mucus layer of the antrum.

METHODS

Male Sprague Dawley rats, 200-250 g, were kept on a 12-12 hr light-dark cycle and allowed food and water *ad libitum* except at the time of dosing. Preliminary investigation showed that between 13:00 and 15:00 hr the rats were somnolent and the stomachs were nearly void of food. During this time period each rat was given a single bolus of 2-3 cc of warmed 2 M NaCl by orogastric tube at 48 hr intervals, placed back into the cage, and deprived of water for 30 min. To verify that the damage produced by 2 M NaCl was confined to the superficial mucosa, rat stomachs were fixed with buffered aldehydes at intervals of 15, 30 and 60 mins and 24 and 48 hrs after one exposure to this necrotizing agent and after one month of dosing.

At four weeks, rats in the experimental group were killed 24 hr after NaCl dosing. The stomachs of anaesthetized rats from the control (no doses of NaCl) and experimental groups were fixed in Bouin's solution for the following histochemical stains [2]: periodic acid Schiffs (PAS), Alcian Blue (AB) at pH 1.0 or 2.5, AB(2.5)-PAS, diastase-PAS, periodate-borohydride/saponification/PAS (Pb/KOH/PAS), high iron diamine-AB at pH 2.5 (HID-AB), or hematoxylin and eosin. Some stomachs were also fixed in buffered aldehydes and embedded in epoxy resins and sectioned for light microscopy of toluidine-blue stained sections and for transmission electron microscopy. Morphometric analyses of cell and mucous granule numbers and sizes were performed on electron micrographs from the luminal surface extending into the gastric pit and isthmus.

Other rats in the experimental group were given 2-3 cc of 6 M NaCl 24 hrs after their last dose (1 month) of 2 M NaCl. Stomachs from these rats were excised and the area of gross hemorrhagic mucosal lesions was determined by planimetry and compared with that of control rats given 6 M NaCl with no prior treatment.

RESULTS

The rat gastric antrum is virtually devoid of parietal and chief cells and the epithelium mainly consists of mucous cells with a few endocrine cells. Nomenclature of the tissue is confusing. Antral "glands" consist of a foveolus (pit) and isthmus region only [3] (Fig. 1). Within the isthmus lies the proliferative zone in which dividing (progenitor) cells and endocrine cells are interspersed among a morphologically different mucous cell type, the mucous neck cells.

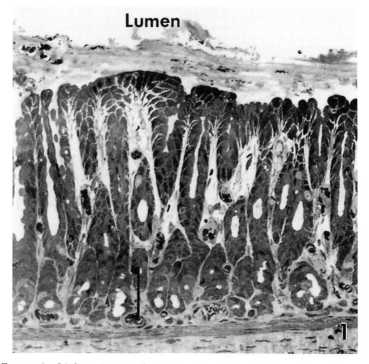

FIGURE 1 *Light micrograph of 1 micrometer thick section of antral mucosa from a rat exposed to chronic 2 M NaCl treatment. Note the uniformly thick mucus layer. The brackets indicate the position of the isthmus. x 300*

CONTROL ANTRAL MUCOSA

Light and electron microscopy showed that the morphology of the mucous cells was not homogenous along the axis of the pit-isthmus but varied according to cell position.   Surface mucous cells constituted those between adjacent foveolae and those lining the gastric pit to the region of the isthmus.   Interfoveolar cells (numbering 3-6) were tear-drop shaped with widely dilated intercellular spaces. The prominent Golgi fields were lateral or apical to the centrally located but highly irregularly-shaped nucleus.   There were fewer mucous granules in interfoveolar cells (21.2 $\pm$ 2.3% of total cell volume) compared with those in mucous cells in the gastric pits (39.2 $\pm$ 5.3%).   The interfoveolar mucous granules were membrane bound and positioned in a thin rim adjacent to the apical plasma membrane which was elaborated into microvilli with a distinct glycocalyx.   These mucous granules were never observed fusing with the plasma membrane but often appeared coalescing with adjacent granules.

From the interfoveolar-pit junction to the base of the isthmus there were 42 $\pm$ 1.5 continuous epithelial (mucous) cells. Surface mucous cells lining the gastric pit constituted 76.2 ($\pm$ 1.4)% of the total epithelial cells and mucous neck cells constituted 23.8 ($\pm$ 1.4)% of the epithelial cells. Although the mucous neck cells constituted about 1/4 of all cells below the opening of the foveolus (gastric pit), they occupied only 19.5% of the total epithelial surface area, indicating that they were slightly smaller than the pit mucous cells which accounted for 81.5% of the total epithelial surface area.

The apical cytoplasm of mucous cells lining the interfoveolar area and the upper gastric pit had densely packed, biphasic mucous granules with a centrally located dense core surrounded by a more lightly staining material (Fig 2). This pattern continued from the foveolus to approximately 1/3 of the mucosal thickness which was about 10 consecutive cells towards the base of the isthmus.   Mucous cells in the middle 1/3 to 1/2 of the mucosa (10-15 cells) had mucous granules whose contents were no longer biphasic but stained homogenously light or dark.   Electron microscopy showed numerous granules in all pit cells fusing with the apical plasma membrane.

Mucous neck cells in the isthmus had irregularly shaped large granules which were not tightly packed in the cytoplasm but more loosely arranged and were routinely observed fusing with the apical plasma membrane.   The granule contents were morphologically distinct in being biphasic but the dense core lay in contact with the granule membrane (Fig 2). Transmission electron microscopy showed a network of fine filamentous material extending from the dense cores into the lighter staining area of the granules (Fig. 2).

Neutral glycoproteins were distinguished from acidic lighter ones (sialo and sulfomucins) by the AB-PAS method.   A thin blue staining pattern indicating acidic glycoproteins at the apical margin of each mucous cell regardless of its position showed the presence of a rich glycocalyx which was particularly prominent over the interfovelar and upper gastric

pit cells.   Acidic glycoproteins within mucous granules were consistently
present in epithelial cells confined to the isthmus where mucous neck cells
were found.   In the transition region between gastric pit and isthmus, some
cells had an Alcian blue (pH 2.5) positive (acidic glycoproteins) apical region
as well as neutral glycoprotein granules nearer the nucleus. Mucous granules
of cells lining the upper pit contained mostly neutral glycoproteins as did
interfoveolar cells.

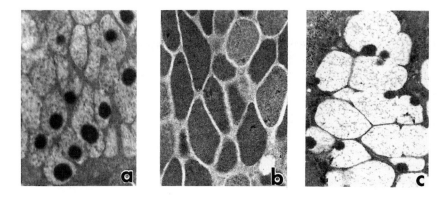

FIGURE 2   *Electron micrographs of mucous granules showing (a) biphasic
granules with a concentric light area surrounding a dense core, (b) a
mixed population of homogenously light and dark granules, and (c)
biphasic granules with the dense core asymmetrically positioned. x
20,000.*

    To distinguish sulfomucins from sialomucins, two methods were used.
The first (D-PAS) showed that upper gastric pit cells had abundant neutral
mucins, as described above.   The second method (HID-AB) showed that the
dark brown to black precipitate indicating sulfomucins was located in
mucous neck cells confined to the isthmus.   The light blue staining pattern
in this method identifying sialomucins was found in about 50% of the cells
within the isthmus.   When the PB/KOH/PAS method was applied to detect
the O-acetyl groups of sialomucins, all slides were negative suggesting that
the sialomucins, found predominantly in the isthmus, were rich in N-acetyl
groups.

    The extracellular mucus layer did not form a continuous sheet over
the mucosal surface.   The maximum thickness observed was 15 micrometers.
Histochemical staining indicated that most of this intermittently present
mucous layer was composed of neutral glycoproteins but there were distinct
strands or layers of sulfo- and sialoglycoproteins incorporated in it.   Within
the lumen of both the isthmus and gastric pit there was strong staining for
both moieties of acidic glycoproteins.

Macroscopic inspection of the mucosal surface showed that the hypertonic insult of luminal 2 M NaCl did not produce hemorrhagic lesions at any time during the four weeks of dosing. In comparison with control rats in which 6 M NaCl caused gross hemorrhagic lesions over 27.6 ($\pm$ 5.8)% of the mucosal surface, experimental rats showed only 1.0 ($\pm$0.4)% of the mucosa occupied by deep lesions.

Light microscopy (epoxy resin sections) of rat gastric mucosae fixed at various time intervals after 2 M NaCl exposure showed consistent and uniform damage to the superficial mucosa that was largely restituted by 24 hr. After damage the interfovelor and upper gastric pit cells exfoliated as a single sheet of necrotic epithelium forming the previously described mucoid layer [4]. Cells deeper in the mucosa showed some evidence of damage but were not exfoliated into the lumen. Subsequently the mucosa went through the typical stages of epithelial restitution in which viable mucous cells in the gastric pits rapidly migrated across the denuded basal lamina and reformed the epithelial surface. By 24 hr, the mucosal surface was re-epithelialized.

The thickness and general organization of the mucosa was not different from that of the control animals (Fig 1). The mucous neck cells occupied the isthmus, which constituted the lower 16.6% of the total mucosal depth compared to 19.5% in the control group, indicating that a slight cellular hypertrophy had taken place in surface cells since the number of isthmus cells remained constant in both groups. Using bromodeoxyuridine immunolabelling [5] there were at least twice as many cells undergoing division (in the proliferative zone) as in the controls.

The average interfoveolar and gastric pit cell volume occupied by mucous granules was 18.2 ($\pm$ 7.5)% and 45.8 ($\pm$ 3.4)%, respectively, which was not statistically significantly different from the untreated rats. Planimetry also showed that there was no difference in the mean diameter of mucous granules in control and experimental animals. However, a major change we observed after four weeks of hypertonic sodium chloride treatment was the contents of the mucous granules. Over half of the samples had no biphasic mucous granules in the interfoveolar cells. Furthermore, in contrast to the control animals, upper gastric pit cells contained only a few biphasic granules mixed in a population of predominantly light and dark granules (Fig. 2). In the middle 1/3 of the mucosa (cells 10-25) there were no biphasic granules and only homogenously light, dark, or a mixture of both granular types were found (Fig 2).

Using the AB-PAS method we observed neutral glycoproteins scattered in mucous cells occupying the lower half of the gastric pits. Adjacent cells in this area were strongly positive for acidic mucin. Those cells lining the upper half of the pit contained abundant mucous granules but stained purple, indicating a mixture of both acidic and neutral mucins in these cells. Each of the interfoveolar cells had few if any mucin granules but, when present, they possessed a mixture of neutral and acidic glycoproteins, as shown by the intense purple staining.   All cells in the isthmus stained for acidic glycoproteins as did long strands of mucus within the lumens of the gastric pits.

The D-PAS method showed a marked reduction in red-pink staining in the isthmus indicating few sialo- or neutral glycoprotein-containing mucous neck cells there. The HID-AB method showed that cells containing sulfomucins occupied 90% of the isthmus and extended into the lower half of the gastric pit. In both regions sulfomucin-rich cells were interspersed with sialomucin-containing cells. It was not uncommon to count 40% of the total cells from foveolus to the base of the isthmus that contained abundant amounts of sulfomucins. The other gastric pit cells that had stained intensely for acidic mucins in the AB-PAS method stained for sialomucins in the HID-AB technique. Sialoglycoproteins were also stained along the apical plasma membrane of all the mucous cells, particularly the interfoveolar and upper pit cells, consistent with the presence of a thick glycocalyx as observed in the control animals. When the PB/KOH/PAS method was applied to detect O-acetyl groups of sialomucins, all slides were negative as in the control animals, indicating that the sailomucins were rich in N-acetyl groups.

The extracellular mucus was much thicker (25-50 micrometers) than in controls and formed a continuous layer over the mucosa as observed in epoxy resin (but not paraffin) sections. This mucus layer consisted almost entirely of sulfo- and sialoglycoproteins, as indicated by the HID-AB and AB-PAS staining, and not of neutral glycoproteins as in the control animals.

DISCUSSION

The phenomenon of "adaptive cytoprotection" was defined as protection of the gastric mucosa against an acute lesion-producing agent (e.g. absolute ethanol) by pretreatment of the stomach with a "mild irritant" [6]. The protection lasted for several hours after a single dose of the mild irritant. The chronic superficial damage induced by the mild irritant (2 M NaCl) in the present study produced a protective response that lasted for at least 24 hours, showing for the first time that "adaptive mucosal protection" can be cumulative.

The histochemical and morphologic results of the present study show that the rat antral mucosa responds to chronic luminal insult of the superficial mucosa by: 1) increased mucous cell production in the proliferative zone; 2) a change from predominantly neutral to a mixture of largely acidic and some neutral glycoprotein synthesis and secretion in gastric pit cells; 3) a marked increase in sulfomucin-secreting cells in the isthmus; 4) a shift to sialomucin synthesis in the lower gastric pit cells; 5) a decrease in the number of concentric biphasic mucous granules in the upper gastric pit and interfoveolar cells;   and 6) formation of a thick, continuous luminal mucus layer largely consisting of acidic glycoproteins.

The unstressed antral isthmus contains proliferating cells interspersed with mucous neck cells which synthesize and secrete sialo- and sulfomucins.

Because these two components of mucus are not produced by other cell types in the normal antral mucosa, it seems likely that acidic glycoproteins in the luminal mucous layer are secreted from the mucous neck cells deep within the mucosa. As in the antral mucus layer, the distinct strands of neutral and acidic glycoproteins in the fundic mucous layer of dogs [7,8] and rats [9] suggest that these two components of mucus do not readily mix and that there may be some as yet undescribed pattern to mucin secretion in the various populations of gastric mucous cells. The heterogenous composition of the luminal mucous layer further suggests that each biochemically distinct component may have a different function in retarding diffusion across this layer [1,9-11].

Although gastric mucus has traditionally been given a role in retardation of acid and pepsin diffusion, there is mounting evidence that its most important role may be after luminal insult rather than preventing the initial damage. The formation of the "mucoid layer" from exfoliated and disrupted surface cells and its subsequent protective role is well documented [9,12]. This layer functions to retard further insult to the mucosa and to trap bicarbonate-rich fluid next to the restituting mucosal surface [4]. It would appear that the synthesis and secretion of greater amounts of mucin in chronically injured (by "mild irritants") rat stomachs, as demonstrated in the present study, would add additional protection to the mucosa, although it is doubtful that the marked reduction in gross lesions following 6 M NaCl could be attributed solely to a thicker mucous layer since endogenous mediators such as prostaglandins probably play a significant role in protection [6]. However, as recent studies of the chronically challenged fundic mucosa showed, protection is acquired against subsequent acute damage when the "mild irritant" was 2 M but not 1 M NaCl [13].

The constant amount of mucin in the gastric pit cells of both experimental and control animals but the marked increase in the thickness and continuity of the mucus layer of experimental animals shown here suggests an increased synthesis and subsequent secretion of mucin fom the mucous cells in challenged stomachs. Furthermore, chronic superficial damage induces a marked shift from neutral to acidic mucin synthesis and secretion, suggesting that sialo- and sulfomucins may be more protective in some as yet undescribed manner than the neutral mucins produced by the unstressed mucosa.

ACKNOWLEDGEMENT

Supported in part by NIH grant DK39074.
We thank Ms. Marion Hinson for excellent secretarial assistance.

REFERENCES

1.   Morris GP. The myth of the mucus barrier. Gastroenterol. Clin. Biol. 1985; 9: 106-7.

2.   Filipe MI. Gastrointestinal tract. In: Spicer SS, ed. Histochemistry in Pathologic Diagnosis, Chapt. 13. New York: Marcel Dekker Inc. 1987: 355.

3.   Ito S. Anatomic structure of the gastric mucosa. In: Code CF, ed. Handbook of Physiology, Section 6, Alimentary Canal, Chapt. 41. Washington DC: Americal Physiological Society, 1968; 705-41

4.   Lacy ER, Ito S. Mechanisms of rapid epithelial restitution of the superficial rat gastric mucosa after ethanol injury. In: Szabo S, Pfeiffer CJ, eds. Ulcer Disease: New Aspects of Pathogenesis and Pharmacology. Boca Raton, FL. CRC Press, Inc. 1989: 65-81.

5.   Lacy ER, Kuwayama H, Cowart K, Deutz A, King J, Sistrunk S. A rapid, accurate immunohistochemical technique for labelling proliferating cells in the gastrointestinal tract: a comparison with tritiated thymidine. Gastroenterology, in press.

6.   Robert A, Nezamis JE, Lancaster C, Davis JP, Field SO, Hanchar AJ. Mild irritants prevent gastric necrosis through "adaptive cytoprotection" mediated by prostaglandins. Am J Physiol. 1983; 245: G113-21.

7.   Zalewsky CA, Moody FG. Mechanisms of mucus release in exposed canine gastric mucosa. Gastroenterology 1979; 77: 719-29.

8.   Zalewsky CA, Moody FG, Allen M, Davis EK. Stimulation of canine gastric mucus secretion with intraarterial acetylcholine chloride. Gastroenterology 1983; 85: 1067-75.

9.   Morris GP, Harding RK, Wallace JL. A functional model for extracellular gastric mucus in the rat. Virchows Arch. (Cell Pathol.) 1984; 46: 239-51.

10.   Williams SE, Turnberg LA. Retardation of acid diffusion by pig gastric mucus: a potential role in mucosal protection. Gastroenterology 1980; 79: 299-304.

11.   Williams SE, Turnberg LA. Demonstration of a pH gradient across mucus adherent to rabbit gastric mucosa: evidence for a 'mucus-bicarbonate' barrier. Gut 1981; 22: 94-6.

12.   Lacy ER. Gastric mucosal resistance to a repeated ethanol insult. Scand J Gastro. 1985; 20 (Suppl. 110): 63-72.

13.   Lacy ER, Cowart K, Smolka A, Hennigar GR. Chronic superficial epithelial damage induces marked cellular changes in rat gastric mucosa. Gastroenterology 1990; 98: A73.

RESTITUTION IN THE INTESTINE

R. Schiessel, M. Riegler, W. Feil, E. Wenzl

Clinic of Surgery 1, University of Vienna, Austria

ABSTRACT

Rapid restitution (RR) after mucosal damage occurs in the entire gastrointestinal tract. This process and its influencing factors were studied in rabbit duodenum and colon and human duodenum in an *in vitro* model. Simultaneous PD, I_{sc}, R and alkaline flux were measured. Morphometric data were obtained by a computerized set up. 10 mM HCl for 10 minutes caused a uniform mucosal damage in rabbit duodenum of $68.3 \pm 0.66\%$ surface area, after 5 hours only $14.01 \pm 1.41\%$ remained damaged. Lack of nutrient bicarbonate inhibited RR at luminal pH (pH_L) = 7.4 ($34.72 \pm 1.31\%$ damage after 5 hours) and completely abolished RR at pH_L = 3. Removal of the post injury necrotic layer covering the mucosa decreased RR only at pH_L = 3, whereas at pH_L = 7.4 RR occurred unaffected. Serosal Ca^{++} free solution entirely blocked RR. Luminal administration of Na-deoxycholate (Na-DOC), sucralfate, EGF, trypsin and pepsin after the damage had no effect on RR. Morphology of RR in human duodenum was not different from that in rabbit duodenum.

Exposure of human colon to Na-DOC (0.5mM for 10 minutes) produced a 50% mucosal damage after 30 minutes. After 5 hours $28.91 \pm 0.36\%$ were still damaged. Luminal Na-DOC or Ca^{++} free solutions suppressed RR ($51.88 \pm 2.79\%$ and $64.61 \pm 2.35\%$ damage after 5 hours). Antifibronectin had no influence on RR whereas antilaminin decelerated RR ($41.66 \pm 1.25\%$ damage after 5 hours). Until now RR can be inhibited as shown, but no stimulatory agents are known.

INTRODUCTION

Rapid restitution (RR) is a repair process by which superficial epithelial defects are covered quickly by migration of intact cells.

This mechanism was first described in the stomach [7] but later also in the duodenum, gallbladder, small intestine and colon [1,2,3,4,5]. We studied factors influencing RR in the duodenum and colon.

403

METHODS

DUODENUM

The proximal duodenum was excised from anesthetized New Zealand white rabbits with an average weight of 3 kg. The mucosa was stripped of its muscular coat and then transferred to a modified Ussing chamber. The solution on the nutrient side contained (in mM/l): NaCl 122.0, KCl 5.0, $CaCl_2$ 2.0, $MgSO_4$ 1.3, Glucose 20.0. It was buffered with $NaHCO_3$ 25.0 mM and gassed with 95% O_2/5% CO_2.

The mucosal side was perfused with a solution containing NaCl 154.0 mM gassed with 100% O_2 prewashed in 1 M KOH. Luminal pH was kept constant at pH = 7.4 by infusion of HCl 100 mM by a pH-stat system in order to measure alkaline flux. In addition we measured PD and 1_{sc} using a Voltage/Current Clamp (World Precision Instruments Inc. Hewhaven, CT, USA, Model DVC-1000). Resistance was calculated using Ohm's law.

HUMAN STUDIES

In order to get information about RR in the human duodenum we used duodenal mucosa from brain-dead organ donors after in situ organ perfusion with Euro-Collins solution. Tissue preparation and measurements were as above.

HISTOLOGY

Tissues were fixed immediately at the end of the experiments in buffered 5% formaldehyde and pinned out on a dental wax plate. For transmission electron microscopy the tissues were postfixed in 1% osmium tretroxyde in 0.1 cacodylate buffer. The further tissue processing was as described previously. To assess the extent of injury and repair we used a computer based morphometry system (MIPSY)[4].

COLON

All studies were performed on human tissues. Small colon segments were excised from patients during surgery for colorectal cancer. The tissues were quickly put into a preoxygenated Euro-Collins solution at 4°C. The mucosa was then separated from the seromuscular coat and transferred into a modified Ussing-chamber with an area of 1 cm^2. The nutrient solution and gassing were the same as in the experiments with the duodenum.

RESULTS

DUODENUM

Rabbit duodenum:

Exposure to HCl 10 mM for 10 minutes caused a significant drop of the PD from -2.41 ± 0.18 mV to -0.55 ± 0.08 mV, there was a recovery within 5 hours to -1.35 ± 0.13 mV.

Histology showed uniform mucosal damage confined to the villi. Morphometry revealed 68.3 ± 0.66% damage of the mucosal surface after 30 minutes. Thereafter the remaining intact cells migrated over the denuded surface along the basal lamina. 5 hours after the injury only 14.01 ± 1.41% of the mucosal surface remained damaged.

The role of nutrient HCO_3^- for restitution:

To investigate the importance of nutrient HCO_3^- for RR we changed the nutrient solution to one containing HEPES buffer instead of HCO_3^- after exposure to HCl 10 mM. This resulted in a significant drop of PD from -3.0 ± 0.08 to -0.66 ± 0.06 mV with no recovery within 5 hours.

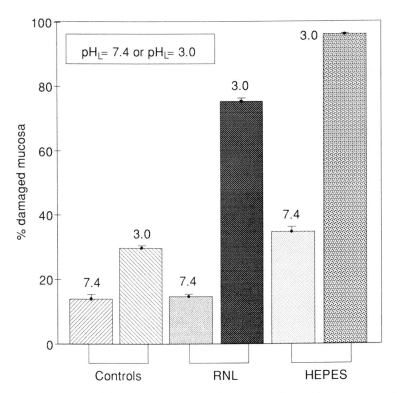

FIGURE 1. *Effects of removal of necrotic layer (RNL), serosal bicarbonate free (HEPES) media and luminal pH on RR in rabbit duodenum 5 hours after mucosal HCl damage. At pH_L = 7.4 controls left over 14.04 ± 1.41% damaged mucosa. This was uninfluenced when the necrotic layer has been removed (14.72 ± 0.77%), whereas lack of nutrient bicarbonate led to a significantly decreased RR (34.72 ± 1.31%). At pH_L = 0.3 RR was also decelerated (29.71 ± 0.73%). This effect was more pronounced after removal of the necrotic layer (75.35 ± 1.01%) or in serosal bicarbonate free media (96.17 ± 0.38)(n=6 each group).*

Alkaline flux decreased from 0.98 $\pm$ 0.03 uEq/cm$_2$/10min. to 0.23 $\pm$ 0.01 uEq/cm$_2$/10 min.   Morphometry showed slight inhibition of RR with 34.72 $\pm$ 1.31% damaged surface after 5 hours when the luminal pH was 7.4. At a luminal pH of 3, however, complete inhibition of RR was observed (Fig.1).

The role of necrotic layer:

After damage the mucosa is covered with a layer of necrotic cells, fibrin and mucus. In order to study the eventual function of this layer we removed it mechanically after mucosal damage. Removal of the necrotic layer had no influence on PD recovery after damage at a luminal pH (pH$_L$) of 7.4 but at pH$_L$ = 3 no recovery occurred. Morphometry showed no additional damage caused by the mechanical irritation. At a pH$_L$ = 7.4 the extent of damage after 5 hours was similar as in controls, but at pH = 3 significant inhibition of RR was observed (Fig. 1).

Ca^{++} free nutrient solution:

When Ca^{++} was removed from the nutrient solution, the PD remained stable for 60 minutes but decreased thereafter. Damage with HCl 10mM and serosal Ca^{++} free medium caused a sudden drop of PD with no recovery. Morphometry showed lack of RR after 5 hours (55.75 $\pm$ 3.85% still damaged after 5 hours)(Fig. 2).

Na-deoxycholate:

Since the duodenal lumen is in contact with bile salt, we studied the influence of Na-deoxycholate (Na-DOC) on RR.   Luminal exposure to Na-DOC 0.05 mM after damage with HCl 10 mM for 10 minutes caused similar changes on PD as HCl alone.   Morphometry showed undisturbed RR after 5 hours (18.8 $\pm$ 1.76%) (Fig.2).   Sucralfate, EGF, trypsin and pepsin had no effect on RR.

Human duodenum:

Up to now restitution was mainly studied in animal tissues.   Our group gave the first demonstration of RR in humans by studying colon mucosa from patients subjected to cancer surgery. However, it is impossible to study duodenal mucosa from pancreatoduodenectomy specimens because the time of ischemia is too long.   To overcome this problem, we used duodenal segments from multiorgan donors after in situ organ perfusion. We were able to study duodena of 2 donors. The tissues were treated in the same way as rabbit mucosa.

60 minutes after damage with the 10mM HCl for 10 minutes clear signs of restitution were seen (Fig.3). After 5 hours RR was demonstrable in both tissues. The morphology was not different to that in rabbit duodenum (Fig. 4)

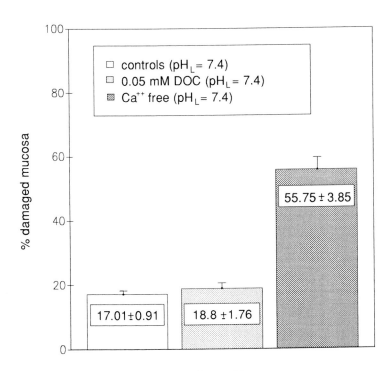

5 hours after acid exposure

FIGURE 2: *Influence of luminal Na-DOC or serosal Ca^{++} free media on rabbit duodenal RR 5 hours after HCl damage. Na-DOC did not affect RR in comparison to controls, whereas serosal lack of Ca^{++} completely blocked RR after 5 hours (n=6 each group, p<0.05).*

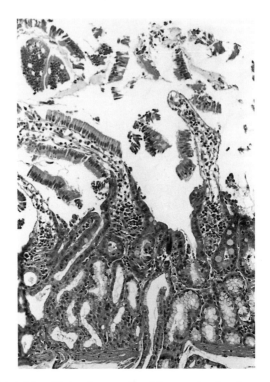

FIGURE 3: *Photomicrograph of human duodenal mucosa 1 hour after HCl damage*

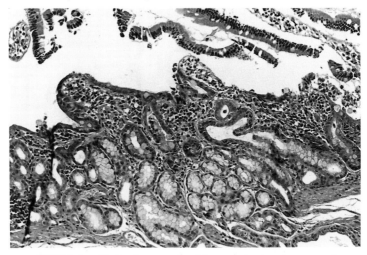

FIGURE 4: *Photomicrograph of human duodenal mucosa 5 hours after HCl damage*

<u>COLON</u>

Effect of mucosal damage with Na-DOC:

Exposure of human colonic mucosa to Na-DOC (0.5 mM for 10 minutes) caused a significant drop of the PD from -26.53 ± 3.23 to -12.22 ± 1.5 mV. The lowest value was reached at 30 minutes after damage and came back to -14.5 ± 2.34 at 5 hours. Morphometry showed 50% damage of surface area after 30 minutes. 5 hours after damage 28.91 ± 0.36% were still damaged (Fig. 5).

In the following experiments we studied the effect of different agents on RR in the human colon.

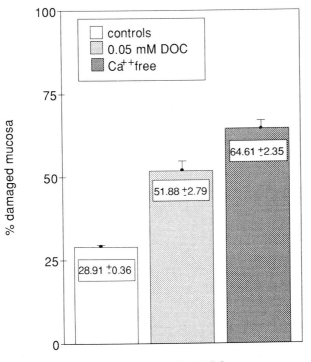

5 hours after NaCl - DOC exposure

FIGURE 5: *Influence of luminal Na-DOC or serosal Ca^{++} free solutions on human colonic RR 5 hours after mucosal Na-DOC damage (0.5 mM for 10 minutes). Luminal Na-DOC slowed RR down, which was more evident bathing in serosal Ca^{++} free solutions (n=6 each group).*

Na-deoxycholate:

In order to study the effect of the bile salt on RR we exposed the mucosa after damage to luminal 0.05 mM Na-DOC for 5 hours. The PD showed no recovery after damage. Morphometry indicated inhibition of RR with $51.88 \pm 2.79\%$ of the surface still damaged after 5 hours (Fig. 5).

Ca^{++} free nutrient solution:

PD dropped from -16.43 ± 2.85 mV to -7.50 ± 1.48 mV 10 minutes after damage. There was no significant recovery after 5 hours (-6.20 ± 3.33 mV). Histology showed inhibition of RR with $64.61 \pm 2.35\%$ surface still damaged after 5 hours (Fig. 5).

ANTIFIBRONECTIN

This agent was added in a concentration of 50 ug/ml to the luminal side after damage. The course of the PD after damage was not significantly different from the control group. Morphometry did not show any effects on RR (Fig.6).

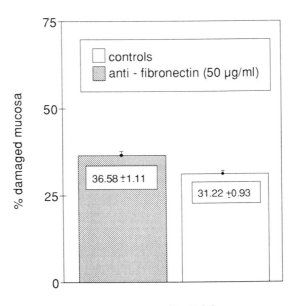

5 hours after NaCl - DOC exposure

FIGURE 6:   *RR in human colonic mucosa remained uninfluenced by antifibronectin 5 hours after mucosal Na DOC damage (0.5 mM for 10 minutes) (paired samples from 6 experiments).*

Antilaminin

Adding antilaminin to the luminal side (50ug/ml) caused a steady decline of the PD after damage. Morphometry indicated inhibition of RR with 41.66 ± 1.25% of surface still damaged after 5 hours (Fig. 7).

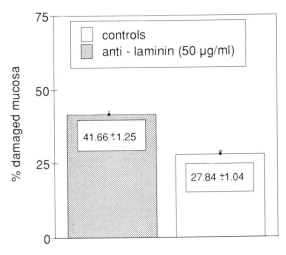

FIGURE 7: *Antilaminin significantly decreased the extent of RR in human colonic mucosa 5 hours after mucosal Na DOC damage (0.5 mM for 10 minutes) (paired samples from 6 experiments).*

DISCUSSION

The presented data confirm previous observations on the stomach that there are many factors which can inhibit restitution, but there is at the present time no agent available that might stimulate this process.

REFERENCES

1.   Argenzio RA, Henrikson CK, Liacos JA.   Restitution of barrier and transport function of porcine colon after acute mucosal injury.   Am J Physiol 1988; 255: G62-G71.

2.   Erickson RA. Effect of 16, 16-dimethyl PGE2 and indomethacin on bile acid-induced intestinal injury and restitution in rats J Lab Clin Med 1988; 112: 735-744.

3.   Feil W, Wenzl E, Vattay P, Starlinger M, Sogukoglu T, Schiessel R. Repair of rabbit duodenal mucosa after acid injury in vivo and in vitro. Gastroenterology 1987; 92: 1973-1986.

4.   Feil W, Lacy ER, Wong YM, Burger D, Wenzl E, Starlinger M, Schiessel R. Rapid epithelial restitution of human and rabbit colonic mucosa. Gastroenterology 1989; 97: 685-701.

5.   Hudspeth AJ. The recovery of local transepithelial resistance following single-cell lesions. Exp Cell Res 1982; 138: 331-342.

6.   Svanes K, Takeuchi K, Ito S, Silen W. Effect of luminal pH and nutrient bicarbonate concentration on restitution after gastric surface cell injury. Surgery 1983; 94: 494-500.

7.   Svanes K, Ito S, Takeuchi K, Silen W. Restitution of the surface epithelium of the in vitro frog gastric mucosa after damage with hyperosmolar sodium chloride. Gastroenterology 1982; 82: 1409-1426.

EFFECTS OF NUTRIENT HCO_3^- AND LUMINAL pH ON RESTITUTION OF COLONIC MUCOSA IN VITRO

P.H. Rowe*, Q. Zhang, D.C. Hanley, R.C. Mason

*Departments of Surgery, Guy's Hospital, London and *Eastbourne District General Hospital, East Sussex*

ABSTRACT

Restitution occurs within 4 hours in Ussing chambered amphibian colonic mucosa following injury by exposure to 10mM sodium deoxycholate (DOCA) for 10 minutes. We investigated the effects of different concentrations of HCO_3^- ($[HCO_3^-]$) in the nutrient solution (N) and different luminal pH (pH_L) during the four hour recovery period, on restitution of the colonic surface epithelium. Tissues exposed to DOCA exhibited an immediate fall in potential difference and resistance and a severe mucosal injury with denudation of the basal lamina. At luminal pH 6.0 tissues with 18mM HCO_3^- and 48mM HCO_3^- in N exhibited histological restitution of the surface epithelium, the process occurring significantly faster in tissues with 48mM HCO_3^- in N ($p<0.05$). In contrast, tissues with no HCO_3^- in N exhibited no electrical recovery or restitution of the surface epithelium with evidence of severe mucosal injury. At luminal pH 4.0 only tissues with 48mM HCO_3^- in N exhibited a normal electrical and histological recovery, however the process of restitution did not occur with a luminal pH 2.0.

We conclude HCO_3^- is necessary in the nutrient solution to facilitate restitution of colonic mucosa in vitro and this process is inhibited by a low luminal pH. This highlights the importance of an alkaline micro-environment for rapid restitution in the amphibian colonic mucosa.

INTRODUCTION

Rapid restitution is a process by which epithelial integrity and continuity are rapidly re-established after superficial injury, before cell proliferation or an extensive inflammatory response occur [1]. Previous studies have described rapid epithelial restitution in the bullfrog [2,3,4] and guinea pig [5] stomach *in vitro* as well as in the rat [6-9] and cat [10] stomach *in vivo* after damage by hypertonic saline solution [2,4,5,10] or ethanol [6-9]. Restitution has been described in the rabbit duodenum *in vivo* and *in vitro* [11], but it was not until recently that cell migration was shown to occur in the porcine colon *in vitro* and *in vivo* [12], in rabbit colon *in vivo* [13] and human colonic mucosa *in vitro* [13].

We have demonstrated restitution of amphibian colonic mucosa *in vitro* after injury by bile salts [14,15]. Restitution in this model is inhibited by application of cytochalasin B [16] and prostaglandins [17]. It has been shown that rapid restitution in the stomach could be affected by the luminal pH and nutrient HCO_3^- [18]. We investigated whether these same effects pertain to the amphibian colonic mucosa *in vitro*.

MATERIALS AND METHODS

American bullfrogs (*Rana Catesbeiana*) were stored in 120mM NaCl at $4^\circ C$. The frogs were not fed but were used within two weeks of purchase. After pithing the colon was removed, divided longitudinally, providing 2 preparations per frog, and each half was mounted between Lucite chambers with an exposed area of $1cm^2$. Nutrient and luminal surfaces were bathed with 15ml of solution at $24^\circ C$ circulated by separate gas-lift systems with 95% O_2 and 5% CO_2; 100% O_2 was the gas used when n-2-hydroxyethyl piperazine -N^1-2-ethane sulfonic acid (HEPES) buffer was in the nutrient solution. The composition, pH and osmolarity of the different nutrient (serosal) solutions and the standard luminal solution are shown in Table 1. The pH of the luminal solution was continuously titrated to the specific pH in each experiment with a Radiometer pH stat (Radiometer A/S, Copenhagen, Denmark) using 50mM HCL as the titrant.

TABLE 1.

COMPOSITION OF SOLUTIONS.

	NUTRIENT SOLUTION $[HCO_3^-]$			Luminal Solution
	18mM	48mM	HEPES	
Osmolarity (mosmol)	289.8	289.8	289.8	289.8
pH	7.3	7.8	7.8	6.0, 4.0 or 2.0
Na^+	102.4	102.4	102.4	102.4
K^+	4.0	4.0	4.0	4.0
Cl^-	91.4	91.4	91.4	91.4
HCO_3^-	17.8	47.8	-	-
$H_2PO_4^-$	0.8	0.8	0.8	-
Mg_2^+	0.8	0.8	0.8	0.8
SO_4^{2-}	0.8	0.8	0.8	10.1
Choline	-	30.0	-	-
Mannitol	60.0	-	60.0	79.3
HEPES	-	-	17.8	-
Ca^{2+}	1.8	1.8	1.8	1.8
Glucose	10.0	10.0	10.0	-

Transmucosal potential difference (PD) and resistance (R) were measured as previously described [19]. Experiments were commenced after a one hour stabilisation period in standard nutrient and luminal solutions. Control tissues were exposed to the standard luminal and nutrient solution containing the $[HCO_3^-]$ relevant to each experiment, and the luminal pH was titrated to the requisite pH for each experiment. A solution of DOCA at luminal pH 6.0 was used to destroy the surface epithelium of the colonic mucosa, the ordinary luminal solution was replaced by 10mM DOCA for a period of 10 minutes, after which the luminal side was washed three times with standard luminal solution. The nutrient solution was also changed twice after the 10mM DOCA treatment. The tissues were then allowed to incubate in the chambers for a period of four hours.

At the completion of the experiments colonic mucosae were removed from the chamber and cut into three pieces. The tissues for light microscopy were fixed in formalin solution. The fixed specimens were dehydrated in ethanol, embedded in paraffin, sectioned at 1uM and stained with haematoxylin and eosin.

Structural analysis was done by two of the authors who had no knowledge of the treatment of the tissue. Statistical analysis was performed using Student's t-test for paired and unpaired variates. Results are presented as means $\pm$ SEM and are regarded as statistically significant if $p < 0.05$.

RESULTS

1. EFFECTS OF DIFFERENT NUTRIENT $[HCO_3^-]$

After application of 10mM DOCA to the luminal chamber, all tissues exhibited a dramatic fall in potential difference (PD) and resistance (R) (Figure 1) with evidence of a severe injury to the surface epithelial cells, exposure of areas of basal lamina and extensive debris in the lumen (Figure 2). After exposure to DOCA, the luminal chamber was washed and the solution changed to standard luminal solution. The nutrient solution was replaced with N containing different $[HCO_3^-]$: 48mM., 18mM, HCO_3^- free using HEPES buffer. In tissues with 18mM HCO_3^- in N, in the next 4 hours the PD returned from -10 ± 4mV to -60 ± 10mV and R from 10 ± 15 ohm cm^2 to 220 ± 40 ohm cm^2 (Figure 1), values not significantly different from PD and R prior to injury. There was complete histological restitution of the surface epithelium. In tissues with 48mM HCO_3^- in N, the PD returned from -6 ± 1mV to -70 ± 15mV and R from 55 ± 10 ohm cm^2 to 210 ± 20 ohm cm^2, values not significantly different from PD and R prior to injury (Figure 1).

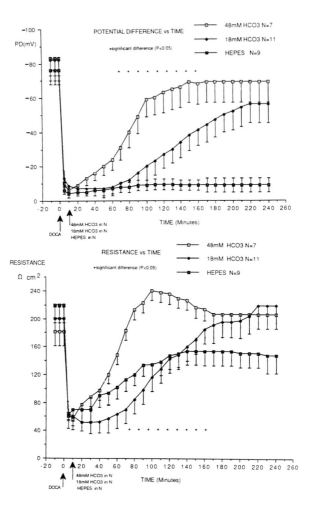

FIGURE 1: *Ten minute exposure of colonic mucosae to 10mM DOCA, in the luminal chamber followed by 4 hour recovery in chambers.   Effects of different [HCO₃⁻] in N during the recovery period.   Luminal pH = 6.0.   Mean ± SEM are presented.   * p <0.05.*

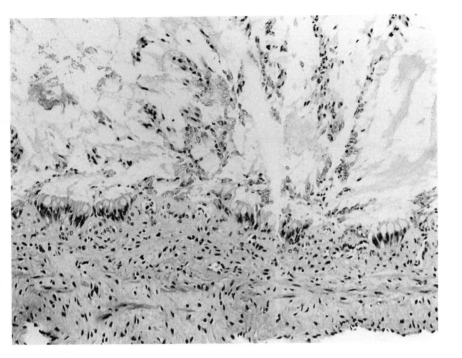

FIGURE 2: *Tissue exposed to 10mM DOCA in the luminal chamber (pH 6.0) for 10 minutes. There is severe damage to the surface mucosal epithelium with exposure of the basal lamina and extensive debris in the lumen.*

This occurred within 2 hours, significantly faster than the restitution process in tissues with 18mM HCO_3^- in N (p<0.05). After only a 2 hour recovery time, tissues with 48mM HCO_3^- in N exhibited complete restitution of the surface epithelium (Figure 3).

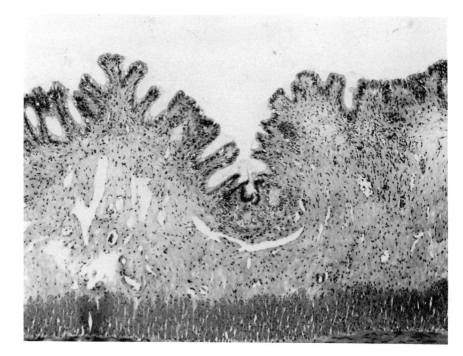

FIGURE 3: *Tissue exposed to 10mM DOCA (pH$_L$ 6.0) for 10 minutes followed by 4 hour incubation in the chambers. 48mM HCO$_3^-$ in N during the recovery period. Restitution of the colonic surface epithelium has occurred producing an intact surface epithelium.*

In contrast, tissues with HCO$_3^-$ free nutrient solution exhibited no significant electrical recovery (Figure 1). Despite a four hour incubation in the Ussing chambers there was still an extensive mucosal injury, the surface only partly covered by a thin, irregular epithelium with exposure of the basal lamina and sloughing of dead cells in the lumen (Figure 4).

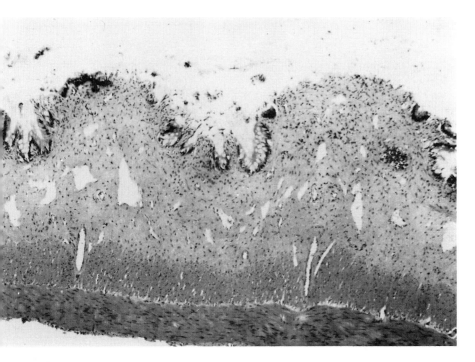

FIGURE 4: *Tissue exposed to 10mM DOCA (pH$_L$ 6.0) for 10 minutes followed by 4 hour incubation in the chambers. HCO$_3^-$ free (HEPES) in N during the recovery period. An extensive mucosal injury is still present.*

2. EFFECTS OF DIFFERENT LUMINAL pH

a) 18mM HCO$_3^-$ in N

After the treatment of 10mM DOCA, replacement of DOCA with standard luminal solution the luminal solution was maintained at luminal pH 6.0 in one group of tissues and luminal pH 4.0 in another group, followed by four hour recovery in the chambers with 18mM HCO$_3^-$ in N. In tissues recovering in luminal pH 6.0, the PD and R returned to values not significantly different from PD and R prior to injury (Figure 5). Histologically complete restitution of the epithelium occurred. In contrast tissues recovering in luminal pH 4.0, did not exhibit the electrical or histological recovery and epithelial restitution had not occurred.

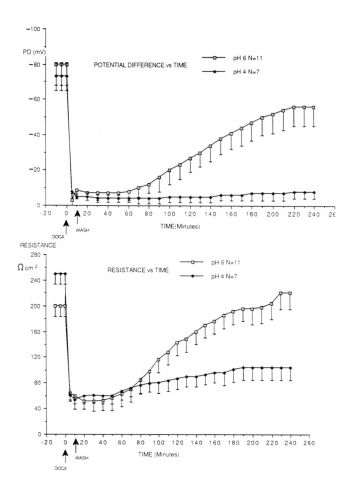

FIGURE 5: *Ten minute exposure of colonic mucosae to 10mM DOCA in the luminal chamber followed by 4 hour recovery in chambers. Effects of different luminal pH during the recovery period. 18mM HCO_3^- in N. Mean $\pm$ SEM are presented.*

b) 48mM HCO$_3^-$ in N

After the treatment of 10mM DOCA replacement of DOCA with standard solution the luminal solution was maintained at luminal pH 4.0 in one group of tissues and luminal pH 2.0 in another group followed by a four hour recovery period in the chambers. In tissues recovering in luminal pH 4.0 the PD and R returned to values not significantly different from control tissues (Figure 6) and histologically complete restitution of the surface epithelium had occurred.

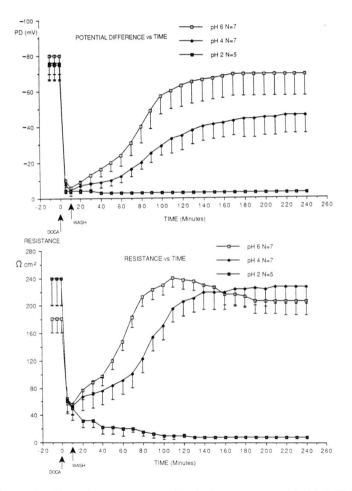

FIGURE 6: *Ten minute exposure of colonic mucosae to 10mM DOCA in the luminal chamber followed by 4 hour recovery in the chambers. Effects of different luminal pH during the recovery period. 48mM HCO$_3^-$ in N. Mean ± SEM are presented.*

However, tissues recovering in luminal pH 2.0 failed to recover electrically or histologically. The surface epithelium remained severely damaged with complete exposure of the basal lamina (Figure 7).

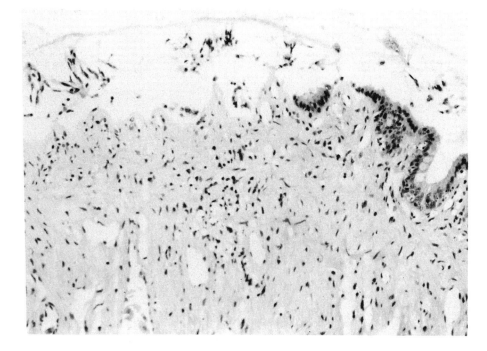

FIGURE 7: *Tissue exposed to 10mM DOCA (pH$_L$ 6.0) for 10 minutes followed by 4 hour recovery incubation in the chambers. 48mM HCO$_3^-$ in N and pH$_L$ 2.0 during the recovery period. Extensive surface mucosal injury and complete exposure of the basal lamina is evident.*

DISCUSSION

The present study shows that the amphibian colonic mucosa responds to superficial injury by bile salts, by re-establishing an intact surface epithelium by restitution. Colonic mucosa of both human and rabbit when damaged by HCl also exhibited restitution but only when the damage was confined to the superficial mucosa [13]. A deeper haemorrhagic lesion heals by processes involving mitosis [19]. The speed of recovery of the electrical parameters *in vitro* and the failure of colchicine to inhibit restitution of colonic mucosa *in vitro* [16] supports the hypothesis that restitution involves cell migration without cell mitosis [1].

Colonic epithelial restitution appears to be highly dependent on the HCO_3^- concentration in the nutrient solution. Similar findings have been reported in the duodenum [13] and stomach [3]. The formation of this alkaline micro-environment occurs at the mucosal surface by transmucosal diffusion of HCO_3^- into the necrotic layer. Luminal alkalinization in the colon is dependent on the presence of bicarbonate in the nutrient solution and is a Na-dependent active transcellular HCO_3^- transport mechanism [20]. Studies on restitution of amphibian gastric mucosa injured by exposure to 1M NaCl, measured the flux of HCO_3^- from the nutrient to the luminal side, and showed increased diffusion of HCO_3^- into the mucosa when the nutrient HCO_3^- concentration is changed from 18 to 48mM. We did not measure HCO_3^- fluxes in this study, but it is likely that the same increased diffusion of HCO_3^- also occurs in the colon with a higher $[HCO_3^-]$ in N.

There is increasing evidence to suggest that ambient HCO_3^- plays an important role in the acid base status of mucosa in the alimentary tract. The migration of the colonic epithlial cells appears to depend on local tissue pH, determined by the diffusion of HCO_3^- from the nutrient solution and the diffusion of H^+ from the luminal solution. The importance of the luminal pH on restitution has been demonstrated in this study. Experiments were initially conducted at pH 6.0, the normal pH value of the colonic mucosal surface *in vivo* [21,22]. When the nutrient $[HCO_3^-]$ was kept at 18mM, epithelial restitution occurred at luminal pH 6.0, but not when the luminal pH was 4.0, in contrast with 48mM HCO_3^- in N, epithelial restitution occurred at pH_L 6.0 and 4.0, but not pH_L 2.0. Rapid restitution of the gastric and duodenal mucosa *in vitro* is also very sensitive to an acid environment [3,5,13]. An intact basal lamina is necessary for rapid cell migration [11,19] but the basal lamina can be extensively damaged by acid [23]. Circumstantial evidence suggests that the lamelli podial membranes projected from the migrating mucus cells possess receptors for one or more components of the basal lamina, thus guiding the migrating cells across the denuded mucosal surface. It is tempting to speculate that a colonic basal lamina damaged by a low luminal pH would not allow this process to occur.

It is generally accepted that damage to the gastric mucosal surface epithelium is associated with a decrease in transmucosal potential difference and resistance and that epithelial restitution after damage is usually accompanied by recovery of the electrical parameters [3]. We have demonstrated similar findings in the amphibian colon. The agreement between structural and functional events has also been described in the porcine colon injured by bile salts *in vitro* [12]. Restitution of the colonic mucosal barrier and ion transport are rapidly restored in sequence after an acute superficial injury. The superficial damage results in a marked decrease in net Na and Cl absorption. In the early stages of recovery, NaCl transport, short circuit current were markedly impaired, but recovered within 2 hours, parallelling the regeneration of the flattened migrating cells to the tall columnar absorptive cells.

In summary, we have demonstrated that restitution of amphibian colonic mucosa *in vitro*, is highly dependent on both the nutrient bicarbonate and the luminal pH. An alkaline microenvironment at the mucosal surface is necessary to facilitate restitution. The similarity in the various factors that affect restitution in different areas in the gastrointestinal tract further supports its role as a probable important basic defense property of these epithelia.

ACKNOWLEDGEMENT

*This research was supported by a grant from the
Special Trustees of Guy's Hospital, London*

REFERENCES

1.   Silen W, Ito S. Mechanisms for rapid re-epithelization of the gastric mucosal surface. Ann Rev Physiol 1985; 47: 217-229.

2.   Svanes K. Ito, S, Takeuchi K, Silen W. Restitution of the surface epithelium of the in vitro frog gastric mucosa after damage with hyperosmolar sodium chloride. Gastroenterology 1982; 82: 1409-1426.

3.   Svanes K, Takeuchi K, Ito S, Silen W. Effect of luminal Ph and nutrient bicarbonate concentration on restitution after gastric surface cell injury. Surgery 1983; 94: 494-500.

4.   Ito S, Lacy E, Rutten MJ, Critchlow J, Silen W. Rapid repair of injured gastric mucosa. Scand J Gastroenterol. 1984; 19(Suppl 101): 87-95.

5.   Rutten MJ, Ito S. Morphology and electrophysiology of guinea pig gastric mucosal repair in vitro. Am J Physiol 1983; 224: G171-82.

6.   Lacy ER, Ito S. Rapid epithelial restitution of the rat gastric mucosa after ethanol injury. Lab Invest 1984; 51: 573-83.

7.   Lacy ER,. Ito S. Ethanol-induced insult to the superficial rat gastric epithelium: a study of damage and rapid repair. In: Allen A, Flemstrom G, Garner A, Silen W, Turnberg LA. eds. Mechanisms of mucosal protection in the upper gastrointestinal tract. New York: Raven 1984: 49-56.

8.   Ito S, Lacy ER. Characteristics of ethanol-induced lesion in rat gastric mucosa. In: Allen A, Flemstrom G, Garner A, Silen W, Turnberg LA. eds. Mechanisms of mucosal protection in the upper gastrointestinal tract. New York: Raven. 1984; 57-63.

9.   Ito S, Lacy ER. Morphology of rat gastric mucosal damage, defence and restitution in the presence of luminal ethanol. Gastroenterology 1985; 88: 250-60.

10.   Dzienis H, Gronbech JE, Varhaug JE, Lekven J, Svanes K. Regional blood flow and acid secretion associated with damage and restituttion of the gastric surface epithelium in cats. Eur Surg Res 1987;19:98-112

11. Feil W, Klmesch S, Karner P, Wenzl E, Starlinger M, Lacy ER, Schiessel R. Importance of an alkaline microenvironment for rapid restitution of the rabbit duodenal mucosa in vitro. Gastroenterology 1989; 97: 112-22.

12. Argenzio RA, Henrikson CK, Liacos JA. Restitution of barrier and transport function of porcine colon after acute mucosal injury. Am J. Physiol 1988; 255: G62-71.

13. Feil W, Lacy ER, Wong YM, Burger D, Wenzl E, Starlinger M, Schiessel R. Rapid epithelial restitution of human and rabbit colonic mucosa. Gastroenterology 1989; 97: 685-701.

14. Rowe PH, Fagg NKC, Mason RC. Restitution of colonic mucosa in vitro. Gut 1987; 28: A1395.

15. Zhang Q, Hanley C, Mason RC, Rowe PH, McColl I. Restitution occurs in colonic mucosa in vitro following bile salt injury. Gut 1988 29: A1485.

16. Rowe PH, Hanley DC, Mason RC. Effects of cytochalasin B and colchicine on colonic restitution. Gut 1988; 29: A1484.

17. Zhang Q, Rowe PH, Hanley C, Mason RC, McColl I. Prostaglandins inhibit resitution of colonic mucosa in vitro. Gut 1989; 30: A747.

18. Takeuchi K, Merhav A, Silen W. Mechanisms of luminal alkalinization by bullfrog fundic mucosa. Am J Physiol 1982; 243: G377-88.

19. Morris GP, Wallace JL. The roles of ethanol and of acid in the production of gastric mucosal erosions in rats. Virchows Arch 1981; 38: 23-38.

20. Sullian SK, Smith PL. Bicarbonate secretion by rabbit proximal colon. Am J Physiol 1985; 251: 436.

21. McNeil NI, Ling KCL, Wager J. Mucosal surface pH of the large intestine of the rat and of normal and inflammed intestine in man. Gut 1987; 28: 707-13.

22. Shiau Y-F, Fernandez P, Jackson MJ, McMonagle S. Mechanisms maintaining a low pH microclimate in the intestine. Am J Physiol 1985; 248: G608-17.

23. Black BA, Morris GP, Wallace JL. Effects of acid on the basal lamina of the rat stomach and duodenum. Virchows Arch 1985; 50: 109-118.

CHRONIC ULCERATION: ROLE OF GASTRIN

F. Halter

Gastrointestinal Unit, University Hospital,
Inselspital, Bern, Switzerland

ABSTRACT

Gastrin represents a causative factor only in rare subgroups on ulcer patients such as in the Zollinger-Ellinson syndrome, the antral G-cell hyperplasia syndrome and in patients where the gastric antrum was erroneously retained following partial gastrectomy. In the pathogenesis of uncomplicated peptic ulcer disease gastrin may play a contributory role insofar as a slight hypergastrinemia appears to be linked to helicobacter colonisation. With the known trophic effects of gastrin this could account for the overall increase in the parietal cell mass of patients suffering from duodenal ulcer disease. Conversely the trophic effects of gastrin have also been linked to ulcer healing, especially since potent acid inhibitors induce a substantial hypergastrinemia. The evidence for such an association is however only circumstantial and potent and selective gastrin receptor antagonists are necessary to fully clarify the role gastrin exerts in ulcer healing.

INTRODUCTION

Since it has be realized that plasma gastrin is an important factor in regulating meal stimulated gastric acid secretion, this peptice has been linked to the pathogenesis of peptic ulcer disease. Conversely the known trophic effects of gastrin and the substantial gastrin release accompanying treatment with potent acid inhibitors has lead to the speculation that plasma gastrin might encourage the helaing of ulcers. It is the aim of this article to discuss the relevance of either hypothesis.

DOES GASTRIN PLAY A CAUSAL ROLE IN PEPTIC ULCER DISEASE?

The hypothesis that gastrin might be causally related to peptic ulcer disease was strengthened when it became apparent that hypergastrinemia is the primary factor in peptic ulcer disease in patients suffering from Zollinger-Ellison syndrome. In this condition excessive amounts of acid are produced as a result of a gastrin producing islet cell tumor [1]. It was later claimed that antral G-cell hyperplasia was another entity in which excessive gastrin production was causally related to peptic ulcer disease [2]. However, doubts remain to date on the existence of the latter syndrome. Similarly, doubts remain whether the slight hypergastrinemia often accompanying pyloric stenosis is causative in the development of gastric ulcers as suggested by Dragstedt et al. [3]. Indeed, when reliable measurements of plasma gastrin levels became available it was soon realised that the majority of patients suffering from peptic ulcer disease have either normal or only slightly elevated plasma gastrin levels [4,5] and that hypergastrinaemia could best be considered to be a contributory factor in peptic ulcer disease. Speculations on whether hypergastrinemia might be related to the severity of the ulcer course [6] were not confirmed in a prospective study on the behaviour of plasma gastrin in so-called non-responders to histamine H_2 antagonist treatment and in patients suffering form ulcer recurrence after vagotomy. Plasma gastrin levels of the responders were not significantly different from those of non-responders [7].

It has also been claimed that the sensitivity of gastrin receptors to the parent hormone may be a causative factor in peptic ulcer disease [8,9] and that failure to subsequently reduce sensitivity during ulcer healing might facilitate an early ulcer relapse [10]. Since such changes are only found in a fraction of subjects suffering from peptic ulcer disease they can at best be considered to exert a contributory role.

The role of gastrin in peptic ulcer disease has recently been revived in conjunction with the discovery of Helicobacter pylori. It is of special interest that in some studies, H. pylori positive duodenal ulcer patients have distinctly higher plasma gastrin levels than H. pylori negative subjects [11-14]. However, this finding has not been confirmed in all studies [15]. Two reports have demonstrated that plasma gastrin levels were significantly reduced when ulcers were healed with a treatment that erradicated the H. pylori colonisation of the antral mucosa [13,14]. This has led to the hypothesis that H. pylori infection could act via the trophic action of gastrin leading to a hyperplasia of the parietal cell mass known to accompany duodenal ulcer disease and thus causally trigger the development of a peptic ulcer [16].

CAN GASTRIN ACCELERATE ULCER HEALING?

The literature supplies some evidence that gastrin could foster the healing of peptic ulcers in conjunction with the growth stimulating effects it exerts on the gastric mucosa [16]. Drugs inhibiting acid secretion promote hypergastrinemia in proportion to their capacity to inhibit gastric acid secretion, which is itself the main determinant of ulcer healing [18]. The question has therefore been posed whether hypergastrinaemia rather than anacidity helps ulcer re-epithelialisation [16]. Some, partially conflicting data is available from animal studies which deal with various aspects of cytoprotective and ulcer healing properties of gastrin.

DOES GASTRIN HAVE GASTROPROTECTIVE PROPERTIES?

A possible role for gastrin in mediating gastroprotection has been documented by Takeuchi and Johnson [19-21]. Using rats depleted of gastrin by a liquid diet, Takeuchi and Johnson [19] found a marked decrease in DNA synthesis in the oxyntic mucosa, which by itself did not lead to ulcer formation but greatly increased the ulcerogenity of restraint stress.

Injection of pentagastrin reversed the decrease in DNA synthesis caused by a liquid diet and significantly protected against stress ulcers, suggesting that regeneration might be an important protective factor. This was indirectly supported by stress ulcer studies performed by Sakamoto et al. [22] but pentagastrin prevention of stress ulcers was attributed to the release of endogenous somatostatin.

Pentagastrin has also been reported to reduce gastric ulceration induced by ASA in a dose-dependent manner in the gastrin depleted model described above [20]. A significant positive correlation was observed between ulcer index and the ratio of DNA loss to DNA synthesis. The damage caused by ASA could be partly reduced by pentagastrin infusion.

Konturek et al. [23] however were unable to confirm the protective effect of gastrin against ASA challenge in normally fed rats. Preliminary results of an ongoing study in our laboratories with blockade of endogenous gastrin in the rat by high doses of a monoclonal antigastrin-antibody, well capable of attenuating gastrin-stimulated acid secretion in the rat, have revealed supportive evidence for a protective effect of endogenous gastrin against strong gastric irritants

GASTRIN AND REPAIR OF SUPERFICIAL MUCOSAL DEFECTS

Mucosal defects which leave the muscularis mucosa intact can be repaired within minutes to hours by migration of viable epithelial cells from the gastric pits, a phenomenon that has been named restitution [24]. This process occurs too rapidly to be accounted for by cell division and no data are availiable which would suggest that gastrin can accelerate restitution or re-epithelialisation in the stomach.

GASTRIN AND REPAIR BY REEPITHELIALISATION

Gastrin can accelerate the growth of gastric corpus mucosa both *in vitro* and *in vivo* [25]. However, the degree to which this trophic effect contributes to the healing of ulcers is not clear. Repair by re-epithelialisation is only one of several important mechanisms contributing to the dynamic process of ulcer healing. The time-course of ulcer healing appers to follow a triphasic course [24] (Figure 1).

During an initial slow lag phase clearance of necrotic tissue debris, angiogenesis and formation of granulation tissue seem to play a major role. In a second phase this granulation tissue is rapidly covered by a primitive flat epithelium much in line with rapid re-epithelialisation of superficial mucosal defects. Only in the third, slow phase is this remodelled into normal gastric tissue. In two studies pentagastrin administration accelerated the reappearance of parietal cells during the remodelling of primitive scar tissue into normal gastric corpus mucosa [27,26].

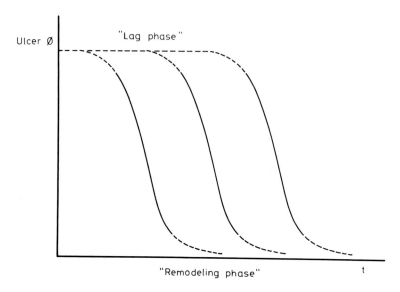

FIGURE 1:   *Hypothetical ulcer-healing model in the form of an inversed growth curve.*

It is less likely that physiologic levels of gastrin exert a role in the initial healing phase. In a study performed in our laboratories covering the two initial healing phases, omeprazole accelerated healing of experimental ulcers following 10 days treatment in conjunction with pronounced hypergastrinemia, but in the absence of an increase in cell proliferation at the ulcer margin [29](Figs. 2 & 3). This data is in contrast with earlier findings of Takeuchi and Johnson [21] who suggested that epithelial cell proliferation is important in the early healing phase of acetic acid-induced ulcers since the process was influenced by pentagastrin application. In their studies, performed in gastrin-depleted rats kept on a liquid diet, the healing of chronic acetic acid-induced gastric and duodenal ulcers was markedly reduced but could be reversed by exogenous pentagastrin. Delayed ulcer healing in gastrin-depleted animals was accompanied by a reduction in DNA synthesis and total DNA and RNA content but all these growth indices returned to normal following pentagastrin. It is, however, difficult to interpret findings in this model since prolonged fasting and liquid diet modify gastric emptying. Furthermore, pentagastrin, the pentapeptide of gastrin used in these studies has biological effects indistinguishable from CCK [30]. Similarly, hypergastrinemia induced by omeprazole in our ulcer model [29] may not be the only hormonal modification resulting from total acid supression. It will not be possible to fully clarify the role of gastrin in ulcer healing until potent and specific gastrin antagonists are available.

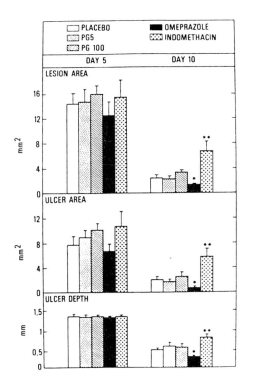

FIGURE 2:   *Microscopic analysis of mucosal injury. Lesion area, ulcer area and ulcer depth were calculated from sectional slides analyzed by light microscopy. Rats were treated for 5 and 10 days with intragastric 16,16-dimethyl prostaglandin E_2 (5 ug/kg body weight, b.i.d. (PG 5) and 100 ug/kg body weight, b.i.d. (PG 100), subcutaneous omeprazole (40 umol/kg body weight), subcutaneous indomethacin (2 mg/kg body weight, b.i.d.) or placebo. Values are given as mean ± SEM (n=8 animals for placebo and n=6 animals for the other treatments). *p 0.05, **p 0.01 vs. all other treatments (one-way analysis of variance).*

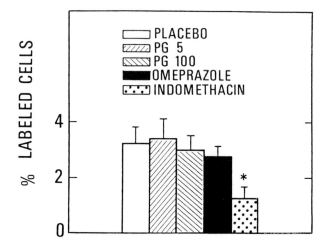

FIGURE 3: *Percentage of radiolabeled cells measured in a 600-um-wide region of corpus mucosa adjacent to the mucosal defect. Rats were treated for 5 days with intragastric 16,16-dimethyl prostaglandin E_2 (5 ug/kg body weight, b.i.d. (PG 5) and 100 ug/kg body weight, b.i.d. (PG 100), subcutaneous omeprazole (40 umol/kg body weight), subcutaneous indomethacin (2 mg/kg body weight, b.i.d.) or placebo. Values are given as mean $\pm$ SEM (n=8 animals for placebo and n=6 animals for the other treatments). *p 0.05, **p 0.01 vs. all other treatments (one-way analysis of variance).*

CONCLUSIONS

Since human peptic ulcers predominantly appear in antral or duodenal mucosa and since physiologic doses of gastrin have not convincingly been shown to have a trophic effect in antral or duodenal mucosa [30], it appears highly unlikely that gastrin plays an important role in healing of genuine peptic ulcers.

REFERENCES

1. Zollinger RM, Ellison EH: Primary peptic ulcerations of the jejunum associated with islet cell tumors of the pancreas. Annals of Surgery, 1955; 142: 709-728

2. Polak JM, Stagg B, Pearce AEG. Two types of Zollinger Ellison Syndrome: immunofluoresecent, cytochemical and ultrastrucural studies of antral and pancreatic gastrin cells in different clinical states, Gut 1972; 13: 501-502

3.   Dragstedt LR, Woodward ER: Gastric stasis, a cause of gastric ulcer. Sand.J. Gastroenterol. 1970; 5 (Suppl. 6):243-252

4.   Lam SK: Pathogenesis of duodenal ulcer. In: Clinics in Gastroenterology, 1984; eds. JI. Isenberg and C. Johansson. W.B. Saunders, London, pps. 447-473

5.   Walsh JH: Pathogenic role for the gastrins. In: Gastrins and the Vagus. eds. Rehfeld JF, Amdrup E. London Academic Press, 1979, pps. 181-198

6.   Primrose JN, Logue F, Ratcliffe JG, Joffe SN. Gastrin and gastric secretion in patients with recurrent peptic ulceration: unexpected correlations. Digestion 1985; 32:30-34

7.   Primrose JN, Naik KS, Blackett RL et al. Is antral gastrin important in the resistance of duodenal ulcers to H_2 receptor antagonists or in recurrent ulceration after highly selective vagotomy? Gut 1990; 31: 763-766

8.   Isenberg JI, Grossman MI, Maxwell V, Walsh JH: Increased sensitivity to stimulation of acid secretion by pentagastrin in duodenal ulcer. J. Clin Invest 1975; 55:330-337

9.   Halter F, Bangerter U, Haecki WH, et al.: Sensitivity of the parietal cell to pentagastrin in health and duodenal ulcer disease: a reappraisal. Scand. J. Gastroenterol 1982; 17:539-544

10. Yanaka A, Muto H: Increased parietal cell responsiveness to tetragastrin in patients with recurrent dudodenal ulcer. Dig Dis Sci 1988, 33: 2459-1456

11. Smith JTL, Pounder RE, Nwokolo CU, Lanzon-Miller S, Evans DG, Graham DY, Evans DJ: Inappropriate hypergastrinaemia in asymptomatic healthy subjects infected with Helicobacter pylori. Gut 1990, 311, 522

12. Levi S, Beardshall K, Haddad G, Playford R, Ghosh P, Calam J: Campylobacter pylori and duodenal ulcers: the gastrin link. Lancet 1989; i:1167

13. McColl KEL,Fullarton GM, Nujumi AME, MacDonald AM, Brown IL, Hilditch TE: Lowered gastrin and gastric acidity after eradication of Campylobacter pylori in duodenal ulcer. Lancet 1989; ii: 499-500

14. Levi S, Beardshall K, Swift I, Foulkes W, Playford R, Ghosh P, Calam J: Antral Helicobacter pylori, hypergastrinemia, and duodenal ulcers: effect of eradicating the organism. BMJ 1989; 299: 1504

15. Hui WH, Lam SK, Chau PY, et al. Persistence of Campylobacter pyloridis despite healing of duodenal ulcer and improvement of accompanying duodenitis and gastritis. Dig. Dis. Sci. 1987; 32: 1255-1260

16. Pounder R, Smith J: Drug-induced changes of plasma gastrin concentration. In: Gastroenterology Clinics of North America: Peptic Ulcer Disease, 1990, ed. RH Hunt. W.B. Saunders Company, London. Vol. 19, number 1, pps.141- 154

17. Card WI, Marks IN. The relationship between the acid output of the stomach following "maximal" histamine stimulation and parietal cell mass. Clin. Sci. 1960; 19: 147-163

18. Jones DB, Howden CW, Burget DW et al: Acid suppression in duodenal ulcer: a meta-analysis to define optimal dosing with antisecretory drugs. Gut 1987; 28: 1120-1127

19. Takeuchi K. Johnson LR. Pentagastrin protects against stress ulceration in rats. Gastroenterology 1979; 76: 327-334

20. Takeuchi K, Johnson LR. Effect of of cell proliferation and loss in aspirin-induced gastric damage in the rat. Am J Physiol 1982; 243; G-463

21. Takeuchi K, Johnson LR. Effect of cell proliferation on healing of gastric and duodenal ulcers in rats. Digestion 1986; 33, 92-100

22. Sakamoto T, Swierczek JS, Odgen D. et al. Cytoprotective effect of pentagastrin and epidermal growth factor. Ann Surg 1985; 201:290-295

23. Konturek SJ, Brzozowski T, Radecki I, et al. Cytoprotective effects of gastrointestinal hormones. In: Gut Peptides and Hormones. Biomedical Research Foundation, Tokyo, 1982, p 411

24. Lacy ER, Ito S. Rapid epithelial restitution of the rat gastric mucosa after ethanol injury. Lab Invest 1984; 51, 573-583

25. Johnson LR. The trophic action of gastrointestinal hormones. Gastroenterology 1976; 70, 278-288

26. Halter F, Barbezat GO, van Hoorn-Hickman R, van Hoorn WA. Healing dynamics of traumatic gastric mucosal defects in the normal and hyperacid stomach. Dig Dis Sci 1980; 25, 916-920

27. Helander HF. Morphological studies on the margin of gastric corpus wounds in the rat. J Submicrosc Cytol 1983; 15, 627-643

28. Blom H, Erkoinen T. Trophic effect of pentagastrin on normal and regenerating parietal cells. Gastroenterology 1984; 87, 537-541

29. Inauen, W., Wyss, P.A., Kayser, A., Baumgartner, A., Schrer-Maly, C.C., Koelz, H.R., Halter, F., Influence of prostaglandins, omeprazole and indomethacin on healing of experimental ulcers in the rat. Gastroenterology, 1989; 95: 636-641.

30. Ryberg B, Axelson J, Hakanson R, Sundler F. Mattsson H. Trophic effects of continuous infusion of [Leu[15]] Gastrin 17 in the rat. Gastroenterology 1990; 98: 33-38

ROLE OF EPIDERMAL GROWTH FACTOR (EGF) AND PROSTAGLANDINS (PG) IN THE PROTECTION AGAINST STRESS-INDUCED GASTRIC ULCERATION

S.J. Konturek, T. Brzozowski, P.K. Konturek, A. Dembinski

Institute of Physiology, Academy of Medicine, Krakow, Poland

ABSTRACT

EGF and PG promote the growth of the gastric mucosa and protect it against various ulcerogens but little is known about their role in the pathogenesis of gastric lesions induced by stress. Rats with intact and resected salivary glands were exposed to water immersion and restraint stress (WRS). The formation of gastric ulcerations increased with the duration of stress and this was accompanied by a decline in the DNA synthesis in the gastric muosa. After sialoadenectomy, a significant increase in the number of stress ulcerations and further reduction in DNA synthesis were observed. Exogenous EGF (100 ug/kg-h s.c.) and dimethyl PGE_2 ($dmPGE_2$, 50 ug/kg p.o.) significantly reduced the ulcerations in the stressed rats with intact salivary glands but this reduction was significantly less pronounced after sialoadenectomy. WRS resulted also in about 50% reduction in mucosal PGE_2 generation and the pretreatment with indomethacin (10 mg/kg i.p.) caused further decrease in PGE_2 biosynthesis (by about 90%) and almost doubled the number of stress ulcerations. Indomethacin abolished the gastroprotective effect of exogenous EGF (but not $dmPGE_2$) against the stress lesions. An inhibition of ornithine decarboxylase activity (ODC) by DFMO (200 mg/kg i.p.) also augmented stress-induced ulcerogenesis and abolished the protective action of EGF while the administration of spermine (50 mg/kg p.o.) almost completely prevented stress ulcerations. This study indicates that stress-ulcers are accompanied by a reduction in mucosal synthesis of DNA and PG and that the presence of salivary glands attenuates the stress ulcerogenesis, probably by releasing EGF which acts, in part, by enhancing ODC activity and maintaining mucosal growth and PG formation.

INTRODUCTION

The mucosa of the gastrointestinal tract is one of the most rapidly proliferating tissues in the body. The constant renewal of epithelial cells is considered as an important mechanism of mucosal protection and repair [1].

Gastric stress ulcerations are common complications following burns, sepsis, major surgery, trauma to the central nervous system and other heterogenous forms of injury [2]. The mechanism of these ulcerations has not been fully clarified and remains controversial - more than 60 years after their original description by Selye [3]. The major factors implicated in the development of stress ulcers include an increase in gastric acid secretion and a decrease in mucosal protection due to the reduction in mucus secretion, mucosal blood flow and prostaglandin (PG) biosynthesis [4]. Whether these are direct aetiologic factors or simply expressions of non-specific stress response is not certain.

Theoretically, gastric ulcers could also develop as the result of an imbalance between the proliferation and the loss of mucoal cells. Indeed, several reports have recently shown that during the exposure to the stress the gastric mucosa exhibits a decreased proliferation of mucosal cells, decreased DNA synthesis and an overall loss of RNA [5-9]. These studies have suggested that the inhibition of DNA and RNA synthesis and cell proliferation with resulting failure to replace the extruded or damaged epithelial cells, might contribute to the development of stress lesions.

During the past few years it became evident that epidermal growth factor (EGF) [9] as well as PG [10,11] exhibit trophic effects on the mucosa of the oxyntic gland area. Administration of exogenous EGF or PG was found to protect the mucosa against various ulcerogens [12-14] and to enhance mucosal cell proliferation [10]. As stress was found to affect salivary production of EGF [15] and gastric mucosal generation of PG [16], the question arises whether EGF and PG are involved in the pathogenesis of stress ulcerations.

This study carried out on rats with intact and resected salivary glands was designed to determine the role of EGF and gastric mucosal PG in cell proliferation and the gastric lesions induced by water immersion restraint stress (WRS).

MATERIAL AND METHODS

ANIMALS

Male Wistar rats weighing 160-200g and fasted for 20 hours were divided into 4 major groups. Animals of group A included rats with intact salivary glands (sham operation) and those with resection of the sublingual-submandibular gland complexes carried out under pentabarbital anaesthesia 7-10 days earlier. All animals were exposed to stress by placing them in a stress cage causing immobilization and immersing into 23°C water to the rat's xyphoid process as described before [17]. Rats with intact or resected salivary glands were stressed for 1.5 or 6 hours without (control) and with the administration of EGF infused subcutaneously (s.c.) at a dose of 100 ug/kg-h 30 min before and throughout the exposure to WRS or dimethyl PGE_2 (dmPGE$_2$) (50 ug/kg) given intragastrically (i.g.) as a single bolus dose 30 min before the start of stress. Group B included normal rats and rats stressed for 6 hours without and with pretreatment with difluoromethylornithine (DFMO) given i.p. 2 hours before WRS as a dose of 200 mg/kg without or with EGF infused s.c. at a dose of 100 ug/kg-h for 30 min before and during WRS and without or with spermine administered i.g. at a dose of 50 mg/kg 30 mins before the stress. In group C, stress ulcerations were induced by 6 hours of WRS without and with pretreatment with i.p. indomethacin at a dose of 10 mg/kg given 1 hour before the start of stress without or with addition of s.c. infusion EGF or i.g. dmPGE$_2$.

DETERMINATION OF DNA SYNTHESIS

Immediately after the stress or other ulcerogens, the animals were killed and the stomach was removed. The number and area of gastric lesions were recorded by computerized planimeter (Morphomat 10, Carl Zeiss, OberKochen, FRG). The lesion number or lesion area from each member of the three groups were summed and divided by the number of rats in each group to give mean ($\pm$ SEM) lesion number or area.

The rate of DNA synthesis in mucosa scraped from the oxyntic gland area of group A rats was measured by incubating the tissue at 37°C for 30 min in Eagle's minimal essential culture medium containing 2uCi/ml of [3H]thymidine (5 Ci/mmol)(Amersham, England) as described before [9]. The incorporation of [3H]thymidine into DNA-containing filtrate was measured in a Beckman liquid scintillation system. DNA synthesis was expressed as disintegration per minute (DPM) per ug DNA.

MEASUREMENT OF MUCOSAL CAPACITY FOR PGE$_2$ BIOSYNTHESIS

The PG biosynthetic capacity of the oxyntic mucosa of both intact and sialoadenectomized rats of group B without or with the pretreatment with indomethacin (10 mg/kg injected i.p. 2 hours before the stress) was determined as described previously [18]. Briefly, the oxyntic mucosa (about 50 mg) was scraped from the musculature, rinsed in a buffer solution containing 50 mM Tris-HCl, pH 8.4, finely minced and incubated on a vortex shaker for 1 min and then centrifuged for 15 seconds. The supernatant was collected and stored at -20°C. PGE$_2$ immunoreactivity was determined using a radioimmunoassay kit (New England Nuclear Munich, FRG). The capability of the mucosa to generate PGE$_2$ was expressed in nanograms (ng) per gram of wet tissue weight.

DETERMINATION OF TISSUE AND PLASMA EGF

In some rats with intact salivary glands without and with exposure to WRS for 6 hours, the samples of gastric content in rats of group A were collected immediately after killing of animals, neutralized with 0.1 M NaOH to pH 7 and frozen at -20°C until EGF radioimmunoassay. Blood samples were also collected from the heart into EDTA containing tubes. Plasma was separated and frozen at -20°C for EGF and gastrin radioimmunoassay as described [19]. The EGF antiserum raised in rabbits against human EGF was used in a final dilution of 1:210000. Iodinated [(3-1251)iodotyrosyl] peptide and rat EGF were calibration standards (Amersham, UK). The detection limit of the assay was 0.01 nmol/l. The interassay and intraassay precisions were about 15% and 10% respectively.

DETERMINATION ON MUCOSAL ODC ACTIVITY

In animals of group C, the ornithine decarboxylase activity was determined in oxyntic mucosa using a modified method described by Haarstad et al [31] by measuring 14CO$_2$ liberated from the (1-14C)-labelled substrate ornithine. The results were expressed as picomoles CO$_2$ formed per milligram of tissue protein per hour.

The results are reported as means $\pm$ SEM. Statistical significance was determined by analysis of variance and where appropriate by the unpaired Student's t-test, a value of less than 0.05 being considered significant.

RESULTS

As shown in Figure 1. the incorporation of labelled thymidine into the oxyntic mucosa in 20 hour fasted rats with intact salivary glands (sham-operation) and without stress, averaged 37.4 $\pm$ 2.4 dpm/ug DNA and no gastric ulcerations were observed. WRS caused a significant reduction in the rate of thymidine incorporation that was significant already after 1.5 hours of exposure to stress and progressed with the duration of stress to reach approximately about 60% of control value after 6 hours of exposure to stress. The number of ulcers also increased with the duration of stress in pattern similar to the decrease in DNA synthesis.

Following sialoadenectomy, the incorporation of thymidine to DNA in fasted rats averaged 20.1 $\pm$ 1.9 dpm/ug DNA and was about 50% of that observed in sham-operated animals but no gastric lesions were observed in these animals. DNA synthesis was significantly decreased after 1.5 and 6 hours, reaching about one half of the control value after 6 hours of stress. All the values of DNA synthesis recorded in sialoadenectomized rats without and with exposure to stress were significantly lower than those obtained in corresponding groups of sham-operated animals with intact salivary glands. In sialoadenectomized rats, the levels of EGF in the plasma (0.15 nmol/l) and gastric juice (3.60 nmol/l) were significantly reduced (by about 70% and 50%) as compared to sham-operated controls. Stress resulted in a significant increase in EGF concentrations in the plasma (1.28 pmol/l) and gastric juice (54 pmol/l) in sham-operated but not in sialoadenectomized animals.

Exogenous EGF infused s.c. at a dose of 100 ug/kg for 30 mins before and 6 hours during WRS reduced by about one-half the number of gastric ulcerations in rats with intact salivary glands but only by about one-fourth in sialoadenectomized animals (Figure 1). Also dmPGE$_2$ administered as a single i.g. bolus dose of 50 ug/kg 30 min before WRS was about twice more effective in reducing stress ulcers in rats with intact salivary glands than in sialoadenectomized animals.

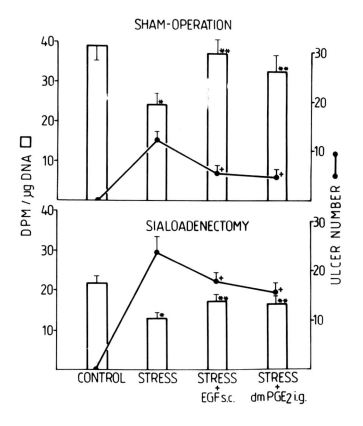

FIGURE 1: *DNA synthesis in the oxyntic mucosa and ulcer number of rats intact (sham-operated) and resected salivary glands after exposure to 6 hours of stress without and with administration of EGF or dmPGE$_2$. Means $\pm$ SEM of 8-12 rats. Single asterisk indicates significant decrease below the control value (in non stressed rats); double asterisks indicate significant increase above the value obtained within stressed rats (without EGF or dm PGE$_2$). Cross indicates significant reduction below the value obtained in rats with stress alone.*

WSR caused a significant reduction in the incorporation of thymidine to DNA both in sham-operated and sialoadenectomized animals. The administration of EGF and dmPGE$_2$ restored the DNA synthesis to the value observed in control rats though in rats with resected salivary glands the value of DNA synthesis was about 50% lower as compared to that in corresponding sham-operated animals.

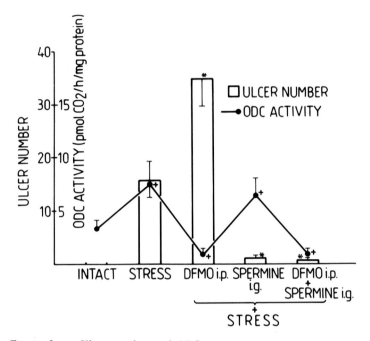

FIGURE 2   *Ulcer number and ODC activity in oxyntic mucosa of intact rats and after 6 hours of stress without and with pretreatment with DFMO, spermine and their combination. Mean ± SEM of 8-10 rats, Asterisk indicates significant change in ulcer number as compared to rats exposed to stress alone. Cross indicates significant change in the ODC value compared to that in intact rats.*

Figure 2 shows the ODC activity in oxyntic mucosa of intact and stressed rats of group B without and with pretreatment with DFMO given i.p. in a dose of 200 mg/kg alone or in combination with spermine (50 mg/kg i.g.). The exposure to 6 hours of stress almost doubled the ODC activity while DFMO caused the reduction in ODC below the value observed in intact rats and this was accompanied by over 2-fold increase in the number of stress ulcerations. Administration of spermine did not affect stress-induced increment in ODC activity but almost completely prevented stress-induced gastric ulcerations. Infusion of EGF significantly increased ODC activity while reducing the number of stress ulcers and the pretreatment with DFMO abolished the EGF-induced rise in ODC activity and mucosal protection against stress lesions. After the addition of spermine to DFMO, the protection of gastric mucosa against stress ulcers was almost complete while the ODC activity in the oxyntic mucosa was suppressed as in tests with DFMO alone.

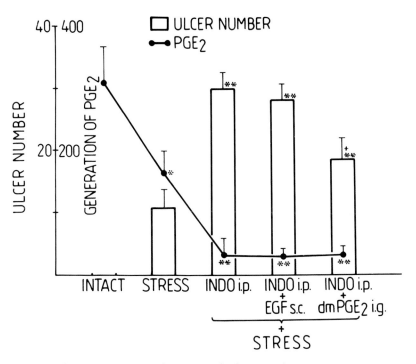

<u>FIGURE 3</u>   *Generation of PGE₂ and ulcer number in oxyntic mucosa of normal rats and those exposed to 6 hours of stress without or with pretreatment with indomethacin alone (10 mg/kg i.p.) or combined with s.c. infusion of EGF or i.g. administration of dmPGE₂.   Mean ± SEM of 8-10 rats. Single asterisk indicates significant decrease below the value obtained in intact rats; double asterisks indicate significant decrease below or above the value obtained in stressed animals.   Cross indicates significant decrease below the value obtained in rats exposed to stress plus indomethacin.*

Figure 3 shows the capacity of the oxyntic mucosa to generate PGE₂ and the ulcer number in rats of group B without and with the exposure to 6 hours of WRS alone and in combination with the pretreatment with indomethacin (10 mg/kg i.p.) alone or indomethacin plus EGF (100 ug/kg s.c.) or dmPGE₂ (50 ug/kg i.g.) Mucosal generation of PGE₂ in oxyntic mucosa of intact non-stressed rats averaged 310 ± 68 ng/g of wet tissue weight. Exposure to 6 hours of stress reduced the generation of PGE₂ by about 50% and this was accompanied by the appearance of gastric ulcerations in all stressed animals. Pretreatment with indomethacin caused further significant decrease in the mucosal PGE biosynthesis to about 20% of the value in 6 hour stressed animals.   The number of stress-induced ulcerations in indomethacin pretreated rats rose about 3-fold compared to stress alone without indomethacin.   Infusion of exogenous EGF

(100 ug/kg s.c.) to indomethacin-treated rats failed to affect the mucosal biosynthesis of PGE_2 or the number of gastric ulcerations induced by 6 hour exposure to stress. In contrast, $dmPGE_2$ reduced signficantly by about one-third the stress-induced ulcerations.

DISCUSSION

The results of this study confirm that sialoadenectomy greatly increased the susceptibility of the stomach to water immersion and restraint stress which caused about twice the number of mucosal lesions than in animals with intact salivary glands [21,22]. Furthermore, exogenous EGF and $dmPGE_2$ afforded significantly less protection against these acute ulcerations in sialoadenectomized rats than in animals with intact salivary glands.

As reported previously by Takeuchi and Johnson [6] we found that the exposure of rats to stress of gradually increasing durations caused progressively increased numbers of ulcerations although this procedure significantly reduced the DNA synthesis. Sialoadenectomy by itself did not cause the formation of gastric lesions though this procedure significantly reduced the DNA synthesis and increased the susceptibility of the mucosa to the development of ulcers in response to stress. The question remains whether the proliferative capacity of the mucosa is of major importance in reducing the stress lesions as originally proposed by Takeuchi and Johnson [6] and Kuwayama and Eastwood [7] or whether the inhibition of cell renewal by stress is the consequence of stress-induced mucosal damage as suggested by Grant et al [23]. According to our data, 1.5 hour stress caused both the significant decrease in DNA synthesis and the appearance of first gastric ulcers. With the prolongation of stress to 6 hours there was further significant decline in DNA synthesis and significant increase in stress ulcerogenesis. This indicates that the DNA synthesis and stress ulcerogenesis are closely related phenomena. The difference in the effects of stress on mucosal growth and integrity reported by various authors could be explained by different species and age of animals used, different techniques of the stress induction and different methods of estimation of mucosal growth and integrity.

The question arises as to what could be the mechanism of the reduction in the epithelial cell proliferation especially in rats deprived of salivary glands. Sialoadenectomy could exhibit an atrophic influence on the gastric mucosa due to the decrease in the release of gastrin which is known to exhibit a potent trophic action on the mucosa but the lack of significant changes in plasma gastrin concentration after this procedure observed in previous report [24] militates against such a possibility Another candidate could be EGF, particularly that salivary glands possess very high capacity to synthesize this peptide and to release it both in an exocrine manner into the saliva and in an endocrine manner into the circulation. Skinner et al [23] reported that the administration of salivary gland extract (containing some EGF-like activity) as well as EGF itself resulted in an increase in DNA synthesis in the oxyntic mucosa of sialoadenectomized rats. Our results show that the sialoadenectomy greatly reduced the content of EGF in the gastric mucosa and this could decrease the cell turnover that might impair the mucosal integrity.

Our finding that the removal of salivary glands increased the stress ulcerogenicity and that exogenous EGF is capable of preventing, at least in part, the formation of stress ulcers indicate that EGF produced by salivary glands provide certain protection for the gastric mucosa against the damage. The mechanism of this gastroprotective action of EGF during the stress probably involves the inhibition of gastric acid secretion that is known to prevent stress-induced ulcerations [2] and the activation of ornithine decarboxylase (ODC), the rate-limiting enzyme in the biosynthesis of polyamines, that appear to be essential for cell division [25]. The implication of ODC in the formation of acute gastric lesions by stress has been recently proposed by Wang and Johnson [25] who also observed an increase in the specific enzyme activity both in the fundic and duodenal mucosa but this increase was accompanied by macroscopic lesions only in the stomach but not in the duodenum. The results of our study confirmed that stress causes the enhancement of ODC activity in the oxyntic mucosa and showed that the pretreatment with DFMO strongly exacerbates the mucosal damage. DFMO also abolished the protective action of EGF against stress ulcerations.

The observation of this and previous studies [25] that stress increases mucosal ODC activity suggests that polyamines may be involved in the pathogenesis of stress ulcerations. This is in keeping with our observation that polyamines such as spermine given into the stomach was highly effective in the protection of gastric mucosa against stress lesions independently whether or not the endogenous biosynthesis of polyamines was intact or suppressed by DFMO. Polyamines were reported previously to afford gastroprotection against ethanol injury [26] but this has been attributed to their antiperoxidative properties due to enhancement of tissue content of free radical scavengers.

The results of this and a previous study [27] demonstrate that sialoadenectomy reduces mucosal PGE_2 synthesis. It is possible, therefore, that the effect of sialoadenectomy on stress ulcerogenesis may be due, at least in part, to a reduction in PG formation in the gastric mucosa. This is supported by our finding that the pretreatment with indomethacin that blocks PG biosynthesis resulted in greatly augmented gastric ulcer response to the stress. Direct determination of mucosal PG generation in animals exposed to WRS alone demonstrated that PG biosynthesis was reduced (by about 50%) by the stress, yet the remaining mucosal PG level has had some protective activity because its further suppression by indomethacin (to about 10% of the normal value) increased by 2-3 folds the severity of stress ulcerations. Moreover, such indomethacin-augmented ulcerations were prevented by $dmPGE_2$ but resistant to the protective action of exogenous EGF. This suggests that the presence of mucosal generation of PGE_2, even at reduced levels, is essential for the protective action of EGF on the mucosa though this peptide does not appear to stimulate directly the generation of PG [15,18,27]. Thus, our results indicate that PG generated in the gastric mucosa and EGF released by salivary glands interact on gastric mucoal integrity, at least in part, by the modulation of the gastric epithelial cell growth. The removal of any of these mechanisms may result in mucosal damage and ulceration.

ACKNOWLEDGEMENTS

*This work was supported in part by Research Grant (MZ-111-15)
of Ministry of Health and Social Welfare.*

REFERENCES

1.   Eastwood GL. Gastroenterology 1977; 72: 962-965.

2.   Robert A and Kauffman GL. In: Sleisenger MH, Fordtran JS (Eds)
Gastrointestinal Disease, Pathophysiology, Diagnosis, Management.
Philadelphia: WB Saunders Co. 612-662.

3.   Selye H. Nature 1936; 138: 32-34.

4.   Moody FG, and Cheung LY. Dig Dis Sci 1976; 31: 148-154.

5.   Kim Y, Kerr RJ and Lipkin M. Nature 1967; 215: 1180-1181.

6.   Takeuchi K and Johnson LR. Gastroenterology 1979; 76: 327-334.

7.   Kuwayama H and Eastwood GL. Gastroenterology 1985; 88: 362-365.

8.   Willems G, and Lehy T. Gastroenterology 1975; 69: 416-426.

9.   Dembinski A, Gregory H, Konturek SJ and Polanski M. J Physiol
(Lond) 1982; 235: 35-42.

10.   Dembinski A and Konturek SJ Am J Physiol. 1985; 248: G170-175.

11.   Reinhart WH, Muller O and Halter F. Gastroenterology 1983; 85:
1003-1010.

12.   Robert A, Nezamis JE, Lancaster C and Hanchar AJ
Gastroenterology 1979; 77: 433-443.

13.   Takeuchi K and Johnson LR Am J Physiol 1982; 243:G463-468.

14.   Konturek SJ, Brzozowski T, Piastucki I and Radecki T. Gut 1981; 22:
927-932.

15.   Gysin B, Muller RKM, Otten U and Fischli AE. Scand J
Gastroentereol 1988; 23: 665-671.

16.   Basso N, Materia A, Forlini A, Jaffe BM. Surgery 1983; 94: 104-108.

17.   Takeuchi K, Okabe S and Takagi K. Am J Dig Dis 1977; 21:742-788.

18.   Konturek SJ, Piastucki I, Brzozowski T, Radecki T, Dembinski-Kiec
A and Gryglewski R. Gastroenterology 1981; 80: 4-10.

19. Konturek SJ, Brzozowski T, Dembinski A, Warzecha Z, Konturek PK and Yanaihara N. Digestion 1988; 41: 121-128.

20. Haarstadt H, Winnberg A, and Petersen H. Scand J Gastroenterol 1985; 20: 530-538.

21. Skinner KA and Tepperman BL. Gastroenterology 1981; 81: 335-339.

22. Olsen SP, Poulsen SS, Kirkergaard P and Nexo E. Gastroenterology 1984; 87: 103-108.

23. Geant P, Delux G and Willems G. Digestion 1988; 40: 212-218.

24. Skinner KA, Soper BD and Tepperman BL. J Physiol (Lond) 1984; 351: 1-12.

25. Wang J-Y, and Johnson LR. Am J Physiol 1989; 257: G259-264.

26. Mizui T, Shimono N, Doteuchi M. Japan HJ Pharmacol 1987; 44:43-50.

27. Tepperman BL, Soper BD and Morris GP. 1989; 97: 123-129.

VASCULAR FACTORS IN MUCOSAL INJURY, PROTECTION AND ULCER HEALING

S. Szabo, J. Folkman*, R.E. Morales, P. Vattay,
G. Pinkus and K. Kato[+]

*Departments of Pathology, Brigham and Women's Hospital, *Departments of Surgery, Children's Hospital Medical Center, Harvard Medical School, Boston, MA 02115,U.S.A. and [+]Takeda Chemical Industries Ltd., Osaka, Japan*

ABSTRACT

Recent studies by us and by other investigators suggest that the microvascular system plays an important role in acute mucosal injury and mucosal protection, as well as in the healing of chronic peptic ulcers. Early damage of vascular endothelial cells precedes hemorrhagic lesions during the development of acute mucosal lesions. Protection of mucosa from acute injury correlates with maintenance of mucosal blood flow. The process of resurfacing of superficial epithelial defects may also require adequate blood flow in mucosal and submucosal capillaries. Endogenous mediators of vascular lesions include leukotrienes (which are approximately 1000 times more potent than histamine in causing endothelial injury as revealed by monastral blue labelling), and endothelins (which are 10-100 times more active than leukotrienes). Angiogenesis also plays an important role in the healing of experimental chronic duodenal ulcers. Drugs which accelerate angiogenesis in the ulcer bed may become useful in the treatment of gastric and duodenal ulcers.

INTRODUCTION

Investigation of the pathogenesis of gastric and duodenal ulceration has been mainly focussed on epithelial cells and their secretory products. Quantitative biochemical methods are available to detect the secreted products of specialized epithelial (parietal, chief and mucous) cells in the stomach. Furthermore, recently developed pharmacologic agonists and antagonists can modify the receptors of endogenous mediators of acid and pepsin secretion (e.g., acetylcholine, histamine, gastrin). All of these developments have facilitated the morphologic, functional and pharmacologic studies of specialised epithelial cells.

The role of vascular endothelial cells in ulcer healing has been more difficult to study. Most experiments have relied on morphologic methods. Thus, intravascular injection of colloidal carbon and monastral blue revealed that early microvascular injury preceded the development of hemorrhagic erosions of the gastric mucosa induced by ethanol, HCl or NaOH [1-3]. Electron microscopy also helped to elucidate vascular changes associated with ingestion of aspirin or ethanol [4,5]. Our understanding of

the role of vascular factors in peptic ulceration has also been limited
because the role of blood flow *per se* was investigated only in relation to its
effect upon gastric secretion.

A broader interest developed in the role of the microcirculation in
ulcerogenesis following reports that "cytoprotection" by prostaglandins,
sulfhydryls and other agents depended partly on their effect upon
submucosal capillary blood vessels [2,3,6-11]. It is also being recognized
that vascular factors play a role not only in protection against acute mucosal
injury, but in the healing of chronic ulcers (Table 1). Many principles
which govern the healing of chronic wounds (e.g. the necessity of
neovascularization induced by angiogenic molecules), also appear to be
essential to the healing of chronic gastric and duodenal ulcers.

In this brief overview, we present preliminary results on the early
appearance of lesions of the vascular endothelium that are associated with
epithelial lesions. We will also describe novel endogenous mediators of acute
gastric mucosal injury. Furthermore, we discuss the possible role of
angiogenesis in the mechanism of ulcer healing, including the effect of basic
fibroblast growth factor (bFGF) and of sucralfate on the induction of
angiogenesis.

TABLE 1

Vascular Factors in Acute Mucosal Lesions and Chronic Ulceration

Acute mucosal lesions:
- **Pathogenesis**: endothelial vs. epithelial lesions
- **Protection**: maintenance of blood flow and epithelial restitution
- **Endogenous mediators**: histamine, leukotrienes and endothelin
Chronic ulceration:
- **Ulcer healing**: angiogenesis, granulation tissue and re-epithelization
- **Angiogenic stimuli**: bFGF and other growth factors.

Acute Mucosal Lesions

It is becoming more generally accepted that reduction or prevention
of microvascular injury in the gastric mucosa results in maintenance of
blood flow which allows rapid epithelial resurfacing to repair early
epithelial defects. Blood flow maintenance and restitution are key elements
in the mechanisms of protection against acute gastric mucosal injury [12,13].

However, in hemorrhagic mucosal lesions the order of appearance of endothelial or epithelial damage, has not been fully elucidated. We thus designed animal experiments using the vascular tracer monastral blue to assess whether endothelial lesions occur before or after early hemorrhagic mucosal erosions induced by chemicals.

PATHOGENESIS OF ENDOTHELIAL AND MUCOSAL LESIONS

In time-response experiments with ethanol and NaOH we used fasted Sprague-Dawley female rats (150-200g). Control and experimental groups consisted of three animals each. Each experiment was performed at least twice and the results pooled.

Groups of rats received 1 ml of vehicle solvent deionized water or 75% ethanol or 0.2N NaOH by intragastric gavage, and the animals were killed by cervical dislocation 5, 15 or 30 sec or 1, 3 or 6 min after ingestion of the damaging agents. All rats also received 0.1 ml/100g of 3% monastral blue B suspension (Sigma) intravenously (i.v.) to label damaged endothelial cells. Autopsy was rapidly performed, the stomach removed, opened along the large curvature, rinsed and pinned flat on a cork board. The area of any hemorrhagic mucosal lesion was measured by computerized planimetry coupled with steromicroscopy [2,3]. The stomachs were then fixed in buffered formalin, cleared in glycerol to visualize deposition of monastral blue particles in the wall of damaged blood vessels and evaluated again by stereomicroscopy and planimetry [2,3].

The results revealed labelling of subepithelial capillaries 5 and 15 sec after i.v. administration of ethanol or NaOH when virtually no hemorrhagic lesions were seen. Subsequently, in the 0.5, 1 and 3 min groups, the area of vascular damage was always greater than that of the hemorrhagic lesions. At later time intervals, in addition to the capillary damage, labelling of mucosal venules was also seen. At 6 min, the area of vascular lesions was almost identical to the density of hemorrhagic mucosal lesions.

We concluded from the experiments that capillary and venular endothelial damage in the gastric mucosa occurs before the appearance of hemorrhagic lesions caused by the intragastric administration of concentrated ethanol or NaOH.

ENDOTHELINS AS ENDOGENOUS MEDIATORS

The rapidly developing microvascular injury in the stomach is due, in part, to the direct toxicity of chemicals such as ethanol, HCl, NaOH or aspirin and to the release of endogenous mediators (e.g. monoamines, leukotrienes) [14,16]. Endothelin (ET), a potent vasoactive peptide, was recently isolated from endothelial cells [17]. We thus tested the hypothesis that endothelin might be a mediator in the chemically induced hemorrhagic mucosal erosions.

We demonstrated earlier that vascular infusion of ER-3 potentiates the damaging action of ethanol [18]. In the new experiments, fasted Sprague-Dawley rats received i.v. the vascular tracer monastral blue 5 min before the celiac arterial infusion of ET-3 0.01, 0.1 or 1.0 ml/100g/min for up to 15 min and were given 1g ethanol (25-50%) or HCl (0.2-0.3N), which alone caused no or mild vascular and mucosal lesions. The peptide potentiated the areas of vascular labelling and hemorrhagic mucosal lesions in a dose-dependent manner. Anti-ER-3 serum (1:2000 or 1:100 dilution) i.v. 1 hr before 1 ml 75% ethanol 1g reduced hemorrhagic mucosal lesions from $12.4 \pm 1.4\%$ to $9.4 \pm 1.3\%$ or $5.1 \pm 1.3\%$ ($p<0.01$).

Thus, ET-3 produced endothelial damage in capillaries and venules and predisposed the gastric mucosa to injury induced by dilute ethanol and HCl. The ET-3 antibody dose-dependently decreased the ethanol-induced hemorrhagic erosions; hence, ER-3 may be important in mechanisms of acute gastric mucosal injury and protection.

CHRONIC ULCERATION

The development and pathogenesis of chronic and duodenal ulcers are multifactorial and incompletely understood. The healing of chronic lesions, however, seems to be controlled by a few processes which govern wound healing such as angiogenesis and proliferation of fibroblasts during the generation of granulation tissue. Recently, we performed two series of experiments to test the hypothesis that angiogenesis and granulation tissue formation might be stimulated by sucralfate whose mechanism of antiulcer effect is very poorly understood [19], and that bFGF, the most potent endothelial mitogen [20], might accelerate the healing of experimental chronic duodenal ulcers.

EFFECT OF SUCRALFATE ON ANGIOGENESIS AND GRANULATION TISSUE

Several mechanisms have been implicated (e.g., enhanced mucus and bicarbonate secretion, reduction of microvascular injury) to explain the acute gastroprotection by sucralfate, but no major unifying and testable explanations are available to elucidate the mechanisms of accelerated ulcer healing by this drug without decreasing gastric acidity [19]. Since angiogenesis is of crucial importance for the generation of granulation tissue and wound/ulcer healing processes, we tested the hypothesis that sucralfate and its active component potassium sucrose octasulfate (SOS) might stimulate angiogenesis and fibroblast proliferation under controlled *in vivo* conditions.

For this purpose, round sterile sponges (8 x 3 mm) which contained 5 or 50 mg of sucralfate, SOS or, as a positive control, bFGF mutein CS23 (Takeda Chemical Industries, Ltd.), 20 or 200ng, were implanted subcutaneously (s.c.). In each rat 2 sponges with vehicle and 2 of each compound with low and high doses were implanted. One week later the animals were killed, the sponges were removed, fixed in formalin and processed for histologic and histochemical evaluation and morphometry. Under high (x200) power field (HPF), the number of blood vessels and the area (mm^2) of granulation tissue surface were measured and the total number of blood vessels calculated.

Mean values for the high doses compared with internal controls are presented in Table 2. Low doses produced results similar to those of controls. The results demonstrate that both sucralfate and SOS increased the number of blood vessels but only sucralfate enlarged the granulation tissue surface. Hence, the total number of blood vessels was 449% and 170% of controls, after sucralfate and SOS, respectively. The positive control FGF increased all the parameters studied and on a molar basis was more active than the other two drugs.

We concluded that sucralfate and its active component SOS increased the number of blood vessels (angiogenesis) in the s.c. implanted sponge assay. The granulation tissue surface was enlarged only by sucralfate, thus in increasing the total number of blood vessels sucralfate was more active than SOS. These processes may have a role in the ulcer healing properties of sucralfate.

TABLE 2

EFFECT OF SUCRALFATE, SOS AND bFGF ON ANGIOGENESIS
AND GRANULATION TISSUE IN S.C. IMPLANTED SPONGES

Treatment	Blood vessels (No./HPF)	(%)	Granulation Tissue Surface (mm^2)	(%)	Total No. Blood Vessels (%)
Controls	30.6+2.1	100	2.9+0.2	100	100
Sucralfate	67.6+2.5	221	5.9+0.7	203	449
Controls	35.8+2.3	100	2.6+0.1	100	100
SOS	58.7+6.6	164	2.7+0.2	104	170
Controls	40.5+2.9	100	3.6+0.5	100	100
FGF	75.9+3.7	187	7.6+0.7	211	396

EFFECT OF bFGF ON HEALING OF CHRONIC DUODENAL ULCERS

The prevention and therapy of gastric and duodenal ulcers have until recently been virtually limited to decreasing the secretion or intraluminal concentration of gastric acid. In addition to this secretory approach, direct cellular pharmacological treatment of ulcer itself is now also possible. Since bFGF is an angiogenic endothelial mitogen which also stimulates the growth of other cell types, we tested the hypothesis that orally administered bFGF might accelerate healing of experimental chronic duodenal ulcers.

Sprague-Dawley female rats (150-200g) received three doses of cysteamine-HCl, 25mg/100g i.g. at about 4 hr intervals. Three days later, rats with penetrating duodenal ulcers (as determined by laparotomy) were randomised into vehicle control and treatment groups. Rats received (a) vehicle alone; (b) wild type recombinant human bFGF; (c) acid-resistant mutein CS23 [21], at 100ng/100g or, for comparison, (d) the histamine H_2 receptor antagonist cimetidine (Smith, Kline & Beecham), 10 mg/100g by gavage twice daily until autopsy on day 21, when ulcers were measured and histologic sections taken.

The results indicate that the incidence, i.e., rats with ulcers, was decreased only by bFGF-CS23 during the 3 week treatment (Table 3). The ulcer crater was reduced by marginal significance by cimetidine, and markedly by bFGF-W and the acid resistant bFGF-CS23. Histology of bFGF-treated rats revealed: prominent angiogenesis, mild mononuclear cell infiltration, dense granulation tissue in the ulcer bed and healed ulcers which were completely epithelized. Morphometric analysis of angiogenesis in histologic sections after immunohistochemical staining for endothelial cell-specific factor VIII revealed hypovascular ulcer craters in comparison with adjacent normal mucosa, and about a 10-fold increase in angiogenesis in ulcer craters of rats treated with CS23.

TABLE 3

INFLUENCE OF CIMETIDINE AND bFGF ON THE HEALING OF CYSTEAMINE-INDUCED CHRONIC DUODENAL ULCERS IN RATS

Therapy	Rats with Ulcers	Ulcer Crater
Vehicle	93%	9.2 ± 3.4 mm^2
Cimetidine	86%	3.6 ± 0.8 mm^2 ($p=0.072$)
bFGF (wild)	80%	2.1 ± 1.3 mm^2 ($p < 0.05$)
bFGF (CS23)	40%	1.6 ± 0.8 mm^2 ($p < 0.01$)

We concluded that oral administration of an angiogenic polypeptide made acid-stable by recombinant site-specific mutagenesis significantly accelerated the healing of chronic duodenal ulcers produced by cysteamine. Treatment with bFGF-CS23 caused a 10-fold increase in angiogenesis in ulcer bed. These findings demonstrate the important role of angiogenesis in ulcer healing and its new pharmacologic modulation.

REFERENCES

1.   Cotran RS, Suter ER, Majno G. The use of colloidal carbon as a tracer for vascular injury. Vasc Dis 1967; 4: 107.

2.   Szabo S, Trier JS, Brown A, Schnoor J. Early vascular injury and increased vascular permeability in gastric mucosal injury caused by ethanol in the rat. Gastroenterology 1985; 88: 228-36.

3.   Szabo S, Pihan G, Trier JS. Alterations in blood vessels during gastric injury and protection. Scand J Gastroenterol 1986; 21(125): 92-6.

4.   Robins PG. Ultrastructural observations of the pathogenesis of aspirin-induced gastric erosions. Br J Exp Pathol. 1980; 61: 497.

5.   Trier JS, Szabo S, Allen CH. Ethanol-induced damage to mucosal capillaries of rat stomach. Gastroenterology 1987; 92: 13-22.

6.   Szabo S, Trier JS. Pathogenesis of acute gastric mucosal injury: sulfhydryls as a protector, adrenal cortex as a modulator, and vascular endothelium as a target. In: Allen A, Flemstrom G, Garner A, Silen W, Turnberg LA. eds. Mechanisms of mucosal protection in the upper gastrointestinal tract. New York: Raven Press, 1984: 287-93.

7.   Guth PH, Paulsen G, Nagata H. Histologic and microcirculatory changes in alcohol-induced gastric lesions in the rat: Effect of prostaglandin cytoprotection. Gastroenterology 1984; 87: 1083-90.

8.   Leung FW, Itoh M, Hirabayashi K, Guth P. Role of blood flow in gastric and duodenal mucosal injury in the rat. Gastroenterology 1985; 88: 281-9.

9.   Pihan G, Szabo S, Trier JS. The role of microvasculature in acute gastric mucosal damage and protection. In: Szabo S, Pfeiffer CJ, eds. Ulcer disease: New aspects in pathogenesis and pharmacology. Florida: CRC Press, 1989: 135-44.

10.   Guth PH. Vascular factors in gastric mucosal injury. In: Szabo S and Pfeiffer CJ eds. Ulcer disease: New aspects of pathogenesis and pharmacology. Florida: CRC Press. 1989;125-34.

11.   Kitajima M. Gastric mucosal microvascular architecture and mucosal blood flow in rats during stress. In: Szabo S, Pfeiffer CJ, eds. Ulcer disease: New aspects in pathogenesis and pharmacology. Florida: CRC Press, 1989: 145-56.

12.   Robert A. On the mechanisms of cytoprotection. In: Szabo S, Pfeiffer CJ, eds. Ulcer disease: New aspects in pathogenesis and pharmacology. Florida: CRC Press, 1989; 417-20.

13.   Szabo S. Critical and timely review of the concept of gastric cytoprotection. Acta Physiol Hung 1989; 73: 115-27.

14.   Galli SJ, Wershil BK, Bose R, Walker PA, Szabo S. Ethanol-induced acute gastric injury in mast cell-deficient and congenic normal mice. Am J Pathol 1987; 128: 11-40.

15.   Peskar BM, Lange K, Hoppe U, Peskar BA. Ethanol stimulates formation of leukotriene C4 in rat gastric mucosa. Prostaglandins 1986; 31: 283-92.

16.   Pihan G, Szabo S. Protection of gastric mucosa against hypertonic sodium chloride by 16,16 dimethyl prostaglandin E_2 or sodium thiosulfate in the rat: evidence for decreased mucosal penetration of damaging agent. Dig Dis Sci 1989; 34: 1865-72.

17.   Yanagisawa M, Kurihara H, Kimura S, Tomobe Y, Kobayashi M, Mitsui Y, Yazaki Y, Goto K, Masaki T. Endothelin: a novel potent vasoconstrictor peptide produced by vascular endothelial cells. Nature 1988; 332: 411-15.

18.   Morales RE, Johnson B, Szabo S. Endothelin induces hemorrhagic gastric mucosal lesions and aggravates the damaging effect of HCl and ethanol. Dig Dis Sci 1989; 34(8):1318 (abstract).

19.   Szabo S, Hollander D. Pathways of gastrointestinal protection and repair: mechanisms of action of sucralfate. Am J Med 1989; 86(6A): 23-31.

20.   Folkman J, Klagsbrun M. Angiogenic factors. Science 1987; 235: 442-47.

21.   Seno K, Sasada R, Iwane K, Sudo K, Kurokawa T, Ito K, Igarashi K. Stabilizing basic fibroblast growth factor using protein engineering. Biochem Biophys Res Commun 1988; 151: 701-8.

EFFECTS OF INDOMETHACIN AND PREDNISOLONE ON CONNECTIVE TISSUE AT THE BASE OF ACETIC ACID-INDUCED GASTRIC ULCERS IN RATS

Y. Ogihara, Y Fuse** and S. Okabe

*Department of Applied Pharmacology, Kyoto Pharmaceutical University, Kyoto, Japan, **Third Department of Internal Medicine, Kyoto Prefectural University of Medicine, Kyoto, Japan*

ABSTRACT

We examined mechanisms by which indomethacin and prednisolone delay the healing of gastric ulcers induced in rats. The ulcers became evident 5 days after the submucosal injection of acetic acid solution into the gastric wall. These animals were killed 1-4 weeks after this ulceration and the ulcerated tissues were examined. Connective tissue (granulation at the time of ulceration) at the ulcer base was isolated from the surrounding mucosa and analyzed for collagen contents (determined as hydroxyproline). Treatment with indomethacin (1 mg/kg) for 2 or 4 weeks significantly delayed ulcer healing and increased the amount of connective tissue and collagen content at the ulcer base. Treatment with prednisolone (5 mg/kg) for 1 or 2 weeks also significantly delayed ulcer healing, yet decreased the amount of connective tissue and collagen content. Histologically, both agents significantly increased length of the rupture of muscularis mucosa. These results suggest that while different mechanisms are involved in the delayed ulcer healing by these agents, the inhibition of contraction of the ulcer base is common to the underlying mechanisms.

INTRODUCTION

Acetic acid-induced gastric ulcer is a well established chronic ulcer model [1,2]. As the healing process closely resembles human gastric ulcers, this model is used for screening anti-ulcer drugs and for studying healing processes. Treatment with anti-inflammatory drugs such as indomethacin, aspirin, prednisolone or cortisone significantly delayed the healing of acetic acid-induced gastric ulcers in rats [3-8]. It was postulated that reduction of hexosamine and hydroxyproline contents [4,5], deficiency of endogenous prostaglandins (PGs)[6-8], inhibition of angiogenesis in the granulation [9], and reduced gastric mucosal blood flow around the ulcers [10] might be involved in the mechanisms related to delayed healing.

It is well known that contraction of granulation tissue is a crucial event in the early stage of wound healing [11,12]. In an attempt to clarify underlying mechanisms of delayed ulcer healing caused by indomethacin and prednisolone, we isolated connective tissue from the base of acetic acid-induced ulcers and analyzed the contents. Histological analysis of the gastric specimens in the control and drug-treated groups was also made.

MATERIALS AND METHODS

Male Donryu rats (Nihon S.L.C. Ltd., Shizuoka, Japan), weighing 240-260g, were used in all experiments. These rats were not fasted before the experiments to facilitate injection of the acetic acid solution [1].

INDUCTION OF GASTRIC ULCERS

Gastric ulcers were produced according to the standardized method previously described [1,2]. Briefly, under ether anaesthesia the abdomen was incised and the stomach exposed. Then, 20% acetic acid (v/v, 0.03 ml) was injected into the submucosal layer of antral-oxyntic border on the anterior wall, using a microsyringe (Terumo, Tokyo, Japan). After closure of the abdomen, the animals were caged and maintained in the usual manner. Since well-defined deep ulcers became evident 5 days after injecting the acid, we defined the 5th day as the day of the ulceration. Rats were administered indomethacin at 1 mg/kg and prednisolone at 5 mg/kg s.c. once daily for 1 to 4 weeks after this ulceration. Preliminary experiments indicated that treatment with prednisolone for more than 2 weeks significantly reduced the body weight of animals and the general physical state was poor. Therefore, experiments concerned with prednisolone were designed only for 1 or 2 weeks treatments. Control animals were administered the vehicle alone. All these animals were eating a regular diet with tap water for drinking. After the final administration of these drugs, the rats were fasted for 24 hours and then killed under ether anesthesia. The stomachs were removed, inflated with 8 ml of 2% formaline and immersed in 2% formalin for 10 min to lightly fix the gastric wall and then opened along the greater curvature. The ulcerated area (mm^2) was determined under a dissecting microscope with a square grid (Olympus, Tokyo, Japan, x10). Some of the stomachs were then immersed in 10% formalin, processed for routine light microscopy and stained with hematoxylin-eosin and azan. As an index of the contraction in the ulcer base, the maximal length of the rupture of muscularis mucosae (mm) was measured under a light microscope (Olympus, Tokyo, Japan, x40) [Figure 1]. Persons who measured the ulcerated area and the histological index were unaware of which treatments the animals had been given.

DETERMINATIONS OF COLLAGEN CONTENT AND CONCENTRATION

After measurement of the ulcerated area, the connective tissue at the ulcer base was isolated from the surrounding tissues under a dissecting microscope (x10) as follows. First, the hepatic tissue adhering to the ulcer base was removed and then about 1 cm^2 of the stomach was dissected away. The gastric mucosa around the ulcers, muscle and necrotic layer covering the ulcer base were then removed using ophthalmic scissors (Figure 1). This isolation was not difficult because the connective tissue forming the ulcer base was harder than the surrounding normal mucosa and muscle. The normal gastric mucosa and muscle layers are very soft and there was no resistances to the scissors at the time of cutting. When the scissors touch the connective tissue, some resistance is felt. Some of the isolated tissues were histologically examined to ensure that the obtained specimens consisted of connective tissue alone.

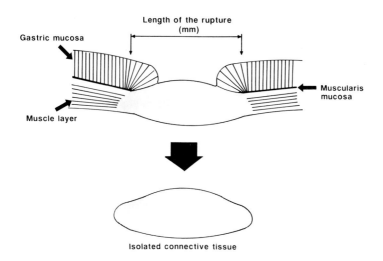

FIGURE 1: *Schematic drawing of the gastric mucosa of a rat with an ulcer and isolated connective tissue. The length of the rupture means the diameter between the muscularis mucosae.*

The isolated tissues were individually put into the test tubes and boiled in ethanol (99.0%, v/v), de-fatted with ether-acetone (1:1,v/v) for 48 hours and dried under a reduced pressure (Eyela, Freeze-Dryer 80, Tokyo, Japan). The dried tissues were weighed and hydrolyzed in 6N HCl for 3 hours and then neutralized with 6N NaOH. The hydrolyzed samples were used for the determination of the amount of collagen [13]. The collagen content and concentration were expressed in terms of the quantity of μg of hydroxyproline and μg hydroxyproline/mg dry tissue weight, respectively.

PREPARATION OF DRUGS

Indomethacin and prednisolone (Sigma Chemical Co, St. Louis, Mo.) were suspended in saline with a trace of Tween-80 and prepared immediately before use. Indomethacin was administered in a volume of 1 ml per 200g body weight and prednisolone in a volume of 0.5 ml per 200g body weight.

STATISTICS

All data represent the mean $\pm$ SEM. Student's t-test was used to determine the statistical significance and value of $P<0.05$ was regarded as being significant.

RESULTS

EFFECTS OF INDOMETHACIN AND PREDNISOLONE ON ULCER HEALING

On the day of ulceration, well-defined deep ulcers were observed with a 100% incidence, the ulcerated area being $33.4 \pm 3.5mm^2$ (N = 15). These ulcers spontaneously diminished in size, i.e., the ulcerated area at 1, 2 and 4 weeks being $8.9 \pm 1.2mm^2$ (N = 15), $4.4 \pm 0.8mm^2$ (N = 20) and $2.7 \pm 0.7mm^2$ (N = 20), respectively. Treatment with indomethacin for 1 week had no effect on healing of the ulcers (Table 1). However, the drug significantly delayed ulcer healing when administered for 2 or 4 weeks. In contrast, repeated administration of prednisolone for 1 week caused a significant delay in ulcer healing as compared to findings in the controls. Similar results were observed after 2 weeks treatment with prednisolone, although the degree of delay was extensive compared to findings in the 1 week experiment.

TABLE 1

EFFECTS OF INDOMETHACIN AND PREDNISOLONE ON HEALING OF ACETIC ACID-INDUCED GASTRIC ULCERS IN RATS AND ON CONNECTIVE TISSUES AT THE ULCER BASE

	Ulcerated area (mm^2)	No. of rats	Dry tissue weight (mg)	Collagen content (ug)	Collagen concentration (ug/mg)
Day 0 of ulceration	33.4+3.5	15			
1 week					
Control	8.9+1.2	15	7.5+1.0	185.2+23.5	25.3+0.7
Indomethacin	10.3+1.8	15	7.7+1.6	192.3+39.2	24.9+1.6
Prednisolone	12.7+1.5*	15	4.8+0.5*	134.9+15.8	28.3+1.6
2 weeks					
Control	4.4+0.8	20	11.0+0.9	289.8+23.6	26.3+0.8
Indomethacin	9.9+0.9*	15	15.1+1.1*	480.8+46.9*	31.2+1.2*
Prednisolone	12.8+1.4*	15	8.1+0.8*	212.7+19.8*	26.6+1.2
4 weeks					
Control	2.7+0.7	20	8.4+ 1.5	217.8+37.3	25.8+0.8
Indomethacin	12.6+1.4*	15	14.9+11.1*	414.9+36.8*	27.8+1.1

Animals were administered indomethacin (1 mg/kg) or prednisolone (5 mg/kg) s.c. once daily for 1,2 or 4 weeks after the ulceration (5 days after the acid injection). Collagen was determined as hydroxyproline.
Data represent the mean $\pm$ SEM.
* Significantly different from the control groups at P<0.05.

EFFECTS OF INDOMETHACIN AND PREDNISOLONE ON CONNECTIVE TISSUES

Histological studies showed that the isolated tissues from the ulcer base consisted primarily of connective tissue (granulation, fibrous tissue and collagen fibers), and did not involve the gastric mucosa and hepatic tissue.

On the day of ulceration, the amount of isolated connective tissue, collagen content and concentration were 16.0 ± 2.0mg, 210.4 ± 33.5ug and 13.6 ± 0.7ug/mg dry tissue weight (N = 15), respectively (Table 1). In the control group, the amount of connective tissue was 7.5 ± 1.0mg, 11.0 ± 0.9mg and 8.4 ± 1.5mg at 1, 2 and 4 weeks, respectively. Collagen content was about 200ug at 1 and 4 weeks later, but the value at 2 weeks was 289.8 ± 23.4ug. Collagen concentration was gradually increased to about 25ug/mg dry tissue weight.

When indomethacin was administered for 1 week, the amount of connective tissue, collagen contents and collagen concentrations did not differ from the corresponding control values (Table 1). After 2 weeks treatment, indomethacin significantly increased the amounts of connective tissue and collagen content, i.e., 15.1 ± 1.1mg and 480.8 ± 46.9ug, respectively. Even after 4 weeks treatment, the amounts of connective tissue and collagen content were significantly larger than in the control groups. Gross appearances of connective tissues isolated were shown (Figure 2).

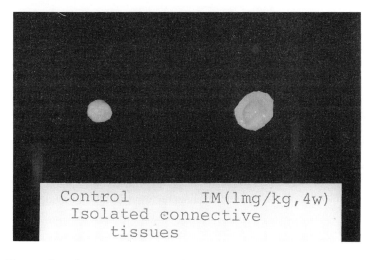

FIGURE 2: *Gross appearances of connective tissues isolated from the stomachs of normal (left) and indomethacin-treated (right) rats. Indomethacin (1 mg/kg) was administered s.c. for 4 wks after ulceration.*

In contrast, treatments with prednisolone for 1 week significantly reduced the amount of connective tissue and tended to reduce the collagen content. After 2 weeks treatment, it significantly reduced the amount of connective tissue and collagen content to 8.1 ± 0.8mg and 212.7 ± 19.8ug, respectively.

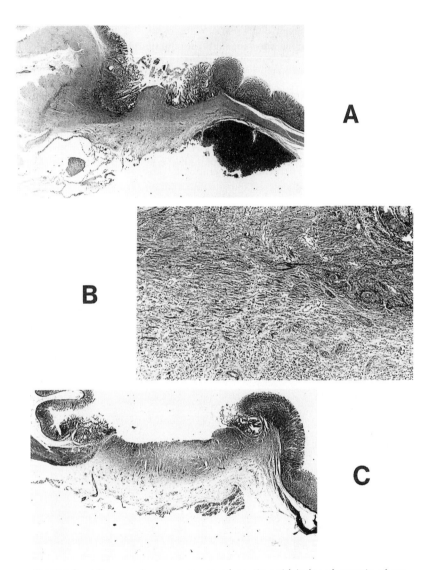

FIGURE 3: *Microscopic appearances of acetic acid-induced gastric ulcers present in rats for 2 wk. A,B: The stomachs in the control group stained with H.E. (A, x 3.3) and Azan (B, x 10). C,D: The stomachs in the indomethacin (1mg/kg)-treated groups stained with H.E. (C, X 3.3) and Azan (D, x 10). E,F: The stomachs in the prednisolone (5mg/kg)-treated groups stained with H.E. (E, x 3.3) and Azan (F, x 10). Note that both indomethacin and prednisolone markedly extended the ulcer area. With indomethacin fibrosis occurred and prednisolone suppressed the formation of collagen fibers at the ulcer base.*

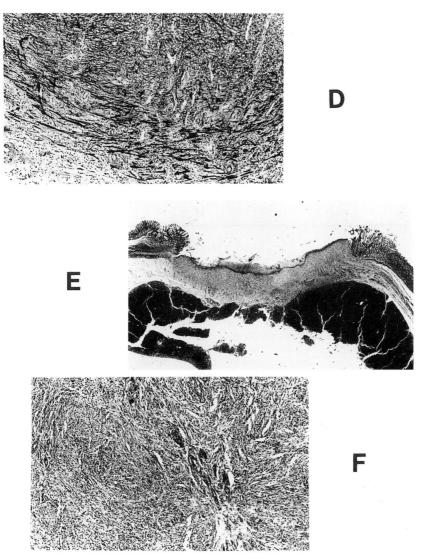

FIGURE 3: *Microscopic appearances of acetic acid-induced gastric ulcers present in rats for 2 wk. A,B: The stomachs in the control group stained with H.E. (A, x 3.3) and Azan (B, x 10). C,D: The stomachs in the indomethacin (1mg/kg)-treated groups stained with H.E. (C, X 3.3) and Azan (D, x 10). E,F: The stomachs in the prednisolone (5mg/kg)-treated groups stained with H.E. (E, x 3.3) and Azan (F, x 10). Note that both indomethacin and prednisolone markedly extended the ulcer area. With indomethacin fibrosis occurred and prednisolone suppressed the formation of collagen fibers at the ulcer base.*

HISTOLOGICAL STUDY

Two weeks after the ulceration, the lesions in the control group diminished in size and granulation tissue enriched capillary vessels were observed at the bottom of the ulcer [Figure 3A, H.E.]. Beneath this granulation tissue, collagen fibers regularly lined up along the horizontal axis [Figure 3B, Azan]. In the indomethacin treated group, large and deep ulcers were observed 2 weeks later [Figure 3C, H.E.] and the tissue in the ulcer base contained irregular, matured collagen fibers and fibrosis developed [Figure 3D, Azan]. Large ulcers, even though the thickness was slightly reduced compared with the one in the control and indomethacin-treated groups, were also observed in the group treated with prednisolone for 2 weeks [Figure 3E, H.E.]. In these tissues, the formation of collagen fibers at the ulcer base was apparently reduced [Figure 3F, Azan]. The length of the rupture of muscularis mucosae of 1- or 2-week old ulcers in the control group was 5.6 ± 0.5 mm or 4.9 ± 0.3 mm, respectively. In groups treated with indomethacin or prednisolone for 1 week, the length was 5.9 ± 0.4 mm or 5.8 ± 0.5 mm, respectively. There was no significant difference between the control and drug-treated groups. After 2 weeks treatment with these drugs, however, the length was significantly larger than that in the control group, i.e. 6.7 ± 0.3 mm for the indomethacin-treated groups and 6.5 ± 0.4 mm for the prednisolone-treated groups.

DISCUSSION

We isolated all the connective tissue at the base of the gastric ulcer. The procedure is readily facilitated because the hardness between the connective tissue and the surrounding tissue differs. This method is applicable when the ulcer is visible under a dissecting microscope. Hase et al [9] removed the granulation tissue from the ulcer base to determine the angiogenesis. However, they excised only the tissue along the margin of the ulcer and did not separate all the whole connective tissues at the ulcer base.

In general, anti-inflammatory drugs are known to inhibit collagen synthesis and granulation tissue formation. Takagi and Abe [4] reported that various anti-inflammatory drugs (including sodium salicylate, phenylbutazone and prednisolone) apparently delayed the healing of acetic acid-induced gastric ulcers in rats. They suggested that the underlying mechanism is related to the reduction of hexosamine contents in the mucosal layer and hydroxyproline contents at the ulcer base. In the present study, we confirmed our previous works [8] that repeated administration of indomethacin for 2 or 4 weeks significantly delayed ulcer healing. Interestingly, we found that the amount of connective tissue at the ulcer base in the indomethacin-treated group was significantly larger than that in the control group when the drug was administered for more than 2 weeks. In parallel to the increased amounts of connective tissue, the collagen content and collagen concentration were also significantly larger than those in the control group. To our knowledge such findings represent the first description of the effect of indomethacin on the connective tissue at the ulcer base.

We did not determine the amount of connective tissue at the time of ulceration as the precise isolation of the tissue was tedious with the base of ulcer consisting of the immature granulation heavily covered by necrotic tissue. Therefore, it is unknown whether the significantly large tissue in response to indomethacin is due to the stimulation of the formation of connective tissue or to prevention of the diminution of the preformed tissue. Fukuhara and Tsurufuji [13] reported that indomethacin significantly inhibited the formation of carrageenin granuloma induced in the dorsum of rats, yet had little or no effect on preformed ones. Therefore, it is most likely that indomethacin prevented the diminution of preformed connective tissue. At the end of experiments, we macroscopically examined the healing of the incised abdomen   There was an almost complete healing of the wound and no evidence for increased connective tissue around the incised area.   Accordingly, it is clear that indomethacin exclusively acts on connective tissue in the ulcerated portion in the stomach.   The difference of our results and those by Takagi and Abe [4] might be explained by the different method of isolation of the connective tissue, the different drugs used and periods of administration (10-20 days before and after ulceration).

Hase et al [9] reported that prednisolone, administered at 20 or 40 mg/kg for 10 days after the acid injection, significantly delayed the healing of acetic acid-induced gastric ulcers, probably by preventing angiogenesis in the granulation tissue at the ulcer base.   We also found that prednisolone, when administered for 1 or 2 weeks after ulceration, significantly delayed the ulcer healing, and reduced the amount of the connective tissue and the collagen contents.   These results suggest that both indomethacin and prednisolone delay ulcer healing, but the mechanism of action of each drug seems to differ.

Contraction of the wounded margin is a prerequisite for wound healing [11,12]. Even in the healing of a gastric ulcer, the contraction of ulcer area, as well as the regeneration of epithelium, is considered to be a crucial event. Majno et al [15,16] reported that the granuloma pouch tissue contracts just like smooth muscle in response to 5-HT, vasopressin, bradykinin or prostaglandin $F_{1\alpha}$, presumably because myofibroblasts are present in the granulation.   Nakamura et al [17] noted the presence of myofibroblasts at the base of acetic acid-induced gastric ulcers in rats. We histologically measured the length of the rupture of the muscularis mucosae, as an index of the contraction of the ulcer base; the length was significantly longer in the groups treated with indomethacin and prednisolone compared with the controls. These results suggest that the drugs might partly prevent the contraction of the connective tissue at the ulcer base, probably by counteracting the action of chemical mediators released or preventing the release of mediators.   Most anti-inflammatory drugs suppress PGs synthesis by inhibiting cyclooxygenase activity and phospholipase A_2 or the release of PGs [18,19].   Szelenyi et al [7] and our group [8] reported that indomethacin markedly reduced PGs contents in the gastric mucosa around the acetic acid-induced ulcers in rats. It is possible that even in the connective tissue at the ulcer area, there is a reduced amount of PGs . Therefore, it is most likely that indomethacin and prednisolone might interfere with the contraction of ulcer area as the results of a reduction in endogenous PGs.   In addition, the well-developed fibrosis observed in the indomethacin-treated group might increase the hardness of the tissue and prevent the contraction of ulcer area.

In the prednisolone-treated group, however, there was a possibility that the ulcer area could not contract because the formation of connective tissue, involving myofibroblasts, was apprently reduced by the drug.

We conclude that while mechanisms by which indomethacin and prednisolone delays the ulcer healing differ, a common mechanism related to the prevention of contraction of connective tissue at the ulcer base can be inferred.

References

1. Takagi K, Okabe S, Saziki R. A new method for the production of chronic gastric ulcer in rats and the effect of several drugs on its healing. Jpn J Pharmacol 1969; 19: 418-26.

2. Okabe S, Pfeiffer CJ. The acetic acid ulcer model - A procedure for chronic duodenal or gastric ulcer. In: Pfeiffer CJ, ed. Peptic Ulcer. Philadelphia: Lippincott 1971; 13-20.

3. Okabe S, Saziki R, Takagi K. Cortisone acetate and stress on the healing process of chronic gastric ulcers in rats. J Appl Physiol 1971; 30: 793-6.

4. Takagi K, Abe Y. Studies on the healing of experimental ulcer in rats II. Influence of anti-inflammatory drugs on the healing of acetic acid ulcer and the components in gastric tissue. Jpn J Pharmacol 1974; 24: 345-56.

5. Suzuki Y, Ito Y, Sudo Y. Changes in connective tissue components in ulcer tissue during the healing process of acetic acid ulcers in rats. Jpn J Pharmacol. 1979; 29: 821-9.

6. Szelenyi I, Engler H, Herzog P, Postius S, Vergin H, Holtermuller KH. Influence of non-steroidal anti-inflammatory compounds on healing of chronic gastric ulcers in rats. Agents and Actions 1982; 12: 180-2.

7. Szelenyi I, Postius S, Engler H. Prostaglandin contents in the rat gastric mucosa during healing of chronic gastric ulcer induced by acetic acid in rats. Agents and Actions 1983; 13: 207-9.

8. Wang JY, Yamasaki S, Takeuchi K, Okabe S. Delayed healing of acetic acid induced gastric ulcers in rats by indomethacin. Gastroenterology 1989; 96 393-42.

9. Hase S, Nakazawa S, Tsukamoto Y, Segawa K. Effects of prednisolone and human epidermal growth factor on angiogenesis in granulation tissue of gastric ulcer induced by acetic acid. Digestion 1989; 32: 135-42.

10. Okabe S, Takeuchi K, Hirose Y. Influence of indomethacin on gastric mucosal blood flow in the rat with acetic acid-induced gastric ulcers. Gastroenterology 1990; 98:A99.

11. Arey LB. Wound healing. Physiol Rev 1936; 16: 327-406.

12. Montandon D, D'Antiran G, Gabbiani G. The mechanism of wound contraction and epithelization. Clinical and experimental studies. Clin Plast Surg. 1977; 4: 325-46.

13. Neuman RE, Logan MA. The determination of hydroxyproline. J Biol Chem. 1950; 184: 299-305.

14. Fukuhara M, Tsurufuji S. The effect of locally injected anti-inflammatory drugs on carrageenin granuloma in rats. Biochem Pharmacol 1969; 18: 475-84.

15. Majno G, Gabbiani G, Hirschel BJ, Ryan GB, Statkov PR. Contraction of granulation tissue in vitro: Similarity to smooth muscle. Science 1971; 173: 548-59.

16. Majno G, Ryan GB, Gabbiani G, Hirschel BJ, Irle C, Joris I. Contractile events in inflammation and repair. In: Lepow IH and Ward PA. ed. Inflammation. New York: Academic press 1972; 13-27.

17. Nakamura M, Oda M, Nishizaki Y, Kaneko K, Azuma T, Tsuchiya M. Fluorescent histochemical study on the localization of myofibroblasts in the healing of acetic acid-induced gastric ulcers in the rat. Scand J Gastroenterol 1989; 24(suppl 162): 150-153.

18. Vane JR. Inhibition of prostaglandins biosynthesis as a mechanism of action of aspirin-like drugs. Nature (New Biol) 1971; 23: 232-5.

19. Lewis GP, Piper PJ. Inhibition of release of prostaglandins as an explanation of some of the actions of anti-inflammatory corticosteroids. Nature (New Biol) 1975; 254: 308-311.

GASTRIC MUCOSAL INJURY AND HAEMOSTASIS:
EFFECTS OF ASPIRIN, SMOKING AND PROPHYLACTIC STRATEGIES

**C.J. Hawkey, A.T. Cole, A.B. Hawthorne, N. Hudson,
Y.R. Mahida, S.G. Mann**

*Department of Therapeutics, Queen's Medical Centre,
University Hospital, Nottingham, U.K.*

INTRODUCTION

Short term studies show that aspirin and non-aspirin, non-steroidal anti-inflammatory drugs (NANSAIDs) injure the gastric mucosa to a greater extent than the duodenal mucosa[1-3]. These studies are complemented by epidemiological observations showing that these drugs increase the relative risk of gastric but not duodenal ulceration. In studies restricted to patients presenting with haematemesis and melaena, a highly significant relative risk is again seen. However, in contrast to studies of "all comers", the risk of presenting with a bleeding duodenal ulceration appears to be enhanced as much as the risk of presenting with a bleeding gastric ulcer.

These observations suggest that an anti-haemostatic effect of aspirin and NANSAIDs may contribute to the risk of presentation with haematemesis and melaena. Such a proposal is supported by data from the US Physicians' Study [4]. In this study healthy subjects took aspirin 325 mg on alternate days. This appeared to protect them against development of myocardial infarction but significantly increased the risk of presenting with upper gastrointestinal ulceration or melaena. This risk was similar to that seen in similarly designed studies of full dose NSAIDs. This raises the possibilities either that low doses of aspirin are more toxic to the gastric mucosa than previously assumed, or that an anti-haemostatic effect is important for presentation with melaena: these possibilities are not mutually exclusive.

There have been considerable efforts to identify effective regimens for the prophylaxis of NSAID induced gastroduodenal disease [3,5-7]. There is evidence that acute gastric lesions can be prevented by misoprostol and (in the case of aspirin) by enteric coating [3,6]. By contrast ranitidine has had little effect on the development of acute gastric ulceration in patients taking NSAIDs although it can prevent duodenal ulceration [7]. For logistical reasons none of these studies has been able to show a reduction in the incidence of life threatening events such as bleeding from peptic ulceration. The suggestions above and evidence presented in this paper imply that haemostasis may be as appropriate a target as mucosal injury for prophylaxis of life threatening events occurring in patients on aspirin or NANSAIDs.

Smoking is also associated with the development of both gastric and duodenal ulceration. However one study suggests that ulcers developing in smokers may be significantly less likely to bleed than those of non-smokers. One possible explanation is that smoking, in contrast to aspirin, can enhance rather than impair gastric haemostasis. There are limited data to suggest that smoking might enhance platelet reactivity, increase thromboxane production by some tissues and reduce gastric mucosal prostaglandin synthesis [8-10]. We therefore postulated that smoking could achieve a differential effect on ulcer development and ulcer bleeding if it enhanced thromboxane synthesis by platelets and other tissues, with secondary inhibition of gastric mucosal prostaglandin synthesis as a result of substrate diversion.

In this paper we present a synopsis of recent studies showing that:

1. gastric mucosal injury and haemostasis are separable phenomena.

2. aspirin both induces mucosal injury and impairs haemostasis in the stomach.

3. aspirin 300 mg daily causes similar injury to aspirin 600mg qds.

4. enteric coating reduces aspirin induced injury but does not reverse the impairment of haemostasis.

5. changes in intragastric pH affect haemostasis. Treatment with ranitidine is shown to promote intragastric haemostasis.

6. smoking inhibits prostaglandin synthesis in the gastric mucosa but not because of increased thromboxane synthesis.

STUDY 1 - COMPARISON OF DIFFERENT DOSES OF ASPIRIN

Three groups of volunteers took aspirin 300mg(n = 12), 1.8g(n = 10), or 2.4g (n = 6) for five days [11]. Endoscopy was used to quantitate mucosal injury, using the modified Lanza scale[7]. Spontaneous bleeding into washings was measured by the orthotolidine reaction. Four biopsies were taken from the greater curve and prostaglandin synthesis stimulated by vortex mixing for one minute. PGE_2 in the supernatant was measured by radioimmunoassay. Serum thromboxane was measured by radioimmunoassay after clotting at $37^\circ C$[12].

RESULTS

Aspirin 1.8g or 2.4g (data pooled) inhibited gastric mucosal PGE_2 synthesis by approximately 100% (median, interquartile range 82-100%, p<0.01). This was associated with significant endoscopic injury (Figure 1). With both doses of aspirin haemorrhagic lesions in the gastric body were most common. Antral lesions were both haemorrhagic and non-haemorrhagic. Aspirin 300mg/day caused less inhibition of gastric PGE_2,

by a median of 58% (interquartile range 30-100%, p<0.01).   However, injury
was not significantly different from that caused by the higher doses of
aspirin (Figure 1).   Both doses of aspirin inhibited platelet thromboxane
production by more than 99%.   However high doses of aspirin enhanced
spontaneous mucosal bleeding by 7(3.1 - 15.7)-fold (p<0.01) compared to a 3.3
(2.1-5.0)-fold enhancement seen with aspirin 300 mg daily.

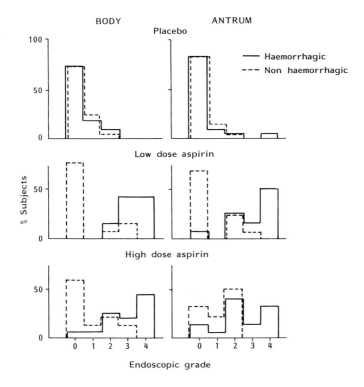

FIGURE 1:   *Frequency distribution of body and antral injury (Classified
by modified Lanza grade [7]) caused by placebo, low doses of aspirin
(300mg daily) and high doses of aspirin (1.8g or 2.4g daily)*

COMMENT

This study suggested that aspirin 300 mg is as gastrotoxic in the short
term as higher doses. However higher doses of aspirin caused more bleeding.
Both doses affected serum thromboxane to a similar extent, suggesting that
the increased bleeding with higher doses of apsirin was due to a platelet
independent mechanism.

STUDY 2 - ASPIRIN 300 MG DAILY AND 600MG QDS IN PLAIN AND ENTERIC COATED (NUSEALS) PREPARATIONS.

The purpose of this study [13] was:

1. to confirm the gastric mucosal toxicity of aspirin 300mg in a formal blinded comparison with aspirin 2.4g.

2. to investigate possible protection by enteric coating.

3. to investigate whether aspirin had an anti-haemostatic effect.

In this study gastric mucosal injury was quantified by counting the number of lesions within the stomach instead of assigning an injury grade. These data could thus be used to relate the level of spontaneous microbleeding to the number of lesions within the stomach, to derive a value for the rate of blood loss per lesion. In addition, bleeding induced by gastric mucosal biopsy - a measure akin to the skin bleeding time was measured, as a second index of intragastric haemostasis.

METHODS

Twenty volunteers each received five days treatment with placebo, aspirin 300mg daily, NuSeals 300 mg daily, aspirin 600mg qds, NuSeals 600mg qds. The order in which the volunteers received each course of treatment was randomised by Latin square design. At the end of each treatment period spontaneous gastric bleeding into washings was measured using the orthotolidine reaction. This was followed immediately by endoscopy when the number of haemorrhagic and non-haemorrhagic gastric mucosal lesions in the oesophagus, body, antrum and duodenum were counted. Four biopsies were taken from the greater curve and ex vivo gastric mucosal PGE_2 synthesis measured. Following endoscopy volunteers were re-intubated with an orogastric tube and biopsy induced bleeding into gastric washings measured five and ten minutes after the biopsy. Blood was taken for serum thromboxane and serum salicylate.

Calculation of derived values

Bleeding per mucosal lesion. This was calculated as:

$$\frac{\text{spontaneous bleeding per 10 minutes}}{\text{total number of gastric lesions}}$$

Biopsy induced bleeding. Blood measured in gastric washings at five munutes and ten minutes after biopsy would include some blood arising as a result of spontaneous (non-biopsy induced) bleeding. A correction was made based on the assumption that spontaneous bleeding occurred at a constant rate throughout the study.

RESULTS

All regimens inhibited gastric mucosal PGE_2 synthesis by 90% or more and in this study there were no significant differences between preparations[13]. Similarly serum thromboxane was suppressed by more than 99% with each preparation.

Plain aspirin 300 mg daily induced significant gastric injury, increasing the number of body haemorrhages to 2 (median, interquartile range 0 - 5). After aspirin 2.4g daily there were 4 (0.75 - 8.75) haemorrhagic erosions in the body.   This was not significantly greater than seen with aspirin 300mg daily. Fewer lesions were seen in the antrum than in the body and only aspirin 600mg qds caused a significant increase in their number.   The numbers of erosions seen when either dose of aspirin was given in enteric coated NuSeals form were not significantly different from placebo.

Table 1 shows that spontaneous gastric mucosal bleeding was increased with both doses of aspirin.   The higher dose of aspirin caused significantly more bleeding than the lower dose of aspirin.   Mucosal bleeding after either dose of aspirin as NuSeals was not significantly different from placebo.

TABLE 1

EFFECTS OF NuSEALS ENTERIC COATING ON ASPIRIN
INDUCED GASTRIC MUCOSAL BLEEDING

	Placebo	Aspirin 300mg daily	NuSeals 300mg daily	Aspirin 600mg qds	NuSeals 600mg qds
Total gastric Mucosal bleeding ul/10mins	0.9 (06.-1.3)	2.8* (1.6-4.8)	1.0+ (0.6-1.5)	7.2**^ (4.8-11.0)	1.5+ (0.8-2.9)

*p<0.01 **p<0.001 compared to placebo
^p<0.05 compared to aspirin 300mg
+p<0.01 compared to plain aspirin

BLEEDING PER MUCOSAL LESION.

This value could only be calculated in subjects where lesions were seen at endoscopy.   Table 2 shows bleeding per lesion for all eleven subjects where lesions were seen on plain aspirin, 300mg daily and 600mg qds. Differences between the two doses approach but do not achieve statistical difference. The effect of enteric coating with NuSeals could be examined in eleven cases where paired data were available for aspirin 600mg qds (eight subjects) or 300mg daily (three subjects).   Table 3 shows that the rate of bleeding per lesion was very similar whether aspirin in plain or enteric form had been received.

TABLE 2

EFFECT OF TWO DOSES OF ASPIRIN ON BLEEDING
PER MUCOSAL LESION

	Aspirin 300mg	Aspirin 600mg qds
Bleeding per mucosal lesion {nl/lesion}	407 (189-879)	933 (468-1862)

$$p \simeq 0.15$$

BIOPSY INDUCED BLEEDING

The effect of aspirin 300mg daily was to increase bleeding by a factor of 1.96 (95% confidence limits, 0.92 - 4.19). Aspirin 600mg qds increased biopsy induced bleeding by 2.65 (1.27 - 5.33)-fold. NuSeals had no effect on biopsy induced bleeding compared to plain aspirin and the data quoted include values for both plain and NuSeals aspirin.

TABLE 3

SIMILAR BLEEDING PER MUCOSAL LESION WITH
PLAIN AND ENTERIC COATED ASPIRIN

	Plain Aspirin	NuSeals
Bleeding per mucosal lesion {nl/lesion}	676 (327-1399)	513 (166-1584)

$$p \simeq 0.616$$

COMMENTS

In this study the differnces between high and low doses of aspirin in their effects on PGE_2 synthesis were less evident than in the first study. There appeared to be somewhat less mucosal injury as measured by numbers of lesions though differences between the doses were not statistically significant. There was more spontaneous bleeding with high dose aspirin than low dose aspirin. It seems likely that this arose both because of a (non-significant) increase in the number of lesions and an increase (also non-significant) in the amount of bleeding per lesion. There was no suggestion that enteric coating had any effect on intragastric haemostasis as measured by the rate of bleeding per lesion or by biopsy induced bleeding.

STUDY 3 - Effect of Changing Intragastric pH

The effect of changing intragastric pH on mucosal injury, spontaneous and biopsy induced bleeding were investigated in two studies, full details of which will be reported elsewhere. In this paper data relating to "bleeding per mucosal lesion" or "biopsy induced bleeding" are presented.

METHODS

Twenty healthy volunteers took aspirin 600mg qds for five days, together with placebo, ranitidine 150mg bd, ranitidine 300mg qds or ranitidine 600mg bd. These manoeuvres resulted in gastric mucosal injury assessed endoscopically and spontaneous bleeding assessed by microbleeding, as in Study 2. Bleeding per endoscopic lesion was derived as described above.

RESULTS

All doses of ranitidine resulted in reduced spontaneous gastric mucosal bleeding, although the effect of ranitidine 150mg bd was of borderline significance. The number of gastric mucosal lesions was significantly reduced by ranitidine 300mg qds and 600mg bd but not 150mg bd. All doses of ranitidine caused a highly significant reduction in the rate of bleeding per lesion (Table 4).

TABLE 4

Effect of Ranitidine on bleeding per
aspirin induced lesion

	Aspirin + Placebo	Aspirin + Ranitidine 150mg bd	Aspirin+ Ranitidine 300mg qds	Aspirin + Ranitidine 600mg bd
Bleeding per mucosal	1230	537*	468**	479**
lesion {nl/lesion}	(752-2014)	(333-867)	(264-828)	(277-826)

*p = 0.011 compared to
**p < 0.01 aspirin and placebo*

COMMENTS

In contrast to enteric coating, elevating the intragastric pH with ranitidine had a greater effect in reducing bleeding than in reducing overall numbers of lesions. This was supported by endoscopic evidence showing reduced numbers of haemorrhagic but not non-haemorrhagic lesions with ranitidine[14].

STUDY 4 - Effect of Intragastric pH on Biopsy Induced Bleeding.

In this study the effects of exogenous acid on biopsy induced bleeding was measured.   No aspirin or NANSAIDs were given[15].

METHODS

Thirteen fasted volunteers underwent unsedated endoscopy. Greater curve biopsies were taken and gastric washings collected every 5 minutes for 25 minutes. On one occasion water was used for washing and on another hydrochloric acid pH 1.5 was used.   Bleeding into aspirated washings was measured by the orthotolidine reaction.

RESULTS

Washing with acid had no significant effect on total biopsy induced bleeding but bleeding was more prolonged than when washing was with water. For acid washings there was 18.19 (geometric mean, 95% confidence limits 11.1 - 32.3)ul/5 minutes between 15 and 20 minutes as compared with 7.2 (4.2-12.3)ul/5 minutes with water (p = 0.016). Values for acid between 20 and 25 minutes were 18.2 (9.4 - 35.4)ul/5 minutes as compared with 5.9 (3.0 - 11.4)ul/5 minutes with water (p = 0.021).

COMMENT

This study complements the results of Study 3 in showing that reducing intragastric pH can prolong bleeding.   It also shows that changes in intragastric haemostasis can be achieved independently of aspirin or NANSAID usage.

EFFECTS OF SMOKING

Similar studies were carried out in smokers.

METHODS

Twelve healthy volunteers were studied on two occasions before and two occasions after smoking. During the smoking period, volunteers smoked two cigarettes at approximately 8 am and were endoscoped immediately after the second cigarette.   During the non-smoking period the protocol was the same except that the subjects did not smoke.   The mucosa was assessed endoscopically and four biopsies were taken from the greater curve. These were used to measure ex vivo prostaglandin synthesis.   Biospy induced bleeding was measured over the subsequent ten minutes.

RESULTS

Urinary cotinine levels showed that subjects stopped smoking during the non-smoking period. Smoking suppressed ex vivo synthesis of PGE_2 by 34.3 (12.5 - 71.6)%. Gastric mucosal thromboxane was also significantly depressed. There was no effect on serum thromboxane. Only a small number of lesions were seen and there was no significant differences between smoking and non-smoking phases. Biopsy induced bleeding was likewise not significantly different between smoking and non-smoking phases.

COMMENT

Smoking inhibited ex vivo production of PGE_2 but to a lesser extent than that seen in Studies 1 and 2 for aspirin 300mg daily. This may explain why, in contrast to aspirin there was little overt mucosal injury. Smoking also reduced gastric mucosal thromboxane synthesis providing evidence against the hypothesis that reduced PGE_2 arose because of substrate diversion to thromboxane. Smoking had no effect on serum thromboxane and biopsy induced bleeding was not, as originally hypothesised, reduced by smoking.

DISCUSSION

We have not been able to show directly that aspirin increases bleeding per mucosal lesion compared to placebo, because lesions are uncommon during the placebo phase. However we deduced that this is the case since bleeding per lesion is reduced by ranitidine. Moreover, aspirin was associated with an enhancement of biopsy induced bleeding. This may reflect the ability of aspirin to interfere with platelet function by acetylating platelet cyclooxygenase and is reflected in a reduction in serum thromboxane. These studies suggest that gastric mucosal injury and haemostasis are separate targets for prophylaxis. We have shown enteric coating can prevent aspirin induced gastric mucosal injury but has no effect on haemostasis. With ranitidine the most striking effect was a reduction in bleeding per mucosal lesion, consistent with a reversal of the impairment of haemostasis which occurs with aspirin.

Changes in intragastric pH were not seen with smoking and there were no differences in biopsy induced bleeding. These represent clear differences between aspirin and smoking which may be relevant to the greater tendency of ulcers on aspirin to bleed and the lesser tendency of ulcers of smokers to bleed. However, our hypothesis that smoking would inhibit PGE_2 synthesis by diversion of arachidonic acid to thromboxane synthesis by enhancement of the activity of thromboxane synthetase has been disproved.

Further studies will need to investigate with larger numbers whether there is a true difference in numbers of lesions and/or bleeding per lesion with high and low doses of aspirin. The observations should be extended to NANSAIDs and it will be important to investigate the effects of enteric coating with these compounds. The effects of H2 antagonists on biopsy induced bleeding both with and without aspirin or NANSAIDs should be investigated to support the blood per mucosal lesion data which suggests that ranitidine promotes intragastric haemostasis.

REFERENCES

1.   Fellows IW, Bhaskar NK, Hawkey CJ.   Nature and time-course of piroxicam-induced injury to human gastric mucosa.   Aliment Pharmacol Therap 1989; 3: 481-488.

2.   Daneshmend TK, Prichard PJ, Bhaskar NK, Millns PJ, Hawkey CJ. Use of microbleeding and an ultrathin endoscope to assess gastric mucosal protection by famotidine.   Gastroenterology 1989; 97: 944-949.

3.   Hawkey CJ.   Non-steroidal anti-inflammatory drugs and peptic ulcers.   Facts and figures multiply, but do they add up?   MBJ 1990; 97: 944-949.

4.   The Steering Committee of the Physicians' Health Study Research Group.   Final report on the spirin component of the ongoing Physicians' Health Study 1989; New Engl J Med 321: 129-135.

5.   Graham DY, Agrawal N, Roth SH.   Prevention of NSAID-induced gastric ulcer with the synthetic prostaglandin, misoprostol - a multicenter, double-blind, placebo-controlled trial.   Lancet 1988; ii: 1277-1281.

6.   Lanza FL, Royer GL, Nelson RS.   Endoscopic evaluation of the effects of aspirin, buffered aspirin, and enteric-coated aspirin on gastric and duodenal mucosa. N Engl J Med. 1980; 303: 135-138.

7.   Ehsanullah RSB, Page MC, Tildesley G, Wood JR. Prevention of gastroduodenal damage induced by non-steroidal anti-inflammatory drugs: controlled trial of ranitidine. Br Med J 1988; 297: 1017-1021.

8.   Benowitz NL.   Clinical pharmacology of nicotine.   Ann Rev Med 1986; 37: 21-32.

9.   Nowak J, Murray JJ, Oates JA, Fitzgerald GA. Biochemical evidence of a chronic abnormality in platelet and vascular function in healthy individuals who smoke cigarettes.   Circulation 1987; 76: 6-14.

10.   McReady DR, Clarke L, Cohen MM.   Cigarette smoking reduces human gastric luminal prostaglandin E_2. Gut 1985; 26: 1192-1196.

11.   Hawkey CJ, Sharma HK, Bhaskar NK, Didcote SM, Hawthorne AB, Daneshmend TK.   High and low dose aspirin: equal gastric damage but impaired haemostasis at high dose. Gut 1989; 30: A1142.

12.   Horn EH, Cooper J, Hardy E, Heptinstall S, Rubin PC.   A cross-sectional study of platelet cyclic AMP in healthy and hypertensive human pregnancy.   Clin Sci (submitted).

13.   Hawthorne AB, Mahida YR, Cole AT, Hawkey CJ.   Aspirin-induced gastric mucosal damage: Prevention by enteric-coating of aspirin and relation to prostaglandin synthesis.   Br Med J (submitted).

14.   Cole AT, Brundell S, Hudson N, Hawthorne AB, Hawkey CJ.   High dose ranitidine prophylaxis of gastric haemorrhagic lesions.   In press (BSG meeting September 1990).

15.   Mann SG, Didcote S, Hyman-Taylor, Hawkey CJ.   Prolongation of intragastric bleeding by acid.   In press (BSG meeting September 1990).

ADAPTATION TO NONSTEROIDAL ANTI-INFLAMMATORY DRUG INDUCED GASTRODUODENAL DAMAGE IN MAN. STUDIES OF MORPHOLOGY, HISTOLOGY AND MUCOSAL BLOOD FLOW

C.J. Shorrock and W.D.W Rees

University Department of Medicine, Queen Elizabeth Hospital, Birmingham, U.K. and Department of Gastroenterology, Hope Hospital, Salford, U.K.

ABSTRACT

To define further the nature of mucosal injury induced by indomethacin we have studied the effect of 28 days continuous administration on human gastroduodenal morphology, gastric histology and gastric mucosal blood flow as measured by laser doppler flowmetry. Indomethacin caused acute gastroduodenal damage in 100% of cases, the damage being maximal at 24 hours of administration. With continued intake damage resolved, although a minority (2 subjects) progressed to discrete ulceration. Biopsies of intact mucosa showed no significant changes in inflammatory or regenerative features and failed to shed any light on the process of adaptation to damage. Gastric mucosal blood flow was reduced by indomethacin and there was a good correlation between the severity of damage and the magnitude of reduction of blood flow. Mucosal recovery was associated with return of blood flow to normal.

In conclusion, mucosal adaptation to acute damage by indomethacin occurs in man. The mechanisms whereby the mucosa adapts in this intriguing way remain unknown but may be dependent on changes in blood flow

INTRODUCTION:

Non-steroidal anti-inflammatory drugs (NSAID's), extensively used as simple analgesics and in rheumatic diseases, have been shown to cause gastrointestinal injury [1-3]. The main sites of this damage are the stomach and duodenum although damage to oesophagus, small intestine and colon have all been reported [4-6]. The damage includes ulceration, bleeding, perforation and stricture formation, complications which may be life threatening [7-9].

The precise mechanisms whereby these agents produce gastroduodenal damage are unknown, although, depletion of mucosal prostaglandins with a corresponding reduction in the competence of mucosal defence mechanisms is widely thought to be of importance [10-12]. The stomach and duodenum are protected from damaging luminal contents - particularly acid and pepsin - by several mechanisms [13]. These include the mucus gel layer, bicarbonate secretion by epithelial cells, surface active phospholipids, the apical membrane itself and the process of restitution. In addition mucosal blood flow plays a vital role in the prevention of injury to the surface epithelium by delivering oxygen, nutrients, bicarbonate and by removing H+ ions which have penetrated the mucus-bicarbonate barrier. Among these the "mucus-bicarbonate barrier" acts as the first line of defence with bicarbonate secretion by the surface epithelial cells into the mucus gel layer setting up a pH gradient, maintaining juxtamucosal neutrality in the setting of low luminal pH's. Such a gradient has been demonstrated in vitro and in vivo in many animal models as well as in man [14-19]. NSAID's have been shown in animal models to reduce both epithelial bicarbonate secretion [20] and mucus synthesis and secretion [21,22] resulting in a reduced pH gradient across the mucus gel layer and exposure of the epithelial cells to a more acidic environment [16,17].

The incidence of serious side effects with NSAID's however is low considering the large quantities of these drugs prescribed [23]. Since endoscopic studies have shown acute gastric mucosal damage in the majority of subjects during the first week of NSAID administration [1,24] these rather contradictory observations suggest that tolerance develops during the course of continued NSAID intake. Such tolerance or adaptation has been documented for gastric mucosa with a variety of damaging agents in animal studies [25] and more recently with aspirin in man [26]. However the mechanisms whereby the mucosa develops tolerance to damage remain uncertain.

The aims of the studies described in this paper were thus twofold; first to document the morphological changes occuring in gastroduodenal mucosa during 28 days of treatment with the NSAID indomethacin and secondly to assess gastric mucosal blood flow during this period of treatment.

METHODS:

SUBJECTS

Studies were carried out on 24 healthy volunteers (15 men and 9 women) with a mean age of 24 years (range 19-37). 6 volunteers were smokers, smoking less than 20 cigarettes daily and who did not change their smoking habits during the study. Alcohol was allowed during the study and subjects followed their normal drinking habits (all subjects consumed less than 80 grammes of alcohol per week). All subjects had no previous history of gastrointestinal disease and had not taken aspirin or any other NSAID in the previous 3 months.

All subjects gave written informed consent for the studies and ethical approval was given by the Salford Health Authority Ethical Committee.

ENDOSCOPY

Standard upper gastrointestinal endoscopy was performed by one investigator throughout (CJS) with a 1% lignocaine hydrochloride throat spray prior to introduction of the endoscope. No sedative or anti-spasmodic drugs were used. All endoscopies were performed between 11am and 12 midday, subjects having a very light breakfast at 7am the morning of endoscopy.

Study Design

Subjects underwent endoscopy at entry into the study. Oral indomethacin 50 mg tid was then taken for 28 days continuously. The indomethacin was taken with meals and with a light breakfast at 7 am the morning of endoscopy. Endoscopy was repeated at 24 hours, 7 days and 28 days while on the indomethacin. At each endoscopy mucosal damage was graded and mucosal blood flow measured in the fundus and antrum of the stomach by a laser doppler technique. At the end of each endoscopy a single biopsy was taken from both the antrum and main body of the stomach, from areas appearing endoscopically normal, for later histological examination.

Prior to each endoscopy subjects were questioned directly about gastrointestinal symptoms and in addition kept a detailed written record of the duration, time of day and severity of any such symptoms between endoscopies. 10 ml of blood was taken randomly during the study from each subject for later detection of indomethacin to confirm compliance.

Three further subjects were used as controls. These subjects underwent endoscopy with mucosal grading, histological examination and measurement of mucosal blood flow as above over a 28 day period but receiving empty indomethacin capsules. The endoscopist was blind to the capsule content.

Blood flow studies

Gastric mucosal blood flow was measured using the technique of laser doppler flowmetry (LDF). The operating principal of LDF has been fully described elsewhere [27] but briefly is based on the principal that light scattered by moving red blood cells undergoes a shift in its frequency, the mean doppler shift providing an estimate of blood flow. Mucosal blood flow measured by LDF correlates well with flow measured by other methods.

In the laser doppler flowmeter used in the present study (Periflux PF2, Perimed Ltd, Stockholm, Sweden) light from a 2mW He-Ne laser is transmitted down an optical fiber (diameter 0.7mm) contained in a PF109 endoscopic probe (Perimed Ltd, Sweden) of outside diameter 2.5mm. The probe is inserted down the biopsy channel of an Olympus Q10 endoscope (Keymed, Southend-on-sea, UK). It became apparent in early experiments that the distance of the probe tip from the end of the endoscope was critical as the magnitude of the laser doppler readings varied with the distance the probe protruded. To get around this problem the probe was marked in such a way that the probe always protruded 3cm from the end of the endoscope. After diffuse scattering of the incident laser light, a portion of the backscattered light is picked up by two further fibres (diameter 0.7mm) contained in the endoscopic probe and transmitted to the flowmeter. The signal is processed giving a low noise output which corresponds to the tissue blood flow beneath the probe. A continuous recording of blood flow is obtained using a chart recorder with a paper speed of 1mm/second. Throughout the studies the upper limit of the signal processor was set to 4KHz with a constant gain of 3 and a time constant of 1.5 seconds.

Measurements of blood flow were made under direct vision in the gastric fundus and antrum from areas appearing endoscopically normal, the tip of the probe being gently abutted against the mucosa by advancing the whole endoscope and not the probe alone. Particular care was taken so as not to dimple the mucosa. A valid reading was one where a constant reading was obtained for at least 5 seconds uninterrupted by any movement artifact of the probe head relative to the tissue or by any loss of optical coupling due to peristalsis. A minimum of three such readings was taken at each site and the mean calculated and recorded.

TABLE 1

ENDOSCOPIC SCORING SYSTEM USED TO GRADE DAMAGE

GASTRIC	DUODENAL
0 = Normal 1 = Up to 5 erosions or submucosal haemorrhages (SMH) confined to one area of the stomach	0 = Normal 1 = Up to 5 erosions or SMH
2 = Erosions or SMH found in more than one anatomical region, or >5 in any one region, no >10 in entire stomach	2 = 6-10 erosions or SMH
3 = Multiple erosions (>10)	3 = >10 erosions
4 = Widespread involvement ± ulceration	4 = Duodenal ulcer

MORPHOLOGY

At endoscopy gastric and duodenal integrity was graded on a standardised scoring system adapted from Lanza et al [1] and recorded (Table 1). The entire stomach and duodenal cap was examined in proximal to distal manner prior to measurement of mucosal blood flow in order to eliminate any errors which might be caused from a misinterpretation of artifacts from either the endoscope or the endoscopic probe.

HISTOLOGY

At the end of each endoscopy a single biopsy was taken under direct vision from antrum and main body from normal looking mucosa, the exact position of the biopsy being noted. Any lesions seen at endoscopy from previous biopsy sites were disregarded and were not included when grading the endoscopic appearances. Specimens were examined by an experienced histopathologist blind to the endoscopic findings and unaware of the nature of the protocol. These were scored for inflammation and regeneration using the scale 0 (not present), 1 (minimal change from normal), 2 (mild), 3 (moderate) and 4 (severe) as previously described by Graham et al [26]. Briefly, inflammation was assessed quantitatively and qualitatively in terms of polymorphonuclear leucocytes, eosinophils, lymphocytes and plasma cells. Regeneration was assessed by examining mitotic rates of the surface and glandular epithelium, the amount of glandular disarray and the presence of enlarged nuclei with prominent nucleoli in the epithelial cells. Other features assessed were mucosal atrophy, flattening of surface epithelium, glandular disorganisation and intestinal metaplasia. The presence of Helicobacter like organisms was evaluated on Haematoxylin and Eosin stained sections, although their presence was confirmed using Giemsa preparations. Immunohistochemical staining by the immunoperoxidase method for kappa/lambda light chains and M, A, G and E heavy chains was performed on those biopsies which had a dense chronic inflammatory cell infiltrate.

STATISTICAL ANALYSIS

Results are calculated as means $\pm$ SE and differences compared statistically using a Students t test for paired data.

RESULTS:

MORPHOLOGY (*Figure 1*)

After 24 hours indomethacin all subjects had evidence of mucosal damage which was more marked in the stomach than in the duodenum (mean scores: 1.7 ± 0.2 in stomach and 0.8 ± 0.2 in duodenum, n=24, p<0.01 for difference between gastric and duodenal damage (unpaired t test)). By 7 days damage had significantly improved in the majority of patients, although 2 subjects had developed discrete ulceration in areas unrelated to biopsy sites - a 6mm antral gastric ulcer and a 7mm duodenal cap ulcer (mean scores: 0.96 ± 0.2 in stomach and 0.58 ± 0.2 in duodenum, n=24, p<0.01 for improvement in gastric damage between 24 hours and 7 days). There was no significant difference between duodenal damage at 24 hours and 7 days (0.80 ± 0.2 and 0.58 ± 0.2, p=0.22) although there was a trend towards improvement. The subjects with ulcers were withdrawn from the study along with 4 others who developed persistent headache and nausea. By 28 days all virtually all macroscopic mucosal damage had resolved (scores: 0.1 ± 0.1 for gastric and duodenal, n=18). No subjects experienced gastrointestinal symptoms during the study and indomethacin was detected in the serum of all subjects. At no time was there any mucosal damage in any of the three control subjects. There was no relationship between endoscopic severity of gastric damage and alcohol intake.

BLOOD FLOW STUDIES

Gastric mucosal blood flow was measured in 14 of our volunteers. Due to major problems with movement artefact in the duodenum, duodenal blood flow was not measured. Gastric mucosal blood flow was significantly reduced in the fundus ($79\pm5\%$ of baseline, p<0.001) and antrum ($72\pm5\%$ of baseline, p<0.002) after 24 hours indomethacin administration - the time of maximal mucosal damage. There was a good correlation between the severity

of mucosal damage and the change in mucosal blood flow after 24 hours
indomethacin administration (r=0.76). By 7 days, gastric mucosal blood flow
had increased but was still significantly below baseline values in fundus
(89±4%, p<0.02) but not in the antrum (93±7%, p=0.08, n=14). Mucosal
recovery by 28 days was associated with return of blood flow to normal
(98±3% in fundus and 93±8% in antrum,p=ns, n=11)

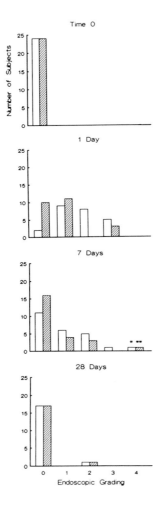

FIGURE 1.   The effect of oral indomethacin (50 mg tid) on gastric (||)
and duodenal (||) morphology over 28 days of continuous administration
in 24 healthy volunteers. * = 6mm gastric ulcer, ** = 7mm duodenal
ulcer.

<u>HISTOLOGY</u>

Biopsies were taken from areas that appeared endoscopically normal in 10 of the 24 volunteers. By strict evaluation, the gastric mucosa of only 3 of the subjects was histologically normal prior to treatment with indomethacin. Of the remaining 7 subjects 4 were found to have HLO's which were associated with at least mild or moderate inflammatory and regenerative changes. The 3 subjects without HLO's and histological abnormalities had minimal to mild inflammatory changes.

During treatment with indomethacin only one subject had mucosa considered histologically normal and this remained normal during the 28 days of the study. In the remaining subjects histological damage was equally severe in the main body and antrum of the stomach, appearances ranging from mild to severe inflammatory and regenerative changes. Unexpectedly, histological grading during treatment with indomethacin was not statistically different from that pre-treatment, although there was a trend towards more severe inflammatory and regenerative changes during indomethacin treatment (Table 2). In addition histological changes during the 28 days of indomethacin treatment did not change significantly.

TABLE 2

THE EFFECT OF INDOMETHACIN (50 MG TID) ON GASTRIC
HISTOLOGICAL INFLAMMATORY AND REGENERATIVE CHANGES.

Biopsy site	Time of biopsy (days)			
	0	1	7	28
Antrum { Inflammation	1.3 ± 0.4	1.5 ± 0.4	1.7 ± 0.5	1.9 ± 0.6
Regeneration	0.8 ± 0.3	1.2 ± 0.3	1.6 ± 0.4	1.6 ± 0.4
Main body { Inflammation	0.8 ± 0.3	1.3 ± 0.5	1.2 ± 0.4	1.5 ± 0.5
Regeneration	0.6 ± 0.3	0.9 ± 0.4	0.8 ± 0.4	0.6 ± 0.4

Values are mean histological grading $\pm$ SE, n=10 (n=8 at 28 days)

The 4 subjects with HLO's had organisms in both the fundus and antrum and they remained positive for these organisms throughout the study. One of these subjects developed a DU at 7 days and was withdrawn. The subject who developed the antral GU was HLO negative and was also withdrawn from the study at 7 days.

Immunohistochemical staining of the specimens demonstrating a dense chronic inflammatory cell infiltrate showed the infiltrate to be polymorphous for both light and heavy chains with no particular subtype of immunoglobulin predominating.

DISCUSSION

Our results show that indomethacin (50 mg tid) produced acute gastroduodenal mucosal damage in all subjects examined. With continued administration the mucosa adapted to this damage in the majority of subjects although a minority progressed to discrete ulceration. Why these 2 subjects failed to adapt is unknown. Both were non-smokers, took little alcohol (GU subject 'teetotal', DU subject <40g alcohol per day) and did not consume other damaging agents. Interestingly, they were at opposite ends of the age range (duodenal ulcer subject 19 years and gastric ulcer subject 35 years). While it is evident that macroscopic adaptation occurs in that focal changes heal with continued administration, the histological findings are surprising and difficult to explain. The histological appearances before and after indomethacin show no statistical change although there is a trend to more severe changes during indomethacin treatment. This observation would fit with other work which has shown no or minimal histological changes in 50% of biopsies taken away from the focal endoscopic damage produced by NSAID's [28] and suggests that indomethacin produces focal damage with little in the way of diffuse change. Alternatively our failure to show a significant histological change in appearance with indomethacin may reflect the small size of the study population. Finally, our grading system may not be a sensitive enough indicator of damage. This is unlikely as we have used the same grading system as Graham et al [26] who did find histological changes in endoscopically normal looking mucosa from subjects taking aspirin. The further finding that histological changes did not alter significantly during the 28 days of indomethacin treatment at a time when visible mucosal injury was resolving implies that further in depth histological studies are needed.

The process of adaptation of the mucosa to damage appears at 7 days and is complete by 28 days. Other authors have shown a similar adaptation to aspirin over 7 days but its mechanism also remains unknown [26]. Adaptation includes healing of the acute mucosal injury and enhancement of mucosal defence to prevent further mucosal damage during continued exposure to the damaging agent. It has been established from animal studies that adaptation can occur in gastroduodenal mucosa to a variety of damaging agents, an effect termed 'adaptive cytoprotection' [25]. This has been attributed to increased generation of 'protective' mucosal prostaglandins [25] - although recently the role of endogenous prostaglandins in this effect has been questioned [29]. With NSAID ingestion however, such a stimulation of endogenous prostaglandins is unlikely since they inhibit mucosal cyclooxygenase activity - which should result in lower mucosal prostaglandin levels.

We have shown a reduction in gastric mucosal blood flow with indomethacin which confirms earlier findings by Konturek et al [30]. In addition we have found a good correlation between the severity of mucosal damage and the magnitude of the reduction in mucosal blood flow. It has been suggested that endogenous prostaglandins contribute to the maintenance of basal gastric mucosal blood flow in animals and man [31]. Thus, reduction of endogenous prostaglandins by the effect of indomethacin on cyclooxygenase activity may explain the reduction in gastric mucosal blood flow seen in our subjects.

In our studies, mucosal recovery was associated with return of blood flow to normal. One would expect endogenous prostaglandins to remain reduced during indomethacin treatment and our preliminary data on mucosal PGE2 during these studies [32] would tend to support this. Thus, it is likely that blood flow returns to normal despite continued reduction of endogenous prostaglandins. How mucosal blood flow regulates itself in this situation remains unclear but an increase in blood flow would enhance mucosal defence and repair to injury and contribute to the adaptive process. However, as mucosal blood flow was not increased above pre-treatment levels it is difficult to envisage its role in preventing further damage during continued exposure to the damaging agent. Clearly, other mechanisms must play an important role in the adaptive process.

The mechanisms of the initial damage by indomethacin and subsequent adaptation to continued intake therefore remain unknown. The clear demonstration of an adaptive response in the majority of subjects should now provide a further stimulus for defining the mucosal mechanisms responsible for it.

REFERENCES

1. Lanza FL. Endoscopic studies of gastric and duodenal injury after the use of ibuprofen, aspirin, and other non-steroidal anti-inflammatory agents. Am J Med 1984; 77 (1A): 19-24.

2. Caruso I, Bianchi-Porro G. Gastroscopic evaluation of anti-inflammatory agents. Br Med J 1980; 280: 75-78.

3. Rees WDW, Turnberg LA. Reappraisal of the effects of aspirin on the stomach. Lancet 1980; i: 410-413.

4. Heller SR, Fellows IW, Ogilvie AL, Atkinson M. Non-steroidal anti-inflammatory drugs and benign oesophageal stricture. Br Med J 1982; 285: 167-168.

5. Bjarnason I, Zanelli G, Smith T et al. Non-steroidal anti-inflammatory drug-induced intestinal inflammation in humans. Gastroenterology 1987; 93: 480-489.

6. Langman MJS, Morgan L, Worral A. Use of anti-inflammatory drugs by people admitted with small or large perforations and haemorrhage. Br Med J 1985; 290: 347-9.

7. Somerville K, Faulkner G, Langman MJS. Non-steroidal anti-inflammatory drugs and bleeding peptic ulcer. Lancet 1986; i: 462-464.

8. Walt R, Katschinski B, Logan R, Ashley J, Langman MJS. Rising frequency of ulcer perforation in elderly people in the United Kingdom. Lancet 1986; i: 489-492.

9.   Armstrong CP, Blower AI. Non-steroidal anti-inflammatory drugs and life-threatening complications of peptic ulceration. Gut 1987; 28: 527-532.

10.   Vane JR. Inhibition of prostaglandin synthesis as a mechanism of action of aspirin-like drugs. Nature New Biol 1971; 231: 232-235.

11.   Whittle BJR, Higgs GA, Eakins KE, Moncada S, Vane JR. Selective inhibition of prostaglandin production in inflammatory exudates and gastric mucosa. Nature 1980; 284: 271-273.

12.   Whittle BJR. Prostaglandin cyclo-oxygenase inhibition and its relationship to gastric damage. In: Harmon JW, ed. Basic mechanisms of gastrointestinal mucosal cell injury and protection. Baltimore, London: Williams and Wilkins 1981: 197-210.

13.   Shorrock CJ, Rees WDW. Overview of gastroduodenal mucosal protection. Am J Med 1988; 88(2A): 25-34.

14.   Takeuchi K, Magee D, Critchlow J, Matthews J, Silen W. Studies of the pH gradient and thickness of frog gastric mucus gel. Gastroenterology 1983; 84: 331-340.

15.   Williams SE, Turnberg LA. Studies of the protective properties of gastric mucus: evidence for a mucus-bicarbonate barrier. Gut 1981; 22: 94-96.

16.   Flemstrom G, Kivilaakso E. Demonstration of a pH gradient at the luminal surface of rat duodenum in vivo and its dependence on mucosal alkaline secretion. Gastroenterology 1983; 84: 787-794.

17.   Ross IN, Bahari HMM, Turnberg LA. The pH gradient across mucus adherent to rat fundic mucosa in vivo and the effects of possible damaging agents. Gastroenterology 1981; 81: 713-718.

18.   Bahari HMM, Ross IN, Turnberg LA. Demonstration of a pH gradient across the mucus layer on the surface of human gastric mucosa in vitro. Gut 1982; 23: 513-516.

19.   Quigley EMM, Turnberg LA. The pH of the microclimate lining human gastric and duodenal mucosa in vivo: studies in control subjects and in duodenal ulcer patients. Gastroenterology 1987; 92: 1876-1884.

20.   Rees WDW, Gibbons LC, Turnberg LA. Effects of NSAID's and prostaglandins on alkali secretion by rabbit fundus in vitro. Gut 1983; 24: 784-789.

21.   Rainsford KD. The effects of aspirin and other NSAID's on gastrointestinal mucus glycoprotein biosynthesis in vivo: relationship to ulcerogenic actions. Biochem Pharmacol 1978; 27: 877-885.

22. Menguy R, Masters YF. Effects of aspirin on gastric mucus secretion . Surg Gynecol Obstet 1965; 120: 92-98.

23. Langman MJS. Epidemiological evidence of the association between peptic ulceration and anti-inflammatory drug use. Gastroenterology 1989; 96,2(2): 640-646.

24. Lanza FL, Royer GL, Nelson RS, Chen TT, Seckman CE, Rack MF. The effects of ibuprofen, indomethacin, aspirin, naproxen and placebo on the gastric mucosa of normal volunteers. Dig Dis Sci 1979; 24: 823-828.

25. Robert A. Cytoprotection by prostaglandins. Gastroenterology 1979; 77: 761-767.

26. Graham DY, Smith JL, Spjut HJ, Torres E. Gastric adaptation: studies in humans using continuous aspirin administration. Gastroenterology 1988; 95: 327-333.

27. Bonner R, Nossal R. A model for laser Doppler measurements of blood flow in tissue. Appl Opt 1981; 20: 2097-2107.

28. Laine L, Marin-Sorensen M, Weinstein WM. The histology of gastric erosions in patients taking NSAID's: a prospective study. Gastroenterology 1988; 94,5(2): A247 (abstract).

29. Hawkey CJ, Kemp RT, Walt RP, Bhaskar NK, Davies J, Filipowcz B. Evidence that adaptive cytoprotection in rats is not mediated by prostaglandins. Gastroenterology 1988; 94: 948-954.

30. Konturek SJ, Kwiecien N, Obtulowicz W et al. Effect of carprofen and indomethacin on gastric function, mucosal integrity and generation of prostaglandins in man. Hepatogastroenterology 1982; 29: 267-270.

31. Guth PH, Leung FW. Physiology of the gastric circulation. In: Johnson LR ed. Physiology of the gastrointestinal tract. Second edition. Raven Press, New York 1987: 1031-1053.

32. Shorrock CJ, Rees WDW. Adaptation to gastric mucosal damage by indomethacin in man - role of local PGE2 metabolism. Gastroenterology 1989; 96, 5(2): A470.

CHRONIC DUODENAL ULCER: THE ABSCOPAL MODEL

R.H. Gompertz, A.S. Michalowski, J.H. Baron

*Royal Postgraduate Medical School, University of London,
Hammersmith Hospital, London, U.K.*

ABSTRACT

A new type of chronic duodenal ulcer model has been developed which seems unique in its similarity to the human ulcer. The ulcer is generated by irradiating the lower mediastinum of mice with a single dose of 18Gy 250Kv Xrays. Ulcers develop in the proximal duodenum of about 45% of animals after 5-8 days. Both acute inflammation and healing take place simultaneously for several weeks without further treatment. No other ulcer model demonstrates such morphological and behavioural similarity to human chronic duodenal ulcer. The ulcer arises as an abscopal effect of irradiation; the duodenum does not receive a significant dose of Xrays. The effect is site specific because irradiation of the upper mediastinum (the adjacent portal) never leads to ulceration. Above a threshold dose (16Gy) the incidence of ulcer rises rapidly to a maximum of 45% at eight days. Ulcers do not increase in frequency with doses above 18Gy. The complications seen in human ulcer of bleeding, perforation and stenosis are also seen in low frequency. The new ulcer model described appears to offer a unique opportunity for the study of the underlying mechanisms of induction of chronic duodenal ulcer and the reasons for chronicity.

INTRODUCTION

Duodenal ulcer is incompletely understood. The reasons for the patient idiosynchrasy, the locality and the singularity of DU are unknown; as is the underlying mechanism of relapse and the reasons for the complications of bleeding and perforation. Since the basic science of duodenal ulcer cannot easily be studied in man an animal model of chronic duodenal ulcer is required. However, even the seemingly best models are, for various reasons, inadequate. Models of mucosal damage in which a noxious agent such as ethanol is employed are not appropriate to chronic duodenal ulcer.

Ulcers induced by causing a deliberate state of hypersecretion [1], such as the histamine-in-beeswax model, assume a hypersecretory aetiology and cannot, therefore, be expected to reveal any new insights into alternative mechanisms.

Cysteamine has been used to induce ulcer [2] and, although an alternative to other models, the cysteamine ulcer could not accurately

491

represent human chronic duodenal ulcer because its chronicity can be induced only by delivering a massive insult which simply takes a long time to heal and which often leads to the death of the animal in the acute phase.

Spontaneous gastric ulcers occur in genetically mast cell depleted mice [3] and duodenal ulcers can occur spontaneously in athymic (nude) mice [4] but the physiological situation is not normal in either case and neither model provides a suitable opportunity for comparisons with human ulcers.

What is needed is an ulcer model which is a single, truly chronic, proximal DU. Ideally such an ulcer would arise in an idiosyncratic way after the induction of an ulcer diathesis, and would behave in a way similar to human chronic DU, sometimes proceeding to the typical complications of bleeding, perforation and stenosis and responding to treatment in a way analogous to man. Such an ulcer is the abscopal model.

THE ABSCOPAL MODEL

Discovery of the Model

The Initial Experiment

The abscopal model of duodenal ulcer was discovered during an experiment to study the dose response relationship of ulcerative oesophagitis (UO) in mice following thoracic irradiation. At the time of this experiment the dose-response relationship in the intact animal was usually established by irradiation of the target with varying doses of the chosen type of ionising radiation with an arbitrary end-point that was easy to assess. For UO the 'oesophageal end points' for the ED 50 were weight loss and for the LD 50 death (systemic manifestations of radiation effect). Whether these observable phenomena correlated closely with oesophageal ulceration (the local manifestation) and were thus appropriate or whether irradiation had other effects which might lead to these changes without affecting the oesophagus was unknown. The time course of UO and the associated changes in body weight were therefore studied after irradiation. Mice were dissected at planned times for morphological assessment of their internal organs. Any mouse that died spontaneously was dissected within 2-3 hours of its death. Although extrathoracic effects were not suspected, all mice underwent full dissection.

Results

Of the 119 irradiated mice 1 died spontaneously on day 12 and was found, on dissection, to be suffering from UO and a duodenal ulcer (DU). The remaining 118 mice were killed and dissected as planned. The incidence of UO assessed microscopically rose from 0% to 100% during the 7th and 8th days after irradiation, remained at 100% until day 9, and subsequently decreased to 10% by day 14. On day 21 all mice were found to be free of UO. From the day of irradiation the mice lost weight at an accelerating rate, decreasing to 80% of their initial weight by day 10 (Fig. 1). During the following 5 days, the animals gained weight at a rate of 2% per day, with little further increase during the third week after irradiation. Because the curve of bodyweight was more diffuse than that for the incidence of UO, it was concluded that both during the lag period and following the healing of UO, radiation lesions in the oesophagus less severe than those defined as UO or lesions affecting other organs (such as duodenal ulcer), or both, were responsible for the weight loss of these mice.

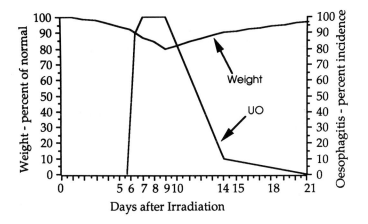

FIGURE 1: *Time course of weight loss and ulcerative oesophagitis after irradiation of the thorax with a single dose. The time course of weight loss and subsequent weight gain is much longer than for the appearance of and subsequent healing of ulcerative oesophagitis suggesting that the weight loss may involve other factors.*

Definition of Target Volume

The experiment

In order to further define the response a further series of experiments in which various thoracic fields (entire thorax, entire mediastinum, lower mediastinum, and upper mediastinum) were irradiated with doses of 14 Gy to 30 Gy of Xrays in 2 Gy increments was performed. Mice were killed on day 9 after irradiation to examine the oesophagus histologically for UO at the peak of its incidence and to look for other effects.

Results

For all portals the incidence of UO increased with radiation dose, however, although the alignment and shielding of mice during thoracic irradiation aimed at, and achieved, good protection of the abdominal organs, these precautions did not prevent the development of lesions in the duodenum [5,6].

Macroscopically, lesions were sharply delineated, with small areas of depression of the luminal aspect of the wall (Fig 2). The surface was flattened, only rarely showing traces of the villous pattern. The floor of the lesion was sometimes covered by a firmly attached film of exudate. The mucous membrane immediately surrounding the lesions appeared either normal or slightly thickened.

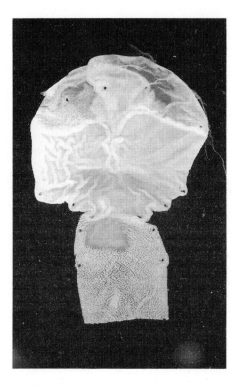

FIGURE 2:   *Photograph of a typical duodenal ulcer induced by thoracic irradiation.*

Microscopically, within the limits of the lesions, the villi and crypts were missing with the mucous membrane replaced by vascularised connective tissue densely infiltrated with mononuclear cells and granulocytes (Fig 3). The luminal surface was, in most instances, covered with a single layer of flat or cuboidal vacuolised epithelial cells deposited presumably by way of long distance migration. Gaps in the epithelial lining were filled with fibrin and leucocytes. The mucous membrane in the vicinity of the lesions was slightly oedematous with hyperplastic crypts, but otherwise normal.

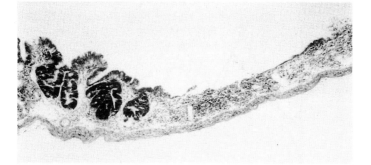

FIGURE 3:   *Microphotograph of typical duodenal ulcer induced by
thoracic irradiation*

Duodenal ulcer is defined in man as a defect in the epithelium
involving the underlying muscularis mucosa. Because the small intestine of
the mouse lacks a well defined submucous membrane (except for Brunner's
glands in the proximal duodenum) the intestinal lesions were considered to
be true ulcers because their abnormal floor abutted onto the circular layer
of smooth muscle which in man would satisfy the criterion for chronic DU.
Only in the proximal duodenum was the luminal layer of the lesions
separated from the muscle by Brunner's glands, and these often showed signs
of inflammatory reaction.   The general shape of the curves for the
frequency of DU was suggestive of heterogeneity in the mice; in the
experimental series only 50% of mice proved to be prone to develop DU [7].

Specific Target

The question of the critical target was then raised. Ulceration due to
a non-specific effect of irradiation was considered, but the consistently
negative results of irradiation of the upper mediastinum with doses as high
as 30 Gy of Xrays demonstrate that duodenal ulcerogenesis is not a
consequence of partial body irradiation *per se* (Fig 4).   In addition there
was no indication in any experiment of DU resulting from radiation damage
to the oesophagus since the appearance of DU preceded the onset of UO,
and continued to be seen long after the healing of the oesophagus was
completed.   DU required lower doses for induction than those necessary to
cause UO and there was no dependence of the incidence of DU on dose
within the range for which the frequency of UO varied between 0 and
100%.   No lesions in the duodenum were found in either the group
irradiated to the upper mediastinum or in 89 control mice: irradiation of
the upper mediastinum led to UO but not DU.   Irradiation of the
oesophagus was not important in the pathogenesis of DU.

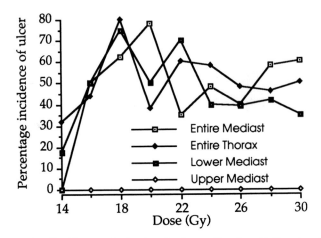

FIGURE 4: *Incidence of duodenal ulcer after irradiation to either the entire thorax, the entire mediastinum, the lower mediastinum, or the upper mediastinum. All fields that include the lower mediastinum lead to approximately the same incidence of ulceration whilst upper mediastinal irradiation never leads to ulcer.*

Because, according to the arguments of conventional radiobiology [8], the target cell line must be one with a mitotic rate sufficient for the expression of damage within 9 days at the latest (the maximum time for DU to appear) the only other obvious target situated within the irradiated volume is the thymus. However, the thymus could be excluded as a factor because irradiation of the upper mediastinum including the thymus did not lead to duodenal ulcerogenesis whereas exposure of the lower mediastinum (largely sparing the organ) elicited proximal DUs as frequently as did irradiation of the entire mediastinum or the entire thorax (which did include the thymus). Therefore DU induced by thoracic irradiation would seem not to be directly dependent on depopulation of a cell lineage contained in the irradiated volume. Instead, the observed effects are by definition abscopal [9]. An abscopal effect being one which is due to irradiation but which takes place at a site remote from the target of the irradiation. Such an effect may be caused by radiation interfering with regulatory mechanisms responsible for the upper GI tract without necessarily causing death of the exposed cells in question [10]. Regulatory pathways known to be included in the irradiated volume are the vagus and the thoracic sympathetic nerves as well as the spinal cord. The vagus was included in both the upper and lower mediastinal fields, yet irradiation of the former never led to DU, in sharp contrast to the exposure of the latter. Since the structure critical for the development of the proximal DU by irradiation has to be contained in the lower mediastinum or the spinal cord at the level of T5-T10, the sympathetic ganglia are a likely specific target because nerve cells are more radiosensitive than nerve fibres and non-myelinated nerves (eg. sympathetic), are more radiosensitive than myelinated (eg parasympathetic) [11]. Thus the ulcer may be induced by imbalance in the autonomic nerve supply to the upper GI tract.

Scattered irradiation

Scatter of radiation must be considered as a possible cause of the induction of DU. The distribution of radiation dosage was therefore checked using lithium fluoride chips implanted into mouse cadavers. Dosimetry showed that only 7.3% of the dose to the mediastinum was received in the duodenum; this dose corresponds to less than 1.5 Gy, an insufficient dose to cause a direct irradiation ulcer (Fig. 5).

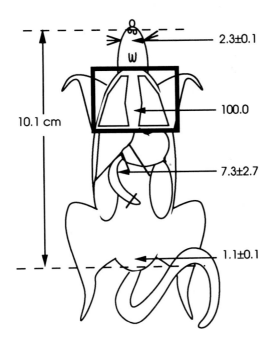

FIGURE 5 *The dose received in various sites after irradiation of the thorax.*

Irradiation of the stomach and duodenum either alone or together with the mediastinum were also investigated to detect whether or not low-dose gastric irradiation might in some way be responsible. It was found that gastric irradiation by itself did not cause ulceration, and that gastric irradiation combined with mediastinal irradiation diminished the incidence of duodenal ulcers, suggesting that gastric irradiation was, if anything, protective against ulceration [6]. This is not surprising, because gastric irradiation has long been known to reduce gastric secretion [12] and has been used in the past, particularly during the 1950s, as a means of treating peptic ulcer [13] probably acting by both direct and indirect parietal cell damage [14]. In a parallel series of experiments we have investigated the effect of direct gastric irradiation with a single dose of 9 Gy of Xrays and found that gastric acid secretion is significantly inhibited for a prolonged period of time [15, 16].

Time Course

The timing of ulcer induction was then studied. Thirty five days after irradiation to the lower mediastinum the incidence of ulceration was found to be the same as at 8 days. Furthermore there were no histological stigmata of healed ulcer amongst animals not bearing active ulcers, and, in some cases, the ulcers had gone on to stenose, perforate or bleed. The inference was thus drawn that mediastinal irradiation led to an ulcer diathesis and that susceptible animals would go on to develop a duodenal ulcer. In those cases where ulcer occurred, it appeared that a chronic lesion ensued and that healing did not spontaneously take place. The potential for a model of chronic duodenal ulcer was thus recognised. The morphological appearance of the ulcer, including scanning electron micrography [17], showed appearances remarkably similar to those of the human ulcer.

APPLICATION

There are two clear avenues for research: first, the explanation, in terms of radiobiological science, of the mechanism of ulcer induction and, secondly, the investigation of the ulcer as a model for the study of DU *per se*. The radiobiological consequences of this abscopal effect are considerable [10] and, whilst radiation damage to the gut is an increasingly significant clinical problem [18], these aspects of the discovery are not addressed in our present studies. We have concentrated on the phenomenon of the experimental model of DU.

Clinical correlate

Duodenal ulcer is more common after spinal irradiation in the treatment of seminoma [19] or teratoma of the testis than after chemotherapy alone [20] and there may thus be a direct clinical application for this research as well as increasing understanding of the basic pathomechanisms of chronic DU.

Scientific application

The abscopal ulcer seems to fulfil the criteria for an appropriate experimental model to study the basic science of DU. It is usually single, it is truly chronic, it is anatomically specific in its site and it arises idiosynchratically after the induction of the DU diathesis. The model is not, however, an ideal one for the pharmacologist precisely because of the idiosynchratic way in which the ulcer arises. This makes comparisons between pharmaceutical compounds much more arduous because of the much larger numbers needed to achieve statistical significance. Perhaps future research will allow the identification of those animals that are ulcer-bearers.

SUMMARY

The abscopal duodenal ulcer is not a direct irradiation phenomenon because:

1.   The dose received by the duodenum is insufficient to cause radiation ulcer.

2.   The time for appearance of the ulcer is too short to be compatible with the chronic radiation ulcer and the site specificity and the histological appearances are not those of acute radiation sickness.

3.   The ulcer is not a non-specific irradiation phenomenon, since irradiation of the adjacent portal (the upper mediastinum), with the same dose to the same irradiated volume of tissue, never causes ulcer.

4.   The dose response relationship is not that of a direct effect, since one would expect that with increasing dose, a 100% yield of ulcer could be achieved. However this was not the case: above a threshold at 16 Gy further increases of dose led to no further yeild of ulcer up to a maximum 30 Gy, at which point direct effects in the thorax are lethal.

CONCLUSION

The abscopal model provides a new means to study the basic mechanisms in duodenal ulcer. It is particularly suited to the basic science of ulcer disease and to the investigation of the mechanisms underlying the idiosynchrasy, singularity, and site of DU and the reasons for chronicity and for complications.

REFERENCES

1.   Robert A, Stout TJ, Dale JE., Production by secretagogues of duodenal ulcers in the rat. Gastroenterology 1970; 59: 95-102.

2.   Selye H, Szabo S. Experimental model for production of perforating duodenal ulcers by cysteamine in the rat. Nature 1973; 244: 458-459.

3.   Shimada M, Kitamura Y, Yokoyama M, Miyano Y, Maeyama K, Yamatodani A, Takahashi Y. Spontaneous stomach ulcer in genetically mast-cell depleted W/Wv mice. Nature 1980; 283: 662-666.

4.   Williams AW, Howie JB, Helyer BJ, Simpson LO. Spontaneous peptic ulcers in mice. Australian Journal of Experimental Biology and Medical Science. 1967; 45: 105-108.

5.   Michalowski AS. Gastrointestinal lesions in thorax irradiated mice. British Journal of Radiology. 1981; 54: 713.

6.   Michalowski AS, Burgin J. Duodenal ulcers as an abscopal effect of thoracic irradiation in mice. In: Karcher KH et al (eds) Progress in Radio-Oncology II. Raven Press, New York, pp 105-110.

7.   Michalowski AS, Uehara S, Yin W-B, Burgin J, Silvester JA. Alternative types of duodenal ulcer induced in mice by partial X-irradiation of the thorax. Radiation Research 1983; 95: 78-86.

8.   Denekamp J, Rojas A. Cell kinetics and radiation pathology. Experientia 1989; 45: 33-41.

9.   Mole RH. Whole body irradiation-radiobiology or medicine? British Journal of Radiology 1953; 26: 234-241.

10.   Michalowski AS. Radiopathology of normal tissues. Are clonogenic survival and cell kinetics all that matter? Berzelius Symposium, XV Umea. 1988; 67-73.

11.   Sasaki H. Causative mechanism of gastric and duodenal ulcer after x-irradiation of the upper thoracic spinal column. Nippon Acta Radiologica. 1943; 4: 692-716.

12.   Palmer WL, Templeton F. The effect of radiation therapy on gastric secretion. Journal of the American Medical Association. 1939; 112: 1429-1434.

13.   Palmer WL, Kirsner JB, Clayman CB, Carpender WJ. Results of treatment. In: Palmer WL (ed) Gastric Irradiation in Peptic Ulcer. University of Chicago Press, London. 1974; 53-61.

14.   Goldgraber MB, Rubin CF, Palmer WL, Dobson RL, Massey BW. The early gastric response to irradiation. A serial biopsy study. Gastroenterology 1954; 27: 1-20.

15.   Gompertz RHK, Man WK, Li SK, Michalowski AS. Gastric secretion in partial-body-irradiated mice. International Journal of Radiation Biology. 1987; 52:487-488.

16.   Man WK, Gompertz RHK, Li SK, Michalowski A, Baron JH, Spencer J. Effect of gastric irradiation on gastric secretion and histamine in mine. Agents & Actions. 1988; 23: 297-299.

17.   Carr KE, Ellis S, Michalowski A. Surface studies of duodenal lesions induced by thoracic irradication. Scanning Electron Microscopy. 1986; 1: 209-219.

18. Galland RB, Spencer JS. Radiation enteritis. Edward Arnold, Sevenoaks. 1990.

19. Hamilton CR, Horwich A, Easton D, Peckham MJ. Radiotherapy for stage I seminoma testis: Results of treatment and complications. Radiotherapy & Oncology. 1987; 10: 85-90.

20. Hamilton CR, Horwich A, Bliss JM, Peckham MJ. Gastrointestinal morbidity of adjuvant radiotherapy in stage I malignant teratoma of the testis. Radiotherapy & Oncology. 1987; 10: 85-90.

THE ROLE OF DIETARY PROSTAGLANDIN PRECURSORS (ESSENTIAL FATTY ACIDS) IN THE PREVENTION OF GASTRODUODENAL MUCOSAL INJURY

D. Hollander and A. Tarnawski

*Division of Gastroenterology, College of Medicine,
University of California, Irvine, California, U.S.A.*

ABSTRACT

The two dietary essential fatty acids, linoleic and arachidonic, can be rapidly converted by the gastroduodenal mucosa into protective prostaglandins such as PGE_2. Chronic feeding of linoleic acid in rats increases the gastroduodenal mucosal synthesis capabilities of PGE_1 and PGF_2 alpha. Rats fed a high linoleic acid diet are more resistant to acute stress induced injury. When these fatty acids are administered together with non-ionic detergents they can penetrate the gastric and duodenal mucosa acutely and promote the rapid synthesis of protective prostaglandins. Rats gavaged with detergent solubilized essential dietary fatty acids show marked resistance to injury by alcohol, aspirin, and thermal damage. In experimental models of gastroduodenal injury, detergent solubilized essential fatty acids are as effective in prevention of injury as any agent available or investigated so far.

Dietary essential fatty acids promote the production of endogenous prostaglandins by the gastroduodenal mucosa. These prostaglandins are removed by first pass through the liver and lungs and therefore do not reach the systemic circulation thus avoiding the systemic side effects caused by the synthetic prostaglandin analogs which are not rapidly metabolized during their first pass through the liver or lungs. As such, they represent a potential therapeutic modality which may not result in the systemic side effects currently observed with the use of synthetic prostaglandin analogs which are not rapidly metabolized during their first pass through the liver or lungs.

INTRODUCTION

Dietary therapy and nutritional manipulation used to occupy a prominent role in the therapy of gastric mucosal injury and peptic ulcer disease. The attention to dietary therapy vanished with the advent of effective and potent pharmacological agents for the therapy of peptic disease [1] which worked by neutralization of acid or the inhibition of acid secretion. More recently, attention has also been given to factors other than intragastric acid in the prevention or the therapy of peptic disease. This new area of physiological and pharmacological investigation has been termed "cytoprotection" or "mucosal protection" [2]. This area of study has

503

concentrated on the stimulation of the defensive capabilities of the gastroduodenal mucosa by mechanisms other than diminishing the concentration of acid in the gastric lumen. Numerous cytoprotective compounds have been investigated which are either endogenously produced or are exogenously administered [3]. Of the endogenously produced compounds, prostaglandins of the E group have been studied most extensively. Prostaglandins have been shown to protect the gastroduodenal mucosa against acute injury by strong acids and bases, alcohol, bile acids, and aspirin. Currently, the evidence is overwhelming that prostaglandins play a key role in maintaining the normal integrity of the gastroduodenal mucosa and the prevention of gastroduodenal mucosal injury. Therapeutically, prostaglandins have a well defined role in the prevention of gastroduodenal mucosal injury by nonsteroidal anti-inflammatory agents [4].

More recently, a number of prostaglandin synthetic analogs have been studied in controlled clinical trials in order to assess their possible efficacy in promoting the healing of acute ulcerations. In controlled trails some of the prostaglandin analogs were found to be superior to placebos in promoting the healing of both gastric and duodenal ulcerations with even greater efficacy in healing duodenal ulcerations [5].

Prostaglandins are synthesized endogenously by virtually all mammalian tissues from the dietary fatty acids - arachidonic and linoleic. Arachidonic acid is stored as a phospholipid in cell membranes of the gastroduodenal mucosa. When the mucosa is damaged, the enzyme phospholipase A2 releases free arachidonic acid from the cell membrane phospholipid pool and provides the free fatty acid for prostanoid synthesis by the cyclo-oxygenase or lipoxygenase enzyme pathways [6-8].

Because arachidonic acid is a relatively uncommon dietary fatty acid in the western diet, we rely predominantly on linoleic acid as the major dietary source of essential fatty acids. Linoleic acid is present in significant amounts in various vegetable oils such as corn or safflower oils. Normally, ingested linoleic acid is absorbed by both mediated transport and passive diffusion in the small intestine [9-11] and is distributed through the circulation to various organs and tissues including the gastroduodenal mucosa. Some linoleic acid is stored directly in the cell membranes. However, most of it is converted by a series of elongase enzymes to arachidonic acid which is then stored in the cell membrane as a structural membrane phospholipid [8]. This process of conversion of dietary linoleic acid to arachidonic acid occurs in most mammals including humans. However, carnivorous animals are unable to convert dietary linoleic acid to arachidonic acid and therefore have to obtain their arachidonic acid by eating meat or liver as the predominant sources for prostanoid precursors [6]. Other dietary sources of fatty acids which are not common in the western diet include evening primrose oil which is rich in gamma linolenic acid and which can be directly converted to prostanoids. In addition, the omega-3 fatty acids which are present predominantly in fish oils can also be converted into prostanoids of the PGI series or into biologically inactive thromboxanes [12-13].

Because of the pivotal role of prostaglandins in gastroduodenal mucosal protection [2] we became interested in the potential use of dietary fatty acids such as arachidonic and linoleic in the prevention of gastroduodenal mucosal injury. Much of the information that we and other groups have generated so far pertains to the use of dietary essential fatty acids, both acutely and chronically in the prevention of gastroduodenal mucosal injury. We will summarise this information and delineate some of the mechanisms by which the dietary fatty acids provide mucosal protection.

PROTECTIVE ACTIVITY OF DIETARY ESSENTIAL FATTY ACIDS AGAINST ACUTE INJURY

Normally, dietary fatty acids are absorbed by the small intestine following micellar solubilization [11]. In initial studies we found that the non-ionic detergent-pluronic F68 is required in order to allow rapid absorption of the fatty acids by the gastroduodenal mucosal cells [14]. When detergent solubilized dietary fatty acids are given to rats by gavage, a rapid synthesis and/or release of prostaglandins with several thousand fold increase in their luminal concentration occurs within 30 minutes [14]. When rats are treated with detergent solubilized arachidonic or linoleic acids we were able to prevent gastric mucosal damage by alcohol or aspirin [15]. As a control, oleic acid (a fatty acid which is not a precursor for prostaglandin synthesis) did not protect the mucosa against acute damage. Similarly, intrajejunal administration of arachidonic or linoleic acid did not offer acute protection in contrast to the intragastrically administered fatty acids [16]. We were able to abolish a large portion of the protective activity of detergent solubilized dietary fatty acids by pretreatment of the rats with indomethacin [14] which inhibits the conversion of arachidonic acid to prostanoids by blocking the activity of the cyclo-oxygenase enzymes. Thus, much of the protective activity of the dietary fatty acids is due to their conversion by the gastroduodenal mucosa to prostanoids. As such, the mechanisms of acute protective effects of dietary fatty acids is due to their conversion to prostaglandins which can protect the mucosal blood vessels, mucosal proliferative zone, and stimulate cell renewal and mucosal restitution [17].

PROTECTION OF THE MUCOSAL PROLIFERATIVE ZONE BY DIETARY ESSENTIAL FATTY ACIDS

In laboratory animals detergent solubilized essential fatty acids can limit the depth of injury if administered prior to onset of mucosal damage by agents such as alcohol or aspirin [14,16,17]. Some superficial injury of the surface epithelium does occur despite fatty acid pre-treatment, but the depth of injury is limited and does not extend into the deeper mucosal regions where cell proliferation occurs [17]. Thus, deep erosions are prevented by pretreatment of the mucosa with detergent solubilized dietary fatty acids. The deeper proliferative zone area of the gastric mucosa is the area where rapid restitution of the superficial epithelium is started. Cells from the proliferative zone migrate from the gastric pits to the surface repairing and renewing the superficial epithelium. Most of the information indicates that the cells which migrate immediately after surface injury of the mucosa are not newly formed cells but rather cells which were already present in the proliferative zone and were available for migration to the surface [17]. Some 12-24 hours after initial injury, cell division does occur in the proliferative zone to replenish those cells which had migrated up to the surface. Thus, the protection of the proliferative zone by dietary fatty acids allows both an immediate migration of cells to repair the superficial epithelium as well as subsequent cell proliferation and division in order to replenish the proliferative zone with cells ready to repair the superficial epithelium [14,15].

THE ROLE OF DIETARY ESSENTIAL FATTY ACIDS IN PROTECTING THE GASTRIC MICROVASCULATURE.

The mucosal arterioles divide into a dense capillary network which surrounds the gastric glands and provides oxygen and nutrients to the surface epithelium and glandular cells. The capillary network coalesces at the surface into a network of collecting venules which form collecting veins which run downward from the mucosal surface to the venular plexus at the bottom of the mucosa. The deep mucosal venular plexus is then drained by submucosal venules which follow the pattern of the submucosal arterial vessels and leads into small submucosal veins which coalesce and connect with the external gastric veins [18]. The rich vasculature of the stomach is essential for maintaining proper oxygenation and nutrient supply to the gastric glands and the superficial mucosal cells. Therefore, the gastric mucosal blood flow is a crucial and essential component of the mucosal resistance to injury.

One of the earliest targets of gastric mucosal damage by a variety of compounds is the endothelial layer of the gastric microvasculature [19]. Both aspirin and alcohol appear to damage the vascular endothelium as one of the earliest sites of mucosal injury [20]. Endothelial damage can occur as early as 15 minutes after the administration of aspirin and is accompanied by edema of the lamina propria, increased vascular permeability, platelet aggregation, fibrin deposition and the formation of thrombi within the vessel lumina leading finally to total occlusion of the microvascular lumina. The resulting microvascular stasis prevents oxygen and nutrient delivery to the gastric mucosa and causes additional secondary mucosal necrosis [21]. The injury may result in the release of many pro-inflammatory mediators which can cause additional venoconstriction and a concomitant arteriolar dilatation [18]. The end result of these changes is hemorrhagic necrosis often seen in the mucosa and submucosal areas following injury. In contrast experiments with protection of the mucosa with detergent solubilized fatty acids show a marked change in the depth and extent of injury. Pretreatment with detergent solubilized arachidonic acid reduces both the extent and the depth of microvasculature injury [14,15]. In mucosa protected with arachidonic acid, only the most superficial capillaries show evidence of damage while the deeper capillaries remain normal with patent lumina and morphologically and functionally intact circulation. At this point, it is not entirely clear whether the detergent solubilized fatty acids protect the gastric microvessels by direct action or through their conversion into protective prostaglandins or a combination of the two. In addition, we do not understand the precise cellular mechanism by which the fatty acids or their prostaglandin metabolites protect the vascular endothelium against damage by diverse compounds such as aspirin or alcohol.

In addition to the direct protective effect of detergent solubilized dietary fatty acids of the gastric microvasculature these fatty acids are also able to promote angiogenesis. Thus, by fostering angiogenesis, detergent solubilized dietary fatty acids can not only protect much of the deeper vasculature but can also promote the repair of the capillaries within the gastric mucosa [22].

The purpose in this discussion is to call attention to the possible importance of dietary fatty acids in the normal protective mechanisms of the gastroduodenal mucosa and in the prevention of damage to the gastroduodenal mucosa. The dietary essential fatty acids, arachidonic and linoleic acids, when administered with the appropriate detergent can be absorbed directly by the gastroduodenal mucosa and can generate the synthesis or release of protective prostaglandins. The prostaglandins which are synthesized by the gastroduodenal mucosa following the administration of dietary fatty acids can be rapidly metabolized and removed from the circulation by both the liver and lungs. Therefore, their prostaglandin metabolites do not reach the systemic circulation and would not result in the systemic side effect seen with the synthetic prostaglandin analogs which are not easily removed from the systemic circulation by the lungs or liver. Thus, dietary essential fatty acids may have a distinct therapeutic advantage over the synthetic prostaglandin analogs.

ACKNOWLEDGEMENT

This work was supported in part by the Goldsmith Family Foundation.

REFERENCES

1. Hollander D. Diet therapy of peptic ulcer disease. Nutrition & the M.D. 1988; 14: 1-2.

2. Hollander D, Tarnawski A. Gastric Cytoprotection - A Clinician's Guide. Plenum Publishing, New York. 1989.

3. Szabo S, Hollander D. Pathways of gastrointestinal protection and repair: mechanisms of action of sucralfate. Amer J Med 1989; 86: 23-31.

4. Holt K and Hollander D. Gastric mucosal injury. In: Annual Review of Medicine. Creger WP, Editor. 1986; Vol 37: 107-125.

5. Wilson DE. Cytoprotective therapy: prostaglandins. In: Gastric Cytoprotection - A Clinician's Guide. Editors: Hollander D, Tarnawski A. Plenum Publishing, New York. 1989.

6. Ramwell PW. Biologic importance of arachidonic acid. Arch Int Med 1981; 141: 275-278.

7.   Gali C, Agrandi E, Petroni A, Tremoli E.   Dietary essential fatty acid, tissue fatty acids and prostaglandin synthesis. Prog Fd Nutr Sci 1980; 4:1-7.

8.   Vane JR, Moncada S.   Polyunsaturated fatty acids as precursors of prostaglandins.   Acta Cardiol (Brux) 1979; 23(Suppl):21-37.

9.   Chow SL, Hollander D.   Arachidonic acid intestinal absorption: Mechanism of transport and influence of luminal factors on absorption *in vitro.* Lipids 1978; 11: 768-776.

10.   Chow SL, Hollander D.   Linoleic acid absorption in the unanesthetized rat: Mechanism of transport and influence of luminal factors on absorption rate. Lipids 1979; 14: 378-385.

11.   Chow SL, Hollander D.   A dual, concentration-dependent absorption mechanism of linoleic acid by rat jejunum in vitro.   J Lipid Res 1979; 20: 349-356.

12.   Grateroli R, Leonardi J, Charbonnier M, Lafont R, Lafont H, Nalbone G.   Effects of dietary corn oil and solmon oil on lipids and prostaglandin E2 in rat gastric mucosa.   Lipids 1988; 23: 666-670.

13.   de la Hunt MN, Hillier K, Jewell R.   Modification of upper gastrointestinal prostaglandin synthesis by dietary fatty acids. Postaglandins 1988; 35: 597-608.

14.   Hollander D, Tarnawski A, Ivey KJ, DeZeery A, Zipser RD. McKenzie WN.   Arachidonic acid protection of rat gastric mucosa against ethanol injury.   J Lab and Clin Med 1982; 100: 296-308.

15.   Tarnawski A, Hollander D, Gergely H.   Protection of the gastric mucosa by linoleic acid - a nutrient essential fatty acid.   Clin Invest Med 1987; 10: 132-5.

16.   Tarnawski A, Hollander D, Stachura J, Krause WJ.   Arachidonic acid protection of gastric mucosa against alcohol injury: sequential analysis of morphologic and functional changes. J Lab and Clin Med 1983; 102: 340-351.

17.   Tarnawski A, Hollander D, Stachura J, Krause WJ, and Gergely H. Prostaglandin protection of the gastric mucosa against alcohol injury - A dynamic time-related process.   Gastroenterology 1985; 88: 334-352.

18.   Oates PJ.   Gastric blood flow and mucosal defense.   In: Gastric Cytoprotection - A Clinician's Guide.   Editors: Hollander D, Tarnawski A. Plenum ublishing, New York, 1989.

19.   Szabo S. Trier JS, Brown A, et al.   Early vascular injury and increased vascular permeability in gastric mucosal injury caused by ethanol in the rat. Gastroenterology 1985; 88: 228-236.

20.   Tarnawski A, Stachura J, Hollander D, Sarfeh IJ, Bogdal J. Cellular aspects of alcohol-induced injury and prostaglandin protection of the human gastric mucosa. Focus on the mucosal microvessels. J Clin Gastroenterology 1988; 10: 35-45.

21.   Tarnawski A, Stachura J, Gergely H, Hollander D. Microvascular endothelium - a major target for alcohol injury of the human gastric mucosa. Histochemical and ultrastructural study. J Clin Gastroenterology 1988; 10: 53-643.

22.   Tarnawski A, Hollander D, Stachura J, Gergely H. Essential fatty acids - arachidonic and linoleic have trophic and angiogenic effect on the gastric mucosa injured by alcohol. Gastroenterology 1988; 94:A455.

UTILITY OF PROSTAGLANDINS FOR PREVENTION OF NONSTEROIDAL ANTI-INFLAMMATORY DRUG-INDUCED ULCERS

David Y. Graham, M.D.

Digestive Disease Section, Department of Medicine, Veterans Affairs Medical Center and Baylor College of Medicine, Houston, Texas, U.S.A.

ABSTRACT

The fact that nonsteroidal anti-inflammatory drugs (NSAIDs) damage the gastroduodenal mucosa is now accepted as a result of the disproportionately high frequency of upper gastrointestinal bleeding and perforation of ulcers associated with NSAID use. More than 10% of patients receiving NSAIDs chronically will have a gastric ulcer on any given day, a point prevalence of ulcer disease 5 to 10 times higher than in patients who are not taking NSAIDs. Endoscopic studies comparing the effects of acute administration of various NSAIDs on the gastroduodenal mucosa in normal volunteers have failed to predict which NSAIDs would be safest when administered chronically. All of the newer NSAIDs appear to be similar in their propensity to cause peptic ulceration. Although antisecretory drugs can ameliorate trivial mucosal damage (petechiae or small erosions) following acute administration of NSAIDs to normal volunteers, recent studies have demonstrated that co-treatment of chronic NSAID users with H_2-receptor antagonists or sucralfate has minimal or no success in preventing the development of the important NSAID-induced gastric ulcers. NSAID-induced gastric ulcers are also not prevented by drug formulations that prevent active NSAID from contacting the gastric mucosa. Co-treatment with the synthetic prostaglandin misoprostol, however has been associated with a marked reduction in gastric ulcer development in osteoarthritis patients receiving NSAIDs chronically, suggesting that inhibition of prostaglandin generation in the gastric mucosa may play a pivotal role in NSAID-induced gastric ulcers.

INTRODUCTION

Rheumatic diseases are among the most common medical disorders. The majority of patients with rheumatic diseases use nonsteroidal anti-inflammatory drugs (NSAIDs) to relieve pain and inflammation and thus remain functional. The introduction of NSAIDs greatly simplified therapy in this group of patients and has led to improved quality of life for countless arthritis sufferers. Unfortunately, NSAID therapy is not without risk as these agents are known to damage the gastroduodenal mucosa [1-3]. The potential importance of this injury is illustrated by the increasingly recognized NSAID-associated upper gastrointestinal bleeding and perforation of ulcers, particularly in elderly women [1,3-5]. Recent studies have suggested that more than 3,000 patients in the United Kingdom are admitted annually because of NSAID-associated gastroduodenal perforation or hemorrhage, and approximately 10% of these patients die as a consequence of their gastroduodenal complications [3].

Almost 70 million NSAID prescriptions are written annually in the United States [6] - twice the number reported in 1984 [7]. Although the incidence of major gastrointestinal problems that can be directly associated with NSAID use is low, the large number of patients receiving these medications has resulted in a significant problem. For example, NSAID-induced gastroduodenal injury is estimated to be responsible for more than 10,000 deaths each year in the U.S. alone [8]. Between 33% and 46% of patients receiving NSAIDs experience some type of gastrointestinal side effect, the most common being indigestion or dyspepsia [9-11]. Between 10% and 20% of patients receiving chronic NSAID therapy will have endoscopically visible gastric ulcers at any one point during treatment [12-15]; this is a point prevalence of ulcer disease 5 to 10 times greater than that of patients not receiving NSAIDs.

NSAID-INDUCED AND OTHER ULCERS

Our concepts concerning the pathogenesis of peptic ulcers are currently undergoing change. We now recognize at least three categories of peptic ulcers: Helicobacter pylori-associated ulcers, NSAID-associated ulcers, and ulcers associated with the hypersecretory states, such as the Zollinger-Ellison syndrome. NSAID-related ulcers may be the most difficult to recognize as some may be acute rather than chronic, others may be H. pylori-associated ulcers that, by chance, occur in NSAID users, and finally, NSAID ulcers may occur in patients with coincident H. pylori infection. The incidence of H. pylori infection increases with age; thus, there is a high probability that H. pylori infection, NSAID use and ulcers will co-exist. There may also be a relationship between NSAID and H. pylori ulcers, as many believe that NSAID use exacerbates H. pylori-associated ulcers. NSAID-related ulcers can be distinguished from H. pylori-related ulcers by histologic examination of the mucosa. H. pylori is associated with acute or chronic inflammation and the presence of H. pylori organisms; NSAID-induced ulcers occur in otherwise normally appearing mucosa.

NSAID ulcers are more likely to be gastric rather than duodenal and they are typically located in the gastric antrum, often prepyloric. NSAID ulcers are also more likely to be associated with other evidence of NSAID gastroduodenal damage such as erosions and mucosal hemorrhage. NSAID-induced ulceration was initially believed to result simply from topical injury to the gastroduodenal mucosa. This concept has been modified over the years to include the view that the major deleterious effects are related to the ability of systemically absorbed NSAIDs to alter the balance of mucosal eicosanoids [1].

The presence of acute topical mucosal damage is now believed to be related to the solubility in gastric acid of these intrinsically corrosive drugs. Thus, NSAIDs that are soluble in an acidic environment are more likely to penetrate gastric mucosal cells, causing cellular damage that is evident in acute endoscopic studies. We now know that the results of studies in healthy volunteers do not provide useful information to help categorize

NSAIDs in relation to safety or to predict which will not cause ulcers [1]. There is a dose-response effect, higher anti-inflammatory activity relates to greater propensity to ulceration independent of the ability to cause acute mucosal damage.

NSAIDs reduce both the secretion of bicarbonate and the synthesis and secretion of mucus in the stomach and duodenum, and this may impair mucosal defense. Studies have shown that NSAIDs reduce gastric mucosal blood flow in both humans and animals [16,17]. NSAIDs have a number of effects that tend to reduce the effectiveness of the mucosal protective barriers. Although it is not yet known which, if any, of these protective mechanisms are critical to maintaining mucosal integrity and which merely represent laboratory curiosities, several recent studies have provided convincing evidence that the systemic inhibition of gastroduodenal prostaglandin synthesis by NSAIDs is the pivotal event in the pathogenesis of NSAID-induced ulcers (reviewed in 1).

PREVENTION OF NSAID-ASSOCIATED ULCERS

A number of studies have investigated the ability of a variety of anti-ulcer agents to prevent acute NSAID-induced gastric mucosal damage. Almost any agent that reduces acid secretion will reduce the frequency and severity of acute lesions such as hemorrhages and erosions. Unfortunately, as noted above, the presence, absence, prevention, or reduction of such acute lesions has little or no predictive value for the prevention of the gastric or duodenal ulcers associated with morbidity and mortality. Studies that have attempted to prevent the more serious lesions associated with chronic NSAID use (e.g., gastric ulcers) have demonstrated H_2-receptor antagonists are ineffective [18-20] (Figure 1).

In contrast, prostaglandin replacement with the synthetic prostaglandin misoprostol has been shown to reduce the incidence of NSAID-induced gastric ulcers in patients with osteoarthritis who were receiving ibuprofen, piroxicam or naproxen [21] (Figure 2).

More recent studies have compared the topical agent sucralfate with misoprostol in patients with osteoarthritis receiving chronic NSAID therapy. Sucralfate proved ineffective for preventing gastric ulcers (Figure 3) or for reducing the frequency of NSAID-induced mucosal erosions (Figure 4) [22].

Duodenal ulcers in NSAID users are more amenable to prevention with acid suppression therapy [18,19]. We believe that this suggests that duodenal complications in NSAID users are often the result of incidental H. pylori-associated ulcers, possibly exacerbated by NSAID use. Misoprostol is as effective in suppressing acid as is cimetidine; 200 ug of misoprostol yields approximately equivalent suppression as does 300 mg of cimetidine. One would expect that the beneficial effects of misoprostol in the stomach would also be evident in the duodenum, and this hypothesis is under study.

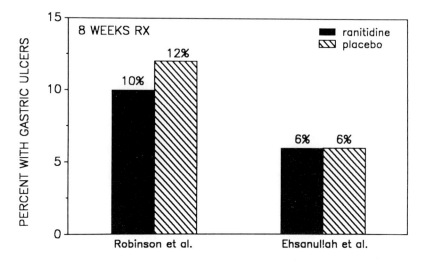

FIGURE 1. *The inability of the H_2-receptor antagonist, ranitidine, to prevent NSAID-induced gastric ulcer is shown. The frequency of gastric ulcers (defined as ≥ 0.5 cm in diameter) in chronic NSAID users was similar whether ranitidine or placebo was given. Data from references 18 and 19.*

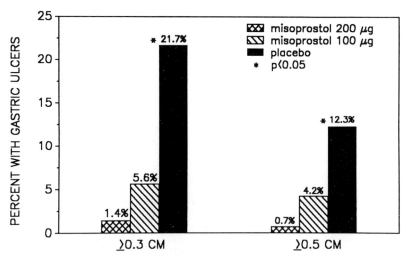

FIGURE 2 *The ability of the synthetic prostaglandin misoprostol to prevent NSAID-induced gastric ulcer is shown. The cumulative percent with ulcers is shown after 3 months of co-therapy of an NSAID and misoprostol in patients with osteoarthritis. Data from reference 21.*

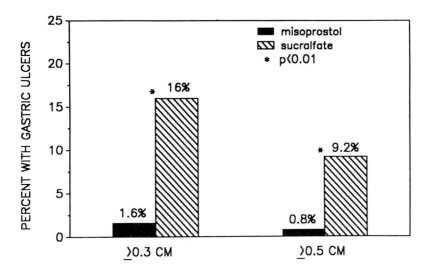

FIGURE 3   *The lack of effectiveness of sucralfate compared to misoprostol for the prevention of NSAID-induced gastric ulcer is shown. The cumulative percent with ulcers is shown after 3 months of co-therapy of an NSAID and misoprostol or sucralfate in patients with osteoarthritis. Data from reference 22.*

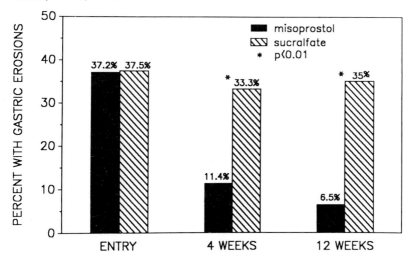

FIGURE 4   *The lack of effectiveness of sucralfate compared to misoprostol for reducing the frequency of NSAID-induced gastric erosions is shown. Data from reference 22.*

Diarrhea, a pharmacologic effect of prostaglandins, has been the side effect reported most frequently following therapy with misoprostol. Most episodes of diarrhea are not severe and are transient. The frequency of diarrhea can be reduced and usually prevented by starting misoprostol at a lower dose (e.g., 100ug bid or qid) and gradually increasing the dose. Studies are in progress to identify dosage schedules that retain the beneficial effects of oral prostaglandin therapy while minimizing diarrhea.

WHO NEEDS PROPHYLAXIS?

There is a poor correlation between the severity of NSAID-induced gastroduodenal damage and symptoms. For example, Armstrong and Blower showed that in 58% of cases of NSAID-associated admissions for bleeding, the first evidence of a problem was the life-threatening complication [23]. The fact that NSAID-induced gastroduodenal ulcerations may be insidious until bleeding and perforation occur represents a serious clinical dilemma.

In addition to the mortality associated with NSAID-induced UGI hemorrhage or perforation, NSAID-related side effects add significantly to the costs of treating rheumatic diseases. A recent retrospective analysis of all direct medical costs related to the treatment of arthritis during a 2-year period in 527 Medicaid patients determined that the management of NSAID-induced GI side effects added 45.5%, or $66 per patient per quarter, to the cost of arthritis treatment [24]. In 1987, approximately $17.5 billion, i.e., 2.5% of total U.S. medical care expenditures, were spent on arthritis treatment and the gastrointestinal side effects associated with this treatment.

Because symptoms are neither reliable indicators of the presence of ulcers nor accurate predictors of gastroduodenal complications in patients receiving NSAIDs, identifying subgroups of NSAID users who are at increased risk of serious NSAID-induced complications would be clinically useful. A number of studies have shown that elderly NSAID users, especially elderly women, are particularly vulnerable to the gastric complications of NSAID therapy [25,26]. Why NSAID gastroduodenal injury seems to be concentrated in this particular patient group is unclear. However, some possible explanations are increased use of NSAIDs in an aging, predominantly female population, or because women receive proportionally higher dosages of NSAIDs than do men because of their smaller size. The problem may be concentrated in the elderly because changes in gastroduodenal physiology associated with aging led to altered healing or altered drug metabolism. Not only are the elderly more likely to develop NSAID-induced gastric side effects, they also seem to be the least likely to experience warning symptoms and the most likely to die from gastroduodenal complications.

We do not have studies separating the group or groups of patients that co-therapy with prostaglandins is mandatory from those in whom it can safely be denied. Most patients do not receive co-therapy. We recommend prostaglandin co-therapy for patients who require chronic NSAID therapy and who are in a high-risk group (Table 1).

TABLE 1.

Factors suggestive of increased risk of NSAID-induced gastrointestinal complications.
Advanced age History of gastric ulcer, GI bleeding or melena Concurrent steroid therapy Recent history of peptic ulcer disease Presence of large ulcers History of severe NSAID gastropathy Recent use of antiulcer medication

Co-therapy adds to the overall cost of arthritis care but theoretically saves by reducing the medical costs associated with major bleeding episodes or gastroduodenal perforation. Simply stopping attempted co-therapy with H_2-receptor antagonists or sucralfate should result in sufficient savings to more than offset the costs of treatment with misoprostol in those who are most likely to benefit from it.

Preventing NSAID-induced gastric ulcers is preferable to treating existing lesions. The most obvious strategy for achieving this end is to review carefully the indications and desired benefits of NSAID use. In many instances, the physician can discontinue NSAIDs and provide simple analgesic therapy with acetaminophen. For those patients who still require NSAID therapy, one should attempt to use the lowest dose possible (such as low-dose ibuprofen or aspirin) to achieve therapeutic objectives. Although no studies have demonstrated that one non-aspirin NSAID is intrinsically more damaging than another, there is ample evidence that the higher the dose (as measured in anti-inflammatory activity), the greater is the risk for serious side effects. Physicians, therefore, should refrain from prescribing the more potent NSAIDs, for example piroxicam, when a high level of anti-inflammatory activity is not needed.

CONCLUSION

The fact that all NSAIDs often induce gastric and possibly duodenal ulceration is no longer a matter for debate. Upper gastrointestinal hemorrhage, perforation and related complications caused by these agents are responsible for a significant number of hospitalizations and for enormous health care expenditures each year. All NSAIDs seem to be equivalent in terms of safety and ulcerogenicity. The prevention of NSAID-induced gastric mucosal lesions is, of course, preferable to treatment, and, therefore, work is in progress to identify individuals at risk of NSAID-associated gastroduodenal complications. A major goal of current research is to determine which patients may benefit most from preventive therapy with synthetic prostaglandins such as misoprostol.

REFERENCES

1.   Graham DY. Prevention of gastroduodenal injury induced by chronic nonsteroidal anti-inflammatory drug therapy. Gastroenterology 1989;96(Suppl):675-681.

2.   Llewelyn JG, Prichard MH. Acute gastric haemorrhage and its relationship to the use of anti-inflammatory analgesics (NSAIDs). Ann Rheum Dis 1983;42:228-229.

3.   Langman MJS. Peptic ulcer complications and the use of non-aspirin nonsteroidal anti-inflammatory drugs. Adverse Drug React Bull 1986;120:448-451.

4.   Alexander AM, Veitch GBA, Wood JB. Anti-rheumatic and analgesic drug usage and acute gastro-intestinal bleeding in elderly patients. J Clin Hosp Pharm 1985;10:89-93.

5.   Griffin MR, Ray WA, Schaffner W. Nonsteroidal anti-inflammatory drug use and death from peptic ulcer in elderly persons. Ann Intern Med 1988;109:359-363.

6.   Roth SH, Bennett RE. NSAIDs and gastropathy: a rheumatologist's review. J Rheumatol 1988;15:912-918.

7.   Paulus HE. FDA arthritis advisory committee meeting: postmarketing surveillance of nonsteroidal anti-inflammatory drugs. Arthritis Rheum 1985;28:1168-1169.

8.   Wolfe E, Kleinheksel SM, Spitz PW et al. A multicenter study of hospitalization in rheumatoid arthritis: frequency, medical-surgical admissions, and charges. Arthritis Rheum 1986;29:614-619.

9.   Giercksky K-E, Husby G, Rugstad HE, Revhaug A. Epidemiology of NSAID-induced gastrointestinal problems and the role of cimetidine in their prevention. Aliment Pharmacol Ther 1988;2(Suppl 1):33-41.

10.   Coles LS, Fries JF, Kraines RG, Roth SH. From experiment to experience: side effects of nonsteroidal anti-inflammatory drugs. Am J Med 1983;74:820-828.

11.   Larkai EN, Smith JL, Lidsky MD, Sessoms SL, Graham DY. Dyspepsia in NSAID users: the size of the problem. J Clin Gastroenterol 1989;11:158-162.

12.   Larkai EN, Smith JL, Lidsky MD, Graham DY. Gastroduodenal mucosa and dyspeptic symptoms in arthritic patients during chronic nonsteroidal anti-inflammatory drug use. Am J Gastroenterol 1987;82:1153-1158.

13.   Silvoso GR, Ivey KJ, Butt JH, et al. Incidence of gastric lesions in patients with rheumatoid disease on chronic aspirin therapy. Ann Intern Med 1979;91:517-520.

14. Morris AD, Holt SD, Silvoso GR, et al. Effect of anti-inflammatory drug administration in patients with rheumatoid arthritis. Scand J Gastroenterol 1981;16:131-135.

15. Farah D, Sturrock RD, Russell RI. Peptic ulcer in rheumatoid arthritis. Ann Rheum Dis 1988;47:478-480.

16. Shorrock CJ, Rees WDW. The effect of indomethacin on human gastric morphology and mucosal blood flow in vivo. Gastroenterology 1988;94:A425.

17. Kauffman GL Jr, Aures D, Grossman MI. Intravenous indomethacin and aspirin reduce basal gastric mucosal blood flow in dogs. Am J Physiol 1980;238:G131-G134.

18. Robinson MG, Griffin JW Jr, Bowers F, Kogan FJ, Kogut DG, Lanza FL, Warner CW. Effect of ranitidine on gastroduodenal mucosal damage induced by nonsteroidal antiinflammatory drugs. Dig Dis Sci 1989;34:424-8.

19. Ehsanullah RSB, Page MC, Tildesley G, Wood JR. Prevention of gastroduodenal damage induced by non-steroidal anti-inflammatory drugs: controlled trial of ranitidine. Br Med J 1988;297:1017-21.

20. Roth SH, Bennett RE, Mitchell CS, Hartman RJ. Cimetidine therapy in nonsteroidal anti-inflammatory drug gastropathy. Arch Intern Med 1987;147:1798-1801.

21. Graham DY, Agrawal N, Roth SH. Prevention of NSAID-induced gastric ulcer with the synthetic prostaglandin misoprostol-a multicenter, double-blind, placebo-controlled trial. Lancet 1988;ii:1277-1280.

22. Agrawal N, Stromatt S, Brown J. Comparative study of misoprostol and sucralfate in the prevention of NSAID-induced gastric ulcers. Gastroenterology 1990;98:A14.

23. Armstrong CP, Blower AL. Nonsteroidal anti-inflammatory drugs and life-threatening complications of peptic ulceration. Gut 1987;28:527-532.

24. Bloom BS. Cost of treating arthritis and NSAID-related gastrointestinal side effects. Aliment Pharmacol Ther 1988;2(Suppl 1):131-139.

25. Langman MJS. Anti-inflammatory drug intake and the risk of ulcer complications. Med Toxicol 1986;1(Suppl 1):34-38.

26. Walt R, Katschinski B, Logan R, Ashley J, Langman MJS. Rising frequency of ulcer perforation in elderly people in the United Kingdom. Lancet 1986;i:489-492.

INDOMETHACIN IMPAIRS QUALITY OF EXPERIMENTAL GASTRIC ULCER HEALING: A QUANTITATIVE HISTOLOGICAL AND ULTRASTRUCTURAL ANALYSIS

A. Tarnawski, J. Stachura, T.G. Douglass, W.J. Krause,
H. Gergely, and I.J. Sarfeh

DVA Medical Center, Long Beach California;
The University of California, Irvine; California State University Long Beach;
The University of Missouri, Columbia, Missouri, U.S.A.

ABSTRACT

The present study was aimed to determine whether chronic administration of indomethacin affects quality of experimental gastric ulcer healing i.e. restoration of mucosal architecture and cellular composition assessed histologically and ultrastructurally. In 60 male Sprague-Dawley rats (225-250 g) standardized gastric ulcers were produced by focal serosal application of acetic acid. The rats were then treated with placebo or indomethacin 1 mg/kg i.p. daily, for 14 days. Ulcer size was meausred under a dissecting microscope. Gastric mucosal specimens from the ulcer area or mucosal scar were obtained for qualitative and quantitative histology. In placebo treated rats, the ulcer size was 1.1 ± 0.1 mm^2. Histologically, the grossly "healed" mucosa demonstrated marked dilatation of gastric glands which were lined predominantly with mature surface epithelial cells, parietal cells constituting less than 6% of all cells. Granulation tissue was rich in collagen and fibroblasts and contained 24 ± 2 vascular profiles/(500 x) per microscopic field. In indomethacin treated rats, the ulcer crater was significantly larger (3.5 ± 0.2 mm^2; $p < 0.001$ vs placebo). Histology and transmission EM demonstrated extensive necrosis, thinning of the gastric wall, poorly developed "healing zone" at the ulcer margin and cystically dilated glands lined with primitive undifferentiated cells. Parietal cells were absent. The lamina propria had increased cellularity with numerous macrophages and lymphoid cells. The number of vascular profiles in granulation tissue was signficantly reduced. We conclude that administration of indomethacin: 1) delays healing of experimental gastric ulcers, 2) impairs the overall quality of ulcer healing, distorting restoration of mucosal architecture and blocking the differentiation and maturation of glandular and surface epithalial cells and 3) inhibits angiogenesis in granulation tissue.

INTRODUCTION

Our previous studies demonstrated that re-epithelializaed mucosa of grossly "healed" experimental gastric ulcers in rats remains histologically and ultrastructurally abnormal [1]. Two patterns of scarring can be distinguished: (a) the mucosa in the area of a healed ulcer is thinner (25% to 45% thinner compared with normal mucosa), with increased connective tissue, poor differentiation and/or degenerative changes in the glandular cells; or (b) the mucosa displays a marked dilatation of gastric glands, reduction in the microvascular network, and poor differentiation of glandular cells. Indomethacin is known to delay healing of experimental gastric ulcers when assessed grossly in rats [2,3]. However, microscopic and ultrastructural effects of chronic indomethacin administration on ulcer healing are unknown. The present study was aimed to determine whether chronic administration of indomethacin affects the quality of experimental gastric ulcer healing i.e. restoration of mucosal architecture and cellular composition.

METHODS

ANIMALS

Sixty male Sprague-Dawley rats (Charles Rivers Labs) 225-250 g body weight were maintained on Purina rat chow. They were fasted for 12 hours, and underwent laparotomy under nembutal anaesthesia (60 mg/kg bw). Acetic acid - 50 ul, 100%, was applied to the serosa of the lower corpus on the posterior wall through a polyethylene tube (3.6 mm i.d.) for 30 seconds as described before [1,4]. The area was then washed with isotonic saline and the abdomen was closed, and all animals fasted for the next 12 hours. For the next 2 weeks rats were treated with indomethacin 1 mg/kg or placebo (isotonic saline, pH adjusted with bicarbonate in a similar manner to indomethacin). These were given once daily (9 am) intraperitoneally. In addition rats received intragastrically 2 ml of isotonic saline twice daily. After 2 weeks, rats were anaesthetized with nembutal 60 mg/kg bw and underwent laparotomy. The stomachs were excised, opened along the greater curvature. The ulcerations or scars were identified under a Nikon SMZ - 2T dissecting microscope (Garden City, N.Y.) and the ulcer size was measured. Standardized, oriented gastric wall specimens with identified ulcers or grossly healed ulcers (scars) were fixed in 10% buffered formalin. Perforated ulcers were excluded from evaluation. After routine processing, perpendicularly cut paraffin sections were stained with hematoxylin and eosin and with Alcian Blue (AB) and periodic acid-Schiff (PAS). Coded mucosal sections were evaluated by 3 investigators unaware of the code. During histological evaluation special attention was paid to the pattern of glandular structures, their restoration, and to the cellular composition of the gastric mucosa and granulation tissue. In addition to the qualitative assessment, the number of PAS positive cells (representing mature surface epithelial cells) and AB positive cells (representing immature mucous cells), the number of total glandular mucosal cells and of parietal cells as well as the number of microvessels in granulation tissue were determined morphometrically under a Nikon Optiphot microscope using a Microplan II video image analyzer.

In 3 rats from each group, gastric mucosal specimens containing ulcers or scars were immediately fixed in 3.5% glutaraldehyde buffered with 0.1 M phosphate buffer pH 7.4 at $4^{o}C$ and processed for transmission electron microscopy [5]. Semi-thin sections were evaluated quantitatively for the number of parietal cells within gastric glands. Silver-gray thin sections were evaluated under a Philips 400 electron microscope at 80 kv by 3 investigators unaware of the code.

The statistical comparison of ulcer size, number of parietal cells in the gastric glands, ratio of PAS positive to AB positive cells and number of microvessels in granulation tissue were made using Student's t-test [6].

RESULTS

ULCER SIZE

In the placebo treated group most of the ulcers were grossly "healed" (Figure 1A) while in the indomethacin treated group large deep ulcers were present (Figure 1D). The ulcer size (mean $\pm$ SE) in the placebo treated group was 1.1 ± 01.1 mm^2 compared with 3.5 ± 0.2 mm^2 in indomethacin treated rats (p < 0.001). This clearly indicates that indomethacin delays ulcer healing.

MUCOSAL HISTOLOGY

A)   **Placebo treated group:**

In the placebo treated group residual necrosis was small or absent. The "grossly" healed mucosa demonstrated re-epithelialization, but the subepithelial mucosa showed marked dilation of gastric glands (Figure 1B) which were lined with mature surface epithelial cells and/or cells resembling mucous neck cells or cells lining pyloric glands.   The ratio of PAS positive to AB positive cells was 2.08 ± 0.22 indicating that the majority of cells were mature surface epithelial cells.   Parietal cells constituted less than 6% of all glandular cells.   The lamina propria and connective tissue replacing granulation tissue were increased and contained numerous fibroblasts.   The number of microvascular profiles in connective tissue replacing granulation tissue at the scar base (Figure 1C) was (mean $\pm$ SE) 24 ± 2 profiles per (500x) microscopic field.

B)   **Indomethacin treated group**

In the indomethacin treated rats residual histologic necrosis was extensive and large ulcer craters were usually present (Figure 1E).   The mucosa at the ulcer margin contained cystically dilated glands (Figure 1E) which were lined with immature cells resembling mucus neck cells or cells lining pyloric glands.   They stained mostly with Alcian blue.   The ratio of PAS positive to AB positive cells was 0.4 (Table 1; p < 0.001 vs placebo) indicating a five-fold reduction in the number of mature surface epithelial cells.   Parietal cells constituted less than 0.14% of all glandular cells (Table 1; p < 0.001 vs placebo). From some of the dilated glands at the base of the ulcer margin, epithelial cells were budding off into the lamina propria and/or granulation tissue and forming tubules. Some of these tubules were undergoing transformation into immature glands.   The granulation tissue consisted predominantly of macrophages, and lymphocytes, while fibroblasts and collagen fibers were scarce. Also the number of vascular profiles in the granulation tissue (Figure 1F) was significantly reduced (p < 0.002 vs placebo; Table 1) indicating impaired angiogenesis.

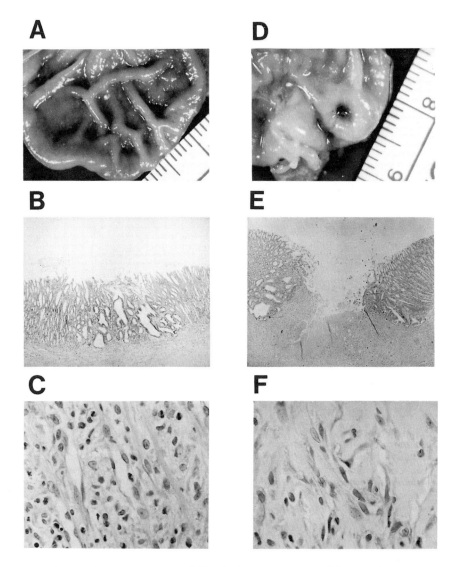

FIGURE 1   *Macroscopic and histologica appearance of the gastric mucosa in rats. In placebo treated rats (A, B & C), the mucosa is grossly healed (A) but histology demonstrates prominent cystic dilation of the gastric glands (B). Granulation tissue contains numerous microvessels (C). In an indomethacin treated rat (D, E & F) a deep ulcer surrounded by elevated margin is seen grossly (D) and histology demonstrates a typical deep ulcer (E). The granulation tissue has fewer microvessels (F).*

TABLE 1

ULCER SIZE AND THE QUANTITATIVE HISTOLOGIC ASSESSMENT

	Placebo	Indomethacin
Size of Ulcer (mm^2)	1.1 ± 0.1	$3.5 \pm 0.2*$
PAS (+) Cells/AB (+) Cells Ratio	2.08 ± 0.22	$0.40 \pm 0.04*$
% of Parietal Cells	5.9 ± 0.2	$0.14 \pm 0.08*$
Microvessels in Granulation Tissue (per $7400u^2$)	24 ± 1.0	$13 \pm 0.8*$

The values represent mean $\pm$ SE. * $p < 0.001$ vs placebo

TRANSMISSION EM

A)   **Placebo treated group** (Figures 2A,B and C)

In placebo treated rats, transmission EM demonstrated that surface epithelial cells covering the gastric mucosa of grossly healed ulcers contained numerous autophagic vacuoles (Figure 2A).   The lumina of cystically dilated glands in the mucosal scar were lined predominantly with mature surface epithelial cells or less frequently with immature cells resembling mucous neck cells (Figure 2B).   The connective tissue (lamina propria) between the cystically dilated glands was abundant, but poorly organized.   Numerous fibroblasts and smooth muscle cells within the lamina propria exhibited a distorted orientation.   Macrophages and lymphocytes were also present.   The extracellular matrix was increased.   In the granulation tissue, undergoing transformation into connective tissue scar, the fibroblasts and the microvessels predominated.

B)   **Indomethacin treated group** (Figures 2D, E and F)

In indomethacin treated rats transmission EM demonstrated deep ulcerations and necrosis.   The surface epithelial cells covering the mucosa at the ulcer margin, displayed prominent folding of the basolateral surface and distended intercellular spaces (Figure 2D).   The mucosa of the ulcer margin contains cystically dilated glands which were lined with poorly differentiated cuboidal cells resembling stem cells or cells lining pyloric glands or immature mucous cells (Figure 2E).   In the lamina propria numerous macrophages were present, some of them undergoing disintegration.   In granulation tissue numerous macrophages and lympho-cytes were seen, endothelial cells and microvessels were fewer than in the placebo treated group, while fibroblasts were virtually absent (Figure 2F).

DISCUSSION

This study demonstrated that indomethacin given daily in a relatively small dose delays healing of experimental gastric ulcer in rats. Moreover it impaired the overall quality of ulcer healing, distorting restoration of mucosal architecture and blocking differentiation and maturation of glandular and surface epithelial cells.   Indomethacin also inhibited angiogenesis in granulation tissue.   While the delay of ulcer healing by indomethacin has been previously observed by gross assessment [2,3], the impairment by indomethacin of the quality of mucosal restoration and angiogenesis in granulation tissue has not been reported upon.

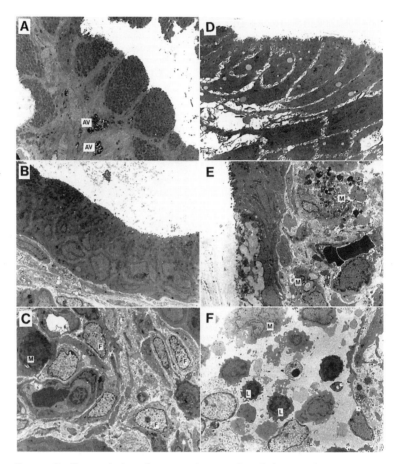

FIGURE 2 Transmission electron micrographs of the gastric mucosa at 3
different levels: surface epithelium, cystically dilated glands and
granulation tissue.   In placebo treated rat (A, B and C), the surface
epithelial cells are columnar and contain numerous mucus granules (A).
Autophagic vacuoles (AV) are present Lumina of dilated gastric glands
are lined with mature surface epithelial cells (not shown) or immature
mucus cells containing less mucus (B).   In granulation tissue (which is
undergoing transformation to connective tissue) fibroblasts predominate
(C).   In indomethacin treated rats (D, E and F), there is a prominent
folding of basolateral surfaces (arrow) and distension of intercellular
spaces (D).   Dilated glands (E) are lined with poorly differentiated
cuboidal mucus cells releasing thick mucus into the lumen.   In the
lamina propria disintegrating macrophages (M) are present.   In
granulation tissue (F) numerous macrophages (M) and lymphocytes (L)
are present, while fibroblasts are virtually absent.   Magnification
(5000x).

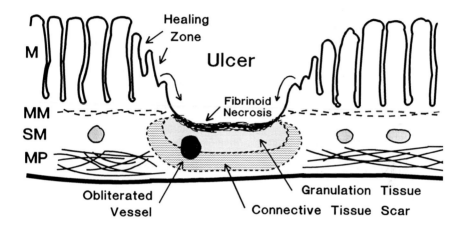

FIGURE 3 *Diagrammatic presentation of ulceration in the gastric mucosa M - mucosa, MM - muscularis mucosae, SM - submucosa, MP - muscularis propria. Healing of the ulcer is accomplished by: a) filling the mucosal defect with cells migrating from the healing zone and replicating (regeneration) and b) by the replacement of the defect with connective tissue which forms a mucosal scar (fibrosis).*

An ulcer is a deep necrotic lesion involving the entire mucosa and penetrating through the muscularis mucosae (Figure 3) [7].   In the acute stage of ulceration, the mucosa and submucosa become necrotic, attracting polymorphonuclear leukocytes and macrophages [4,7].   Eventually the necrotic portions of the mucosa detach and/or are removed by scavenging macrophages [4,7].   During the chronic stage, the base of the ulcer becomes covered by granulation tissue (Figure 4) consisting of proliferating connective tissue cells, i.e. fibroblasts, endothelial cells (which form microvessels) and macrophages. [4,7].

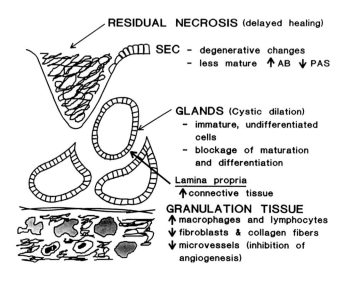

FIGURE 4   *Diagrammatic summary of the effect on indomethacin on healing of acetic acid-induced gastric ulcers in rat.*

Ulcer healing is a very complex process, requiring interaction between different structures and cellular systems [7-10]. Two distinct structures are known to play a major role in ulcer healing: (a) the mucosa at the ulcer margin [8-10], and (b) granulation tissue at the ulcer base [7-11]. Mucosa at the ulcer margin forms a "healing zone" which undergoes striking changes in structure and cellular composition. The glands become cystically dilated and their portions lean toward the ulcer crater [1,4,10]. The epithelial cells at the ulcer margin de-differentiate and proliferate [9,10,12], supplying cells for re-epithelialization of the mucosal surface and reconstruction of the mucosal glandular structures. The poorly differentiated cells appear to migrate from the ulcer margin to cover (re-epithelialize) the ulcer base as soon as the connective tissue infrastructure permits [9,10]. As shown in our present study, the poorly differentiated cells from the cystically dilated glands at the base of the ulcer margin (healing zone) bud off into the lamina propria and/or granulation tissue forming tubules. These tubules undergo transformation into glands that eventually communicate with the gastric lumen. This process resembles the normal morphogenesis of primitive gut during development [13].

Granulation tissue is an important component of the healing process because it supplies (a) connective tissue cells to restore the lamina propria and (b) endothelial cells to restore the microvasculature within the scar [7].

A part of the connective tissue component may also originate from the ulcer margin. An increased number of mitoses has been reported in lamina propria fibroblasts at this site [9]. Granulation tissue undergoes continuous remodelling with changes in its cellular composition. Initially inflammatory cells and macrophages are abundant while at the later stages fibroblasts predominate. The final outcome of the healing process reflects a dynamic balance between the epithelial component from the "healing" zone at the ulcer margin and the connective tissue component (including microvessels) originating from granulation tissue.

A number of factors modulate ulcer healing: a) luminal factors: H^+ ion secretion, pepsin, mucus and bicarbonates; b) growth factors, most notably epidermal growth factor [7,14,15] from salivary glands or that produced locally by cells of regenerating glands [16]; c) the blood supply delivering oxygen and nutrients [7,11]; d) macrophage activity for removal of necrotic debris and stimulation of angiogenesis [7,17]; e) unstirred mucus and bicarbonate layer [18] to protect newly formed cells from acid and pepsin injury; and f) generation of prostaglandins. The importance of the latter is stressed by the fact that inhibition of endogenous prostaglandins with indomethacin significantly delays ulcer healing [3], and that administration of exogenous prostaglandin E_2 reverses this deleterious effect of indomethacin [3].

Formation of new microvessels (angiogenesis) plays an important role in morphogenesis, wound healing and tissue regeneration [7,19]. It probably plays a role in healing gastroduodenal ulcers and in repairing of acute gastric mucosal injury; however, this subject remains unexplored. Our preliminary studies demonstrated that following acute gastric mucosal injury there is an angiogenic response: within 24 hours 6% of the microvessels in injured (but non-necrotic) mucosa sprout of new endothelial cells forming the vascular tubes, basement membranes and ultimately microvascular lumina [20]. We have also shown that angiogenesis in injured gastric mucosa is stimulated by arachidonic acid (prostaglandin precursor) and 16, 16 dimethyl prostaglandin E_2 [20]. Further, we found that indomethacin (which inhibits prostaglandin synthesis) completely blocks the angiogenic response (spontaneous or stimulated by arachidonic acid) of acutely injured gastric mucosa [21]. However, indomethacin does not block the angiogenic response stimulated with 16, 16 dm prostaglandin E_2 [21]. All these indicate a possible role of prostaglandins in mediation gastric mucosal angiogenesis in response to acute injury.

In the present study we showed that there are significantly less microvessels in granulation tissue of indomethacin treated rats than in the placebo treated rats, indicating impaired angiogenesis. We postulate that this effect of indomethacin is due to inhibition of prostaglandin synthesis and/or inhibition or interference with other factors which stimulate angiogenesis. Such factors include a basic fibroblast growth factor, platelet derived growth factor, transforming growth factors and/or interleukin - 1 or tumor necrosis factors - mitogenic mediators, that are chemotactic for fibroblasts [7,18,22]. Indeed, we observe a virtual absence of fibroblasts in granulation tissue of indomethacin treated rats.

In summary, our present studies demonstrate that chronic administration of indomethacin 1) delays healing of experimental gastric ulcers, 2) impairs the overall quality of ulcer healing, distorting restoration of mucosal architecture and blocking the differentiation and maturation of glandular and surface epithelial cells and 3) inhibits angiogenesis in granulation tissue.

ACKNOWLEDGEMENT

*This work was supported by the Research Service
of the Veterans' Administration.*

REFERENCES

1.   Tarnawski A, Hollander D, Krause WJ, Dabros W, Stachura J, Gergely H.   "Healed" experimental gastric ulcers remain histologically and ultrastructurally abnormal.   J Clin Gastroenterol   1990; 12 (Suppl 1):S139-147.

2.   Inauen W, Wyss PA, Kayser S, Baumgartner A, Schurer-Maly CC, Koelz HR, Halter F.   Influence of prostaglandins, omeprazole, and indomethacin on healing of experimental gastric ulcers in the rat. Gastroenterology 1988; 95: 636-641.

3.   Wang JY, Yamasaki S, Takeuchi K, Okabe S.   Delayed healing of acetic acid-induced gastric ulcers in rats by indomethacin. Gastroenterology 1989; 96:393-402.

4.   Tarnawski A, Hollander D, Stachura J, Krause WJ, Eltorai M, Dabros W, Gergely H.   Vascular and microvascular changes - key factors in the development of acetic acid-induced gastric ulcers in rats. J Clin Gastroenterology 1990; 12(Suppl 1):S148-157.

5.   Spurr A.   A low viscosity epoxy resin embedding medicine for electron microscopy. J Ultrastruct Res 1969; 26: 31-5.

6.   Glantz SA.   Primer of Biostatistics.   2nd Ed. McGraw-Hill Book Co, New York, 1987.

7.   Robbins SL, Cotran RS, Kumar V, eds. Healing and Repair in Robbins Pathologic Basis of Disease.   Philadelphia: W.B. Saunders, 1989, pp 71-86.

8.   McMinn RMH, Johnson FR.   The cytology of mucosal regeneration in experimental gastric ulcer. In: Pathophysiology of peptic ulcer. Ed. Skoryna SC. Lippincot, Philadelphia 1963, pp. 369-385.

9.   Helpap B, Hattori T, Gedigk P.   Repair of gastric ulcer. A cell kinetic study. Virchows Arch (Pathol Anat) 1981; 392:159-170.

10. Helander HE. Morphologic studies on the margin of gastric corpus wounds in the rat. J Submicrosc Cytol 1983; 15: 627-643.

11. Szabo S, Hollander D. Pathways of gastrointestinal protection and repair: mechanisms of action of sucralfate. Am J Med 1989; 86(6A): 23-31.

12. Eastwood GL. Epithelial cell renewal. In: Gastric Cytoprotection. Eds. D. Hollander and A. Tarnawski, Plenum, New York 1989, pp 109-124.

13. Krause WJ, Cutts JH, Leeson CR. The postnatal development of the alimentary canal in the opossum. II. Gastric mucosa. J Anat 1976; 122: 499-519.

14. Skov Olsen P, Poulsen SS, Therkelsen K, Nexo E. Effect of sialoadenectomy and synthetic human urogastrone on healing of chronic gastric ulcers in rats. Gut 1986; 27: 1443-9.

15. Konturek SJ, Dembinski A, Warzecha Z, Brzozowski T, Gregory H. Role of epidermal growth factor in healing of chronic gastroduodenal ulcers in rats. Gastroenterology 1988; 94: 1300-1307.

16. Wright NA, Pike C, Elia G. Induction of a novel epidermal growth factor - secreting cell lineage by mucosal ulceration in human gastrointestinal stem cells. Nature 1990; 343: 82-85.

17. Leibovich SJ, Polverini PJ, Shepard HM, Wiseman DM, Shively V, Nuseir N. Macrophage-induced angiogenesis is mediated by tumour necrosis factor-a. Nature 1987; 329:630-632.

18. Allen A, Hunter AC, Mall A. Mucus section. In: Gastric Cytoprotection. Eds. D. Hollander and A. Tarnawski, Plenum, New York, 1989, pp 75-90.

19. Klagsbrun M. Angiogenesis factors in endothelial cells. In: Endothelial Cells, Vol II. Ed. U.S. Ryan, CRC Press, Inc. Boca Raton, Fla 1988, pp. 37-50.

20. Tarnawski A, Hollander D, Stachura J, Sarfeh IJ, Gergely H, Krause WJ. Angiogenic response of gastric mucosa to ethanol injury is abolished by indomethacin. Gastroenterology 1989; 96:A505.

21. Tarnawski A, Hollander D, Stachura J, Sheffield M, Gergely H, Kasuse WJ. Angiogenic response of damaged gastric mucosa - a prostaglandin mediated process? Gastroenterology 1990; 98: A136.

22. D'Amore PA, Braunhut SJ. Stimulatory and inhibitory factors in vascular growth control. In: Endothelial Cells, Vol II. Ed. U.S. Ryan, CRC Press, Inc. Boca Raton. Fla 1988, pp13-36.

1,10-phenanthroline, 55
14C-aminopyrine, 253-267
16,16-dmPGE$_2$, see Prostaglandin
^{51}Cr-EDTA clearance, 91-99,141, 142,145,146
6 Keto PGF$_{1\alpha}$, see Prostaglandin

A

αsubunit, 187-198
α2 receptors 223,227,228
AA-861, 301,306,307
Acetic acid-induced gastric ulcers, 456
Acetylcholine, 299-307
Acetylsalicylic acid, see Aspirin
Acid
- acetic, induced gastric ulcers, 456
- acidification, 247-250, 271-278
- acidosis, 47,52,277,278
- back diffusion, 82,83,108-109
- luminal, 1-5
- secretion, 1-5,19,24,37-44,61,104
- suppression, 1-5
Acridine orange quenching, 177, 179,180
Actin, 53
Adaptation
- and acid secretion, 367
- and gastric mucosal blood flow, 481
- gastric, 357-370
- to injury, 395
- prevention by indomethacin, 365
- to necrotizing agent, 357-370
- to NSAIDs, 479-490
Adrenal 223,227
Adrenergic, 223,227
Afferent neuron, 103,127-128
Aged rats, 310-317
Aging, 310-317
Alcohol, 175,181,183
Alkaline secretion, 91-99
Allopurinol, 53,54,152, 159-174
Ambient chloride, 81-87
Amiloride, 181,182,183,248, 249, 253-267,271,272,273
Amoxycillin, 211,216
Amphibian mucosa, 247-250
Anastomosis, 292,293
Angiogenesis, 450
- effect of dietary fatty acids, 507
Angiotensin, 167,169

Anion exchange, 262, 267
Anoxia, 47-56,82,84,159-174
Anti-neutrophil serum (ANS), 139, 140,142,146,155,156
Antrum
- contact angle, 207-218
- mucosal microvascular architecture, 292-297
- mucous cells, 395-403
Apical
- cell membrane,, 271-278
- membrane, 199-205
- membrane vesicles, 175-185
- surface, 175-185, 187-198
Arachidonic acid, 503, 160,169
Aspirin
- and gastric mucosal injury, 467
- and haemostasis, 467,469
- PGE2 synthesis rate, 469-472
- prevention by fatty acids, 505
ATP, 47,52,53,55,56
Atrial natriuretic peptide (ANP), 227
Atropine, 37,39,43,224,225,238,240

B

β-subunit, 187-198
bFGF, 450
b-fibroblast growth factor (bFGF), 450
- and ulcer healing, 452
Back diffusion, 175,250,276
Back titration, 238
Barrier breaking agent, 271-278
Barrier, 175,184 see Mucus layer
Basolateral membrane, 247-250
Bethanechol, 238
Bicarbonate (HCO$_3^-$)
- barrier, 1
- inhibition, 29-35
- secretion, 29-35,61,223-232, 237-244,271-278,292-297
- HCO$_3^-$/Cl$^-$ exchanger, 247-250
Bile
- acid, 210,213,214
- reflux, 208,217
- salts, 61-68,175,181,183
Biphenylacetic acid, 29-35
Bismuth, 211,216
Body temperature, 37-44
Bombesin, 224
Brunner's gland, 292-297

SUBJECT INDEX

C

Calcitonin
- and capsaicin-sensitive
  neurones, 388
- and ethanol injury, 387
- and inhibition of vagal
  outflow, 385,386
- and gastric mucosal
  blood flow, 387
- gene related peptide, 103,
  105-109,128,227,383-393
- intracisternal injection, 383
Calcium, 54,56,61-68
cAMP, 240,253,265
Capillary
- network, 292,297
- fenestrated, 292-297
- plexus, 292,293,297
- unfenestrated, 292,297
Capsaicin, 103-106,108-110,
  115,116,119,122,127-135
Carbachol, 37,38,42-44
Catalase, 53,54,139-147,153,159-174
Celiac artery clamping, 323
Cell
- bleb formation 49,53,56
- death, 47-56
- gastric mucosal, 61,62,64-67
- injury, 47-56,61-68
- swelling, 53
- suspension, 62,64,65
- viability, 47-49,61,66
CGRP - see calcitonin - gene
  related peptide
Chamber - ex-vivo, gastric, 372
Chemiluminescence, 163
Cholecystokinin, 225
Cholinergic, 223,240
Chronic ulcer model,456,491
- abscopal model, 491
- acetic acid-induced
  gastric ulcer, 521
- effects of indomethacin, 458
- effects of prednisolone, 458
- induced by acetic acid, 455
- induced by irradiation, 491
Cimetidine, 3,39,249,327,333
Cl$^-$/HCO$_3$ exchanger, 253-267
Clonidine, 39
CO$_2$/HCO$_3^-$, 253-267
Colchicine, 53,54

Cold
- exposure, 37,38,42,43
- restraint, 37,43,44
- restraint stress, 384
Colloidal Bismuth Subcitrate
  (CBS), 71,72,74-76,327
Confocal laser scan
  microscopy, 281-287
Connective tissue, 343
Contact angles, 207-218
Corticotropin releasing
  factor (CRF), 224
CV-3988, 301,305
Cyanidanol, 52,54
Cyanide toxicity, 47,51,52,56
Cyclo-oxygenase, 371
- inhibition, 29
Cytochalasin B, 53,54
Cytoprotection, 61-68
- adaptive, 371
- local, 371-382
- prostaglandin-independent, 371
- referred, 371-382

D

Deep necrotic lesion, 527
Deglycosylation, 187-198
Denol, 211,216
Deoxycholate (DC), 61-68
Desferrioxamine, 52,54,153,165
Dibucaine, 55
Duodenum, 91-99
- distal, 207, 213,238
- human, 237,240
- proximal, 237,238,241
DMSO, 153, 159-174
DNA synthesis rate, 437
Duodenal, 175-185
- bulb, 207,213,238
- ulcer, 207-218,237-244
Duodenogastric reflux, 31,33
Dyspepsia, 19,21,24,209,218

E

EDRF, 301,304,307 *see also*
  Nitric oxide
Electrical resistance (R), 175-185,
  199-205

Electron
- spin resonance, 163
- spin trapping, 163
Electrophysiology, 81-87,199,200
End arteries, 295
Endoscopy
- samples, 207-218
- scoring of injury, 482
Endothelial cell, 71,159-174
Endothelins, 449
Endothelium, 159-174
- vascular, 139-147
- derived relaxing factor, 127-135
Enprostil, 328,332
Enteric nervous system (ENS), 223,
    225,226
Epidermal growth factor
- and stress-induced
    gastric ulceration, 435
- radio immunoassay, 437
Epithelial cell permeability, 175-185
Esophageal, 199-205
Essential fatty acids
- and gastric microvasculature, 506
- and PGE_2 synthesis rate, 504,505
- and resistance to
    stress-induced injury, 505
Ethanol induced injury, 271-278,
    299-307
- adaptation to, 357
- time for expression, 333-336
- fixation of tissue, 327-328
- prevention by fatty acids, 505
Evans Blue, 38

F

Fenbufen, 29-35
Fibrin gel, 11,15
Flunarizine, 54,56
Fluorescent dye
- FURA 2/AM, 61-64,68
- pH sensitive, 281-287
- fluorometric assay, 281-287
- for cell viability, 47-51
Forestomach, 296
Free radical 48,52,53,159-174
Fructose, 54,56

G

Gastric
- acid secretion
- adaptation, 357-370
- basal, 310-317
- biopsy, 207-218
- body (contact angle), 207-218
- carcinoma, 19,21,24
- chamber, 311,312,313
- cytoprotection, 327
- juice (surface tension), 207-218
- metaplasia, 19,22,24
- stimulated, 310-317
- mucosal blood flow,71,75-77,
    103-110,321-328
    and adaptation to NSAIDs, 483
    and protection against
    acute injury, 448
    reduction by indomethacin, 483
- mucosal defence, 29
- ulcer, 207-218
Gastrin releasing peptide (GRP), 224
Gastrin, 427-434
- and Helicobacter pylori, 428
- and ulcer healing, 428,429
- and restitution, 429
- causation factor in
    peptic ulcer, 427
- gastroprotective
    properties, 428,429
- secretion, 24,25
Gastritis, 207-218
- antral type B, 19-27
Gastropathy, 139-147
Glucagon, 238,239
Glucose, 54,56
Glycoproteins, 187-198,343,397-398
- neutral, 397
- acidic, 398,399
- glycosylated, 187-198
- glycosaminoglycans (GAGs), 343
Goniometer, 209,211
Granulation tissue, 528
Granulocytes, 141,149-157

H

H. pylori, see Helicobacter Pylori
H^+, see Hydrogen Ion
H,K-ATPase, 187-198

SUBJECT INDEX

Haemostasis
- and ranitidine, 473
- and smoking, 475
- effect of aspirin, 471-474
H_2O_2, see Hydrogen Peroxide
HCT-8, 175-185
Healing, see Ulcer
Helicobacter pylori
- adherence, 20,24
- and chronic peptic ulcer, 572
- antibody detection, 21
- chemotactic factors, 20,24-26
- eradication, 19,27
- mode of transmission, 21,22
- mucosal effects, 25
- pathogenesis, 22,24,26
Hepatocyte, 47-56
HEPES buffer, 415
Hexamethonium, 39,43,224,231,232
Histamine, 310-317
Histology
- assessment of injury, 329
- quantitative, 327-341
Hormonal, 223-232
Human duodenum, see Duodenum
Hydrochloric acid, 92,93,96,98,99
Hydrogen
- gas clearance, 104-106,
    299-307,311,315
- ion (H^+), 199-205
- H,K-ATPase, 187-198
- receptor antagonist, 2,3,4
- peroxide (H_2O_2), 149,155,159-177
- peroxide (H_2O_2) scavenger,
    139-147
Hydrophobic, 276
- hydrophobicity, 207-218
Hydroxyl radical (OH)159-174
Hyperemia, 323
Hyperemic response to injury, 323
Hypertonic saline, 323
Hypothermia, 37-44
Hypovolemia, 226,227,228
Hypoxia, 47-56,167

I

Ibuprofen, 513
Image analysis, 105
In vivo microscopy, 299-307
In-vitro chamber, 30

Indomethacin, 29-35,61-68,91-93,95,
    98,127,131-134,238,239,240,
    299-307
- and gastric adaptation, 359
- delay in healing of ulcer, 523
- effect on gastric mucosal
    blood flow, 483
- effect of gastric ulcer
    healing, 523-525
- inhibition of angiogenesis, 529
- injury to human gastric
    mucosa, 481
- on chronic ulcer healing, 458
- on connective tissue
    in ulcer base, 459
Inflammation - mediators, 19,20,25-26
Injury
- by ethanol, 325
- by hydrochloric acid, 323
Intercellular matrix, 343
Interfoveolar cells, 397
Intra cerebroventricular
    (ICV), 224,227
Intracellular
- buffering capacity, 253-267
- edema, 86,87
- pH, 247-250,271,278
- pH regulation, 281-287
- resistance, 272-275
Ion transport systems, 253-267
Iron, 165,166
Ischaemia, 71-77,149-157,159-174,
    301-304
Isolated duodenal enterocytes, 281-287
Isolated rabbit parietal cells, 253-267

K

K^+, 175-185

L

Lactate dehydrogenase (LDH), 48-52
Lamina propria, 343
Laser doppler flowmetry (LDF),
    127-131,134,299-307,311,315
Lectins, 195
Leukocyte, 139-147
- adherence, inhibition of,
    141,143,146
Leukotrienes, 307,447

SUBJECT INDEX

Lidoflazine, 54,56
Linoleic acid, 503
Lipid
- dynamics, 177,178,183
- peroxidation, 162,163
Local anaesthetic, 223-232
Luminal acid, *see* Acid
Luminal alkalinisation,
29,31,91,92,94-96,98
Lysophosphatidylcholine, 207,217,218

M

Mannitol, 53,54,159-174
Matrix - intercellular, 343
MDCK, 175-185
Membrane, 175-185
Meta-analysis, 3,4,5
Mg2+ precipitation method, 176
Microangioarchitectural, 293,295
Microcirculation, 299-307
Microelectrode, 271,272,274
Microfilament, 53
Microinjection, 286
Microtubule, 53
Microvascular, 159-174
- casting, 72,75
- capillary network, 72,74
- density in granulation tissue, 525
- permeability, 149-157
- structure, 72,74
Microvasculature, 292-297
Misoprostol, 511-520
Mitochondral dysfunction, 47,48,52,53
Monastral blue, 449
Morphine, 115-123
Mucoid coat, *see* Mucus Layer
Mucolytic activity, 7-16
Mucosal blood flow, 29,127-135,
140,299-307,310-317,321-328
Mucosal injury, 29-35,37-44,81-87
- by ethanol, 2,7,11-13,15,71-77,
105,107-108,115-122,139
- by hypertonic saline, 2,8,11-13,15
- by Indomethacin, 139-147
- histological assessment, 1,2,9-13,
105,144
- macroscopic, 116,117,119,129,
132-133,140,143-145
- mucosal protection, 115-123
Mucosal permeability, 9,11,91-99,145

Mucosal protection, 71-77,103-110,
115-123
Mucus layer, 11-13,15,395
- and protection against
injury, 395-403
- barrier, 7-16
- bicarbonate barrier, 29,35
- gel thickness, 9,13,14,29
- gel thickness measurement, 373
- granules, 397,399
- secretion, 13,14
- soluble, 13-15
- thickness and protection, 377-378
Mucus neck cells, 363
Multiple organ failure, 167
Muscarinic, 223,225,240
Myeloperoxidase (MPO), 154,155
- reduction of levels, 141,143,146
- enhancement of, 141,143,146

N

N-glycosylation, 187-198
N-methyl nalorphine, 115,116,119
Na   - channels, 199-205
- dependent, 285,286
- ion Na^+, 253-267,271-278
- Na^+/H^+ exchange, 175-185,
253-267,271-278,281-287
- Na_2SO_4, 238
- NADPH oxidase, 159-174
- $NaNO_2$, 299-304
-NaOH - as injurious agent, 358
Naloxone, 115-119
Naproxen, 513
Necturus antral mucosa, 271
Neuro, 223-232
- endocrine, 223,226
- peptide, 103-110,127-135
Neutropenia, 140,142
Neutrophil, 159-174
- adherence, 139-147,155,156,157
- extravasation, 155, 156, 157
N^G-monomethyl-L-arginine
(L-NMMA), 127-135
NH_4Cl prepulse technique, 199,201,203
Nicardipine, 54,56
Nicotinic, 223,225,231
Nigericin, 179,180,257
Nisoldipine, 54,56
Nitrendipine, 54,56

Nitric oxide
- biosynthesis inhibition, 127
Nocodazole, 53
Non-cholinergic, 223,224,240
Non-steroidal anti-inflammatory drugs
- see NSAIDs
NSAIDs, 139-147
- and chronic gastric ulcer, 511-512
- prevention of ulcers, 513
- tolerance, 357
Nuclear magnetic resonance, 163

O

O_2^-, see Oxygen
OH, 149,155
Oligosaccharide, 192-196
Omeprazole, 3,248, 249
Opioid-sensitive, 115-123
Ornithine decarboxylase activity, 438
Osmotic agent
- polyvinylpyrolidone (PVP), 53
- albumin, 53,54
- glycerol, 53,54
Osmotic reflection coefficient, 150
Ouabain, 258
Oxygen (O_2), 159-174
- consumption, 61,64-66
- derived free radicals, 140,145-146
- O_2^-, 149,153
Oxynticopeptic cells, 247-250
Oxyradical, 149-157
- generated chemoattractants,
156,157
- scavenger, 149-157

P

PAF, 156,301,304,305,307
Pancreatitis, 167
Papaverine, 299-307,310-317
Paracellular, 199,200,275,278
Parietal cells, 176,179,187-198,223
PD, see Electrophysiology
Pentagastrin, 310-317
Pepsin secretion, 310-317
Pepsin, 1-5,7-16
Pepstatin, 55
Peptic ulcer, 1-5,7-16,29
Permeability, 175-185
- junctional, 199-205

PGD_2, see Prostaglandin
PGE, see Prostaglandin
pH - determination, 29-31,34
- gradient across mucus layer, 373
- luminal, 81-87
- relevance to protection, 377-378
- sensitive fluorescent dye,
247,248,253,255
Phalloidin, 53,54
Phenamil, 199-205
Phosphatidylcholine, 207,217,218
Phospholipase, 207,208,218
- inhibition, 55
Phospholipid, 207-218,271-278
Pirenzipine, 327,333
Piroxicam, 513
Plasma membrane, 48,49,53
Poly-N-acetyllactasinine, 187,195,196
Polyethylene glycol (PEG), 30,31,53,54
Prednisolone
- effect on chronic ulcer
healing, 458
- effect on collagen content
of ulcer base, 459
Prophylaxis
- of gastric ulcers with
misoprostol, 516
Propidium iodide - fluorescence, 47-52
Prostaglandin, 29,43,61-68,71,72,74-76,
115,116,119-123,223,224,226
- PGD_2, 301,307
- PGE, 237-244
- PGE_2, 175,180,181,183
- 16,16-dimethyl PGE_2, 61-68
- 6-Keto-$PGF_{1\alpha}$, 357,365,366
- and stress-induced ulceration, 435
- and cytoprotection, 332
- biosynthesis rate, 437
- effect of dietary fatty acids on
synthesis rate, 504
- synthesis rate, 357, 365,366
Prostanoid, 127-135
Protease inhibition, 55
Protection by hyperemia, 323
Protein kinase C, 55
- inhibition, 55
Proteoglycans, 343
- assay, 345-346
- biological functions, 348
- heparan sulphate, 348
- Chondroitin sulphate, 349
- dermatansulphate, 349
- localization, 353

Proton
- buffering, 258,267
- extrusion, 260,267
- permeability, 253-267
- permeability coefficient, 177,178
Proximal duodenal 237,238,241
Pylorus - ligated stomach, 7,8

Q

Quantitative histology, 327-341
- and ethanol injury, 331
- technique for, 329-331

R

Rabbit
- chief cells, 253-267
- surface cells, 253-267
Radio immuno assay - for TSH, 38
Ranitidine, 3,31,211,216
Reactive oxygen metabolites, 159-174
Rectum, 209,210
Reoxygenation, 168
Reperfusion, 149-157,159-174,301-304
Respiratory burst, 159-174
Restitution, 336,403-412, 413-426
- and antilaminin, 411
- and bile acids, 406,409
- antifibronectin, 410
- duodenum, 404,
- colon, 409-411, 413-426
- effect of luminal pH, 413-426
- intestinal, 403-412
- role of calcium, 406,410
- role of nutrient HCO_3^-, 405, 413-426
Restraint stress, see Cold

S

Scanning electron microscopy, 293
Secretin, 238,239
Secretion
- acid, 61
- bicarbonate, 61
Sham feeding, 238,240
Shock, 149-157,159-174
Short circuit current, (Isc), 199-205
Sialomucins, 397-398
Smoking
- and haemostasis, 468

SOD, 149-153,303,304
Sodium, see Na
Sodium deoxycholate, 413
Soluble mucous, see Mucus layer
Splanchnic nerves, 227,228,232
Splanchnicotomy, 223-232
Stress, 226,232,301,303,304
Stress-induced ulcers, 166
- and epidermal growth factor, 435
- and prostaglandin E_2, 435
- biosynthesis rate, 437
- ornithine decarboxylase, 440
- spermine, 440
Substance P, 103,105-107,109
Sucralfate, 71,72,74-76,327,332,333,513
- and angiogenesis, 450
Sucrose, 53,54
Sudden potential drop (SPD), 84
Sulfomucins, 397-398
Superoxide (O_2^-), 159-174
- dismutase (SOD), 53-54,159-174
Surface mucosal blood
- oxygenation, 299-307
- volume, 299-307
Sympathetic nerves, 226,227,232

T

T84, 175-185
Taurocholate, 271-278
Taxol, 53,54
Theophylline, 238,240,241
Thromboxane B_2, 357,365,366
Thyroid stimulating hormone (TSH), 37,42-43
- radio immuno assay for, 38
Thyrotrophin - releasing hormone, 385
Transcellular, 199,205
Transmucosal potential difference, 7,11,30,31,81,87.
see also Electrophysiology.
Trypan Blue, 61,64,66
Tubulovesicles, 187-198

U

Ulcer base
- collagen content, 456,457
- connective tissue in, 455
- hydroxyproline, 457

Ulceration
- duodenal, 2,3,19-21,24
- gastric, 1-5,7-16,19,21,25,37-44,
    139,140,146,207-218,455,456,458,
    467,491,521,523,527
- healing, 1-5
- stress, 37,43,44,166
Unfenestrated, *see* Capillary
Urea breath test, 20
Ussing chamber, 82,199-205,413,

V

Vagal, 240
- nerve, 223,224,226
- nerve stimulation, 310-317
Vagotomy, 37-39,42-44,223-232
Valinomycin, 181,257, 258
Vascular factors in ulcer healing, 447
Vasoactive Intestinal Peptide, see VIP
Vasoactive mediators, 127-135
Verapamil, 54,56
Vinculin, 53
VIP, 91-94,98,238,239,240
- antagonist, 224,225

W

Water immersion, 436

X

Xanthine oxidase, 149-157,159-174
- derived oxidants, 149-157